# *Complementary and Alternative Medicine in* REHABILITATION

# Complementary and Alternative Medicine in
# REHABILITATION

## ERIC LESKOWITZ, MD

Staff Psychiatrist
Pain Management Program
Spaulding Rehabilitation Hospital;
Instructor
Department of Psychiatry
Harvard Medical School;
Senior Clinical Instructor
Department of Psychiatry
Tufts University School of Medicine
Boston, Massachusetts


*Series Editor* **MARC S. MICOZZI**, MD, PhD
Executive Director
The College of Physicians of Philadelphia
Adjunct Professor of Medicine and Rehabilitation Medicine
University of Pennsylvania
Philadelphia, Pennsylvania

*with 42 illustrations*

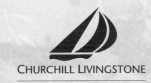

CHURCHILL LIVINGSTONE

An Imprint of Elsevier Science
New York   Edinburgh   London   Philadelphia

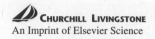
**CHURCHILL LIVINGSTONE**
An Imprint of Elsevier Science

11830 Westline Industrial Drive
St. Louis, Missouri 63146

---

**NOTICE**

Complementary and alternative medicine is an ever-changing field. Standard safety precautions must be followed, but as new research and clinical experience broaden our knowledge, changes in treatment and drug therapy may become necessary or appropriate. Readers are advised to check the most current product information provided by the manufacturer of each drug to be administered to verify the recommended dose, the method and duration of administration, and contraindications. It is the responsibility of the licensed prescriber, relying on experience and knowledge of the patient, to determine dosages and the best treatment for each individual patient. Neither the publisher nor the editors assume any liability for any injury and/or damage to persons or property arising from this publication.

---

**International Standard Book Number 0-443-06599-3**

*Acquisitions Editors:* Kellie White, Inta Ozols
*Developmental Editor:* Jennifer Watrous
*Publishing Services Manager:* Karen Edwards
*Design:* Renée Duenow

TG/MVB

Printed in the United States of America.

Last digit is the print number:   9   8   7   6   5   4   3   2   1

# Contributors
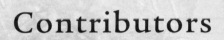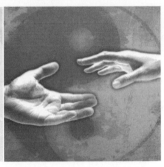

**DOUGLAS ALEXANDER, BSc, RMT**
Professor
Massage Therapy Program
School of Health and Community Studies
Algonquin College
Ottawa, Ontario CANADA

**PHILIP R. APPEL, PhD, FASCH**
Past President and Fellow of the American Society
   of Clinical Hypnosis;
Chair, Behavioral Science Section of the Medical Staff
National Rehabilitation Hospital
Washington, DC

**PAUL ARNSTEIN, RN, PhD**
Assistant Professor
Community Health Nursing
Boston College
Chestnut Hill, Massachusetts

**JOSEPH F. AUDETTE, MD**
Instructor
Harvard Medical School
Department of Physical Medicine & Rehabilitation;
Medical Director
Outpatient Pain Service
Spaulding Rehabilitation Hospital
Boston, Massachusetts

**HERBERT BENSON, MD**
Associate Professor of Medicine
Mind/Body Institute
Department of Medicine
Harvard Medical School
Boston, Massachusetts

**VINCENT BREWINGTON, MA**
Grants Management Officer
Lincoln Medical and Mental Health Center
Bronx, New York

**EDWARD H. CHAPMAN, MD, DHt, DABFP**
Former President
American Institute of Homeopathy;
Private Practice
Newton, Massachusetts

**OLIVIA CHEEVER, EdD, GCFP, LCMT**
Faculty and Co-Founder
Mind/Body Department
Longy School of Music
Cambridge, Massachusetts

**EFFIE POY YEW CHOW, PhD, RN, Lic Ac, Dipl Ac, NCCAOM**
Member, White House Commission on CAM;
Qigong Grandmaster;
President
East West Academy of Healing Arts
San Francisco, California

**LISA JANICE COHEN, MS, PT, OCS**
Adjunct Professor
MGH Institute of Health Professions
Graduate Programs in Physical Therapy
Boston, Massachusetts

**AGATHA COLBERT**
Newton, Massachusetts

**PATRICIA CULLITON**
Alternative Medicine Clinic
Minneapolis, Minnesota

**RAM DASS**
San Anselmo, California

**HARRIS DIENSTFREY**
Freelance writer/editor
Sharon, Connecticut

**CHARLOTTE ELIOPOULOS, RNC, MPH, PhD**
Specialist in Holistic Chronic Care Nursing;
President
American Holistic Nurses Association
Glen Arm, Maryland

**LYN W. FREEMAN, PhD**
Senior Research Associate
Institute for Circumpolar Health
University of Alaska, Anchorage;
President
CompMed Alaska
Anchorage, Alaska

**FRED P. GALLO, PhD**
Clinical Psychologist
Private Practice
Hermitage, Pennsylvania

**RICHARD T. GOLDBERG, EdD**
Associate Clinical Professor of Psychology
Harvard Medical School;
Senior Clinical Psychologist
Spaulding Rehabilitation Hospital
Psychiatry Department
Boston, Massachusetts

**ELMER GREEN, PhD**
Director Emeritus
Center for Applied Psychophysiology Menninger Clinic;
Founder, Past President, and Board Member
International Society for the Study of Subtle Energy and
    Energy Medicine
Ozawkie, Kansas

**LAURO S. HALSTEAD, MD**
Clinical Professor of Medicine
Georgetown University;
Director Post-Polio Program
National Rehabilitation Hospital
Washington, DC

**PRISCILLA IVIMEY, RN, LMHC**
Psychotherapist
Private Practice
Newton, Massachusetts;
Adjunct Faculty
Boston College
Boston, Massachusetts

**YOUNG SOO JIN, MD, PhD**
Professor of Sports Medicine
University of Ulsan College of Medicine;
Director
Sport & Health Medicine Center
ASAN Medical Center;
Vice President
The Korean Society of Sports Medicine
Seoul, Korea

**JON KABAT-ZINN, PhD**
Professor of Medicine
Center for Mindfulness in Medicine, Health Care, and
    Society
University of Massachusetts Medical School
Worcester, Massachusetts

**GARY KAPLAN, DO**
Medical Director
Kaplan Clinic
Department of Family Medicine
Georgetown University School of Medicine
Washington, DC

**DHARMA SINGH KHALSA, MD**
President and Medical Director
The Alzheimer's Prevention Foundation
Tucson, Arizona

**MICHAEL J. KUDLAS, DC**
Chiropractic Advisor
American Holistic Health Association;
Diplomate and Peer-Review Panel Member
American Academy of Pain Management;
Board of Governors
World Chiropractic Alliance;
Founding Member
Michigan Chiropractic Society;
Desert Hot Springs, California

**G. FRANK LAWLIS**
Chair
Department of Transpersonal Medicine
Greenwich University
Norfolk, Australia

**SARA LAZAR**
Department of Psychiatry
Massachusetts General Hospital
Charlestown, Massachusetts

**ERIC D. LESKOWITZ, MD**
Staff Psychiatrist
Pain Management Program
Spaulding Rehabilitation Hospital;
Instructor
Department of Psychiatry
Harvard Medical School;
Senior Clinical Instructor
Department of Psychiatry
Tufts University School of Medicine
Boston, Massachusetts

**MAY LOO, MD**
Assistant Clinical Professor
Stanford Medical Center;
Director
Neurodevelopmental Program
Santa Clara County Valley Medical Center
Santa Clara, California

**CHARIS F. MENG**
Instructor of Medicine
Rheumatology
Weill Medical College of Cornell University
New York, New York

**MARGARET A. NAESER, PhD, LAc, Dipl Ac**
Research Professor of Neurology
Boston University School of Medicine
Boston, Massachusetts

**ADAM PERLMAN, MD, MPH**
Assistant Clinical Professor of Medicine
Mount Sinai School of Medicine;
Director of Integrative Medicine
Saint Barnabas Health Care System
Livingston, New Jersey

**ROBYN ROSS, RYT**
Advanced Certification, Integrative Yoga Therapy
    and Kripalu Yoga;
Co-Director, Integrative Yoga Therapy Teacher
    Certification Training;
Co-Director, Prana Yoga Teacher Certification Training;
Former Credentialed Yoga Therapist, Columbia
    Presbyterian Medical Center;
Certified Holistic Health Educator;
Founder and Co-Director, Living Yoga
New York, New York

**GLENN S. ROTHFELD, MD, MAC**
Medical Director
WholeHealth New England
Arlington, Massachusetts;
Clinical Assistant Professor of Medicine
Department of Family Medicine and Community Health
Tufts University School of Medicine
Boston, Massachusetts

**Sr MARY SAMSON, SHCJ**
Director of Pastoral Care
Spaulding Rehabilitation Hospital;
Certified Chaplain Advanced
National Association of Catholic Chaplains;
Supervisor of Field Education
Boston Theological Institute
Boston, Massachusetts

**C. NORMAN SHEALY, MD, PhD**
Founder and Former President
American Holistic Medical Association
President and Professor of Energy Medicine
Holos University for Graduate Studies
Springfield, Missouri

**RICHARD A. SHERMAN, PhD**
Director of Orthopedic Research
Madigan Army Medical Center
Tacoma, Washington

**SAMUEL C. SHIFLETT, PhD**
Director of Research
Continuum Center for Health and Healing
Beth Israel Medical Center
New York, New York

**ANDREW DAVID SHILLER, MD**
Medical Director
Outpatient Rehabilitation
Kent Hospital
Warkwick, Rhode Island

**BERNIE S. SIEGEL, MD**
Founder
Exceptional Cancer Patients Therapy Program
Woodbridge, Connecticut

MICHAEL O. SMITH, MD, Dr Ac
Director
Lincoln Hospital Recovery Center
Bronx, New York
Assistant Clinical Professor
Department of Psychiatry
Cornell Medical College
New York, New York

JOHN E. UPLEDGER, DO, OMM
President
Medical Director
Upledger Institute
Palm Beach Gardens, Florida

SCOTT WALKER
Albuquerque, New Mexico

JOHN WEEKS
Co-Founder
Collaboration for Healthcare Renewal Foundation;
Publisher/Editor
*The Integrator* for the Business of Alternative Medicine
Seattle, Washington

REBECCA REYNOLDS WEIL, MS, OTR/L
Executive Director
Seabury School
Animals As Intermediaries
Concord, Massachusetts;
Faculty Associate
Tufts Center for Animals and Public Policy
Tufts University School of Veterinary Medicine
Grafton, Massachusetts

MICHAEL I. WEINTRAUB, MD, FACP, FAAN
Clinical Professor of Neurology
New York Medical College
Valhalla, New York

HARVEY ZARREN, MD, FACC
Medical Director
Department of Cardiac Rehabilitation
Union Hospital
North Shore Medical Center
Lynn, Massachusetts

*To the patients of Spaulding Rehabilitation Hospital*
*for their inspiring blend of courage, compassion,*
*and patience in the face of very long odds.*

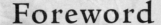

Foreword

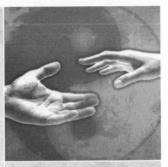

# Mindfulness: The Heart of Rehabilitation

JON KABAT-ZINN

This volume presents the work and insights of many prominent and dedicated proponents of complementary and alternative therapeutic approaches in rehabilitation medicine, as well as their visions of the future in this rapidly growing field. It is in large measure a product of the abiding vision and passion of the editor, Dr. Eric Leskowitz. Dr. Leskowitz and I have had numerous conversations about developmental trends in this field, and I am delighted to have been asked to write the foreword to this seminal text, which appears at a critical moment in the emergence of the medicine of the twenty-first century.

Dr. Leskowitz and I share a passion for the origins of words. He encouraged me to base this foreword on some of my own investigations and experiences regarding the very words we use to name the work we do, and how such an inquiry might expand the boundaries of our understanding of the scope of the possible in rehabilitation medicine.

In my experience, it can be illuminating to ponder the origins of those words that name our professional fields of endeavor and calling. Doing so sometimes reveals novel dimensions of meaning and potentially relevant interconnections that may ordinarily go unnoticed or unexamined. For instance, in the nascent field of mind/body medicine, I find it intriguing that the words *meditation* and *medicine,* which are clearly related by superficial inspection, share the same root meaning of "right inward measure" or "wholeness."[1] From this perspective, medicine is the attempt to restore right inward measure when it is disturbed or compromised, and meditation can be thought of as the direct perception or realization of right inward measure. In seeing such a link, new avenues of thought and investigation may open up that can give rise to novel insights and practical clinical and teaching applications, as well as to fresh ways of reconceptualizing the growing edges of a rapidly changing field.

Thus it was natural to pursue the origin of the word "rehabilitation" some years ago when Dr. Leskowitz invited me to speak at a symposium he organized at the Spaulding Rehabilitation Hospital on CAM in rehabilitation. I consulted the Appendix of Indo-European Roots[2] in the *American Heritage Dictionary of the English Language* in part to follow up on a hunch that the word seemed to contain two French verbs: "habiter" (to live in, to inhabit, to dwell) and "habilitier" (to qualify, to enable). As it turns out, there is an interesting and telling association that may be of considerable relevance to those of us who work in rehabilitation.

The first meaning of *rehabilitation* is given as: "to restore to good health or useful life, as through therapy and education." This is the meaning we all commonly think of and the usage we conventionally employ in our discourse, based on the Latin "re" + "habilitare," to enable, thus to re-enable, make well again, to restore to a former state or capacity.

If, however, one probes a little deeper, following the suggestion to "*see HABILITATE,*" one notices immediately that this word is situated among a bevy of words: habile, habiliment, habit, habitable, habitant, habitat, habitation that all derive from the deep Indo-European root, **ghabh-e,** and its core meaning: to give or receive. Here, we discover that the English words *able* and *inhabit,* among many others, are indeed linked. Rehabilitation carries deep in its core not only the meaning "to re-enable" but also (and tellingly) "to re-inhabit." Rehabilitation is thus a process of learning how to reinhabit one's life and body, a process that can be furthered by various therapies, as well as education, as noted in the first definition, but which is ultimately one of interior angst: felt, lived, and embodied experience.[3,4] After all, we grow into a dwelling and it grows on us over time, like our clothes, which is another meaning (habillier) from the same root.

And this is where the giving and receiving comes in.* One cannot truly inhabit a space without *giving* one's self over to it—to the light, shadows, colors, sounds, layout of the rooms, texture of the space, to what the Chinese call its "feng shui"—touching it through our senses and through our awareness and in this way, *receiving* its unique qualities. It takes time for us to "feel" our way into a new home, to sense its energies and how they might be worked with and modulated. That happens through just such a reciprocal process of giving and receiving, of dwelling in and honoring our senses and sense impressions.[5]

The revelation of "to learn to live or dwell inside again" reminds us that rehabilitation from injury, trauma, disease, or insult of any kind involves a kind of learning, a "moving in" to, a taking up residence in dimensions of one's life, one's body, and one's being, dimensions that may—whether we like it or not, or wanted it or not—now need to be rediscovered or perhaps, in some cases, encountered for the first time if one hopes to heal and recover optimally. We feel our way, working at the edges of how we find things in this moment, exploring our boundaries, giving ourselves over to our attempts, and listening carefully for and receiving the feedback from foot, or leg, or hip, or heart, or lungs, or mind. We learn as we go, by seeing how our efforts and expectations (predictions) accord with the feedback the body (and mind) give us and by then making appropriate adjustments in our efforts and attitudes and beginning again. Out of this often slow and sometimes painful process comes the re-enabling, the recovery of whatever degree of capacity might be realizable, moving toward a limit that usually remains unknown and mysterious.

Rehab professionals are continually surprised at what people are capable of and by how the body and mind can sometimes respond to a strong determination to take up residence again and to work with self-compassion and gentleness at the boundaries of what one can and cannot do at any given moment, even in the face of what may sometimes seem like insurmountable obstacles or challenges. This interface is where the learning takes place, and the growing into oneself, as one feels one's way into what will be inevitably and to a large degree a new territory within one's own interior landscape of being.

Note that the root meaning of "to learn to live inside again" carries a strong energy of agency. It is the person himself or herself who is taking up residence again and going through the learning process, not the physician or the therapist. The terrain of this learning process is the inner landscape of the body and the

---

*I am indebted to Barbara Gates, editor of *Inquiring Mind,* Berkeley, Calif, for this insight.

mind, one's entire sense of self, and thus includes whatever we mean when we speak of heart and soul, and spirit, the reflections of our completeness and interconnectedness as a human being, as a person, our *right inward measure.*

This sense of personal agency and interiority on the part of the patient is not so much in evidence in the more conventional definition of *rehabilitation,* which emphasizes the perspective of the support system that is assisting in the re-enabling by providing the therapies and the context in which the work and the learning can unfold. Yet we all know that both outer and inner agency are vital for true and full rehabilitation to take place. The person who is patient needs the help of a very special holding environment, a setting in which well-chosen and well-monitored treatment programs and therapies can take place, and in which the staff can provide technical expertise, ongoing emotional support, counseling, and encouragement. Such an environment serves as the crucible in which the outer and inner work and the learning can begin and then unfold over time. But optimal rehabilitation also clearly requires the full engagement of the patient as a participant in the process of this intimate giving and receiving. It is after all the person himself or herself who is moving in and who will have to engage directly with whatever heat is generated in the crucible in the slow and sometimes long-term process of taking up residence once again in one's body, as it is in any given moment and in one's life.

The richness of meaning embedded within the word *rehabilitation* invites us to be exquisitely sensitive to both the outer and the inner domains in which the work of rehabilitation unfolds, their intimate reciprocal interconnectedness, and to the various roles that health professionals and patients are called to in furthering that work and optimizing potential outcomes. "Learning to live inside again" necessitates a high degree of focused and sustained attention and awareness rooted in the present moment, as well as a high degree of sensitivity to boundaries and limits and a willingness to dwell at them, *inhabit them,* in inner stillness, beyond the reactivity of thought and judgment but with great discernment and intentionality. This embodied attention, this consciousness *in* the body, this willingness to work at the boundaries of what one finds in this moment when one looks and then makes an intentional effort to be with, accept, and work with things as they are is a condition of body and mind known as *mindfulness.*[6]

If rehabilitation is above all a participatory process that involves mobilizing the full repertoire of inner and outer resources of the individual patient for the learning, growing, healing, and transformation, that, over time, comprise the experience of "giving and receiving" and "living inside again," then mindfulness and its embodiment from moment to moment might be said to constitute the heart of rehabilitation. By the same token, the process of rehabilitation also requires a high degree of mindfulness on the part of rehabilitation professionals in the sense of a continual keeping in mind what the interior and exterior contexts of the therapies involve, a sensitivity to the sacred trust of the relationship with the patient (who is often in a state of high vulnerability), and a continual titrating of the treatment protocol to the changing status of the patient.[7] And what is that relationship if not a compassionate and embodied engagement in giving and receiving on the part of rehabilitation professionals?

To frame mindfulness as a participatory process in more concrete terms, consider the ways it has been integrated into medicine at the University of Massachusetts Medical School. The medical patients who participate in the Department of Medicine's Stress Reduction Clinic are all engaged in learning, to one degree or another, to inhabit their lives and their bodies anew, whether they are traditionally classified as rehabilitation patients (i.e., suffering from chronic pain conditions, heart conditions, lung conditions, and so on) or not. In this case, the rehabilitation is catalyzed through intensive training in and practice of formal and informal mindfulness meditation (including mindful hatha yoga, which is a rich and gentle meditative discipline of mind/body interiority and exploration) and their applications to the situations and circumstances in which the patients find themselves in their daily lives.[8,9,10] Mindfulness practices have been integrated to varying degrees into the standard cardiac and pulmonary rehabilitation programs in our hospital as well. From the perspective of the consciousness disciplines,[11] such as meditation, tai chi, qigong, and yoga, we may all—patients and professionals alike—suffer from a lack of intimacy with our experience of the present moment and would stand to benefit significantly from learning to live inside again. A rough but accurate paraphrasing of a line in James Joyce's *Dubliners* makes the point and seems sadly to have quasi-universal applicability: "Mr. Duffy lived a short distance from his body."

With a recalibrated perspective on rehabilitation from our etymological exploration, it becomes clear than there may be many valid pathways to effect the learning to live inside again. These pathways include those that emphasize what the patient can do for himself or herself (with appropriate and on-going support, training, and classes), such as meditation, exercise, yoga, tai chi, physical therapy, occupational therapy, biofeedback, stress reduction, and those that require direct treatment (and/or prescription) from skilled therapists and physicians, such as chiropractic, massage, craniosacral therapy, acupuncture, or naturopathy.

This book addresses a major need on the part of practitioners, patients, and students alike to have together in one place comprehensive expertise on the vast range of so-called complementary and alternative practices and approaches currently finding their way into use and investigation in the field of rehabilitation. It appears at a time in which all of medicine is experiencing a rising tide of consumer and physician interest in alternative approaches and its massive economic implications for health care.[12,13] Ultimately, as has been observed many times in recent years,[14,15] the terms *complementary* and *alternative* are likely to dissolve in the face of new research results and clinical experience, and we will have a larger, evidence-based *integrative rehabilitation*, part of the larger phenomenon of an expanded-modality, evidence-based *integrative* medicine that is currently developing. Beyond that, we may be able at some point to drop the term *integrative* and just have these approaches be an intimate and common-sense part of medicine, *good* medicine, and of rehabilitation, *good* rehabilitation.

This unique volume in the series, *Medical Guides to Complementary & Alternative Medicine*, is likely to be an important catalyst in that unfolding. The visionary editorial leadership of Dr. Leskowitz has gathered together an impressive array of experts across a broad spectrum of disciplines, many of which are not commonly integrated within mainstream medicine and rehabilitation at this particular moment in time. The result is a forward-looking and valuable resource for evaluating what is known about specific interventions and therapies and how

they might be utilized when appropriate to meet the profound and multidimensional needs of the specific individual rehabilitation patient and further his or her returning to a fuller, healthier life. Many people, professionals and patients alike, for years to come, will be the beneficiaries of this pioneering contribution.

## References

1. Bohm D: *Wholeness and the implicate order,* London, 1980, Routledge & Kegan Paul.
2. *The American Heritage Dictionary of the English Language,* ed 3, Boston, 1996, Houghton Mifflin.
3. Toombs SK: *The meaning of illness: a phenomenological account of the different perspectives of physician and patient,* Dordrecht, Netherlands, 1993, Klewer.
4. Varela FJ, Thompson E, Rosch E: *The embodied mind: cognitive science and human experience,* Cambridge, 1991, MIT Press.
5. Abrams D: *The spell of the sensuous,* New York, 1996, Random House.
6. Gunaratana H: *Mindfulness in plain English,* Boston, 1991, Wisdom.
7. Epstein RM: Mindful practice, *JAMA* 282:833-839, 1999.
8. Kabat-Zinn J: *Full catastrophe living: using the wisdom of your body and mind to face stress, pain, and illness,* New York, 1991, Dell.
9. Kabat-Zinn J: *Wherever you go, there you are: mindfulness meditation in everyday life,* New York, 1994, Hyperion.
10. Santorelli S: *Heal thy self: lessons on mindfulness in medicine,* New York, 1999, Bell Tower.
11. Walsh RN: The consciousness disciplines and the behavioral sciences: questions of comparison and assessment, *Am J Psychiatry* 137:663-673, 1980.
12. Eisenberg DM, Kessler RC, Foster C, et al: Unconventional medicine in the United States, *N Engl J Med* 328: 246-252, 1993.
13. Eisenberg DM, Davis RB, Ettner SL, et al: Trends in alternative medicine use in the United States, 1990-1997, *JAMA* 280:1569-1575, 1998.
14. Jonas WB: Alternative medicine—learning from the past, examining the present, advancing to the future, *JAMA* 280:1616-1618, 1998.
15. Fontanarosa PD, Lundberg GD: Alternative medicine meets science, *JAMA* 280: 1618-1619, 1998.

# Series
# Introduction

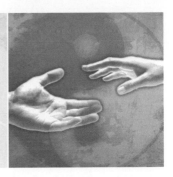

The aim of this Series is to provide clear and rational guides for health care professionals and students so they have current knowledge about:

- Therapeutic medical systems currently labeled as complementary medicine
- Complementary approaches to specific medical conditions
- Integration of complementary therapy into mainstream medical practice

Each text is written specifically with the needs and questions of a health care audience in mind. Where possible, basic applications in clinical practice are explored.

Complementary medicine is being rapidly integrated into mainstream health care largely in response to consumer demand, as well as in recognition of new scientific findings that are expanding our view of health and healing—pushing against the limits of the current biomedical paradigm.

Health care professionals need to know what their patients are doing and what they believe about what has been called alternative medicine. In addition, a basic working knowledge of complementary medical therapies is a rapidly growing requirement for primary care, some medical specialties, and throughout the allied health professions. These approaches also expand our view of the art and science of medicine and contribute importantly to the intellectual formation of health professions students.

This Series provides a survey of the fundamentals and foundations of complementary medical systems currently available and practiced in North America and Europe. Each topic is presented in ways that are *understandable* and that provide an important *understanding* of the intellectual foundations of each system—with translation between the complementary and conventional medical systems, where possible. These explanations draw appropriately on the social and scientific foundations of each system of care.

Rapidly growing contemporary research results are included whenever possible. In addition to providing evidence indicating where complementary medicines may be of therapeutic benefit, guidance is provided as to when complementary therapies should not be used, as well.

This field of health is rapidly moving from being considered *alternative* (implying exclusive use of one medical system or another), to *complementary* (used as an adjunct to mainstream medical care), to *integrative medicine* (implying an active, conscious effort by mainstream medicine to incorporate alternatives on the basis of rational clinical and scientific information and judgment).

Likewise, health care professionals and students must move rapidly to learn the fundamentals of complementary medical systems in order to better serve their patients' needs, protect the public health, and expand their scientific horizons and understandings of health and healing.

MARC S. MICOZZI
Philadelphia, Pennsylvania
1997

# Series Editor's Preface

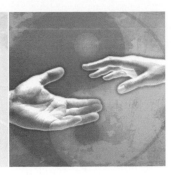

This volume represents an important contribution to the series, *Medical Guides to Complementary & Alternative Medicine,* wherein we address topics in CAM by their application to the practice of various medical specialties, in this case Rehabilitation Medicine. There is much discussion currently about the progression of "alternative," then "complementary," and now "integrative" medicine. The professional practice of medicine is organized today along medical specialty lines, with roughly half of practitioners representing primary care (family medicine, general internal medicine, as well as alternative fields such as naturopathic medicine) and the other half the full range of medical specialties. Most medical conditions are ultimately diagnosed and treated, and health care delivered, in the context of medical specialty practice today. True integration of CAM will come when alternative and complementary medical modalities are recognized and respected as part of the range of therapeutic options available to practitioners for treating medical conditions in which they specialize.

Rehabilitation lies at the end points, or final common pathways, of many medical conditions where the integrity of the structure and function of the body has somehow been impaired by disease or injury. In this regard, a full-range of alternative medical therapies may be applied to the full spectrum of human disability. In fact, rehabilitation medicine has been (often quietly) a leader for many years in the application of alternative medicine to mainstream medical practice as evidenced by the presence of so many alternative practitioners affiliated with academic departments of physical and rehabilitation medicine. These academic affiliations, sometimes decades in duration now, challenge one operational definition of alternative medicine made popular by workers at Harvard University, as "therapies which are not in the mainstream health care system."

There was a time in history when rehabilitation hospitals and practices were focused on patients and conditions known as "incurable." Despite the therapeutic pessimism explicitly manifest in such terminology, it is important to recognize in rehabilitation when the patient must learn to live with, rather than be cured from, a medical condition. Our twentieth century emphasis on cure and the therapeutic expectations made possible by "miracle" drugs such as antibiotics have often skewed our modern expectation and evaluation of newly popular complementary therapies. As the evidence comes in, our definition of "cured" may not always be achievable even with the best "new" complementary medicines. However, even where cure is not possible, there is always room for healing.

Complementary medicine today combines some of the best modalities for health and healing "outside the mainstream medical system." Applying these modalities to rehabilitation yields proven benefits and holds much promise for the future.

MARC S. MICOZZI
Bethesda, Maryland
November 2001

# Preface

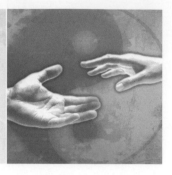

Physical medicine and rehabilitation (PM&R) may be the most widely misunderstood branch of contemporary medicine. As it is most commonly used, the term *rehab* refers to celebrities going into detox programs for their substance abuse problems or to professional athletes "rehabbing" after knee surgery. But, as Jon Kabat-Zinn points out in the Foreword to this book, to "re-habilitate" means to regain abilities, to be able to re-inhabit one's life again. The real focus of rehabilitation is on the recovery of function after illness or injury. Some day in the future, we may be able to regenerate amputated limbs or restore brain function after a stroke, but for now there are no miracle cures in rehab, just the day-to-day heroism of progressing from wheelchair to walker to crutches to independent ambulation. It is that life-affirming emphasis on functional ability, rather than on the antagonistic elimination of symptoms that characterizes most other medical specialties, which gives rehabilitation its special, if unglamorous, power. This patient-oriented emphasis on function rather than symptom suppression, on empowerment rather than dependency also puts rehabilitation in alignment with an important wave of change that is sweeping through today's health care system.

I am referring to the practice of a multidimensional form of medicine that encompasses all levels of the human being—body, mind, and spirit. This approach is both ancient and modern and is called by many names—alternative, holistic, complementary, and integrative are the most commonly heard. But they all share a common belief that if the innate healing abilities of the human being can be tapped, dramatic clinical benefits will occur.

"Holistic" physicians are appearing everywhere these days, including the cover of *Time* magazine and as the subject of PBS specials. Much as a rising tide lifts all boats, this trend has of course impacted PM&R but without the fanfare of such media favorites as Dr. Andrew Weil or Dr. Dean Ornish. This book is an attempt to outline the current state of knowledge in the area of complementary and alternative medicine (CAM) as it relates to the field of rehabilitation. Ironically, rehabilitation has quietly anticipated this trend with its long-standing emphasis on patient empowerment, teamwork, and deep compassion.

My interest in the field comes from over 10 years work as a psychiatrist in the Pain Management Program at Spaulding Rehabilitation Hospital in Boston, where I have seen how numerous CAM modalities and philosophies can have a significant impact on the challenging condition of chronic pain. As an outgrowth of this clinical experience, I organized a course for Harvard Medical School in 1998 and 1999 called "Complementary and Alternative Medicine in Rehabilitation." This course demonstrated both the high level of expertise gained by CAM practitioners in the field of rehabilitation and also the high level of interest in this sort of material by rehabilitation clinicians of all stripes. Physician attendees were in fact in the minority, outnumbered by occupational therapists, physical therapists, registered nurses, chiropractors, social workers, and so on.

It was with this multidisciplinary approach in mind that I set out to expand the course offering into a textbook. As a psychiatric consultant to a rehabilitation pain program, I have learned that rehabilitation is above all else a team effort. So any text that hopes to serve the field of rehabilitation well must be addressed to all members of the team. As text editor, I attempted to keep this goal in mind when I assembled my team of contributors from all of the major clinical rehab disciplines.

I also faced the challenge of trying to highlight a field known for its proliferation of therapies. By some estimates there are over 300 distinct techniques and therapies that come under the umbrella of CAM, and each modality is potentially applicable to each of the dozens of common clinical rehabilitation conditions. So rather than end up editing an encyclopedia, I decided to wield my editorial hatchet and simplify along the following lines.

In the first section of the book, several representative therapies from each of the four main categories or dimensions that mark our human body/mind/spirit nature are considered. I chose five or six therapies from each realm: the body-oriented treatments (ranging from chiropractic to massage), the mind/body therapies (including biofeedback, hypnosis, and so on), the energy-based therapies (acupuncture, homeopathy, etc), and the emergent or transcendent categories (spirituality, nature as healer, and several other hard-to-categorize topics). My charge to these contributors was to expand on their topic for an audience of open-minded and curious but skeptical clinicians who may not be well-versed in the practice of CAM but who wanted to learn about the state of the art and the state of the science in CAM as it relates to rehabilitation. Thus the emphasis here is on evidence-based medicine. Each chapter provides enough research citations for further study but without expanding into a series of in-depth academic literature reviews, while at the same time recognizing that some of these important new modalities have at present only a rudimentary supporting scientific literature. Most important, in addition to addressing the history and theory underlying these many novel and ancient approaches, I asked each author to describe in some depth several clinical examples, to anchor their presentation in the real world of clinical experience.

The second section of the book deals with some of the most widely encountered clinical conditions in rehabilitation. Again, the emphasis here is on clinical practice, and while some of the chapters have a solid research base to build on, others are admittedly more anecdotal in nature. However, the power of a sustained series of clinical experiences (for example, Bernie Siegel's work with exceptional cancer patients) gives us all pause when we weigh the relative impor-

tance of double-blind trials compared to actual patient stories. I have tried to keep a balance between analysis and experience, between research and practice in these chapters.

The third section is called "Research Directions." Basically, it provides an opportunity for cutting edge researchers in CAM to look into their crystal balls and outline where they see their current research pathway leading them in the near future. A very exciting vision certainly emerges for the future of CAM in rehabilitation. Surely there is room for some educated guesses and inspired hunches in a medical textbook!

The fourth section acknowledges that CAM does not operate in a vacuum. Liscensure, insurance coverage, and the politics of the medical literature are all addressed here.

Finally, the fifth section presents the patient's perspective. Nothing that has been described in the first 40 chapters of the book would have happened without the participation of patients, who are the main characters in this dramatic story. So to complete the book, I have included three in-depth patient accounts of the rehabilitation process, all of which have been leavened by exposure to various holistic attitudes or practices. They include the perspectives of a manual laborer who suffered a spinal cord injury and a freelance journalist whose equilibrium was destroyed by a skeletal imbalance, each writer brings a unique perspective to the challenge of rehabilitation, and each story reminds us that rehab is by, for, and about human beings.

So this book is fairly wide-ranging: it includes a large but not all-inclusive array of topics and a variety of writing styles that range from the dryly academic and scientific to the joyfully personal and experiential. It is an attempt to show that a holistic approach to health care can be not only enjoyable to read about but also enjoyable to practice and to experience. Hopefully, the training resources that are included with each chapter will encourage you to take the next step by pursuing some personal exposure to a modality or approach that interests you. The transformative power of CAM becomes most apparent through personal experience. The impact of CAM on the providers who master these skills is just as powerful as its impact on patients: we all become more complete healers and more complete humans in the process.

ERIC LESKOWITZ
Boston, Massachusetts

# Acknowledgments

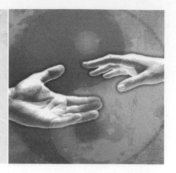

In no particular order, I would like to thank

- The chapter authors, for kindly contributing their time and expertise to make a book that will be of benefit to many
- Series Editor, Marc Micozzi, for maintaining his commitment to this book through so many daunting waves of corporate mergers
- The staff at Elsevier Health Sciences, including Kellie White, Carol Weis at Top Graphics, and especially Developmental Editor, Jennifer Watrous, for keeping track of a nearly infinite number of production details
- My colleagues in the Pain Management Program (Inpatient unit and Outpatient/Medford) at Spaulding Rehabilitation Hospital, for making difficult work enjoyable, and the Monday night healer's group for their support and enthusiasm as we explore the unknown together
- My family, for tolerating all my hours of poring distractedly over manuscripts and emails, and especially my wife, Doreen, for her unconditional love

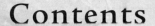

# Contents

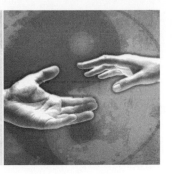

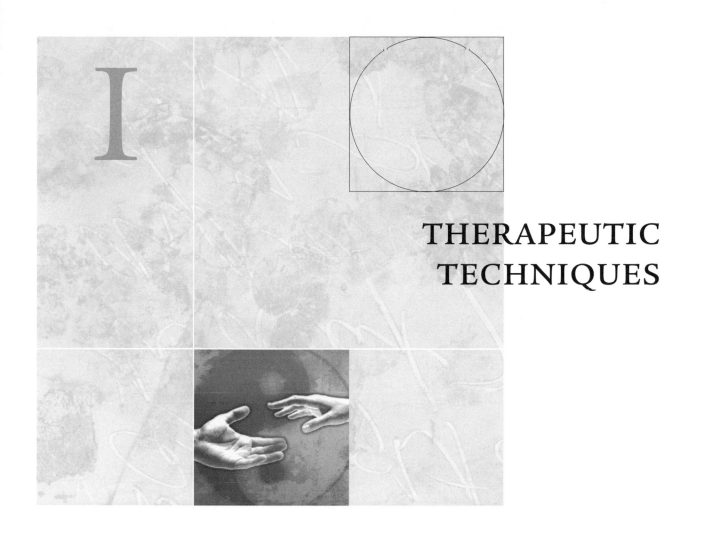

# THERAPEUTIC TECHNIQUES

1

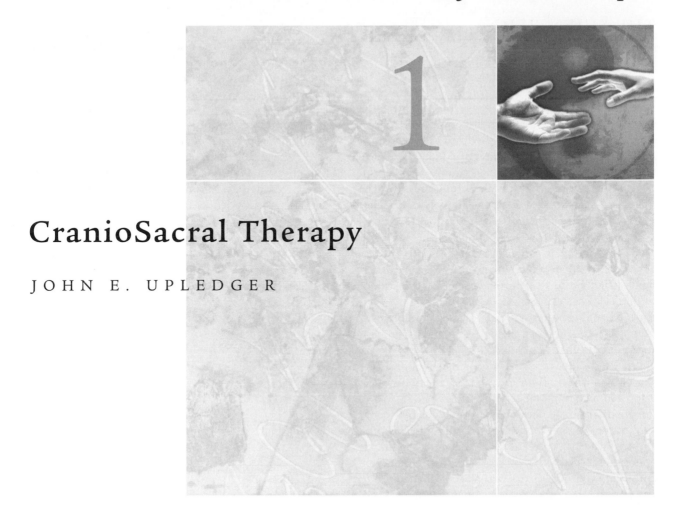

# CranioSacral Therapy

JOHN E. UPLEDGER

CranioSacral Therapy (CST) is a gentle, hands-on method of whole-body evaluation and treatment that may have a positive impact on nearly every system of the body. Whether used alone or with more traditional healthcare methods, it has proven clinically effective in facilitating the body's ability to self-heal. CST often produces extraordinary results.

CST helps normalize the environment of the craniosacral system, a core physiological body system only recently scientifically defined. The craniosacral system extends from the skull, face, and mouth down to the sacrum and coccyx. It consists of a compartment formed by the dura mater membrane, the cerebrospinal fluid contained within, the systems that regulate the fluid flow, the bones that attach to the membranes, and the joints and sutures that interconnect these bones.

Because the craniosacral system contains the brain, spinal cord, and all related structures, any restrictions or imbalances in the system may directly affect any or all aspects of central nervous system performance. Fortunately, these problems can be detected and corrected by a skilled therapist using simple methods of palpation.

By using about 5 gm of pressure, or roughly the weight of a nickel, the CST practitioner evaluates the system by testing for ease of motion and the rhythm of cerebrospinal fluid pulsing within the membranes. Specific treatment techniques are then used to release restrictions in sutures, fasciae, membranes, and any other tissues that may influence the craniosacral system. The result is an improved internal environment that frees the central nervous system to return to its optimal levels of health and performance.

## THE SCIENTIFIC FOUNDATION OF CRANIOSACRAL THERAPY

In its most basic sense the craniosacral system functions as a semi-closed hydraulic system that bathes the brain and spinal cord and their component cells in cerebrospinal fluid pumped rhythmically at a rate of 6 to 12 cycles per minute. To accommodate these pressure changes, the bones of the cranium and sacrum must remain somewhat mobile throughout life. The joints and their sutures do not fully ossify as was once believed. William Sutherland, DO, introduced this premise in the 1930s.

In the mid-1970s, Michigan State University (MSU) asked me to uncover a scientific basis for Dr. Sutherland's belief. From 1975 through 1983, I was Professor of Biomechanics at MSU's College of Osteopathic Medicine, where I led a team of anatomists, physiologists, biophysicists, and bioengineers to test and document the influence of the craniosacral system on the body. Together we conducted research—much of it published—that formed the basis for the modality I went on to develop and name CranioSacral Therapy, or CST.

We discovered that corresponding changes occur in dura mater membrane tensions as cerebrospinal fluid volume and pressure rises and falls within the craniosacral system. These changes in turn induce accommodative movements in the bones that attach to the dura mater compartment. When the natural mobility of the dura mater or any of its attached bones is impaired, the function of the craniosacral system and the central nervous system enclosed may be impaired as well.

## RESEARCH SUPPORTS THE EXISTENCE AND SIGNIFICANCE OF THE CRANIOSACRAL SYSTEM

Studying bone specimens from live surgical patients ages 7 through 57 years, the MSU team was able to demonstrate definitive potential for movement between the cranial sutures.[1-5] Several other studies then laid the foundation for developing a model to explain the mechanism of the craniosacral system.

One important factor contributing to the MSU research was the discovery of what appeared to be fascia hanging from the free border of the falx cerebri on some of the cranium dissections that were performed on both embalmed and unembalmed cadavers. Under the microscope these tissues appeared to be nerve tracts running out of the falx cerebri with brain tissue attached to their free end.

Further research indicated they were components of a nerve impulse/message delivery system between these identified intrasutural nerve receptors and the walls of the ventricles of the brain in which the choroid plexuses were located. This research provided the basis for what our team named the Pressurestat Model, which explains the function of the craniosacral system as a semi-closed hydraulic system (Figure 1-1). Our findings supported those published in *Anatomica Humanica*[6] by Italian Professor Guiseppi Sperino, who noted that cranial sutures fuse before death only under pathological circumstances.

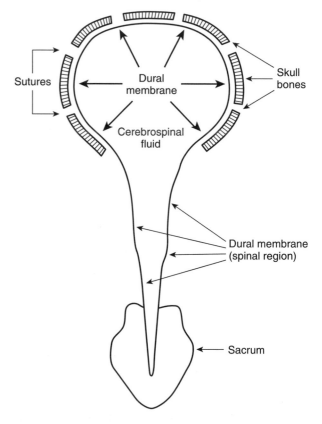

*Figure 1-1* Semi-closed hydraulic system of the cerebrospinal fluid and dural membrane. (From Upledger JE: *CranioSacral therapy II: beyond the dura,* Seattle, 1987, Eastland Press.)

As a springboard toward the clinical application of therapy on the craniosacral system, an interrater reliability study was devised. Twenty-five nursery-school children were examined by two of four examiners on each of 19 parameters. The percentage of agreement varied from 72% to 92%, depending on the examiners and the allowed variance of either 0% or 0.5%.[7]

Subsequently, this same 19-parameter evaluation protocol was used to examine 203 additional school children. A technician recorded the orally reported data for a statistician, who collected information from each child's school file and historical data from parent interviews. This information was compared with the craniosacral system examination findings.

The results of these studies showed that the standardized, quantifiable craniosacral system motion examination represents a practical approach to the study of relationships between craniosacral system dysfunctions and a variety of health, behavior, and performance problems.[8] Other researchers have done similar studies related to psychiatric disorders[9] and symptomatology in newborns.[1]

## CRANIOSACRAL THERAPY ENCOURAGES THE BODY TO SELF-CORRECT

CST is based on the idea that each patient's body contains the necessary information to uncover the underlying cause of any health problem. The therapist communicates with the body to obtain this information and helps facilitate the patient's own self-healing processes.

Thus the usual sequence of events carried out in conventional medicine is reversed in a CST session. Rather than taking a verbal patient history, the therapist begins through palpation, that is, touch. If the therapist is familiar with the patient's history before the session, he or she may find only what is expected rather than sensing the subtle clues offered by the patient's body, energies, and psyche. For that reason, patients are generally asked to write their medical histories and bring them to the clinic for their files. The therapist can then review the history later when he or she feels safe from the issue of suggestibility.

Although avoiding initial history taking is controversial, CST has been practiced this way successfully by tens of thousands of therapists since these concepts were first taught at MSU in 1976.

CST also diverges from conventional medicine in its approach to symptoms. Rather than trying to simply relieve symptoms, CST practitioners work to find and resolve the primary dysfunction underlying the presenting symptom complex. For instance, rather than seeing strabismus as a diagnosed condition to be corrected by surgery, the therapist searches for a cause within the intracranial membrane system and the motor control system of the eyes. In this case the cause is often found to be an abnormal tension pattern in the tentorium cerebelli. Quite often these tension patterns are referred from the occiput or from the low back and/or the pelvis.

The CST "diagnosis" would be intracranial membranous strain of the tentorium cerebelli due to occipital and/or low back and pelvic dysfunctions resulting in secondary motor dysfunction of the eyes. Clearly in such a case the therapist would focus on the sacrum, pelvis, occiput, and then the tentorium cerebelli. Correct evaluation and treatment would be signified by a "spontaneous correction" of the strabismus.

A similar approach is used for almost any presenting problem, from TMJ disorders to recurrent bronchitis and spastic colitis. The nature of the presenting problem is usually of secondary importance unless immediate amelioration is critical, or if the patient does not understand CST. If this is the case, the therapist may attend to immediate complaints while patient understanding is developing.

## HOW CRANIOSACRAL THERAPY DIFFERS FROM CRANIAL OSTEOPATHY

CST is often compared with cranial osteopathy, which was developed by Dr. William Sutherland, the "father of cranial osteopathy." Although Dr. Sutherland's discoveries regarding the flexibility of skull sutures led to the early research behind CST and while both approaches affect the cranium, sacrum, and coccyx, similarities end at this point.

Today, as in the beginning, cranial osteopathy remains focused on the sutures of the skull. However, CST, as developed at MSU, focuses on the dura mater membrane system as the primary cause of dysfunction. The bones of the skull are involved only as they serve as "handles" for the practitioner to use to access and affect the membrane system that attaches to those bones.

Another major difference between the two approaches is in the quality of touch. CST practitioners generally evaluate and often correct imbalances in the system by using a light touch that has been scientifically measured between 5 and 10 gm, which is approximately the weight of a nickel resting in the palm of the hand. CST involves no invasive or directive forces but uses a gentle quality that often belies the effectiveness of the therapy. Most patients say they feel nothing more than subtle sensations during a typical session. In general, the manipulations used in cranial osteopathy are often heavier and more directive.[10]

## PERFORMING THE CRANIOSACRAL EVALUATION

During an initial CST evaluation, the therapist senses subtle motions while looking for any restrictions impeding free motion of the craniosacral system and various body regions, tissues, and organs, as well as the body's energies (Figures 1-2 to 1-4). The whole body responds to the rhythmical activity of the craniosacral system, which is evaluated for amplitude, quality, rate, and symmetry/asymmetry of response. Similar evaluations are conducted on the vascular and respiratory systems. The bodily responses, or lack thereof, to these systemic activities are significant factors in the search for the primary dysfunction.

Another integral part of the initial CST evaluation involves the myofascial system. Fascia runs like a continuous web of tissue throughout the body and re-

mains somewhat mobile under normal circumstances. Gentle traction applied on the fascia in arbitrary directions from various positions helps localize restricted areas. These areas of restricted mobility are then interpreted to be sites of either current problems or residue from previous lesions or problems.

Active lesions/problems are differentiated from inactive residual effects by a technique known as "arcing," which I developed with biophysicist Zvi Karni at MSU. By using mechano-electrical monitoring, we discovered that energies both within and off the body are

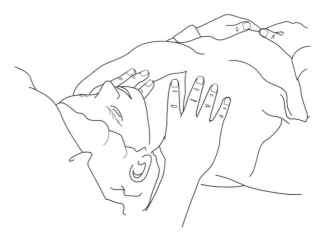

*Figure 1-3* Palpating craniosacral rhythm at the thorax. (From Upledger JE: *CranioSacral therapy II: beyond the dura,* Seattle, 1987, Eastland Press.)

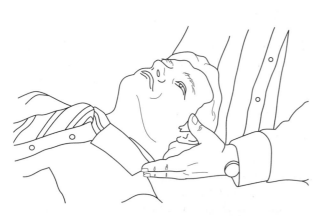

*Figure 1-2* Palpating craniosacral rhythm at the head. (From Upledger JE: *CranioSacral therapy II: beyond the dura,* Seattle, 1987, Eastland Press.)

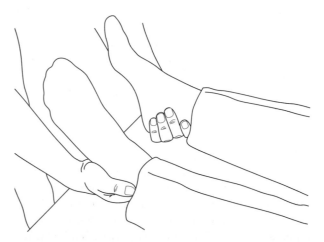

*Figure 1-4* Palpating craniosacral rhythm at the feet. (From Upledger JE: *CranioSacral therapy II: beyond the dura,* Seattle, 1987, Eastland Press.)

palpable to the skilled therapist.[12] Arcing requires the therapist to sense the energetic waves of interference produced by the active lesion/problem; these waves tend to be superimposed over the normal subtle physiological motions of the body, organs, tissues, and energies. Practitioners then trace these waves to their source by manually sensing the arcs that they form.[12-14]

The source of the waves is considered to be the core site of the underlying problem or lesion, which may actually be quite distant from the location of the patient's symptoms. Usually the active lesion/problem disrupts gross physiological activities, as well as more subtle energy functions and patterns, such as acupuncture meridians.

As sites of dysfunction and disruption are discovered, the therapist may attempt to restore mobility to the involved tissues and energy fields. More often than not these attempts will be partially if not completely successful. In either case the result is often the appearance of a deeper problem or lesion for which the dysfunction just treated has served as an adaptation. The therapist then follows these clues layer by layer until the primary problem is disclosed. This may occur during the first evaluation or it may require more than one visit to bring the deepest underlying problems to the surface. In CST, it is necessary to clear the entire body of any mobility restrictions to achieve the highest level of craniosacral system function.

Most of this evaluation is carried out before the complete evaluation of the craniosacral system itself. Skilled therapists are encouraged to move in and out of the various body systems and regions, including the craniosacral system, as their judgment and intuition suggest. Peripheral body problems often refer into the spinal cord via their nerve root connections. The effect of these referrals on related spinal cord segments includes an effect on the dura mater, which is key to the function of the craniosacral system.

## CORRECTING THE FACILITATED SEGMENT

CST includes the concept that the dura mater membrane within the vertebral canal (dural tube) has the freedom to glide up and down within that canal for a range of 0.5 to 2 cm. The slackness and directionality of the dural sleeves allow this movement as they depart the dural tube and attach to the intertransverse foramina of the spinal column.

When nerve roots refer increased levels of impulse activity into the spinal cord from their peripheral domains, a facilitated condition of the related spinal cord segment occurs. A condition of hyperactivity in that facilitated spinal cord segment sends out impulses to the related dural tube and dural sleeves. The result is a tightening and loss of mobility of the dural tube related to the involved segment(s).

Clinical observation suggests CST is effective in releasing dural tube restrictions to normalize the activity of facilitated spinal cord segments. To locate these areas of restricted mobility, the evaluator tests the mobility of the dural tube and releases restrictions as they are found using gentle traction techniques. These releases are mandatory: if a peripheral restriction is released but the dural tube restriction and facilitated spinal cord segment are not, the peripheral problem usually reoccurs.

Once the peripheral body and the dural tube have been treated for restrictions, the therapist can focus on the cranium and sacrum. During this time the therapist also helps correct both primary and secondary dysfunctions of the skull bones, facial bones, hard palate, and sacrococcygeal complex. All related sutures and joints are very gently mobilized through the use of the bones as handles on the dural membranes inside the skull and spinal canal.

After mobilizing bony restrictions, the therapist then focuses on correcting abnormal dural membrane restrictions, irregularities in cerebrospinal fluid activities, and dysfunctional energy patterns and fluctuations related to the craniosacral system. At this stage the patient often moves from a phase of having obstacles removed to one of self-healing with the therapist simply facilitating the process. In essence the patient moves out of the realm of "fighting disease" into one of enhancing health. This self-healing is why CST is such an excellent preventive medicine modality—it mobilizes natural defenses rather than focusing on the etiological agents of disease.

## *A Case Study*

### *Vertigo in an Olympic Diver*

Mary Ellen Clark was a world-class platform diver who had won several major competitions, including a bronze medal in the 1992 Olympic games in Barcelona, Spain.

Not one to rest on her accomplishments, she had set her sights on making the 1996 Olympic diving team and bringing home another medal. She was in the best physical shape of her career. In spite of her age (she turned 33 in 1996), experts gave her excellent odds at accomplishing her goal.

Suddenly, Mary Ellen began experiencing vertigo, a condition that had ended the careers of several other divers she knew. Vertigo is a devastating condition for anyone and particularly for a platform diver. Each time Mary Ellen stood at the edge of the diving platform she felt off balance. Once she hit the water, she would become confused and disoriented, occasionally causing her to mistakenly swim to the bottom of the pool.

Mary Ellen saw many doctors and specialists and tried both traditional and unconventional treatment methods to find relief. Yet there seemed to be no solution to her problem. She was unable to train for 9 months because of the devastating effects of the vertigo, and she had all but given up her dream of remaining on the Olympic team.

In September 1995, Mary Ellen came to see me at The Upledger Institute HealthPlex Clinical Services in Palm Beach Gardens, Florida. I started our first session by conducting a whole-body evaluation using my hands to test the mobility of the tissues and areas of restriction throughout her body. I quickly found several significant "energy cysts," or concentrated areas of foreign, disruptive, or obstructive energies, that likely resulted from traumatic blows to her body. Mary Ellen often did 50 dives a day from the 10-meter platform, and she hit the water at speeds of about 35 miles per hour. I used simple CST techniques to release her energy cysts manually without difficulty.

In the second session the CST evaluation pointed to Mary Ellen's left knee. She confirmed she had seriously wrenched it during a trampoline accident while practicing a new dive. At the time she paid little attention to the injury; she was accomplished at denying any presence of pain. As the evaluation continued, however, it became clear that the knee injury had caused a chain of compensation through her pelvis and lower back. Her spine had twisted to support her, which in turn caused her head to be improperly positioned on her neck.

As I helped Mary Ellen correct these problems, she began to improve. I continued to see her for at least one session each week for a straightforward combination of CST, knee and spine manipulation, pelvic rebalancing, and myofascial release. Within 30 days of her first treatment, Mary Ellen resumed her physical conditioning. Within 90 days she experienced a complete correction of the problem and was able to return to a full training schedule.

At the Olympic games in Atlanta, in July 1996, Mary Ellen Clark captured another bronze medal.[15,16]

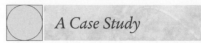

## A Case Study

### Intracranial Hemorrhage in a Newborn

Onar Bargior was born prematurely in Moscow, Russia, on February 7, 1991. He suffered severe cerebral circulation impairment, intracranial hemorrhage, and encephalopathy. He was diagnosed with infantile cerebral paralysis, spastic diplegia, and hypertension-hydrocephalic syndrome. Any stimulation produced muscle spasms that made his legs rigid and scissored, causing hyperextension of his truck and neck. His arms became rigid with clenched fists crossed in front of his body. Having almost no hip flexion, it was difficult for him to assume a sitting position.

In March 1992, Onar was registered as an invalid who could neither stand nor sit without direct assistance. His mother, Maiga, had tried to find help for her only son, yet medical treatment in Russia was limited and sporadic. Onar spent much of his life merely lying on a bed. Then a nonprofit medical relief agency in Waterville, Ohio, the International Services of Hope (ISOH), offered Onar and Maiga hope. ISOH specializes in bringing Third World children to the United States for donated medical treatment not available in their own countries. The organization has had remarkable success in securing life-saving and life-enhancing surgical and medical care for physically impaired or compromised children.

The agency arranged to fly Onar and his mother to New York for treatment at the Division of Pediatric Neurosurgery of New York University's Medical Center. Their clinical team evaluated Onar in October 1994. However, the doctors determined he was not an appropriate candidate for surgery and the subsequent rehabilitative care because of his extreme spasticity and psychomotor delays. The birth trauma and accompanying cerebral palsy had left his body too rigid to crawl or walk and had severely restricted the use of his right hand.

Onar's mother's hopes were shattered. Acutely aware of what this treatment meant to Onar, ISOH began to explore the availability of other medical care. In their investigations a representative consulted with a New York physician who had heard of an innovative program of care available through The Upledger Institute. ISOH contacted the Institute with the plea that the Institute was their "last resort." The alternative was to return Onar and his mother to Moscow without assistance.

The Upledger Institute accepted Onar into a 2-week intensive therapy program beginning March 13, 1995. This specialized treatment program is built around the use of CST complemented by physical therapy, Visceral Manipulation, acupuncture, massage therapy, play therapy, family counseling, and education. Onar's therapists consisted of a multidisciplinary team of physical therapists, occupational therapists, massage therapists, osteopathic physicians, and psychologists.

During Onar's first session, one of his therapists found severe restrictions in his dural membrane system—the falx cerebri, falx cerebelli, and tentorium cerebelli membranes inside the skull and the dural tube inside the spinal canal. She also found a compression of the sphenobasilar synchondrosis with a right sheer, ethmoid/frontal restriction with bilateral maxillary impaction and restrictions in the right temporoparietal suture, as well as the coronal suture. There were fascial restrictions in the cervical area relating to the hyoid bone, the sternocleidomastoid, and the suboccipital triangle muscles. The thoracic inlet and entire rib cage was restricted and rigid. There were also respiratory diaphragm restrictions with a visceral component into the stomach, and pelvic diaphragm restrictions with compression at the L5-S1 vertebral juncture. Treatment was applied to all of these areas.

On the second day of treatment, Maiga reported that Onar had slept soundly, which was an unexpected and pleasant surprise, since he normally woke three or four times a night. On awakening in the morning, he asked when he would be returning to the clinic. Throughout the program, Onar continued to show tremendous daily improvement, including an increased appetite, decreased spasticity, awakening without crying each morning, and increased range of movement of all joints.

Originally, the staff in Moscow and New York described Onar's psychomotor delays as so pronounced as to indicate mental retardation. Consequently, we were expecting a child slow to respond, both interpersonally and intellectually. What we found was quite the contrary. He impressed us from the beginning with his ability to communicate—initially through smiles, laughter, and emotional engagement. As he became more comfortable he began reacting in his native language, which was peppered with growing numbers of English words and phrases.

Coming into the program, Onar preferred to move by logrolling across the floor. The day he struggled to push himself up on his knees was another great milestone. He also began reaching for toys, and he developed the skills needed to play with stickers, little cars, and trucks.

The intensity of these programs and the systemic nature of the therapy they provide usually results in physiological gains continuing for several months after the program has ended. Because CST removes the restrictions that prohibit the body's natural inclination toward health, the body experiences a period of reorganization. Encouraged by such remarkable gains in Onar after just one treatment program, our staff decided to provide a second 2-week intensive treatment program after a 2-week period of rest.

The second treatment program began on April 10, 1995. To the delight of all involved, Onar demonstrated continued gains of physiological movement and decreased spasticity. On the second day of the program, when asked, "How are you today, Onar?" he answered in English: "I feel soft." On the fourth day of the program he was able to place his feet flat on the floor. By the end of the program he was crawling on all fours.

One of our physical therapists noted that, after the second 2-week session, Onar was using his right hand to reach and grasp objects with relative ease and accuracy. With minimal to moderate assistance, he was able to get into sitting, kneeling and high-kneeling positions. He had not been able to perform any of these developmental gross motor movements before coming to the United States. Overall, his contracted musculature or spasticity had greatly relaxed.

When Onar first came to the clinic, his entire cranial system was extremely restricted and compromised. By the end of his second intensive-treatment program his cranial system was moving with greater amplitude and symmetry. This indicated that Onar's system was operating more efficiently and fluidly without many restrictions in and around his central nervous system. In time Onar was able to sit for longer periods, crawl with reciprocal movement, crawl in high kneeling position with moderate assistance, and use his right hand without verbal prompting. He also began speaking more clearly and displaying a clarity of emotion and projection of love—traits most healthy children display.

By the time Onar completed his treatment programs he had also finished the necessary testing and inoculations to begin attending school. Maiga had worried that Onar might not be intelligent enough to get along in the world. But school testing showed that Onar has a fine mind. With opportunities for education, there is no telling what this child will do. He has already contributed in a profound way to the lives of his therapists and friends.[17,18] ∽

## CLINICAL APPLICATIONS OF CRANIOSACRAL THERAPY

CST is well known for its multiple applications and positive results in thousands of cases like those of Mary Ellen and Onar. By facilitating and enhancing the body's self-corrective mechanisms, it has proved useful as both a primary and adjunctive treatment modality for a wide variety of dysfunctions, from coronary insufficiency to Crohn's disease.

The number of sessions required to achieve results depends on the complexity of the adaptive layers, patient defense mechanisms, and other factors. After an initial hands-on evaluation is conducted, a recommendation can be made. In general, if there is no change in condition after five or six sessions, CST may not be effective for that individual.

Following is a partial list of condition types that have shown response to CST in clinical applications. While research conducted at MSU proved the existence of the craniosacral system and its effect on health and disease, this information is based primarily on clinical observations over the last 15 years of practicing CST. Although no formal outcome studies have been conducted, thousands of patients have reported their results to us, and what is noted here are observations of clear and compelling results and trends.

## Chronic Pain Syndromes

### Arthritis: Degenerative and Inflammatory

CST enhances fluid motion, releases muscle tonus and desensitizes facilitated segments, all of which contribute to joint rejuvenation. Excellent responses have been reported, including some results that have shown normalized blood studies.

### Headache Syndromes

CST is excellent at identifying and treating a wide variety of underlying causes for headaches, including migraine, tension cephalalgia, fluid congestion, and hormonally related syndromes. Sutural immobility seems to be a contributing factor in migraines for many patients. CST addresses this problem, as well as autonomic and neuromusculoskeletal dysfunctions, both of which may be underlying causes of the migraine syndrome.

### Pain Syndromes

All pain syndromes, including myofascial, neuromusculoskeletal, and radicular pain syndromes, have shown response to CST. Because of its effects on the autonomics, CST desensitizes facilitated segments and enhances fluid exchange throughout the body and psychoemotional effects. CST also addresses many of the neuromusculoskeletal, myofascial, and psychoemotional factors that may serve as contributing factors to chronic neck and back pain.

### Reflexive Sympathetic Dystrophy

Reflexive sympathetic dystrophy (RSD) is a painful condition that results from the sympathetic nervous system going out of control. The cause could be an injury, entrapped nerve, inflammation, toxicity, or any circumstance that might feed an abnormal amount of energy into the sympathetic nervous system. Conservative medical treatment for this condition, which in extreme cases includes amputation of the painful area, has proven rather ineffective. The key to helping the RSD patient is discovering and resolving the underlying source of the excess energy. CST is well suited to finding and treating the underlying causes of RSD and subsequently resolving pain.

### Spinal Dysfunctions

Spinal dysfunctions, including scoliosis, low-back (lumbar and lumbosacral) instability, disc compression, postoperative complications, and others, have shown response to CST. Once the underlying cause is determined, CST is effective in solving biomechanical, neurogenic, and facilitated segment problems.

### Temporomandibular Joint Syndrome

Temporomandibular joint syndrome (TMJ) is a painful problem caused by the joints of the lower jaw becoming dysfunctional for any number of reasons. Surprisingly, TMJ can originate from a craniosacral system restriction that results in an imbalance between the temporal bones on each side of the head. Other causes include nervous tension that results in tooth grinding and/or jaw clenching, whiplash injury to the neck, or a malocclusion of the teeth. CST is highly effective at locating and alleviating the underlying problems. It is also highly effective at mobilizing temporal bones.

## Traumatic Injuries

CST practitioners treat a multitude of traumatic brain and spinal cord injuries, including closed-head injuries, spinal cord injuries, whiplash and other spinal ligament strains, and nervous system sequelae due to injuries. Success varies, depending on the extent and severity of the injury. I usually do well with patients who suffer seizures subsequent to their head injuries, often eliminating the need for further medication. Although a small number of cases do not respond to CST, I have been treating seizure patients since 1975 and have yet to see an adverse reaction.

I have seen moderate improvement in the movement of paralyzed limbs due to head injuries. The greatest improvement usually appears in the area of intellect and social responsiveness. Some patients have had remarkable improvement in vision, hearing, smell and taste, and in secondary autonomic dysfunction such as disequilibrium, cardiac pulmonary function, bowel function, urinary tract function, sexual function, and related conditions. The positive results are probably due to the effect of CST on the autonomics and related spinal cord segments, as well as its ability to reduce stress and anxiety.

## Degenerative Diseases of the Central Nervous System

Until a few years ago it was thought that cerebrospinal fluid simply bathed the surface of the brain. All that changed with the use of radioactive tracers that flow with the fluid. It has since been observed that when tracers are injected into the ventricular system of the brain, they are distributed throughout the brain substance within minutes. Since cerebrospinal fluid carries all sorts of messenger molecules that facilitate communications between cells of different systems, it stands to reason that improving cerebrospinal fluid circulation may explain the success seen when CST is used to treat degenerative diseases such as Parkinson's disease.

Another recent discovery is that cerebrospinal fluid contains molecules that attach to metallic atoms that are deposited in the brain. These metallic atoms are then carried away and excreted from the body in a process known as *chelation*. Metal atoms deposited in the brain tissue are thought to be contributing factors in problems such as Alzheimer's disease and senility. Thus the improvement of cerebrospinal fluid circulation through CST may be considered preventive therapy.

Elderly patients who have trouble concentrating and putting words together have responded with increased mental alertness and brain function. By improving the circulation of blood, cerebrospinal fluid, and interstitial and intracellular fluid, CST helps clear toxic wastes accumulated in the brain cells and tissues.

## Cerebrovascular Insufficiency Problems

CST has been shown to be effective in both preventing and recovering from stroke when thrombosis or arterial insufficiencies are causative agents. As soon as a patient's condition has stabilized after stroke and the danger of hemorrhage passes, CST can effectively help wash away toxic byproducts of blood cell deterioration to help enable a speedier recovery.

## Postoperative Rehabilitation

CST is an excellent addition to any postsurgical rehabilitation program. It restores the movement of body fluids to areas traumatized by surgical procedures, which enhances the healing process and holds the potential for reducing the formation of adhesions and scar tissue. CST also helps remove residual toxicity of anesthetics and pain medications.

From about 1973 to 1974 I treated several postoperative neurological patients as early as the first postsurgical day with very good results. The neurosurgeon felt these patients demonstrated a decreased number of complications, lowered morbidity rates, and shortened recovery times. In general, the sooner the therapy begins, the better it is at helping to prevent complications.

## Brain Dysfunctions

### Autism
CST has shown great promise in cases of autism, a complex set of symptoms with no known origin. While it is not clear precisely which mechanisms are at work in either causing or "curing" the condition, it has been widely noted that patients generally inflict much less pain on themselves, display more affection toward others, and show improved social behavior after CST.

### Cerebral Palsy
*Cerebral palsy (CP)* is a general term that means the brain is not working correctly. Because CST often has a positive effect on the motor control system, including relief of muscle spasticity, we do well with a majority of CP patients. There is occasional remarkable

improvement, although sometimes there is little or no change. Either way it deserves a trial of approximately 10 sessions, although the rule holds true—the sooner we treat them the better these patients usually do. For example, if we treat a patient as an adolescent and can correct the underlying problem, the nerve pathways necessary for proper functioning may not be present because they never had a chance to form in the first place.

### Learning Disabilities

I have treated a great number and variety of learning-disabled children. In my experience, over half of these children had problems with the craniosacral system. In cases like this, when the problem in the craniosacral system is resolved, the child has up to a 90% chance of overcoming his learning disabilities, especially in cases such as dyslexia and hyperkinesis. Quite often the disability simply disappears.

### Motor System Problems

CST can almost invariably improve motor and speech problems. Even in the case of eye-motor problems, a skilled practitioner can tell in a matter of minutes if the problem is caused by tension in the membranes through which the nerves to the eyes pass. When this is the case, especially in children, the problem can often be permanently corrected in two or three sessions. Surgery for problems such as convergent strabismus (cross-eyed) can often be avoided. Patients treated with CST have also reported great success in cases of olfactory dysfunction and vertigo, although we have seen only moderate success with tinnitus.

## Endocrine Disorders

Many endocrine disorders, including premenstrual tension, pituitary dysfunction, pineal gland problems, and related emotional problems, often respond favorably to CST. It enhances the mobilization of fluids and autonomic balancing, improves endocrine control, and relieves neuromusculoskeletal and psychoemotional symptoms. Releasing the dural sleeves that may be restricting nerve outflow to the adrenals, the thyroid, the spleen, the liver, the thymus, and the reproductive glands has also been very helpful in some patients.

## Many Other Conditions

The most important thing to remember about CST is that it is extremely gentle and often resolves conditions in a shorter timeframe than many other approaches. Quite simply, it can almost always help in some fashion, even if simply to improve the chance of long-term success of other therapies used.

## CONTRAINDICATIONS OF CRANIOSACRAL THERAPY

Even in the most critical cases, CST has wide applications when used in conjunction with conventional treatment programs. However, the following are contraindications for the use of CST[13]:

1. *Acute intracranial hemorrhage:* Affecting the craniosacral system membranes may significantly change intracranial fluid pressure dynamics, which could interrupt the tenuous progress of clot formation and prolong the duration of the hemorrhage.
2. *Intracranial aneurysm:* Changing intracranial fluid pressure dynamics could potentially precipitate a leak or rupture of a dangerous, already present intracranial aneurysm.
3. *Recent skull fracture:* A very careful approach should be applied in the case of recent skull fracture, lest an increase in cranial bone motion leads to bleeding or a membranous tear.
4. *Herniation of the medulla oblongata:* A herniation of the medulla oblongata through the foramen magnum is a life-threatening situation. You would not want to alter fluid pressures within the craniosacral system by any means.

## HOW TO LEARN CRANIOSACRAL THERAPY

The Upledger Institute was developed in 1985 to educate the public and healthcare practitioners about the value of CST. Since that time, these techniques have been taught to more than 50,000 therapists in some 56 different countries.

Today the Upledger Institute is dedicated to teaching CST as it was originally developed. Its curriculum offers a full range of workshops totaling more than 500 hours of training.

In addition to providing a sound academic foundation, the training helps therapists develop the subtle senses of touch, motion, and energy perception necessary to become effective CST practitioners. The Upledger Institute also offers a two-level certification program to help ensure the quality of skills.

Because it was originally developed as a complementary modality for healthcare professionals, there is currently no single license to practice CST. Thanks to its rapid increase in practice and acceptance, however, plans are underway to create a separate and distinct professional license program.

## PROSPECTS FOR THE FUTURE

Over the last decade, positive clinical results and the public's growing acceptance of nontraditional healthcare methods have caused a surge in the demand for CST. It is continuing to become well known as an effective facilitator for the inherent healing processes with which every human being is endowed.

Its future in the field of rehabilitative care is bright. Yet its greatest value may be seen even earlier in the cycle of health: in the newborn nursery.[19] CST appears to be an efficient neutralizer for all types of birth traumas and their potential effects on the brain and spinal cord, including autonomic nervous function, endocrine function, and immune function. Research strongly suggests that the birth process alone may be responsible for numerous brain dysfunctions and central nervous system problems. CST carried out within the first few days of life could potentially reduce a wide variety of difficulties, many of which might not become apparent until later in life.

CST is also viewed as a successful method of integrating the body, mind, and spirit. This focus on "holistic" health may result in a significant reduction in disease and a great improvement in the quality of life.

## References

1. Retzlaff EW et al: Nerve fibers and endings in cranial sutures research report, *J Am Osteopath Assoc* 77:474-475, 1978.
2. Retzlaff EW et al: Possible functional significance of cranial bone sutures, Report of the 88th session of the American Association of Anatomists, 1975.
3. Retzlaff EW et al: Structure of cranial bone sutures, research report, *J Am Osteopath Assoc* 75:607-608, 1976.
4. Retzlaff EW et al: Sutural collagenous and their innervation in Saimiri Sciurus, *Anat Rec* 187:692, 1977.
5. Retzlaff EW, Mitchell FL Jr: *The cranium and its sutures,* Berlin, 1987, Springer-Verlag.
6. Sperino G: *Anatomica humana* 1:202-203, 1931.
7. Upledger JE: The reproducibility of craniosacral examination findings: a statistical analysis, *J Am Osteopath Assoc* 76:890-899, 1977.
8. Upledger JE: Relationship of craniosacral examination findings in grade school children with developmental problems, *J Am Osteopath Assoc* 77:760-776, 1978.
9. Woods JM, Woods RH: Physical findings related to psychiatric disorders, *J Am Osteopath Assoc* 60:988-993, 1961.
10. Upledger JE: Differences separate craniosacral therapy from cranial osteopathy, *Massage & Bodywork* X(4): 20-22, 1995.
11. Upledger JE: Mechano-electric patterns during craniosacral osteopathic diagnosis and treatment, *J Am Osteopath Assoc* 1:49-50, 1979.
12. Upledger JE, Vredevoogd J: *CranioSacral therapy,* Seattle, 1983, Eastland Press.
13. Upledger JE: *CranioSacral therapy II: beyond the dura,* Seattle, 1987, Eastland Press.
14. Upledger JE: *SomatoEmotional release and beyond,* Berkeley, Calif, 1990, North Atlantic Press.
15. Lyttle J: An Olympian comeback, *Columbus Monthly* 1:105-107, 1996.
16. Murphy J: Olympic diver sinks vertigo with CranioSacral Therapy, *Adv Phys Therap* 7(42):5, 1996.
17. Bourne RA Jr: To Onar, with love, *Massage Ther J* 35(2): 68-70, 72,74, 1996.
18. Hammond F: The Upledger Institute offers Russian boy hope for more active life, *Nurse's Touch,* 6(2):12, 1995.
19. Frymann VM: Relation of disturbances of craniosacral mechanisms to symptomatology of the newborn: a study of 1,250 infants, *J Am Osteopath Assoc* 65:1059, 1966.

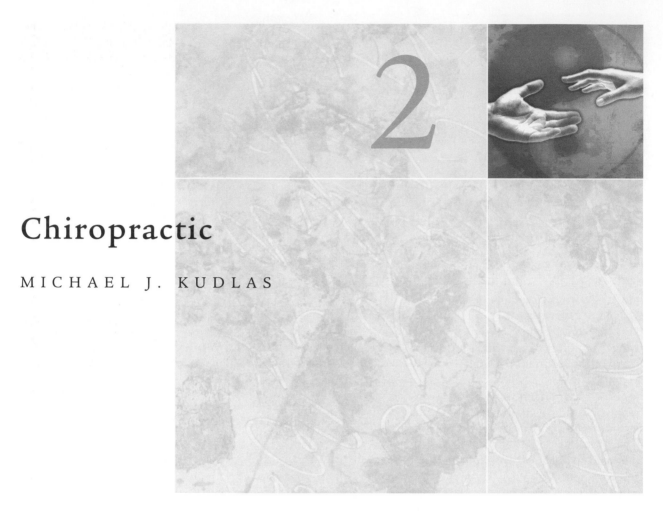

# Chiropractic

MICHAEL J. KUDLAS

Chiropractic is a uniquely American approach to health and wellness grounded in certain ancient principles and developed as a clinical model of healthcare.

Chiropractic has grown from modest beginnings in Iowa to become a drug-free/surgery-free healing profession practiced throughout the world.[1] Because it has sometimes healed those whom allopathic medicine could not, chiropractic has a strong grass roots appeal. Chiropractic's cost effectiveness, coupled with its rehabilitative capacity, promises a greater role in today's healthcare arena.

## HISTORY AND DEVELOPMENT

Hippocrates enunciated foundational principles of chiropractic 20 centuries ago. He said, "Get knowledge of the spine for it is the requisite of many diseases."

He also taught that there is a physis, or vital spirit, in all living things and that healing comes from within.[2] Hippocrates presaged some essentials of chiropractic care. First, identify and correct vertebral misalignments, which create and maintain nerve interference (vertebral subluxation), thus allowing the recuperative powers of the body to restore full function. In rehabilitation, as in all chiropractic treatment, this combination translates to a holistic approach of caring for the whole person, rather than addressing a disease process, simple symptom suppression, or a single presenting condition. Chiropractors draw on a rich history, ongoing research, and strong clinical results.

### Ancient History of Spinal Care

Spinal manipulation dates back thousands of years. In southern France, cave paintings dated at 17,500

BCE depict crude forms of manipulative care. Records from Japan, Assyria, Tibet, Babylonia, India, and Egypt all provide evidence that spinal manipulation was practiced in those cultures. In the Americas, the Toltecs, Incas, Mayans, and Aztecs all routinely used manipulation of various body parts in their health-care systems.

In Rome during the second century AD, Galen was teaching the proper relationship of the spine and vertebrae. He was given the title of "Prince of Physicians" when he realigned the neck of a famed scholar who had lost use of his right arm, allowing function to return.[3] Other Western and Eastern cultures have histories replete with village "bonesetters" renowned for their ability to heal by straightening the spine.[1]

## Early Chiropractic— D.D. and B.J. Palmer

It was in 1895 when Daniel David Palmer, then a practicing magnetic energy healer, delivered the first chiropractic adjustment, in what today could be a workers' compensation case, to Harvey Lillard, an African-American who operated a janitorial service for the building that housed Palmer's office. Lillard had been deaf for 17 years as a result of an injury he suffered while exerting himself in a cramped, stooping position. According to Lillard, he felt something give, heard a "pop," and soon lost all hearing. Palmer's examination revealed a lump in Lillard's cervical spine, which he reasoned was a misaligned vertebra. Palmer thought that if the vertebra was returned to its normal position, Mr. Lillard's hearing might return. After some persuasion, D.D. Palmer performed the first chiropractic adjustment to Harvey Lillard on September 18, 1895. Within a short while, Mr. Lillard's hearing returned.[3,4,5]

Palmer continued what he called "hand treatments," observing great clinical success in a wide variety of ailments including heart problems, lumbago, seizures, flu, and stomach disorders. With his friend and patient Reverend Samuel Weed, a Greek student and Presbyterian minister, they coined the term *chiropractic* (done by hand) on January 14, 1896 (Figure 2-1).[3] "Being an intensely practical man and having much experience with human nature during his 50 years, Palmer conceived this new practice to be so simple that he was afraid that someone else might at-

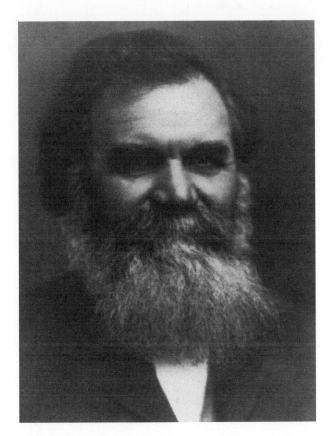

*Figure 2-1* David Daniel (D.D.) Palmer, the Founder of Chiropractic. (Courtesy David D. Palmer Health Science Archives, Palmer College of Chiropractic, Davenport, Iowa.)

tempt to steal it from him. He therefore sought to keep his discovery and method of practice a family secret only for him and his descendants."[3]

Fortunately, the profession outgrew Palmer's earliest plans for it. Since then, more than 30 chiropractic colleges have been established, and today it is the third largest healthcare profession (behind medical doctors and dentists), with over 57,000 practicing chiropractors in the United States.[1]

D. D. Palmer's son, Bartlett Joshua Palmer (B.J.) (Figure 2-2) is known as the developer of chiropractic. His many innovations in the profession include the first use of x-ray for spinal studies in 1910 at the Palmer College of Chiropractic in Davenport, Iowa. B.J. later developed numerous instruments and analytic devices, many of which are still used today in modern form, for the analysis and correction of vertebral subluxation.

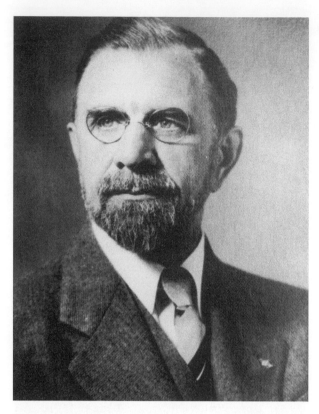

*Figure 2-2* Bartlett Joshua (B.J.) Palmer. (Courtesy Sherman College of Straight Chiropractic, Spartanburg, South Carolina.)

## Modern Chiropractic— Modern Battles

Because the rise of chiropractic paralleled the rise of organized medicine's efforts to monopolize healthcare treatment in the United States,* many chiropractors were arrested and spent time in jail and prison on charges of practicing medicine without a license. In the 1930s and 1940s, B.J. Palmer often traveled across the country testifying in defense of the profession and the arrested doctors, establishing chiropractic as a separate and nonduplicating form of healthcare. He wrote numerous books establishing and clarifying his father's initial vitalistic approach of chiropractic as a separate philosophy, science, and art. This led to the licensing of chiropractors throughout all 50 states and the acceptance of chiropractic as a separate and distinct form of healing.

Unfortunately it did not deter the AMA from its attempts to restrain the competitive forces of the chiropractic profession. In 1963 the AMA formed an anticompetition committee, interestingly called the "Committee on Quackery," with its prime mission as "first the containment of chiropractic and ultimately the elimination of chiropractic."[7]

This organized illegal activity against chiropractic and the public welfare continued unrestrained until 1976, when five chiropractors filed a lawsuit against the AMA and seven other medical coconspirators for restraint of trade under the Sherman Anti-trust Act. The case lasted 11 years with the chiropractic profession prevailing, and the AMA appealing all the way to the United States Supreme Court. At each and every level of appeal by the AMA, the 1987 decision of Judge Susan Getzendanner was upheld. "Evidence at the trial showed [the AMA and defendants] took active steps, often covert, to undermine chiropractic educational institutions, conceal evidence of the usefulness of chiropractic care, undercut insurance programs for patients of chiropractors, subvert government inquiries into the efficacy of chiropractic, engage in a massive disinformation campaign to discredit and destabilize the chiropractic profession, and engaged in numerous other activities to maintain a medical monopoly over healthcare in this country." Judge Getzendanner ruled, "The AMA never acknowledged the lawlessness of its past conduct," and issued a permanent injunction against the conspirators,[8] which included the American College of Surgeons, the American College of Radiologists, the American Association of Orthopedic Surgeons, the Joint Commission on Accreditation of Hospitals, the American College of Physicians, the American Hospital Association, and the Illinois State Medical Society. The American Academy of Physical Medicine and Rehabilitation and the American Osteopathic Association settled out of court before the decision. The surgeons and radiologists groups, after being found guilty but before the federal injunctions were imposed, also settled with the chiropractors.

---

*The AMA has been convicted three times for anti-trust activity. "In 1943, the AMA was convicted for criminal violation of the anti-trust laws for its attempt to destroy an innovative and cost cutting health care insurance and delivery system in Washington, DC. Again, in 1982, the AMA was found guilty by the Federal Trade Commission of a decades-long systematic violation of the anti-trust laws for restricting informative advertising practices and banning innovative group practice and physician hiring practices." The third conviction came in 1987, the AMA against the chiropractic profession.[6]

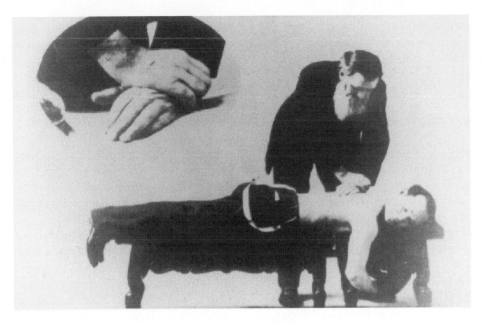

*Figure 2-3* D.D. Palmer—Adjusting with one of his early "hand treatments." (Courtesy Sherman College of Straight Chiropractic, Spartanburg, SC.)

## THEORY AND PRACTICE OF CHIROPRACTIC

### The Holistic Philosophy

Since its professional birth in the American Midwest in 1895, chiropractic has maintained its focus on restoring nerve function by adjusting misaligned vertebrae (vertebral subluxations). What may appear at first glance to be a very narrow view of health and well-being is, in practice, a profound multidimensional healing approach that directly addresses the musculoskeletal and neuromuscular systems and indirectly affects all others systems via the nervous system connections, mental/emotional levels, and biochemistry of the individual (Figure 2-3).

Based on clinical success, B.J. Palmer realized the importance and practicality of this approach, but it has taken years of scientific study to understand and expand the theory behind it. Christopher Kent, DC, researched three basic operational clinical models for vertebral subluxation: the segmental model, the postural approaches, and the tonal model.[9] Scott Walker, DC, defined and delineated the mental/emotional factors affected by the neuro-emotionally induced subluxation patterns from the work of Pavlov, Riddler,

Frank, and Goodheart.[10,11] However, underlying the science is a fundamental holistic philosophy from which other facets of the profession have developed.

This philosophical perspective makes chiropractic useful in rehabilitation settings because it results in the rehabilitation of the entire person during the normal course of care. From a chiropractic perspective this is only natural. After all, if a person is suffering from an acceleration/deceleration cervical injury (whiplash), he or she must be seen "in toto" and cannot be separated from his or her injury; the effects of the subluxation damage are not limited to just the injury site, but effect the entire person. In chiropractic, there is no mind/body "connection" because chiropractors understand that there cannot be a mind/body "separation." We are all one, in one.

In 1907 D.D. Palmer explained, "Life is the result of the combination of intellectual spirit and unintelligible matter. Life expressions are made manifest by acts, functions performed."[5] This "triune of life"—intelligence, expressed through matter by forces—is a fundamental unifying tenet in chiropractic philosophy, science, and art, and led to further development and refinement by his son, B.J. Palmer, into the concept that, "Chiropractic is based upon a major philosophical premise: There is a Universal Intelligence in all matter constantly giving to it all its property and activities, thus maintaining it in existence."[12,13] It is through this vitalistic philosophy that the holistic clinical chiropractic approaches have developed.

## The Triune of Life

From D.D. Palmer's early writings, B.J. Palmer developed the vitalistic chiropractic philosophy and clinical concepts that are the basis of today's chiropractic. "Triune of life" refers to the basic elements necessary for living things to exist—intelligence, force, and matter. The Palmers totally refuted the Western medical disease model, particularly through their philosophy and partially through the necessity to differentiate the profession from medicine. "Chiropractic is not evolved from medicine or any other method."[5] Neither could they work without the holistic philosophy, which was based on their understanding of the universe and life. "Man is not a machine—a mechanical contrivance run by mechanical power. The bodily functions are carried on by an energy known as vital force. [B.J. would later refer to this as *Innate Intelligence*.] Mental impulses are not power; they do not run the body. They are a production of Innate, spirit. Power and mental impulses are not synonymous."

"Vital force furnishes the energy, [mental] impulses direct them."[4] "The basis of Chiropractic is the identification of God with Life-Force. The Intelligent Life-Force of Creation is God. It is individualized in each of us. It desires to express itself in the best manner possible."[4] Although expressed in the language and reflecting the belief in the spiritualism of the times, these early concepts of mind/body integration would be considered advanced even by today's standards. From these concepts we can see that D.D. and B.J. Palmer's philosophy was health oriented, not disease oriented. Even in those formative days, they recognized the role of consciousness and its health influence over the body. A case could be made that chiropractic is the first Western mind/body profession because the care rendered in chiropractic is "health enhancing" rather than "disease treating," and the enhancing portion is consciousness based.

Today these concepts of vital intelligent forces (consciousness) directing the processes of living things are being reinforced by the applied discoveries in quantum physics. Consider physicist Henry Stapp, who said, "The message of quantum nonlocality is that the fundamental process of Nature lies outside space-time but generates events that can be located in space-time,"[14] or Goswami, professor at the Institute of Theoretical Science at the University of Oregon, who puts the chiropractic major premise even more clearly from the quantum physics viewpoint when he states, "The success that Democritus's materialism has enjoyed in science for the past three hundred years may only be an aberration. Quantum theory interpreted according to an idealist metaphysics is paving the road for an idealist science in which consciousness comes first and matter pales to secondary importance."[15]

The view that there is a "vital force" in man is not new or specific to chiropractic. Chiropractic has updated that idea with its philosophy that there is an Innate Intelligence in all living things, healing comes from above-down-inside-out, and this process is accomplished via an optimally functioning nervous system free of interference.

From this holistic viewpoint, the rehabilitative care rendered by a chiropractor is based on working with the natural inherent recuperative powers of the body (as intelligence expressing through matter via force), addressing the structural, biochemical, and mental/emotional aspects of the person. This approach is referred to as the Triangle of Health.

## The Triangle of Health

Because D.D. Palmer was interested in the cause of a problem, he resisted all forms of palliative treatment that only sought to cover up the patient's symptoms. "Chiropractic is not a method of treatment or a process of treating diseases." Instead, chiropractors replace the parts that are not in apposition into their normative relative position. "The determining causes of diseases," Palmer wrote in 1907, "are traumatism, poisons, and autosuggestion."[16] Walker has modernized the language and formatted the truth of this Palmer principle, updating the "Triangle of Health" (originally from Walther and Applied Kinesiology Systems) in which, "Each equilateral side of the triangle represents aspects of those factors affecting man's health. One side is structural (traumatism), the second side is biochemical (poison), and the third emotional (autosuggestion) (Figure 2-4)."[10]

Walker states, "In practice, chiropractors as a group are without parallel in their expertise and tech-

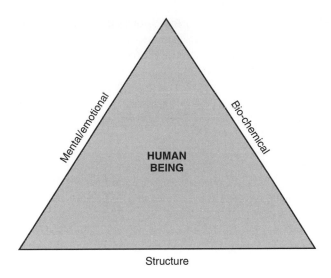

*Figure 2-4* Triangle of Health.

nology of the structural and biochemical sides of the health triangle. The various chiropractic techniques have provided unparalleled sophistication in the treatment of these imbalances."[10] This is supported by Manga in his research for the Ontario Ministry of Health, who found "on the evidence, particularly the most valid clinical studies, spinal manipulation applied by chiropractors is shown to be more effective than alternative treatment for LBP (Low Back Pain). Many medical therapies are of questionable validity or are clearly inadequate."[17] Numerous other studies[18,19,20] strongly support Manga's findings.

The unique aspect of this triangle has been the finding by Walker that about one third of patients' problems can be emotionally caused, leading to his refinement of the "neuro-emotional subluxation complex—the NEC." Further studies by Peterson[21,22,23] and Monti, et al,[24] plus the clinical findings of Walker[25] and thousands of practicing clinicians, have demonstrated that the nervous system can house an elusive but chiropractically correctable emotionally based interference pattern that is symptomatically displayed physically and that with chiropractic intervention by spinal adjustment, the pattern, with symptoms, disappears.

Because chiropractic is health-enhancement oriented, its approach to health is open-ended and, with its vitalistic philosophy, attempts to answer the question, "How healthy can we become?" Consequently, when a chiropractor cares for an injured patient, he or she looks at the patient from an open-ended

health perspective, seeking to build on the natural inherent recuperative powers of the body to return homeostasis to the person. In rehabilitation, to appropriately do this, the chiropractor will often address the patient as if he or she were a triangle, made up of these structural, biochemical, and mental/emotional components.

The chiropractor evaluates not only the extent of the injury but, in a measure, what is right with the patient as well. This procedure leads to impressive cost-effective treatment statistics by building on the remaining levels of health the patient has and not merely by attempting to suppress the patient's symptoms. The evaluation includes, but is not limited to, those aspects of the triangle as seen in Figure 2-4.

Using various chiropractic techniques (discussed below), the adjustments made by the chiropractor address the various sides of the triangle by correcting the subluxations related to each side, thus allowing health and stability to return naturally to the patient. Depending on the severity of the injury, one or more of the sides of the triangle may be involved. If we take into account the injury of a patient, the Triangle of Health can be seen as a treatment plan for the rehabilitative process, with each side receiving particular attention at the appropriate time (Figure 2-5).

## Chiropractic Techniques

Chiropractic has thrived because of its unique approach to the human frame and relationship to the nervous system. Chiropractors have long maintained that the bones of the spine can and do impinge on the nervous system and cause a form of nerve interference called a vertebral subluxation, which interferes with the homeostasis of an individual.

Today there are over 130 chiropractic adjusting techniques devoted to the correction of the vertebral subluxation complex,[3] each technique having been developed over the years to meet a specific patient need. Some techniques are complete adjusting systems, addressing all areas of the spine with a specific adjusting style (Gonstead, Diversified, Thompson Terminal Point Technique). Other techniques address a specific side of the health triangle and are designed to be incorporated into the overall rehabilitative approach of the doctor (i.e., Neuro Emotional Technique [NET]—emotional, Contact Reflex Analysis—biochemical). Other techniques address a specific system of the body

MENTAL/EMOTIONAL       BIO-CHEMICAL

Neuro-emotional complexes

Diet

Self-esteem

Nutrition

Altered brain chemistry

**HUMAN BEING**

Supplementation

Trauma residuals

Drug side effects

STRUCTURE

Gait   Posture analysis   Structure

Special senses   Spine   Pelvis   Skull/cranial   Sutures

Muscle physiology   Neurolymphatics   Stress receptors

Discs   Dura mater   Righting reflexes   Etc.

*Figure 2-5* Expanded Triangle of Health with many but not all components evaluated by a chiropractor during patient rehabilitation.

(Neuro Organizational Technique, Neuro Vascular Reflex Technique, Neuro Lymphatic Reflex Technique). Still others employ energetic approaches in correction (Bio-Energetic Synchronization Technique, Chiroenergetics, Touch for Health). Many use the entire body for analysis and correction (Total Body Modification, Applied Kinesiology, Applied Spinal Biomechanical Engineering). Even though a technique is used to address one side of the treatment triangle, its influence will be translated throughout the body within the healing process via the nervous system.

Many adjusting techniques employ a short-lever, high-velocity, doctor-generated impulse, creating the corrective force for the body to use (Gonsted, Pierce-Stillwagon, Diversified) and may cause cavitation of the joint. Some techniques use lower force, either through low mass instruments rapidly accelerated mechanically to generate the force or by specific rapid hand movements (Activators, Atlas Orthogonality Technique, HIO Toggle Recoil) with no cavitation. Other techniques rely on extremely slow acceleration of large mass to produce the generated force, either by the application of specially shaped blocks to lever the body over time into the correction, or by gentle light hand placement (Sacral-Occipital Blocking Technique, Logan Basic Technique) (Figure 2-6).

 *A Case Study*

### Chronic Shoulder Pain

Bob, a 49-year-old mechanical engineer, has chronic right shoulder pain and loss of motion. He is unable to raise his arm forward to abduct it above his shoulder without noticeable pain. The original onset of pain occurred 2 years prior when he was handing groceries to his wife from their car trunk.

Bob is very fit at 6 foot tall and 220 pounds, although he complains of "about 20 pounds" of weight gain since the reduction of his fitness program because of the injury. His main concern is his chronic pain and inability to successfully lift weights and stay in shape. He has had to give up recreational softball and has not lifted weights in 9 months.

Previous relevant history reveals that Bob was a professional minor league baseball player with an extensive ball-playing career and minor injuries to his arm and shoulder associated with playing baseball at that level. He also boxed in the military and suffered peroneal nerve damage in the right leg as a result of a stab wound.

According to Bob, unsuccessful medical treatment included treatment by two MDs who prescribed Flexeril and Motrin and then medications, which were "other variations on that theme." The second MD, "injected me with a cortisone shot, which helped for 2 weeks," and ordered physical therapy consisting of general range-of-motion

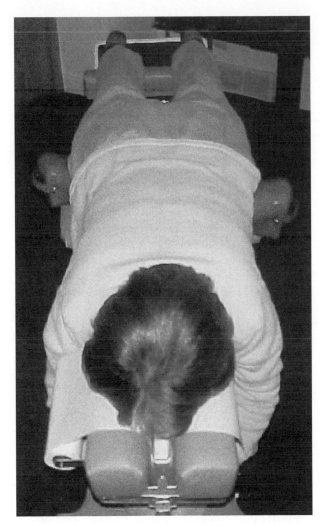

*Figure 2-6* Patient receiving Sacral-Occipital Blocking Adjustment for a lumbar subluxation involving a disc herniation. (Courtesy Kalamazoo Community Chiropractic, Kalamazoo, Michigan.)

(ROM) shoulder exercises with no relief. He was first seen 1 year after the accident.

Chiropractic examination revealed positive orthopedic findings in the lumbosacral spine, with palpable muscle tightness and spasm from T3 to occiput. Spinal ROM elicited painful responses and reduced cervical ROM and pain in the dorsolumbar motions of flexion (which was increased). Deep tendon reflexes were 2+ normal, except for the Achilles, which was bilaterally absent. Applied Kinesiology Manual Muscle Testing demonstrated both right rhomboids and the entire right shoulder girdle muscles to be weak to testing, as were the right arm extensors.

With the use of Total Body Modification Protocol (TBM), Bob demonstrated a dysinsulinism pattern. He demonstrated a Cranial Injury Complex with the use of Neuro-Organizational Testing (NOT) procedures, demonstrating failure of the righting reflexes of the head and neck.

With the use of Gonsted analytical techniques, radiographic studies of Bob's spine indicated vertebral misalignments at C1, C5, T2, T3, T4, T5, T7, T8, T11, L5, and sacrum. Disk degeneration was noted at C5 through C7, and T7 through T10. Posterior weight bearing as calculated from the lateral lumbar view, and using Applied Spinal Biomechanical Engineering Techniques (ASBE), lateral flexion failure of the lumbar spine was noted bilaterally from L1 through L5, which was correctable with ASBE anterior ileum maneuvers.

A computer analysis of a paraspinal surface EMG scan using the Insight 7000 Subluxation Station and protocol demonstrated significant heat imbalances at C1, C3, C5, T1, T2, L3, L5, and S1.

Based on these findings, a regimen of twice weekly corrective care was instituted that included subluxation correction in the cervical, thoracic, and lumbosacral spine using standard TBM, NOT, and Gonsted adjusting protocols for the structural subluxations, and Neuro Emotional Technique (NET) for the emotionally based subluxations. Bob was also instructed on corrective ASBE spinal maneuvers for the lateral bending lumbar spine failure. In addition, with the use of a specific Applied Kinesiology (AK) protocol called Total Integration of Muscles (Tim Francis, DC, developer), the subluxations associated with shoulder muscle failures were corrected and specific ROM and shoulder strengthening exercises targeting external rotation, shoulder retraction, hyperextension, and the supraspinatus muscle were instituted.

Within two visits, Bob indicated "the old Bob is back." He demonstrated complete normal circumduction of the shoulder with complaints of "mild pain" on forward and lateral abduction. Even with a reduced care schedule, within 2 months (eight visits), Bob was back at the gym working out and even the mild pain continued to decrease. Total visits: 13 over 4 months. Total cost: $761. ∾

In each case, only after the necessary informed consent has been made, with a thorough case history, examination (including instrumentation; physical; x-ray examination; and possibly lab, orthopedic, and neurological reports), patient report of findings, and proper technique selection based on the findings, will the necessary rehabilitative adjustment along with any supporting ancillary care be given. This criterion for patient safety has long been a cornerstone in chiropractic care and has lead to extremely safe rehabilitative procedures in chiropractic.

## A Case Study

### Degenerative Lumbar Scoliosis

Mabel is an 84-year-old female, former RN, with Alzheimer's disease and a degenerative lumbar scoliosis (21 degree Cobb's), with immobilizing pain, unable to walk, and confined to a wheelchair. She is living in an assisted care facility. Family reports continuous self-destructive thoughts and statements from her resulting from the severe pain, which is unmodulated by medication.

At presentation, Mable's medications are Procardia, Zoloft, Vasotec, Antivert, Naprosyn, and Aricept. Previous history: Cobalt treatment for uterine cancer 30 years ago, laminectomy 15 years ago (ruptured L5 disk), and cholecystectomy 10 years ago. Mable has had no previous chiropractic care.

Chiropractic examination reveals positive orthopedic tests in SI joint and positive Neuro-Organizational Technique (NOT) scoliosis test.* SEMG reveals significant temperature variation beyond one or more standard deviations in the cervical, thoracic, and lumbar spine.

Radiological studies reveal spinal misalignments in the cervical, thoracic, and lumbopelvic spine.

Care began with specific adjustments in thoracic and lumbosacral spine, with biochemical support, anti-inflammatory homeopathic support, and a homeopathic systems drainer. Four days later, patient walks into office under assistance but without wheelchair. Specific adjustments continue in cervical, thoracic, and lumbosacral spine three times per week for 2 weeks. NOT scoliosis test was positive on sixth visit, and patient is corrected for a right scoliosis pattern. Therapeutic massage is ordered twice weekly, and assisted care facility offers hydrotherapy twice weekly to support chiropractic care.

By the third month and sixteenth visit, patient can walk to the office without assistance (¼ mile). Patient still remains under care because of advanced degeneration of spine but is seen every 3 to 4 weeks now. Total cost (through acute phase): $1047. Continuing care $100/month : $60 for DC, $40 for massage.  ᴥ

---

*NOT, developed by Dr. Carl Ferreri in Brooklyn, New York, is a specialized applied kinesiological technique that corrects the aberrant neuromuscular reflexes and other components that cause the distortion pattern known as *idiopathic scoliosis*. Chiropractors, specially trained in scoliosis correction techniques, do not recognize scoliosis as "idiopathic" because they have long corrected the cause of the biomechanical distortion leading to it, i.e., the subluxation. This is one technique that addresses portions of that distortion pattern. It has been successfully used clinically for many years to stop advancing scolioses, while other techniques (Barge, Logan Basic) have clinically reduced the curvature.

## Patient Safety

Again, we return to Hippocrates' principle "First, do no harm." Terrett discusses the lingering effectiveness of the AMA disinformation campaign at length, observing that cases of cervical stroke by "manipulation" attributed to chiropractors in the medical literature were in fact, on examination, not performed by chiropractors at all, but by kung fu instructors; osteopaths; physiotherapists; general practitioner medical doctors; massage therapists; and in one case, someone's wife! Terrett also noted that the medical authors had complete access to all the original documentation in these cases when they assigned the damage erroneously to chiropractors.[26]

Dabbs reported a risk assessment of 0.00025% for cervical manipulation vs. NSAIDs for the treatment of neck pain,[27] while Myler reported the National Center for Health Statistics places the risk of stroke in the general population to be 0.00057%. He concluded, "If these data are correct, the risk of fatal stroke following 'cervical manipulation' is less than half the risk of fatal stroke in the general population."[28]

Jaskoviak reported that no stroke complications occurred in approximately 5 million cervical "manipulations" in the National College of Chiropractic Clinic from 1965 to 1980.[29] This is in keeping with the findings of Vick, et al, osteopathic researchers who found only 185 cases of injury from 1923 to 1993 associated with several million treatments.[30]

In addition, one must differentiate between a chiropractic adjustment and manipulation. The Council on Chiropractic Practice (CCP) defines an adjustment as "the correction of a vertebral subluxation" and a manipulation as "the taking of a joint past its passive range of motion into the paraphysiological space, but not past the anatomic limit, accompanied by articular cavitation (Kirkaldy-Willis). It is not synonymous with chiropractic adjustment, which is applied to correct a vertebral subluxation."[31] In fact, the CCP "Panel found no competent evidence that specific chiropractic adjustments cause strokes."[31]

## The Vertebral Subluxation Complex

The term *subluxation* has a long and extensive history in healing, maybe dating back as far as Hippocrates. The earliest English definition is attributed to Randall

Holme in 1688, who defined it as "a dislocation or putting out of [joynt]." The large array of alternative terms for the subluxation in the medical literature leads to complexity rather than clarity. Rome found 296 variations used by chiropractic, medical, and other professions and concluded that, "with so many attempts to establish a term for such a clinical and biological finding, an entity of some significance must exist."[32] Stephenson, in his classic 1927 chiropractic text, defined a subluxation as having four components.

1. Loss of juxtaposition of a vertebra with the one above, the one below, or both
2. Occlusion of an opening
3. Nerve impingement
4. Interference with the transmission of mental impulses[46]

Further research has included some form of kinesiological dysfunction; neurological involvement; soft tissue involvement such as muscles, ligaments, or tendons; plus other spinal structures. Various models of subluxation have arisen: the component model, the segmental model, the postural approaches, a three-dimensional model, and tonal models.

Component models of subluxation developed and popularized by Dishman and Lantz contain five components.

1. Spinal Kinesiopathology
2. Neuropathology
3. Myopathology
4. Histopathology
5. Biochemical changes[33]

This leads to the vertebral subluxation complex, which includes specific components as described by Herfert in 1986.

1. An osseous component
2. Connective tissues including the disk, ligaments, fascia, and muscles
3. Altered biomechanics including kyphosis, lordosis, scoliosis, and spondylosis
4. The neurological component including nerve roots and spinal cord
5. Advancing complications in the innervated tissues resulting in the patient's symptoms, sometimes referred to as the "end tissue phenomenon" or distal tissue damage[34]

Lantz has since expanded his model to include nine components so that the model can be used to integrate every aspect of clinical management. He refers to this as sort of a "unified field theory" of chiropractic.

1. Kinesiology
2. Neurology
3. Myology
4. Connective tissue physiology
5. Angiology
6. Inflammatory response
7. Anatomy
8. Physiology
9. Biochemistry

"Each component can, in turn, be described in terms of precise details of anatomic[al], physiologic[al], and biochemical alterations inherent in subluxation degeneration and parallel changes involved in normalization of structure and function through adjusting procedures."[35]

The segmental models of subluxation are described in terms of specific intervertebral motion segments. In these approaches radiographic procedures are used to identify and list the disrelationships between the segments. Clinical examination procedures such as static and motion palpation, surface electromyography, or dermathermographs will also be used to define the subluxation.

Postural models of subluxation evaluate "global subluxation patterns" that have created measurable postural distortion patterns. Aragona's Applied Spinal Biomechanical Engineering (ASBE) uses radiographs to determine both the aberrant spinal motion patterns and the appropriate therapeutic maneuvers to correct those distortion patterns. Pettibon Spinal Biomechanics and Harrison Biophysics use a mathematical spinal model of "normal" and through specific adjustive and ancillary procedures return the spine to that predetermined norm.[36]

Kent proposes a unique three-dimensional model for the subluxation, which is outcome assessment based, with all components easily measurable and functionally defined via the correction of the subluxation. In this model there are only three components.

1. "Dyskinesia, which refers to distortion or impairment of voluntary movement. This may be readily measured by inclinometry since regional ranges of motion are associated with subluxations."
2. Dysponesis, or abnormal involuntary muscle activity. "Dysponesis refers to a reversible pathophysiologic state in which errors in energy expenditure are capable of producing functional disorders. These disorders are usually the result of covert errors in action potential from the motor and premotor cortex and those output consequences.

These neurophysiological reactions may result from responses to environmental events, body sensations, and emotions. The resulting aberrant muscle activity may be evaluated using surface electrode techniques. Typically, static surface electromyography (SEMG) with axial loading is used to evaluate innate responses to gravitational stress."

3. Dysautonomia or autonomic dysfunction. Kent states, "Acquired dysautonomia may be associated with a broad array of functional abnormalities. Autonomic dystonia may be evaluated by measuring skin temperature differentials. Uematsu, et al, determined normative values for skin temperature differences based upon asymptomatic "normal" individuals."[37]

Tonal approaches of subluxation date all the way back to D.D. Palmer in 1910, who stated, "Life is an expression of tone. Tone is the normal degree of nerve tension. Tone is expressed in function by normal elasticity, strength, and excitability—the cause of disease is any variation in tone."[38] In tonal approaches, a variety of adjusting techniques may be used to achieve the clinical objective of increased functional performance.

Each of these models includes a progressive form of spinal degeneration as a result of the degenerative affects of the abnormal spinal biomechanics, leading to various pathological tissue changes. Although Kent has described this separately as the subluxation degeneration model, it is usually found in the latter stages of other models.

These different approaches in the theory of chiropractic subluxation are the result of the extensive array of results-driven adjusting techniques within the chiropractic profession. They help to explain subluxation and to detail the consistent successful clinical outcomes achieved since Harvey Lillard regained his hearing as the result of a chiropractic adjustment in 1895.

# CHIROPRACTIC IN REHABILITATION

## Chiropractic's Unique Approach

Chiropractic serves a tremendous role in the course of almost all rehabilitation programs because of its unique and nonduplicating service of subluxation correction. Kudlas states, "While chiropractic does not re-

ally 'treat anything' but instead raises a person's health level, a large number of traditional study designs continue to demonstrate its safety, effectiveness, and superiority over medical treatment."[2] In this line of raising levels of health, it is not unusual to find that nonrelated secondary complaints of patients are also improved under chiropractic care. Leboeuf-Yde et al found that nearly one in four chiropractic patients experiences some form of nonmusculoskeletal improvement after being adjusted. These secondary improvements clustered around ease of breathing, better vision, improved digestive function and circulation, heart rhythm and blood pressure changes, and improved hearing.[39]

 *A Case Study*

*Gastroesophageal Reflux Disease, Food Allergies, and Unrelated Mild Low Back Pain*

Susan is a 20-year-old college student and restaurant hostess with a chronic history of gastroesophageal reflux disease (GERD) and occasional low back pain. Her medications are Prevacid, Lo Ovral for birth control, and Keflex for strep urinary tract infection at the first visit.

Food allergy testing had revealed allergies to tomatoes, citrus, and chocolate. Previous history was unremarkable except for infectious mononucleosis at 9 years of age, and a car accident 2 years before seeking treatment, in which she was a passenger and left "very sore" afterward but for which she sought no treatment.

Chiropractic examination revealed positive orthopedic findings in the cervical spine and pelvis. Palpable spasm and tender muscle fibers were elicited in the right SI joint, L5, and C5 through C2. AK muscle testing revealed weaknesses in the omohyoid and myohyoid muscle groups, a Cranial Injury Complex, positive findings for hiatal hernia, and a sugar metabolism problem.

Cervical ROM was restricted in lateral flexion but hypermobile in lumbar lateral flexion. Radiological studies demonstrated spinal misalignments in the cervical, thoracic, and lumbopelvic spine.

Treatment along the structural side consisted of specific spinal adjustments to the areas of subluxation, with ancillary muscle balancing AK techniques, and along the biochemical side with proprietary nutritional protocols and homeopathic remedies supporting gut detoxification and tissue repair. In addition, the mental/emotional side of care utilized extensive NET adjusting protocols.

In this case it was necessary to eliminate her food allergies, using the TBM allergy elimination protocol* so that healing could occur. After 15 visits and 2 months of care, Susan reported with a visual analog scale that she was 7 to 9 out of 10 better with her GERD (with 10 being "completely healed") with some days "a 7" with stress causing mild gut distress, but the remaining days "9 out of 10 better." Total visits: 16. Total cost: $1030, including supplements and homeopathic remedies.

NOTE: At follow-up 2 years later, patient remains asymptomatic of all presenting complaints. ∾

---

*Total Body Modification Technique (TBM), developed by Dr. Victor Frank et al (Sandy, Utah), has an allergy elimination technique that is clinically 85% effective for eliminating subluxation-induced allergies. This technique examines the cascade of reactions that occur when a patient is exposed to an allergen. Each step along the cascade is then systemically evaluated for subluxations and the proper sequence adjusted. Once the 2- to 4-minute correction is complete, the allergy has been completely eliminated—no reactions, no drugs, no additional treatment is usually required.

## Cost Effectiveness

Joint or back pain, which is one of the most common presenting complaints in the healthcare arena today, accounts for almost $60 billion annually, or 8% of national healthcare expenditures.[40] Research by Quo et al found back pain in the workplace at 17.6%, with almost 25% of that number resulting in lost work days. In this study, depending on the age group, men lost an average of 5.4 to 8.5 days of work, while women lost an average of 4.4 to 8.8 days. Based on the research, chiropractic offers great benefit to individuals with joint or back pain.[41]

James Zechman, CEO of Alternative Medicine, Inc. (AMI), an Illinois-based healthcare provider organization that utilizes chiropractors instead of medical doctors as primary care "gatekeepers" in their managed care health plan, indicates from insurance data supplied by Blue Cross Blue Shield of Illinois that in the first 18 months of its operation, AMI, in comparison to normative values in the greater Chicago area, reduced hospitalizations by nearly 60%, outpatient surgery by 85%, pharmaceutical use by 56%, and had no Cesarean deliveries over a 2-year period compared with a network average of 22%. From his viewpoint, "We are truly the 'best medicine of both worlds': the prevention-oriented skills of well-trained chiropractic physicians and emergency skills of allopathic physicians on an 'as needed' basis."[42]

In a retrospective statistical study of 395,641 patients, economist Myron Stano found a total cost difference on the order of $1,000 total savings per patient for those using chiropractic care as little as once per month over those using medical or osteopathic care. Further, those cost differences remained statistically significant after controlling for demographics and insurance plan characteristics.[40,43]

With these figures in mind, research into the affect of chiropractic on these huge costs must be weighed. Kirkaldy-Willis and Cassidy studied 283 patients with total medical disability (Grade 4 disability). Patients were grouped according to various syndromes. All the groups had radicular signs and "most presented with leg pain." Of the studied patients, 25% had undergone previous back surgery, which had failed. The length of disability of the participants was between 5.6 and 16.9 years. All groups were given only a 2- or 3-week daily regimen of chiropractic care by an experienced chiropractor and the results were independently assessed by a neutral observer at 1 month and then followed up at 3-month intervals. In each group, at least 50% were returned to a Grade 1 (symptom free—no work restrictions) or Grade 2 (mild intermittent pain with no work restrictions). The results of the study were that 202 of the 283 patients in the study, or 71%, were graded as able to return to work without restrictions.[60]

The following is a brief review of further workers' compensation case studies.

- A 1960 study by First Research Corporation in Florida found that chiropractic care costs less than medical care and returns nonoperable injured workers to gainful employment 12 times faster than if they were treated by orthopedists or neurologists (30 days' medical treatment compared with 2.5 days' chiropractic treatment).
- In a 1972 California study of 1,000 (500 MD, 500 DC) workers' compensation cases, the chiropractically treated group lost an average of 15.6 days of work[45] while the medically treated group lost an average of 32 days. In addition, only 34.8% of the medically treated group reported "complete recovery," compared with 51% of the chiropractically treated group. Of the chiropractically treated group, 47.9% reported "no lost work days," while only 21% of the medically treated group reported similarly.[46]

- In a 1971 Oregon study, 82% of patients treated chiropractically returned to work within 1 week, compared with 4.1% of the medically treated group. A follow-up study revealed that 13% of a medically treated group received total disability awards, while only 6% of the chiropractically treated group was classified as totally disabled.[46]
- A 1972 Kansas study found 40% cost savings in the chiropractically treated group over the medically treated group and a work day loss of 5.8 for the chiropractically treated group vs. 13.1 for the medically treated group.[48]
- Patients under chiropractic care in Wisconsin returned to work faster and had lower overall healthcare costs ($145.64) than their medically treated counterparts ($267.58).[49]
- In a 3-year Montana study, chiropractic care reduced both time lost in the workplace and net compensation savings over medical treatment of similar injuries.[43]

These early studies of workers' compensation claim savings were only heralding the cost savings in the general population made by Zechman. In addition, in 1995, Stano did a follow-up retrospective statistical study based on total insurance payments and total outpatient payments, each adjusted for sociodemographical characteristics, and found that the chiropractic group had significantly lower total healthcare costs as represented by adjusted third-party payments in the fee-for-service sector. Total adjusted cost differences ranged from $291 to a significant $1,722 over a 2-year period.

# SUMMARY

The cost effectiveness of chiropractic is enhanced by studies that demonstrate that chiropractic patients are more satisfied with their care than with medical treatment.[50] As a result, it must be concluded that chiropractic inclusion into rehabilitation programs is not only prudent and cost effective, but in the best interest of the patient as well. "Chiropractic first, drugs second, and surgery last" has been a chiropractic axiom for over 60 years. As chiropractic grows into the twenty-first century, the benefits of its unique health-enhancing approach to rehabilitation are reaching new levels of public awareness and demand, requiring and accompanying expansion of inter-professional acceptance and cooperation.

## References

1. Rondberg T: *Chiropractic first: the fastest growing healthcare choice—before drugs or surgery,* Chandler, Ariz, 1996, Chiropractic Journal Publications.
2. Kudlas M: Chiropractic. In Jacobs M (ed): *The encyclopedia of alternative medicine,* London, 1996, Carlton Books.
3. Peterson D, Wiese G: *Chiropractic: an illustrated history,* St Louis, 1995, Mosby.
4. Dye A: *The evolution of chiropractic: its discovery and development,* Philadelphia, 1969, Dye.
5. Maynard JE: *Daily meditations of D. D. Palmer,* Marietta, Ga, 1982, Maynard Institute of Applied Chiropractic Philosophy.
6. Motion Palpation Institute: Public service announcement, 1987.
7. Wilk et al *v* AMA: Exhibit #172, December, 1962.
8. Getzendanner S: Memorandum opinion and order, Wilk *v* AMA, Order #76C3777.
9. Kent C: Component models of subluxation, *Chiropr J* March, 1997.
10. Walker S: The triangle of health: once more with feeling, *Digest Chiropr Econ* May/June, 1990.
11. Walker S: Ivan Pavlov, his dog and chiropractic, *Digest Chiropr Econ* March/April, 1992.
12. Stephenson RW: *Chiropractic text book,* 1948 edition, Davenport, Iowa, 1948, Palmer School of Chiropractic.
13. Gold R: *The triune of life,* Philadelphia, 1989, AIDO Institute of Chiropractic.
14. Stapp HP: Are superluminal connections necessary? *Nuovo Cimento* 40B:191-199, 1995.
15. Goswami A et al: *The self-aware universe: how consciousness creates the material world,* New York, 1993, Tarcher/Putnam.
16. Palmer, DD: *The chiropractic adjuster,* Davenport, Iowa, 1907, Palmer School of Chiropractic.
17. Manga P et al: *The effectiveness and cost-effectiveness of chiropractic management of low back pain,* Toronto, 1993, Ontario Ministry of Health.
18. Jarvis KB, Phillips RB, et al: Cost per case comparison of back injury claims of chiropractic versus medical management for conditions with identical diagnostic codes, *J Occup Health* 33(8):347-852, 1991.
19. Wolk S: Chiropractic versus medical care: a cost analysis of disability and treatment for back-related Worker's Compensation cases, *FCER* Sept 1988.
20. Schifrin LG: *Mandated health insurance for chiropractic treatment: an economic assessment with implications for the Commonwealth of Virginia,* Richmond, Va, 1992, Medical College of Virginia.
21. Peterson K: Two cases of spinal manipulation performed while the patient contemplated an associated stress event: the effect of the manipulation on serum cholesterol levels in hypercholesterolemic subjects, *Chiropr Tech* 7:2, May 1995.

22. Peterson K: A preliminary inquiry into manual muscle testing response in phobic and control subjects exposed to threatening stimuli, *J Manipulative Physiol Ther* 19(5):310-316, 1995.

23. Peterson K: The effects of spinal manipulation on the intensity of emotional arousal in phobic subjects exposed to a threat stimulus: a randomized, controlled, double-blind clinical trial, *J Manipulative Physiol Ther* 20(9):602-606, 1997.

24. Monti D et al: Muscle test comparisons of congruent and incongruent self-referential statements, *Percept Motor Skills* 88:1019-1028, 1999.

25. Walker S: *NET basic manual,* Encinitas, Calif, 1994, NET Inc.

26. Terrett AG: Misuse of the literature by medical authors in discussing spinal manipulative therapy injury, *J Physiol Manipulative Ther* 18(4):203-210, 1995.

27. Dabbs V, Lauretti WJ: A risk assessment of cervical manipulation vs NSAIDs for the treatment of neck pain, *J Manipulative Physiol Ther* 18(8):530-536, 1995.

28. Myler L: A risk assessment of cervical manipulation vs. NSAIDs for the treatment of neck pain (letter to the editor), *J Manipulative Physiol Ther* 19(5):357, 1997.

29. Jaskoviac P: Complications arising from manipulation of the cervical spine, *J Manipulative Physiol Ther* 3:213, 1980.

30. Vick D, McKay C, Zengerle C: The safety of manipulative treatment: review of the literature from 1925 to 1993, *J Am Osteopath Assoc* 96:113, 1996.

31. Council on Chiropractic Practice (CCP): *Clinical practice guideline, No 1: vertebral subluxation in chiropractic practice,* Phoenix, 1998, Council on Chiropractic Practice.

32. Rome PB: Usage of chiropractic terminology in the literature: 296 ways to say subluxation—complex issues of the subluxation, *Chiropr Tech* 8(2):49, 1996.

33. Lantz CA: The vertebral subluxation complex part 1: introduction to the model and the kinesiological component, *Chiropr Res J* 1(3):23, 1989.

34. Herfert R: *Communicating the vertebral subluxation complex,* East Detroit, Mich, 1986, Herfert Chiropractic Clinics.

35. Lantz CA: The subluxation complex. In Gatterman MI (ed): *Foundations of chiropractic subluxation,* St Louis, 1995, Mosby.

36. Kent C: Clinical models of vertebral subluxation, *Chiropr J* March 1998.

37. Kent C: A three dimensional model of vertebral subluxation, *Chiropr J* June 1998.

38. Palmer DD: *Textbook of the art, science, and philosophy of chiropractic: the chiropractor's adjustor,* Portland, 1910, Portland Publishing House.

39. Leboeuf-Yde C et al: The types and frequencies of improved nonmusculoskeletal symptoms reported after chiropractic spinal manipulative therapy, *J Manipulative Physiol Ther* 22(9):559-564, 1999.

40. Stano M: A comparison of health care costs for chiropractic and medical patients, *J Manipulative Physiol Ther* 16(5):291-299, 1993.

41. Quo HR et al: Back pain prevalence in US industry and estimates of lost work days, *Am J Public Health* 89:1029, 1999.

42. Zechman J: Interview, *Dynamic Chiropr* 19:4, Feb 2001.

43. Stano M: Further analysis of health care costs for chiropractic and medical patients, *J Manipulative Physiol Ther* 17(7):442-446, 1994.

44. Kirkaldy-Willis WH, Cassidy JD: Spinal manipulation in the treatment of low back pain, *Can Fam Phys* 31: March, 1985.

45. Wolfe R: A comparison of patient reported time loss treated by medical doctors and chiropractors, *Industrial Back Injury* December, 1972.

46. Martin RA: *Back injury study of workman's compensation records: State of Oregon,* personal communication, 1972.

47. Kansas Workman's Compensation Board, 1972.

48. University of Wisconsin commissioned study by the Wisconsin Chiropractic Association, 1979.

49. Montana Worker's Compensation Study commissioned by the American Chiropractic Association, 1975-1978.

50. Cherkin DC: Patient satisfaction as an outcome measure, *J Chiropr Tech* 2(3):138, 1990.

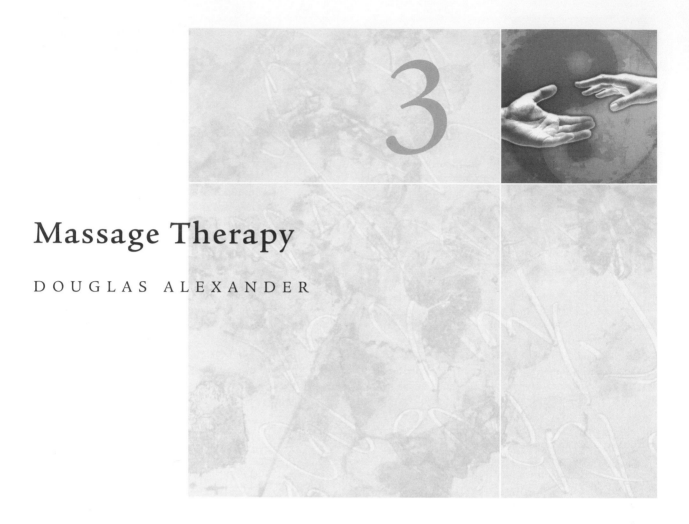

# Massage Therapy

## DOUGLAS ALEXANDER

Massage Therapy uses touch to help people relax and normalize their physiology. However, massage affects the body and mind in many ways beyond relaxing stubborn, stuck muscles. This chapter explores how Massage Therapy works so that you, as a Rehabilitation Clinician, can decide whether it might be helpful for a particular client.

## THE CORE RESPONSES TO MASSAGE THERAPY

Massage Therapy is a health profession created around and within a natural impulse to touch for comfort and caring. Although Massage Therapy interventions can be very technical, they build on the basic psychological and physiological response to caring touch.

Primates can often be seen in the act of social grooming. They take turns stroking and attending to each other's fur. The context of this touching speaks without words, "I know you and care about you." This comforting social context is at least as important as the pragmatic concerns of bug and dirt removal. Similarly, the context of Massage Therapy is as important as the mobilization of a particular joint or nerve, a heroic stretching campaign, or a gently ruthless search for trigger points (TrPs).

The massage experience is unique. During the treatment—whether it lasts 15 minutes or 1 hour and 15 minutes—the Massage Therapist covers and uncovers, picks up and sets down, pushes, pulls, and kneads the client's flesh. Words are seldom spoken as the Massage Therapist responds to nonverbal cues of held and released breath, muscle guarding, and letting go. Most of us have not had this much physical attention since we were infants. This nurturing experience is at the core of any Massage Therapy intervention and is extremely valuable at any stage in the lifespan.

Tiffany Field pioneered studies of simple soothing massage routines for premature babies, who tend to be denied regular handling. The babies massaged in intensive care neonatal units demonstrated increased weight gains and alertness and accelerated discharge time from the ward.[1] These studies have been duplicated in a number of centers with similar results.[2]

Field has gone on to study the basic physiological responses to simple, soothing massage for people with a wide variety of health problems, such as those living with HIV, Parkinson's disease, chronic fatigue syndrome, depression, diabetes, or bulimia. An exhaustive set of research abstracts is available at the website for the Touch Research Institute.[3]

In almost all situations the basic physiological response to a soothing massage is decreased stress hormone levels, elevated immune response, better sleep patterns, better self-image, and less body pain. For people living with HIV and other immunosuppressive diseases, the psychoneuroimmunological effects of Massage Therapy can only be helpful. In addition, some diseases/conditions have attendant social isolation, which Massage Therapy can often help alleviate.

The simplest guideline would be to consider Massage Therapy for anyone who has been or is under stress or who has impaired immune function, sleep disturbance, poor body image, or body pain. To get a better understanding of how people may benefit from Massage Therapy, let's examine further how it works.

## MASSAGE THERAPY AS MANIPULATION OF CONSCIOUSNESS

The seemingly simple shift of consciousness from goal-directed thoughts and feelings to an inner-directed reflective state is fundamental to the massage experience. It is a behavioral skill or quality that many people have forgotten. Many of us live our lives like Indianapolis 500 race car drivers, without thorough between-race maintenance. After the 500 mile race, the car is totally disassembled and rebuilt with new parts before it is ready to race again. During the metaphorical race we all pause for an occasional pit stop, but most of us never do this fundamental between-race

maintenance. We mistake a pit stop for thorough maintenance. It is amazing that our bodies hold up as well as they do.

The metaphor of the race car driver can easily be extended. Most of us have forgotten how to shift gears in our consciousness to a state of deep rest and relaxation. In a state of rest and relaxation, muscles naturally relax, and the body heals itself.

The behavioral pattern of not giving the body time to rest and the psychological/cognitive inability to slow consciousness to a rest and recovery state creates a vulnerability to sickness and/or injury. Most of the clients I have seen that fail to recover from light-impact, seemingly innocuous car accidents have this vulnerability. They may be able to knock sense out of a complex spreadsheet but not have a clue how to stop and relax long enough to allow a simple and minor muscle injury to heal.

Several years ago I arrived at the home of a feisty older woman to perform a Massage Therapy house call. She had been a nurse in the Second World War and was now housebound as a result of severe degenerative changes in her body. When I arrived I was shocked to find two police cars with their lights flashing. As I approached the house I was met by a policeman who let me in.

I was worried for my client, but I should have known better. She was in the process of telling off two towering policemen, "You have enough information for now, she must rest." I soon found out that the person who "must rest" was a young woman whom my client had placed in her own bed. The young woman had had a minor car accident just outside the house. My client had ascertained that the woman was safe, but shaken up, so she had put her to bed. She then had put on soothing music and made some herbal tea before calling the police.

As a result of my client's intervention, the young woman was relaxed and calm. Her physiology was normalized and primed for healing. One wonders how well people would recover from accident/injury if only they would fully relax directly afterward.

Massage Therapy allows people to relearn this fundamental shift to rest and recovery that many of us have forgotten. People often suffer from a nonspecific, functional complaint for which a physician has been unable to identify pathology. Although massage treatment is very general, usually consisting of a full body relaxation massage, the client gradually makes gains in measurable functional outcomes such as improved sleep, better concentration, and increased ability to function at work. When this happens, the client is usually accessing deeper, reflective states of consciousness during the massage treatments, as well as bringing some of the qualities of these states into his or her life.

It is generally accepted that "massage is relaxing," but how are these changes maintained after someone gets off the massage table and reenters the maelstrom of his or her life? Relaxation is not a skill to be practiced only on massage tables, or in meditative postures. Relaxation is a state of calmness and equipoise that one brings to the cry of children or the work required to meet a deadline.

## SOMATOSENSORY NOISE— OR LISTENING TO THE SYMPHONY

The key to understanding the carryover effects of massage is to appreciate the considerable muscle tension that most people carry around from day to day. For example, a first-time massage client may arrive with considerable tension in the upper trapezius muscles and compression of the cervical spine. The tension in the client's trapezius escalates toward the end of the day, causing a temporal headache through TrP referral.[4] The compression of the neck through muscle tension and poor posture irritates facet joints in the client's cervical spine.[5]

The client senses tension in his or her body but lacks a clear awareness of just where the tension is and what the effects are of the body use choices he or she makes. The client may hold the telephone with the shoulder instead of using the hand, for example. This just adds to the tension.

During the client's first massage he or she becomes acutely aware of how sore his or her neck is in terms of the precise location and quality of soreness. Think of when you heard a symphony for the first time. It probably seemed like a richly textured sea of sound. It took a few listening experiences to begin to pick out various instruments and to appreciate how they play together to weave beautiful and stirring harmonies.

When people receive their first massage, they are often surprised to find that their flesh resembles a discordant symphony. As one client once remarked, "I've got sore spots in places I didn't even know I had places!" The more massage the client participates in, the more the client senses a rich variety of feelings in his or her flesh. For example, it is common to feel areas that are dense and tense in close proximity to areas that are stretched and tired feeling, as well as other areas that may feel raw and bruised.

The client often comes to an awareness of his or her flesh as a rich, three-dimensional tapestry. The Massage Therapist is not a bulldozer that plows through all this variegated tissue but a caring, sensitive biofeedback device that allows the client to become aware of the exact state of his or her myofascial tissue.

The physical state of the muscle—muscle tone or tonus—is a product of physical factors such as elasticity, viscosity, and plasticity, as well as the idling contraction of motor units within the muscle.[6] This sense of there being two components—physical and neuromuscular—that contribute to the texture of a muscle is one of the central keys to effective Massage Therapy. We will address physical factors later in this chapter. For the moment, let's focus on neuromuscular tension.

## NEUROMUSCULAR TENSION

Muscles are designed to contract and shorten, as well as to lengthen in controlled ways. They do this through the contraction of subvolumes of muscle called motor units.[7] In an ideal erect posture the sustained, weak contraction in muscles such as those in the neck is achieved through the rotating contraction of a number of motor units. After one motor unit within the neck muscles contracts, it relaxes and another motor unit contracts. This rotation, or sharing, of the work allows the muscle to be working and takes care of all its nutritional and other needs. A muscle that is contracting strongly will have more motor units activated, with shorter rest periods before any one motor unit is called on to work again.

A muscle that is tense will have many motor units contracting at once and/or fail to rotate motor unit activation. It is probable that a tense muscle is prone to ischemia, resulting in a buildup of metabolic waste products, as well as simple physical wear and tear.

The relative activity of working motor units in a muscle is sensed by the Massage Therapist as a "rubbery" quality in the muscle. As a muscle relaxes, the rubbery spot or region is felt to melt or deflate. This is one of the key events in a massage treatment that is specifically addressing neuromuscular tonus. If the spot has been a source of myofascial pain, then the pain will be felt to melt or dissolve to the same extent that the knot melts or dissolves.

This melting or dissolving of tension is accompanied by a lovely feeling within the client of letting go or release. It may vary from a subtle, barely noticeable feeling to a significant change of consciousness that reflects a fundamental shift in the client's thoughts and feelings. When a Massage Therapist feels the melting or release of a rubbery spot that the client has identified as painful and the client reports no change in sensation consequent to the tissue softening, then the therapist knows that there are more than neuromuscular pain factors at play. If this pain point was a key feature of the client's inital presentation, then referral to another healthcare professional probably needs to be considered at this point.

The resting tonus, or idle, of a muscle is set in a largely unconscious way. The massage process allows the client to sense tonus directly. Simply by attending to the sensations in his or her flesh, the client often finds the "tonus control switches," and resetting of the tonus of the muscles automatically follows. This is one of the profound pleasures of Massage Therapy; simply by attending to our flesh, our flesh normalizes.

We often carry so much tension around with us that we don't know when we are adding more. If we are lucky, at one point in our lives we had a healthy body. For a variety of reasons, tension can build up over the years. Muscle tension in the body can be compared with water filling a bathtub. If the bathtub is empty, then we are quite aware of adding a thimbleful of water to it. However, once the bathtub is half full, it is not obvious when a thimbleful of water has been added. In other words, if tension keeps getting added to the system, additional quanta (or units) of tension may be invisible.

The Weber-Fechner Principle describes this phenomenon. It states that the smallest perceptible change in a sensory stimulus is a fraction of the stimulus that is already there.[8] This means that if you are carrying a paperback novel and someone adds another one on top of it, you will feel a change in the perceived weight you are carrying. However, if you are carrying a refrigerator and someone places a paperback on top of it, you won't notice any difference in weight.

Similarly, when our muscles are relaxed with a normal resting tonus, we feel the effects of our body use decisions. For example, we will notice the tension in our neck or shoulder within seconds of holding the telephone with our shoulder. However, if our muscles are rocklike with tension already, we won't notice the increase in tension from holding the telephone with

our shoulder. When the muscles finally complain loudly through activation of one or several myofascial TrPs, the ache seems to have "come out of nowhere!"

Massage Therapy works to systematically release each person's characteristic pattern of tension. When the somatosensory noise—the backdrop level of sensory input—from tense muscles, active and latent TrPs, joint compression, etc., drops to a certain level, the client often becomes aware of creating tension through certain habitual actions. It is at this point that the client can become more self-correcting. As a client once said, "No one ever has to tell my dog that he is tense. He knows it and changes position or stretches right away. Before massage I lacked this skill. However, after receiving Massage Therapy I have developed the same awareness that my dog has naturally!"

The ability of the client to develop somatic awareness is part of the foundation of successful Massage Therapy. It is important for the Massage Therapist to help the client find effective postures in which to stretch tight muscles and to teach the client how to strengthen weak and inhibited muscles, as well as improve posture.

A recent study by Preyde[9] demonstrated that Massage Therapy can help a significant number of people with subacute low back pain. As a population, 60% of subjects had experienced low back pain before the current episode. The average duration of the current episode was greater than 3 months. Preyde had four pools of approximately 25 subjects. The comprehensive Massage Therapy group received Massage Therapy coupled with exercises tailored to each client. The soft tissue manipulation group received Massage Therapy manipulations alone, with no exercise prescription. A third group received only exercise prescription, and a fourth group received a placebo of sham laser. Each subject received six treatments/interventions over the course of roughly a month. Outcome measures consisted of the Roland Disability Questionnaire, the McGill Pain Questionnaire, the State Anxiety Index, and the Modified Schober test (lumbar range of motion).

The comprehensive Massage Therapy group had improved function, less intense pain, and a decrease in the quality of the pain relative to the other three groups. Both the comprehensive Massage Therapy group and the soft tissue manipulation group had a significant change in function. However, 1 month after the interventions were finished, 63% of the comprehensive Massage Therapy group reported no pain, compared with 27% of the soft tissue manipulation group, 14% of the exercise group, and 0% of the sham laser group.

Preyde's is a landmark study because it studies Massage Therapy as it is practiced: treatments and exercise/postural advice tailored to the client with a treatment frequency of roughly one to two treatments per week. Massage Therapy without the inclusion of exercise prescription was only half as effective as Comprehensive Massage Therapy in terms of pain reduction. In the profession, such a form of therapy (without exercise/postural advice) is considered incomplete. A Massage Therapist reading this study feels that the blending of the effects of the massage and the somatic awareness of the client work together with targeted exercises and postural advice to make for a potent intervention.

# MYOFASCIAL TRIGGER POINTS

One of the specific ways Massage Therapy can help people beyond psychoneuroimmunological change and reduction of somatosensory noise is through the resolution of myofascial trigger points (TrPs).

Myofascial TrPs are hyperirritable spots within taut bands of skeletal muscle that refer pain, and sometimes autonomic phenomena, in predictable patterns. Travell and Simons[4] are responsible for bringing the phenomena of TrPs into broad awareness. Numerous authors and clinicians have furthered the process through treatments, seminars, and publications.[10,11]

Simons has devoted the majority of his professional life to exploration of myofascial TrPs. He has recently published a picture of TrPs based on clinical evidence and electromyographic and microscopic study. The palpably dense and sensitive "knot" within a taut band of muscle is now thought to be a cluster of electrically active loci in the motor endplate zone of the muscle.[12]

Myofascial TrPs are caused by acute or chronic overload, direct trauma, and chilling. Chilling in this case is not the act of relaxing, but exposure to a cold draft! Finding the exact location of a TrP that is causing myofascial pain often involves a bit of detective work. This is because the hallmark of TrPs is their tendency to refer pain (usually distally) to their actual physical location. Working backward from published TrP referral maps and the client's history, the Massage Therapist carefully explores for palpably taut bands of muscle. When taut bands are found, the therapist further explores for hyperirritable loci, which may be causing all or part of the client's pain experience.

It is important to have the hands-on skills to identify TrPs in a client's muscles and to release them with an appropriate strategy. It is just as important to understand the context that created a TrP and is maintaining it. TrPs may be caused by different stressors and may interact with other clinical problems.

The following case studies show two very common low back pain scenarios.

 *A Case Study*

*Low Back Pain from TrPs and Facet Joint Dysfunction*
The client's erector spinae and multifidi muscles in his low back are tight with several trigger points (TrPs) from an old ice hockey injury. These TrPs are often quiescent (latent) but also are often reactivated by the heavy lifting he performs at work. The client's somatic experience is a chronic feeling of shortness and a dull ache in the low back as he fatigues over a long day of work. This is punctuated by stronger ache and more fatigue in the region when the TrPs are activated by lifting. Once or twice a year he gets a facet joint jamming because of the chronic approximation of the facet joints in the region of the tight multifidi muscles. At this time he also has a precise, sharp pain in the region of the facet joint, which takes a few days to a week or 2 to abate.

Care for this client will involve normalizing the inflammation, pain, and articular restriction associated with the facet joint jamming, followed by progressive stretching of the thoracolumbar fascia and normalization of the TrPs in his erector spinae and multifidi muscles. This can be done through precise compression and stripping manipulations. He will find that drawing his knees up to his chest while lying on his back is relieving and therapeutic.  ☙

 *A Case Study*

*Low Back Pain from Muscle Imbalance, Fatigue and Disk Compression*
A client with chronic low back pain has excessively tight abdominal and hamstring muscles. His erector spinae muscles are overstretched from an unbalanced stretching program. He has a feeling of chronic fatigue and weakness in his low back because his erector spinae and multifidi work overtime when he is lifting and bending.

When the Massage Therapist touches this client's low back muscles on the massage table, they feel tight and achy to the client. There may actually be some trigger points (TrPs) in the erector spinae and multifidi, but the muscles are mostly in pain from postexercise soreness from being overloaded. The client will get some relief out of stretching his low back, but it will not feel like his back is getting all the help it needs. This is because he needs to strengthen his low back and change the pattern of how his muscles are recruited during daily activities. He must bend so that his buttock muscles help the erector spinae and multifidi muscles with the lifting. The only way he will be able to do this is if he and the Massage Therapist can get adequate length out of his hamstrings.

If the client does not stop this chronic pattern of loading the lumbar spine in a flexed position, then over the years his lumbar disks will deteriorate and he will get a new pain from the disks being strained. This will feel like a central or nearly central pain in his spine. If this is not recognized and measures taken, then it will probably gradually, or even quickly, progress to sciatica. This process has been graphically illustrated by McKenzie.[13]

When sciatic pain expresses itself, the client will find that flexion of the low back is not helpful, or actually makes things worse. Extension, or backward bending, will often be more helpful.

Treatment of TrPs is usually stock-in-trade for Massage Therapists. However, it is important for clients, and some Massage Therapists, to realize that not all sore spots in people are TrPs. It is common to find areas that are overstretched, strained, twisted, weak, congested, and/or adhered. These areas need to be treated appropriately and self-care steps taken to normalize function.

## Trigger Points Vs. Tender Points

Myofascial TrPs should not be mistaken for the tender points of fibromyalgia. The tender points of fibromyalgia are hypersensitive spots within or above skeletal muscle or over bone that usually do not meet the criterion of occurring within a taut band of muscle. They also don't refer pain in characteristic patterns and are usually only locally sore. For the Massage Therapist the muscle usually feels "empty" of TrPs and even tension and is often weak feeling and hypotonic. Gerwin[14] differentiates between TrPs and tender points through these and other criteria.

The tender points of fibromyalgia are best thought of as signs of a centrally mediated hypersensitivity rather than local tissue abnormalities. The Massage Therapist is most helpful with these clients through the systemic physiological normalizing effects of Massage Therapy, as opposed to "squishing the fibromyalgia out of the person." If the massage intervention helps to normalize and deepen sleep patterns, then it might be very helpful for the client with fibromyalgia. That being said, it is true that fibromyalgia clients can also have true TrPs, which will then need to be carefully and thoroughly treated as well.

## An Exercise in Releasing Neuromuscular Hypertonicity

The following exercise illustrates how common neuromuscular hypertonus is in the body, as well as how quickly it can change when precisely targeted.

Allow your head to fall toward your chest just to the point at which you feel tension building up at the base of your skull where the skull joins the neck. Holding your head in this position, look up into your eyebrows and take a deep breath in. Hold your breath for a comfortably long period while you study the sensation of tension at the base of the skull. Then exhale, allowing your eyes to relax and unfocus.

Notice how your head spontaneously drops further toward your chest. Allow it to continue to fall until tension again prevents it from falling further. Again look up into your eyebrows and take a deep breath in. Again feel the tension at the base of the skull and how it dissipates as you release the breath and relax your eyes. Repeat a third time.

This is a simple exercise that can show the effects of breath inhibition and static muscle contraction. It can also show the difference between neuromuscular tonus dysfunction and physical change in the muscle. If there is still tension at the base of the skull after this exercise, the region is likely going to have a more fibrous texture than the previously rubber quality.

## CONNECTIVE TISSUE RESTRICTION—OR GULLIVER IN THE LAND OF THE LILLIPUTIANS

TrPs and other neuromuscular restrictions in which the nervous system has set the tonus of the muscle too high feel rubbery and have a certain spring-like feeling. However, it is also common for Massage Therapists to find dense, fibrous, and inelastic areas as well. This fibrous feeling often coincides with a neuromuscular tension feeling in the same tissue. When this occurs, it is important to reset the tonus or resolve the TrP before addressing the fibrous tissue. If the fibrous tissue is still a problem, it requires a different approach.

To resolve fibrous proliferation or adhesion, it is important to understand how it came to be present in the tissue. It is usually present after an injury that caused postinflammatory adhesions, and/or through immobilization or altered use of the tissue. When a muscle, tendon, ligament, joint capsule, or fascial sheet is immobilized, placed in shortened positions, or simply not used through a normal full range of motion, the normal maintenance/repair processes of connective tissue still carries on. This means that collagen fibers continue to be fabricated and laid down, but their fiber direction and adherence to each other and other tissues is not dictated by the normal therapeutic motion. As a result, collagen cross-links are formed that prevent the tissue from moving normally when motion is called for. It is not a matter of simply relaxing this tissue because it is physically stuck together, knitted in nonfunctional ways that prevent the tissue from lengthening properly.[15,16]

This shortening phenomenon occurs within the planes of connective tissue ensheathing muscles, as well as within the muscles themselves. While any one restrictive fiber is threadlike, the overall effect of these fibrous elements acting three dimensionally is considerable. This is often analogous to Gulliver's experience in the Land of the Lilliputians. A single thread could not have held Gulliver down. However, the gestalt of several hundred or several thousand threads, which a person engages all at once, proves impossible to break. Similarly, if one holds one's arm to the chest in a sling after injury, the joint capsule of the shoulder shortens, as do all the adjacent muscles and the connective tissue sheets overlying them.

It might take a force of 20 pounds operating through each square inch of this tissue to achieve length. This is easily achieved through the application of precise force in the context of a massage. The therapist leans (carefully!) into the client's pectoral fascia and slowly strips through the tight tissue with a gently ruthless thumb or two. If the client tries to do this by self-stretching, he or she might need to stretch an area of 10 to 15 square inches at once. As a result, the necessary force to achieve length in the connective tissue overlying the pectoral muscles would be in the realm of 200 to 300 pounds. Attempting to put such force through one's shoulder would cause injury to weaker links in the kinetic chain.

This is a little-appreciated dynamic in many rehabilitation cases. As a result of pain avoidance and disuse, clients often have several shortened areas (or global tightness—think of scleroderma) that restrict certain movements and/or breathing. To try to free themselves is to strain against an invisible straitjacket or several layers of plastic wrap. This is fatiguing and depressing, to be held down by the very tissue that one uses to move. In addition to the challenge of engaging these physical restrictions, one also struggles with the deconditioning, which naturally occurs with lack of normal motion and exercise.

The Massage Therapist works as a soft tissue homogenizer, picking up thick, fibrosed bands of tissue and kneading, torquing, and stretching them. Educated hands naturally gravitate toward tight tissue, and while they will give normal tissue a caress, they tend to not challenge it. Tissue that is overstretched and incompetent feeling is often coalesced and repacked by the intuitive therapist. Such an approach is a key feature of interventions, which sometimes return normal length and properties to overstretched and torn ligaments.[17]

Weintraub[17] has formalized four palpatory states that are common to injured fibrous tissue in tendon and ligament injury. He states that he often finds fibers that feel lax, torn, adhered, or misaligned and that chronic injuries usually have at least two of these factors at play. This is a very helpful typology that can guide therapists toward stretching, condensing, ungluing, and realigning manipulations rather than just going on "hunt-and-squish" or stretch journeys.

## THE NERVOUS SYSTEM AND DOUBLE CRUSH PHENOMENA

For a long time Massage Therapists have been treating myofascial tissue and the nervous system indirectly through creating therapeutic sensations. It is just beginning to be appreciated that the nervous system is an organ that is amenable to hands-on treatment as well. CranioSacral Therapy[18] and Nerve Mobilization[19] are two common and contrasting approaches to the nervous system. See Chapter 1 for a discussion of CranioSacral Therapy. However, Butler's work on Nerve Mobilization is also very important to Massage Therapists.

Much of a person's pain experience may be coming from the sheaths of the spinal cord and the peripheral nerves, as well as the neural tissue itself. The myofascial system is in a particularly effective position to adversely affect the nervous system and its sheaths. Tight muscles and/or connective tissue can compress nerve sheaths, causing a type of pain that feels almost myofascial (i.e., aching, pulling, and tight feelings). If the compression is sufficient, then the nerve itself and its conduction properties can be affected, causing altered sensation resulting in burning, tingling, numbness, and hyperalgesia or hypoalgesia.

The way in which the nervous system is affected by the myofascial system is seldom clear because it is often the combination of several subclinical compromises that give rise to sheath irritation and/or conduction change. The double crush phenomenon was first identified by Upton and McComas.[20] Briefly stated, a client with a nerve compromise is more vulnerable to another nerve compromise more proximally or distally along the same nerve.

From a Massage Therapy perspective, multiple subclinical impairments of the nervous system can give rise to neural symptomatology. This goes against the grain of conventional wisdom, which looks for a single source for the symptomatology, such as compression of the median nerve in the carpal tunnel. A "single" source for much pain and dysfunction in the body is hypertonicity and lack of elasticity in the myofascial system that is creating multiple subclinical compromises of the nervous system.

The Massage Therapist's approach to the treatment of carpal tunnel syndrome is a good example of treating multiple subclinical impairments. Treatment usually starts with a relaxing massage to the neck and shoulders, which decreases somatosensory noise and teaches the client how to attend to muscle tension in the body and how to find the metaphorical "control knobs" to turn down alpha motor neuron firing. The therapist examines for muscle tension in a global sense, as well as for a specific pattern of tension that will tend to compromise the median nerve. This would include tension in the scalene muscles through which the nerve roots of the brachial plexus pass, under the clavicle and pectoralis minor, in the forearm where the median nerve passes under the pronator teres muscle and flexor digitorum superficialis and the flexor retinaculum at the wrist. By normalizing the tension and length of muscles and connective tissue at neural interface points, the health of the median nerve is optimized. Consequently, it is common for signs of neural dysfunction to be gradually alleviated over the course of a treatment series.

In an ideal situation the client gradually learns how to stretch the muscles of the neck, shoulders, forearms, and hands. The client also learns how to breathe using the abdominal muscles because the scalenes are often hypertonic and short due to constant recruitment during breathing. This tense pattern of breathing needs to be gradually dismantled, and the client needs to begin to breathe predominantly with the diaphragm.

Once again it is clear how the generalized, holistic approach of Massage Therapy often has serendipitous outcomes.

For clients suffering from frank neurological disease/trauma, Massage Therapy is not curative but often is helpful. For many of these clients, touch has been withdrawn as a result of people's reaction to their condition and/or attendant isolation and loneliness. Massage Therapy can be a nurturing link to the world of human touch and can facilitate touch in the person's relationships.

In terms of technical benefits, massage has not been shown to be a consistent therapy for alleviation of spasticity, but it does help clients to relax and maintain range of motion. Stroke clients suffering from unilateral neglect may benefit from having stimulation and awareness drawn toward the neglected side of their body. It is common in Massage Therapy education to talk about massage interventions that are designed to maintain the nutritional status of denervated tissue, but I don't know of any literature that supports this contention. Clients with neurological problems often have functional body parts that are working overtime. Massage Therapy can help overworked body parts adapt to the necessary challenges, usually through stretching, release of TrPs and help in adjusting to increased workloads.

In all clients with neurological dysfunction, Massage Therapy helps with relaxation and adaptation of functional parts that may be working overtime, and it helps people remain connected to the mainstream of life.

## BODY IMAGE, SELF-CONNECTEDNESS, AND SELF-CARE

One of the most common subjective outcomes during a massage is a feeling of "returning home" to the flesh. Stressful thoughts and ideas are gradually set aside, and a comforting and grounded sense of awareness of the body often occurs. Massage Therapists encourage clients to cease talking and to pay attention to their breath and somatic awareness during the treatment.

The acceptance and nurturing of the client's body by the Massage Therapist can be a powerful factor in healing and prevention of disease. People who have undergone disfiguring surgeries (or any surgery) often cut off their awareness from the part of their body that was treated. Similarly, people who have been traumatized physically, sexually, and/or emotionally often dissociate from the traumatized body part (or the entire body). This can have far reaching repercussions on their quality of life, relationships, and self-care.[21]

It is common for touch of a traumatized region to activate memories of the traumatic experience. Many people do not perform breast self-examinations or basic dental hygiene or have Pap smears performed as a result of posttraumatic reactions.

While Massage Therapy is not psychotherapy, it is vital that the Massage Therapist be aware that possible posttrauma situations may be encountered during Massage Therapy care. Well-trained, well-intentioned therapists employ the psychological equivalent of universal precautions for infectious disease when interacting with clients. The massage interaction itself must feel safe to the client, and the Massage Therapist must be boundary conscious at all times. The therapist must seek informed consent for treatment from the client, which can be withdrawn or modified whenever the client wishes. Although the Massage Therapist is not performing psychotherapy, he or she must be trained in some type of emotional first aid to know how to deal with touch-triggered emotional responses (see case study). Haldane[22] is a good reference in this regard.

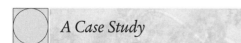

## A Case Study

### Psychological Impact of Cancer Surgery

I once massaged a woman who had a skin cancer lesion removed from her left arm several months prior. She was cleared by her physician and surgeon for Massage Therapy care. Her entire left shoulder and neck were much more dense and inelastic than the right, although she was strongly right dominant. As I approached the arm, the texture of her skin and muscle tissue became increasingly dense and inelastic.

I asked her for permission to touch her arm where the cancer lesion had been removed. She acquiesced somewhat nervously, not for any medical reason but from a sense of anxiety about my touching her arm. As I got closer to the spot, she reported that the area felt "dead," or at least "numb." I asked her if I could help her "bring it back to life" and she agreed to let me give it a try. I gently held her arm and slowly kneaded the triceps region where the lesion had been removed. Very slowly it began to soften and differentiate into a palpably distinguishable muscle mass with softer and more pliant fibers. As this happened, she silently wept. She reported that she felt that we were massaging "life" back into a part of her body that she had vacated. After the treatment she told me what a relief it was to connect to her arm again and how she had wept with sadness at her sense of loss, as well as released fear over how part of her body could attack itself. She felt that she had returned to "herself."

This type of change has often happened in my office with clients who have had various surgical interventions such as mastectomies and lumpectomies, as well as physical and emotional traumas. ∾

Return to a normal somatic awareness is a commonly discussed outcome amongst Massage Therapists and is increasingly being paid attention in the scientific literature. Bredin[23] showed how massage helps women cope with body image challenges after mastectomy. Hart, Field, and Hernandez-Reif[24] report that anorexic patients' body dissatisfaction was improved after a trial of Massage Therapy, and Hernandez-Reif, Field, and Theakston[25] reported how multiple sclerosis patients have improved body image after a Massage Therapy treatment series.

This "soft outcome" of Massage Therapy interventions is perhaps one of the most important effects of Massage Therapy. Massage Therapy accepts the client and the client's body, nurturing the person and modeling what is sometimes a new relationship of trust, warmth, and affection between the client and his or her body.

Feeling at home and trusting of their body is often quite a struggle for people with chronic recurrent diseases such as multiple sclerosis and lupus, as well as those with functional disorders such as irritable bowel syndrome. Massage Therapy helps these people deal with the stress of the uncertainty of their situation, and it often helps them to feel more connected to their body and state of health, which often seem unpredictable and precarious.

## SUMMARY

Massage Therapy is both a simple and a complex intervention. Built around the natural impulse to touch a person to provide comfort and to bond, it has powerful effects simply on the basis of providing caring, respectful, and boundary-conscious touch. It has the systemic effects of immune system enhancement and physiological normalization, and it lessens excessive muscle tonus in the body. By reducing the somatosensory noise of muscle tension and compression in the body, as well as quieting the chattering of the mind, Massage Therapy often makes it possible for people to notice the effects of their body use choices and to make changes that are not of a recipe nature but that arise spontaneously from an accurate awareness of how their body feels.

Precise clinical effects are achieved through the normalization of tension in specific problematic muscles and resolution of myofascial TrPs. Shortened connective tissue is lengthened, and often numerous subclinical nervous system compromises are alleviated.

There are numerous other affects that Massage Therapy may have on, for example, swelling, constipation, and concentration that space precludes us from exploring in this chapter. The interested reader is referred to the texts of Clifford and Andrade[26] and Rattray and Ludwig.[27] Perhaps the most important effects are those of body acceptance and feeling at home in the flesh.

## FINDING A MASSAGE THERAPIST

The best way to find a Massage Therapist is through referral from a trusted source. If you can't get a referral that way, then you might have to find a therapist through a referral service. Most fraternal organizations run a referral service, and the most reputable and effective therapists tend to be registered with such an organization. Regardless of how you find a Massage Therapist, speak to the therapist before you consider going for a treatment or sending a client/patient for one.

Massage Therapy is variably regulated throughout the world. In the United States and Canada, regulation is on a state-by-state or province-by-province basis.

- In the United States, the American Massage Therapy Association runs a referral service. Call (847) 864-0123, or visit the website at: http://www.amtamassage.org/.
- The National Certification Board for Therapeutic Massage and Bodywork certifies Massage Therapists and body workers to a uniform level throughout the United States. Call (800) 296-0664, or visit the website at: http://www.ncbtmb.com/.
- In Canada, Massage Therapists are regulated in Ontario, British Columbia, and Newfoundland. The Ontario Massage Therapist Association runs a referral service. Call (800) 668-2022. To contact the British Columbia Massage Therapist Association, call (888) 413-4467, or visit the website at http://www.massagetherapy.bc.ca/.

## References

1. Field T, Scafidi FA, Schanberg SM: Factors that predict which preterm infants benefit most from massage therapy. *J Dev Behav Pediatr* 14(3):176-180, 1993.
2. Field T: Massage therapy for infants and children, *J Dev Behav Pediatr* 16(2):105-111, 1995.
3. Touch Research Institute Database: http://www.miami.edu/touch-research/.
4. Travell J, Simmons D: *Myofascial pain and dysfunction,* Baltimore, Williams & Wilkins, 1983.
5. Aprill C, Bogduk N: The prevalence of cervical zygapophyseal joint pain: a first approximation, *Spine* 17(7):744-747, 1992.
6. Smith LK, Weiss EL, Lehmkuhl LD: *Brunnstrom's clinical kinesiology,* ed 5, Philadelphia, FA Davis, 1995, p 115.
7. English AW, Wolf SL, Segal RL: Compartmentalization of muscles and their motor nuclei: the partitioning hypothesis, *Phys Ther* 73(12):857-867, 1993.
8. Rywerant Y: *The Feldenkrais Method: teaching by handling,* San Francisco, Harper & Row, 1983.
9. Preyde M: Effectiveness of massage therapy for subacute low-back pain: a randomized controlled trial, *CMAJ* 162(13):1815-1820, 2000.
10. Prudden B: *Pain erasure,* New York, Random House, 1982.
11. Chaitow L, DeLaney JW: *Clinical application of neuromuscular techniques,* New York, Churchill Livingstone, 2000.
12. Mense S, Simons DG: *Muscle pain: understanding its nature, diagnosis and treatment,* Philadelphia, Lippincott Williams & Wilkins, 2001.
13. McKenzie R: *Treat your own back,* Waikanae, New Zealand, Spinal Publications, 1997.
14. Gerwin RD: A study of 96 subjects examined both for fibromyalgia and myofascial pain, *J Musculoskeletal Pain* 3(Suppl 1):121, 1995.

15. Akeson WH, Amiel D, Woo SL: Immobility effects on synovial joints: the pathomechanics of joint contracture, *Biorheology* 17(1-2):95-110, 1980.

16. Beaupre LA, Davies DM, Jones CA et al: Exercise combined with continuous passive motion or slider board therapy compared with exercise only: a randomized controlled trial of patients following total knee arthroplasty, *Phys Ther* 81(4):1029-1037, 2001.

17. Weintraub W: *Tendon and ligament healing: a new approach through manual therapy,* Berkeley, Calif, North Atlantic Books, 1999.

18. Upledger JE, Vredevoogd J: *Craniosacral therapy,* Seattle, Eastland Press, 1983.

19. Butler D: *Mobilisation of the nervous system,* London, Churchill Livingstone, 1991, pp 65-68.

20. Upton ARM, McComas AJ: The double crush in nerve entrapment syndromes, *Lancet* 2:359-362, 1973.

21. Fitch P, Dryden T: Recovering body and soul from post-traumatic stress disorder, *Massage Ther J* 39(1):40-68, 2000.

22. Haldane S: *Emotional first aid: a crisis handbook,* Barrytown, NY, Barrytown Ltd, 1998.

23. Bredin M: Mastectomy, body image and therapeutic massage: a qualitative study of women's experience, *J Adv Nurs* 29(5):1113-1120, 1999.

24. Hart S, Field T, Hernandez-Reif M et al: Anorexia symptoms are reduced by massage therapy, *Eat Disord* 9:217-228, 2001. Abstract published at Touch Research Institute website: http://www.miami.edu/touch-research/.

25. Hernandez-Reif M, Field T, Theakston H: Multiple sclerosis patients benefit from massage therapy, *J Bodywork Movement Ther* 2:168-174, 1998.

26. Clifford P, Andrade CK: *Outcome-based massage,* New York, Lippincott Williams & Wilkins, 2001.

27. Rattray F, Ludwig L: *Clinical massage therapy,* Toronto, Talus Inc, 2000.

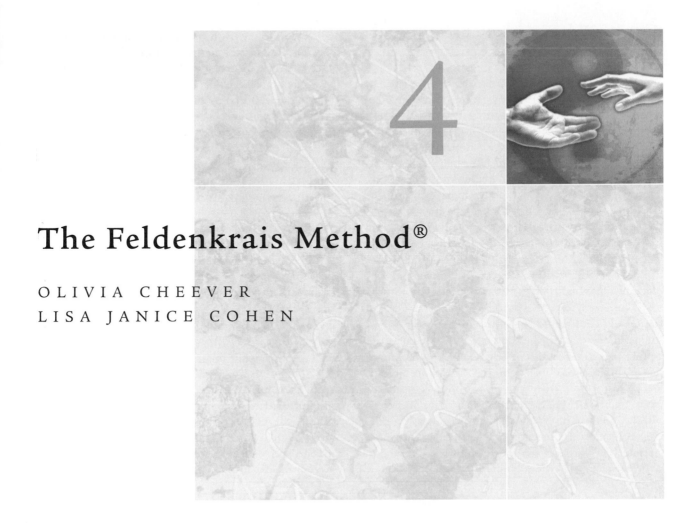

# The Feldenkrais Method®

OLIVIA CHEEVER
LISA JANICE COHEN

## THE NAGI MODEL: REHABILITATION IN A DISABLEMENT MODE

Traditional rehabilitation is based on the World Health Organization (WHO)[1] model of the relationship among impairments, functional limitations, and disability. Simply stated, *impairments* are problems at the tissue level and include sprains and strains, fractures, and disease processes. *Functional limitations* are problems manifesting in the inability of an individual to complete a task. Asthma is an impairment. Shortness of breath climbing stairs is a functional limitation. *Disability* is defined in terms of an individual's life role. For example, *Mr. Smith is unable to work as a pri-* *mary school teacher because of uncontrolled asthma*. In a traditional rehabilitation setting, clinicians would likely identify and attempt to directly ameliorate and/or teach compensations for impairments, functional limitations, and disability.

This is primarily a deficit model: problems are identified and the individual categorized by what he or she cannot do. This construct is also best suited to an allopathic medical model where health is defined by the absence of disease. Although the relationship among impairments, functional limitations, and disability is not linear, the Nagi model is limited in its ability to include the rich background of skills, abilities, and feelings that an individual brings to the healing process.

## Somatic Education: Rehabilitation in an Empowerment Mode

*Somatic education* is the term used to describe somatosensory, kinesthetically based body-centered learning practices that developed at the beginning of the twentieth century from the work of F.M. Alexander[2,3] (The Alexander Technique), Elsa Gindler[4] (Gymnastik), Charlotte Selver[4] (Sensory Awareness), Ida Rolf[5] (Rolfing), and Moshe Feldenkrais[6-10] (The Feldenkrais Method®), among others. All of these are educational learning models. Other forms of somatic education have continued to develop with the work of Thomas Hanna[11-15] (Somatics), Judith Aston[16] (Aston-Patterning®), Bonnie Bainbridge Cohen[16a] (Body Mind Centering), Emily Conrad[4] (Continuum Movement), Ilana Rubenfeld[17] (Rubenfeld Synergy), and Marion Rosen[18] (Rosen Method), among others. The term *somatic education* comes from *soma*, the Greek word for body. Hanna referred to soma in the specific context of "the body as perceived from within by first-person perception."[14] He heralded "a new manner of thinking of ourselves in the breadth of our biological history and the depth of our physiological reality."[13] Hanna believed that one's self-image and one's physical self are intertwined: "Self-awareness (or self-consciousness) is a function of experiencing the whole state of one's organic structure, [and] as that organic structure changes, so does our basic self-awareness—and vice versa."[11] Others have referred to similar holistic neurobiologically based views of embodiment.[19-22]

Somatic Education develops an individual's self-awareness and is a process that educates the *whole* person. The somatically educated self is an embodied, aware, whole self that participates fully in both the secular and spiritual domains. In the Feldenkrais model of somatic education, students delve into their own rich background of skills and abilities and learn how to move out of pain and into ease, pleasure, and spontaneity. Adding a form of somatic education such as the Feldenkrais Method® to a program of recovery from injury, disability, or illness can speed up the process of learning self-knowledge, self-care, self-repair, and personal empowerment.

## MOVING FROM IMPAIRMENT TO EMPOWERMENT

An impairment model with its focus on the patient as a passive recipient of care is appropriate to physiological trauma and acute medical conditions. However, when working with chronic conditions such as hypertension, myofascial pain, or asthma, for example, the clinician must alter his or her therapeutic relationship to focus on education, self-care, and patient empowerment. The clinician must also alter his or her professional role from one who cures or "fixes" to one who mentors or guides the healing process. This enables the patient to become an equal partner in the healing process and to take responsibility for his or her own wellness. Somatic Education can furnish a missing integrative link in rehabilitation by involving individuals more actively in their process.

Somatically based approaches such as the Feldenkrais Method may help to unravel the often puzzling findings in patients with abuse histories presenting with nonanatomically based pain syndromes.[23] In a traditional allopathic medical paradigm, such patients are referred for psychiatric care with the unspoken assumption that there is no somatic (anatomical) basis to the patient's pain and therefore the pain must be solely of psychiatric origin. This extreme separation of psyche and soma is in itself nonanatomic as the scientific world begins to confirm the intimate connections between brain structure, brain chemistry, emotions, behavior, and physical functioning in the discipline termed psychoneuroimmunology.[24-27]

## SOMATIC EDUCATION WITH THE FELDENKRAIS METHOD®

Several philosophies underlie all methods of somatic education: the integration of mind with body, the integration of structure (anatomical architecture) with function (purposeful movement), and self-directed learning within the individual's milieu. Modalities may vary as to the degree to which they emphasize each component. The Alexander Technique and the Feldenkrais Method® exist at one end of the spectrum in which function and functional movement is emphasized with structure in the service of function. At the other end of the continuum, Aston-Patterning® and Rolfing emphasize a bodywork approach where structure is emphasized and function serves structure. Somatic Education includes aspects of emotional intelligence[28] such as self-awareness and empathy, somatic empathy,[29,30] kinesthetic intelligence, spatial intelligence,[31] and the care of the soul.[32] Somatic Education is an emerging discipline, and consensus regarding its taxonomy has yet to be established. Ongoing dialogue among somatic educators will undoubtedly clarify which modalities fall under the rubric of somatic education.

## The Feldenkrais Method®

The Feldenkrais Method® is a form of somatic/movement education that integrates body, mind, and psyche. It has two complementary components: hands-on individualized Functional Integration (FI) sessions (in which the Feldenkrais Practitioner individually guides a student's movements through touch) and a verbally guided movement exploration called Awareness Through Movement (ATM). A Feldenkrais student does not disrobe while being guided into nonhabitual movement sequences by the touch and/or voice of a certified Feldenkrais Practitioner. Both components are based on sensorimotor developmental learning.[33,34] Feldenkrais practitioners refer to this as organic learning.[35,36]

Moshe Feldenkrais, DSc (1904-1984), the method's originator, considered it a teaching rather than a treatment paradigm. He thought of his clients as "students" and his sessions "lessons." This is an important distinction. The Method is not a therapeutic technique to be applied to a set of impairments; rather it is a process of self-exploration by which individuals consciously reconnect with their unconscious sensorimotor selves. This results in increased awareness, new connections created within the self, and increased movement repertoire and cognitive flexibility. The method empowers individuals to *learn how to learn* to regain, maintain, or find new, more efficient functioning through reducing extraneous effort. Within this process, students often begin to see changes in old restrictive habits and find new functional abilities, but the method itself is not primarily for treatment of specific impairments.[6-10,36-39]

## Feldenkrais: The Man and the Method

Moshe Feldenkrais trained in the disciplines of mathematics, engineering, physics, and martial arts. He earned an advanced degree in electrical engineering, as well as a doctorate in physics from the Sorbonne in France. A dedicated scientist (he was Joliot-Curie's research assistant in the area of nuclear fission), he was also a "renaissance man" with a voracious interest in learning. He was one of the first Europeans to earn a black belt in Judo.

As an adult, Feldenkrais sustained serious knee injuries playing soccer. Surgery was recommended, but his prognosis was extremely poor with the surgical technique available at the time. Feldenkrais declined surgery and instead applied his scientific acumen to the problem. This led him to thorough investigations in anatomy, physiology, neurobiology, developmental movement, psychology, hypnosis, learning theory, cybernetics, philosophy, judo, Zen, yoga, exercise, movement therapies, and acupuncture. Feldenkrais incorporated a developmental focus, systematically observing how babies moved through their first 2 years of life. He explored his own movement patterns, recreating developmental milestones, and found ways to decrease unneeded effort in his own body. Despite marked degeneration of his injured knee joints, Feldenkrais was ultimately able, through his careful observations and discoveries, to experience a full recovery of function. He used his experience in the development of what was to become the Feldenkrais Method®. One of Feldenkrais' vital contributions was teaching the importance of movement awareness as a way to improve efficiency and increase one's moving, sensing, feeling, and thinking. Feldenkrais' sensorimotor approach also helped to promote and teach self-care and independence. He believed that Westerners, especially, had been taught to look outside themselves to authorities rather than trust their own knowledge and experience.

Refining the learning processes of FI and ATM, Feldenkrais devised a 4-year, 800-1,200 hour professional training program through which individuals can become certified Feldenkrais Practitioners. (The professional trainings are administered under the nonprofit Feldenkrais Educational Foundation of North America [FEFNA]. See www.feldenkrais.com.) He deliberately designed the training with time between segments for integration of sensorimotor learning and reorganization of the self. Guild Certified Feldenkrais Practitioners must also complete 40 hours of continuing education credit every 2 years to keep their certification current.

In recent years there has been a trend toward more healthcare professionals, including physical and occupational therapists, becoming certified Feldenkrais Practitioners. This has created several dilemmas within the Feldenkrais community as the method becomes more widely applied in therapeutic rather than purely educational venues. There are a plethora of short workshops, seminars, and conferences on the Feldenkrais Method® available for the practicing rehabilitation professional. However, the method is not simply a tool or technique to be applied for a particular patient problem. It is a process and paradigm of somatic education that is mastered by the Feldenkrais Practitioner during his or her training. When modalities are mixed, the unique Feldenkrais learning outcomes may be compromised. Integrating rather than subsuming the philosophies of somatic education into a more traditional rehabilitation perspective is a vital and necessary paradigm shift. The authors have benefited from referring patients/students to each other in an integrative program of rehabilitation and somatic education.

## Recurrent Themes in the Feldenkrais Method®

### Non Goal-Directed Learning

The Feldenkrais Method® is a synthesis of what Feldenkrais learned from the fields of engineering, physics, martial arts, and other domains he had mastered. His carefully chosen words on audiotapes with his written instructions reflect this synthesis.

In the phrase "We do not say at the start what the final stage will be," Feldenkrais is setting the stage for non–goal-directed learning. In so doing, Feldenkrais concurred with F.M. Alexander's notion of avoiding "end-gaining."[2,3,40] When the learner focuses on the goal of movement in this construct, he or she loses focus on the internal processes of awareness that create movement. When focusing exclusively on the goal, learning can be negatively impacted.

### Organic Learning

The Method teaches one the links between perception of sensation, intention, and action. The student learns to remain mindful and attentive to proprioceptive and exteroceptive sensations throughout the body while moving and is taught to notice relationships and patterns of relationships between parts of the moving self. Feldenkrais stated, "Our self-image consists of four components: movement, sensation, feeling, and thought."[6] Organic learning is nonreductionistic in that it does not separate the organism into its anatomical parts but joins those parts into one continuous feedback loop. This feedback loop contains the sensory domain, the motor domain, the affective domain, the cognitive and the spiritual domain. It builds on dimensions such as pleasure and spontaneity.

### Skeletal Support

The Feldenkrais student learns in the initial body scan beginning every movement sequence how to sense the skeleton in relation to the resting surface in all positions. This pressure indicates our relationship to gravity. When our movement is light and easy, skeletal support is at its maximum and movement is most efficient. Feldenkrais believed that using the least amount of effort while moving allows for awareness of greatest connectivity between contiguous joints and across several joints. This use of the kinetic chain in function further increases ease and efficiency. Unlike forms of biofeedback where the relaxation component is separated from movement, Feldenkrais students learn how to move while reducing the effort. Thus they are able to bring an awareness of muscle effort, support from the skeleton in relation to the ground, and connectivity into function.

### Differentiation/Nondifferentiation

This refers to Feldenkrais' sense of the importance of learning through making distinctions. In ATM and FI a student experiences how to increase ease and efficiency by repeating movements each time with less effort. Students learn to differentiate between necessary and unnecessary contraction of muscles, or "parasitic" movements.

Differentiation also occurs when we choose to move parts of the self either separately in "differentiated" movement or together as a whole in "nondifferentiated" movement. In the Feldenkrais parlance, students through trial and error learn to improve the use of individual body segments as they combine and recombine in new patterns in response to a given task. An example of differentiated movement is glenohumeral movement without scapulothoracic movement, or ankle dorsiflexion with toe flexion/ ankle plantar flexion with toe extension. Nondifferentiated movement is movement of body segments in more primitive patterns of logrolling of the trunk, for example, where the shoulder and hip girdles move as one functional unit. Another example of nondifferentiated movement is ankle dorsiflexion with toe extension/ankle plantar flexion with toe flexion.

### Habitual/Nonhabitual

Like F.M. Alexander, Feldenkrais believed that we develop problems as we become increasingly out of touch with and automated in our movements. Most people lose spontaneity and alternatives in their movements as they age. This loss of repertoire may be a risk factor for falls in the elderly. Feldenkrais also believed that we learn best when we are presented with novel stimuli. He emphasized nonhabitual movements to provide learners with new stimuli and novel sensations. Exploring new ways of moving theoretically offers new options to the brain, which reorganizes itself and rewrites the sensory motor cortex, facilitating new, more efficient ways of moving. Also, with stroke[7] or injury, parts of the brain that were not directly involved in the original movement can learn to perform an action. The brain pathway for the original movement is not exactly reproduced, but an auxiliary pathway is forged.

## Whole Body Focus

Feldenkrais emphasized sensing each part of the self in relation to the whole. After scanning their body contact with the floor, students are often amazed to observe how there are missing pieces to their kinesthetically based homunculus. Thomas Hanna,[15] referred to this as *sensorimotor amnesia*. Others have termed it *kinesthetic dystonia*.[41] Through the ATM and FI learning process, students learn to reestablish kinesthetic links to all parts of their bodies. This facilitates the linking of body segments into a kinematic whole for improved function. Students then experience a "river of movement"[42] that expands throughout the body. Learning to move toward pleasant and away from unpleasant sensations while moving is important for learning in this model. As students experience greater ease in movement reducing effort, they increasingly experience greater connectivity with their skeletal structure.

## Proximal Initiation of Movement

From his martial arts, biomechanical, and developmental perspectives, Feldenkrais emphasized the importance of increasing awareness and mobility of the "power center" comprising the pelvis, upper thighs, and hip joints in movement. Other disciplines such as Pilates[43] also emphasize strengthening the body from the center outward through certain exercises focusing on the trunk. Proprioceptive Neuromuscular Facilitation (PNF), a form of therapeutic exercise widely used in the physical therapy community, also focuses on the role of the pelvis and trunk in motor control and function. This "strengthening from the inside out"[44] is a key component of many of the ATM lessons Feldenkrais and his colleagues devised.

## Less is More/Least Noticeable Difference

In using the phrase "It is easy to tell differences when the effort is light," Feldenkrais was drawing on his background as a physicist. The Weber-Fechner law in physics describes the different ratios for stimuli necessary for an individual to detect a difference for each of the senses. For example, when outdoors where there is so much light already, if one lights a match, it is not noticed the way it is when one strikes a match in a darkened room. For an individual to perceive a difference relative to muscular effort, the change must be at least $\frac{1}{40}$ of the original stimulus.[45] Feldenkrais used the example of how when carrying a refrigerator one would not notice if a box of matches were added or removed, whereas "everybody can tell with closed eyes when a fly alights on a thin match-like piece of wood or straw [one is holding] or when it takes to the air again."[8] It is only when we are able to reduce the effort in the neuromuscular system that we are able to pick up more subtle differences through sensing. "The lighter the effort we make, the faster is our learning of any skill; and the level of perfection we can attain goes hand in hand with the finesse we obtain."[8] Feldenkrais' focus on reducing effort through ATM and FI was based on this notion. Through ATM and FI students learn to decrease effort and are able to make finer and finer distinctions when choosing how to move. The less effort expended, the more sensing becomes refined.

Students are also taught the value of imagining movements. Biofeedback has since confirmed that motor neurons fire when the individual is simply imagining the movement.

## Active Dynamic Stability

Feldenkrais focused on the dynamic nature of posture. He realized that even when we are standing still we are continually making minor adjustments to maintain our balance. Feldenkrais coined the term "acture"[10] rather than "posture" to convey this constantly moving nature of posture. Many ATM lessons explore subtle movements around the center of gravity through the fluid loss and recovery of balance.

## Scientific Support for the Feldenkrais Method®

### Neurodevelopmental Underpinnings of the Feldenkrais Method®

There is significant support for the Feldenkrais Method® when we examine its scientific underpinnings. It draws heavily on neurodevelopmental theories in emphasizing a person's sensorimotor and somatically based modes of learning. Recent findings regarding neurodevelopment in the burgeoning field of embodied cognition,[46] as well as developmental psychology,[47] point toward a dynamic, experientially based notion of the self. Research in these fields shows that during the first few months of life there is simultaneous development of several senses in crossmodal processing as babies increasingly interact with the world/environment in a global way, using several senses at once. Stern, a psychoanalytically trained child psychiatrist, after extensive video analysis of infants' behavior, revises the old psychoanalytically based view of a passive infant whose nascent self is symbiotically intertwined with that of its mother and concludes that "The sense of self is not a cognitive construct. It is an experiential integration."[47]

The Feldenkrais Method® assumes this integration between sensorimotor learning and neurologically based self-image. ATM and FI lessons help the individual improve his or her sense of self and subsequent patterns of movement. The Method also builds a foundation for emotional intelligence because it involves such human qualities as self-awareness (recognizing a feeling as it happens) and empathy (recognizing emotions in others).[28] The Feldenkrais Method® fosters the development of a particular kind of somatically attuned empathy in both practitioner and student—somatic empathy whereby we learn to feel into our own experience, as well as to sense and observe others' somatic experience.[30] Learning kinesthetically with somatic empathy can help mental health counselors develop empathy by better sensing their somatic sensations as they empathically attune to their clients.[48]

Sensorimotor learning shows whole body involvement in relating to the world on a nonverbal, nonanalytical level. This is also called *procedural learning* or knowing "that."[49] With the development of language, a baby's sense of self undergoes a transformation that results in bringing him or her farther away from pure procedural learning into *declarative learning*—or "know-ing what." Declarative learning is language based, memory dependent and analytical.[50] Thus it is susceptible to cognitive distortions that can impair functioning. The Feldenkrais Method® relies not primarily on verbal feedback but on kinesthetic and sensory feedback in the learning process. This focus on procedural rather than declarative knowledge is presumably less prone to conscious interference or distortions. From the Feldenkrais perspective, "Language breaks the body into separate parts: the hand, the wrist, the arm, etc., [that] create a fragmented 'body of thought' apart from our unified organismic body."[51]

### Somatic Education and the Embodied Mind

Findings in neuroscience and embodied cognition[19,21,22,52] have challenged the mechanistic model of the brain as the central processor, or "software" with the body as the output generator.[21] Just as Lashley could not localize the engram of a given memory in the brain, neither is there a specific geographical location of any given motor plan.[53] Organization is distributed throughout the brain holonomically.[54] Part of Feldenkrais' genius was in recognizing the nonlinear nature of human development. We transition back to an earlier developing part of the brain—the sensorimotor cortex and bring it to the fore again in recalibrating ourselves toward balance and homeostasis. Sensorimotor learning modes do not become obsolete as we develop. Thelen and Smith[20] in observing the development of motor learning in infants, argue for a model of nonlinear dynamic systems constantly in flux. Thus in this view, the embodied human self is continually changing in interaction with its context, and development is not linear and stage-like as in Piaget's view. Behaviors appear and then recede into the background until they reappear in a more sophisticated form later on. As Thelen states, "The grand sweep of development seems neatly rule driven. In detail, however, development is messy."[20] In essence, the mind and the self emerge from that complex, messy interaction between the brain and the body in a constantly shifting environment.[19,21,22,52]

Learning requires both internal and external feedback in the context of environmental cues. The strength of the Feldenkrais Method® is in teaching the student to remain fully aware of the interaction between external feedback (environment) and internal feedback (self) while sensing and directing movement. In this way our sense of self is always developing in relation to our movement, and as our movement changes so does our sense of self. In using another computer analogy, it's as if the software rewrites itself and reconfigures the hardware both in relation to the output and the quality of its own process.

## The Feldenkrais Method®, Neuroscience, and Motor Learning

### Research

Areas that are virtually exploding in the literature are those of neuroscience and motor learning.[55] A recent Medline search showed over 17,000 citations referencing motor learning alone since 1977. If we examine the literature, there is much to indicate basic scientific support of the underlying principles of the Feldenkrais Method®.

Georgopoulos[56] presents compelling evidence of the involvement of both motor and cognitive processes in the production of motor tasks. He cites numerous studies using electroencephalography (EEG), magnetoencephalography (MEG), positron emission tomography (PET), functional magnetic resonance imaging (fMRI), and transcranial magnetic stimulation (TMS) that have clearly demonstrated that the motor cortex is involved in all aspects of motor learning, motor memory, and motor imagery. There is strong research support for the engagement of the motor cortex with imagined movements in the absence of movement execution. Further research on rats, primates, and humans shows that learning can change the motor cortex throughout the lifespan. Bizzi and Mussa-Ivaldi[57] postulate that motor learning requires the building of internal models in the brain/central nervous systrem (CNS) and that the model is distributed throughout many structures including sensorimotor cortex, basal ganglia, cerebellum, and spinal cord. This model highlights the connectivity between elements in the CNS and shows that one's learning takes place in the context "of repeated exposure to sensory signals coming from [ ] moving limbs while [ ] interact[ing] with the environment," (pp. 97-98, emphasis added). Their work implies that highly complex motor skills can be learned through the formation of new complex internal models built from interactions of more simple ones.

To investigate the complex relationship between learning, pain, and anxiety, Sieve et al[58] conducted a study exposing rats to varying doses of a presumed anxiogenic in various adversive learning situations.

Their findings indicate that panic undermines learning in Pavlovian fear conditioning. They suggest that panic inhibits pain and that some pain sensitizes the organism to prepare for and respond to danger. If we extrapolate their findings to humans, this panic state may be elicited by abuse and may inhibit somatic learning and appropriate self-protection in patients with abuse histories.

### Evidence for Efficacy

Because the Feldenkrais Method® is not considered by its core practitioners to be a therapy, there is very little in the research literature on its application in rehabilitation. In the English language literature on MEDLINE, there are only a handful of relevant references to the Feldenkrais Method® between 1977 and 2001.

Johnson et al[59] compares the Feldenkrais Method® to sham (nontherapeutic) bodywork on the physical status, mood, and ADLs of individuals with multiple sclerosis (MS). Results in this small sample showed significant decrease in anxiety with the Feldenkrais sessions as compared with the sham bodywork sessions. There were no significant differences seen in any other markers, including MS symptoms, function, or UE performance. There was some evidence for a trend to higher self-efficacy with both the Feldenkrais and the sham bodywork. This may reflect the powerful effect of touch even in the absence of "therapeutic" work. However, apart from the generic effect of touch, The Feldenkrais group experienced decreased anxiety. It would be of interest to repeat this study with a larger sample size and additional functional markers.

Bearman and Shafarman[60] sought to assess the efficacy and cost effectiveness of the Feldenkrais Method® in the treatment of chronic pain. In this pilot study, a group of seven patients with refractory chronic pain with pain-related medical costs in excess of $1000 per year was enrolled in a program consisting entirely of the Feldenkrais Method®. The program was primarily composed of group ATM lessons, with a limited amount of individualized FI. Patient mobility, perception of pain, and total healthcare and pharmacy costs were measured. The authors used the American Academy of Pain Management's National Pain Data Bank (NPDB) test instrument prestudy, immediately poststudy, and 1 year poststudy. Per member per month healthcare costs decreased from an average of $141 (for the year preceding the study) to an average of $82 (for the year following the study). This was primarily a descriptive study with a small population and no true control group (although the authors did compare their patients to like patients enrolled in small, multidisciplinary pain management programs who had also completed the NPDB instrument). Nonetheless, it is an interesting first step in assessing the potential effectiveness and cost effectiveness of intervention with the Feldenkrais Method®.

In 1999 Lunblad et al[61] compared the Feldenkrais Method® with physical therapy or no treatment on head and shoulder complaints in a population of female industrial workers with neck and shoulder pain. In this study 97 workers were randomized into the three groups. Participants were treated for 16 weeks and a posttest was conducted one year after the conclusion of treatment. Results indicated that the Feldenkrais group showed significant decreases in neck/shoulder pain and disability during leisure time. The physical therapy intervention group showed no change in base complaints. The control group showed worsening of symptoms.

Gutman et al[62] showed no significant difference between the FM and conventional exercises in an elderly population. In this study, tenants in a retirement community were assigned into three groups: a Feldenkrais intervention group, a conventional intervention group, and a no-exercise group. There were no significant differences seen among groups on any measure, including blood pressure, heart rate, balance, flexibility, morale, perception of health, ADLs, and pain. It is likely that the measures used here were not sensitive enough to detect difference in this population because some difference between the two intervention groups and the no-exercise group just as a byproduct of the Hawthorne effect would be expected. Small sample size and insufficient randomization of the groups were problematic as well.

In general, the research literature on the effectiveness of the Feldenkrais Method® is sparse and poorly designed. Most of the literature that exists on the Method is in the form of anecdotal reports, nonscientific publications, and books written by Feldenkrais Practitioners.[36,37,63] This dearth of peer-reviewed, scientific literature does not mean that the FM does not have value but merely that, as in many other arenas, it has had little systematic study. In addition, the researcher must choose appropriate instruments that will do justice to the experience of somas. Different qualitative research approaches lend themselves to capturing the subjective and phenomenological experience of a soma than those measuring range of motion.[64]

Much of what Feldenkrais postulated in the 1940s until his death in 1984 is being borne out through basic science research on the brain in the fields of neuroscience and motor learning. Now that the tools exist to track changes in the brain with learning, we are able to see what Feldenkrais saw in his detailed and meticulous observations of human movement so many decades ago: We can continue to learn and change through our whole lives, we constantly access both internal and external cues in our movements, we have the capacity for much higher skill and discrimination in our movement than we usually use, and our movement patterns and our self-image are inexorably linked. These ideas are illustrated in the case study that follows.

## A Case Study

### Chronic Myofascial Pain

This case illustrates how the Feldenkrais Method® enables change in perception and sensation of anxiety and pain. The student develops awareness through creative exploration of movement and regains function while learning self-empathy and self-esteem.

A is a 37-year-old right hand dominant unmarried female who is a professional string player currently working part-time as a freelance musician. Chief complaints: Pain in the left side of her neck and shoulder blade, both hips, and thighs; constant pain (6/10), which increases when playing and performing (10/10); and sitting and walking increase pain.

### History

Pain began in 1995 without specific physical event.

### Functional Limitations

1. Inability to manage chronic pain and anxiety
2. Limited ability to hold and play her viola/violin and to use bow without increased pain
3. Inability to sit without pain
4. Inability to lie down without pain (10/10)
5. Difficulty walking more than 5 minutes

### Psychological Limitations

1. Heightened anxiety, depression, and low self-esteem resulting from persistence of
   • Myofascial pain and dissociation from her somatic experience
2. Hypercritical negative self-talk (". . . pray that I would somehow be able to hold on until the end of the piece not knowing how to play the correct notes in the correct rhythm and feeling stupid and self-critical.")

3. Inability to improve musically according to her and her teacher's perception of her potential ability to play her instrument
4. Parents' denial of her being sexually abused by family friend at 5 years of age

*Previous Medical History*
Surgical removal of left parotid gland resulting from swelling and calcium deposits in 1995.
1. Physical treatment (without success)
   • Physical therapy, occupational therapy
   • Chiropractic, acupuncture, Massage Therapy, Alexander Technique of Somatic Education, Medical Intuitive
   • Yoga
2. Psychological treatment
   • Several courses of psychotherapy (before onset of her myofascial pain) for inability to express herself emotionally or musically and difficulty with sexual relations
   • Psychotherapy focusing on issues of sexual abuse (weekly, 6 years); psychotherapy group for survivors of sexual abuse (1½ years)
   • Psychiatric consultation for psychopharmacological workup resulted in her referral to OC for Feldenkrais in summer 2000
3. Medications: Tylenol prn

*Posture*
1. Static
   • Head held anterior to pelvis
   • Both shoulders internally rotated, left : right
   • No clear standing leg
   • Tendency to hyperextend both knees when standing
2. Dynamic
   • Habitually initiating movement with head
   • Little sense of support of movement from below (base of support)
3. Palpation
   • Excess effort in both left and right trapezius and rhomboids and erector spinae and serratus
   • Excess effort of upper and lower arm muscles bilaterally
   • Excess effort of upper and lower leg muscles bilaterally
4. Body scan (supine)
   • Midthoracic spine, left and right rib cage not contacting the table surface
   • Breathing movement only in upper chest
5. Initial movement exploration (supine)
   • Head turns easier to left than right
   • Difficulty rolling legs medially and laterally and tilting knees
   • Intrusion of abuse memories, especially when OC touched upper left shoulder

6. Goals
   • Reduce anxiety and depression in playing instruments
   • Reduce pain in playing instruments
   • Develop more confidence in playing and performing
   • Increase her stamina in playing and performing
   • Sit more comfortably
   • Walk more comfortably
   • Eliminate tendency to dissociate from physical sensation in playing and performing
   • Lessen and/or alleviate intrusion of abuse memories

*Feldenkrais Somatic Learning Course*
1. Weekly, then biweekly Feldenkrais lessons with A in summer 2000
   • OC recommended consultation with rheumatologist to rule out fibromyalgia
   • Rheumatologist diagnosed myofascial pain
   • OC supported A's taking a break from all playing and performing for 5 months
2. Feldenkrais Lesson Plan: Functional Integration (FI) and individualized Awareness Through Movement (ATM) lessons
   • Help A to sense different body parts in motion through differentiated and undifferentiated movements
   • Help A to increase her ability to move as a whole self, including the pelvis
   • Help A to reduce effort (less is more) through FI and ATM lessons
   • Help A to observe self and nurture self without overly self-critical judgment
3. Progress report after 1 year of Feldenkrais lessons: FI (1½ hours) with individualized ATM sequences twice a week for 4 months; FI/ATM once a week and occasionally twice a week for 8 months, supplemented by ATM group class for last 6 months. Student reports she is able to
   • Lessen her pain when playing and performing
   • Practice and perform for longer duration
   • Remain present and not dissociate from her body while playing and performing
   • Sit more comfortably at her computer
   • Walk without pain for periods of longer duration
   • Decrease negative self talk and hypercritical stance
   • Experience a greater sense of self-efficacy
   • Experience lessening of her depression and anxiety
   • Control intrusion of memories of abuse so as not to feel overwhelmed by them
   • Engage in ATM to alleviate her pain when holding and not holding her instruments
   • Participate in OC's weekly group ATM class since January 2001 (Student was unable to participate when she initially tried to join a class in October 2000

because of anxiety, pain, and intrusion of memories of abuse)

Student has seen her psychotherapist for four sessions since beginning Feldenkrais work with OC up through December 2000.

### Recommendations

A hopes to resume a full schedule of playing and performing. OC suggests that she continue weekly or bi-weekly FI lessons and continue participating in weekly ATM classes over the next 3 months. ❧

This case illustrates the importance of an integrative approach including somatic education for effective recovery from psychophysical symptoms of sexual abuse. The patient was able to return to employment after not having played publicly for 5 months. After her first two concerts, she experienced a pain level of 6/10. She then stopped and engaged in her ATM movements, reducing her pain considerably and was able to play three performances the next day with an increasing sense of competence and self-efficacy. She has reported successfully

---

 ## Sample ATM Lesson

### The Pelvic Clock

*This lesson is done while lying on your back.*

Begin by bending your knees with your feet flat on the floor. Visualize a clock face painted on the back of your pelvis: 12 o'clock is at the center of the lumbar curve, 6 o'clock is at the center of the tailbone, 9 o'clock is at the right side of the pelvis, and 3 o'clock is at the left side of the pelvis.

1. Gently, slowly, and easily press your pelvis toward 12 o'clock, then rest.
   - Does the low back flatten?
   - Is this the same as doing a pelvic tilt?
   - Can you continue to breathe while moving to 12 o'clock?
   - Do you breath in or out as you move to 12 o'clock?
2. Gently and easily, using small slow movements, press your pelvis toward 6:00, then rest.
   - Does the low back arch?
3. Gently and easily, press your pelvis toward 9 o'clock, then rest.
   - Do your legs tilt to the side? Do they have to?
   - Does the left side of your pelvis lose contact with the mat?
   - What happens if you gently push on your left foot while moving your pelvis to 9 o'clock?
4. Repeat to 6 o'clock.
   - Notice whether you move with ease or with difficulty to each of the four cardinal points on the clock.
5. Stretch out your legs and take a break.
6. Return to bending your knees with feet standing.

7. Gently press your pelvis toward 12 o'clock, then allow your pelvis to roll toward 1 o'clock. Swing back to 12 o'clock, then rest.
8. Gently press your pelvis toward 12 o'clock. Roll to the 1 o'clock position, then to the 2 o'clock position, then rest.
9. Continue to expand the movement until you are rolling from 12 o'clock to 3 o'clock. Return to 12 o'clock, then rest.
   - Notice if there are points of the clock that are more difficult to feel than others.
   - Is the movement smooth, like the sweep second hand of a clock? Or jerky and ratchet-like?
10. Now begin by gently pressing your pelvis toward 6 o'clock. Allow your pelvis to roll toward 5 o'clock. Swing back to 6 o'clock, then rest.
11. Continue to expand on the movement as before, first to 4 o'clock, then 3 o'clock. Keep the movements smooth and light.
12. Allow the pelvis to move in a continuous arc from 12 o'clock to 6 o'clock.
    - Notice if there are points of the clock that are more difficult to feel than others.
    - Is the movement smooth, like the sweep second hand of a clock? Or jerky and ratchet-like?
13. Repeat this sequence for the other side of the clock.
    - Allow yourself sufficient resting time. Do not move through pain.
14. Conclude the clock exercise by moving around the entire circle.
    - Can you allow the movement to mimic the sweep second hand (i.e., smooth and continuous)? ❧

rehearsing for 4 hours with no pain. A sample ATM lesson is contained in the box on p. 48.

In FI lessons, the patient became aware of her fear that the perpetrator would attack her when she was playing her instrument. In learning how to independently engage in ATM movement sequences, she was able to alleviate discomfort during and after performances. She was able to improve her performing and her ability to nurture and care for herself. The patient realized that she had first learned to feel safe in her body with OC while receiving FI. She was able to take this sense of safety into other situations when she was without OC. Through the Feldenkrais Method,® the patient learned a different way of listening, sensing, and empathizing with her own somatic experience. She also began to validate her own sensing and feeling in an embodied way.

## ACKNOWLEDGMENTS

Feldenkrais, The Feldenkrais Method,® Awareness Through Movement, Functional Integration, and The Feldenkrais Guild are registered service marks of The Feldenkrais Guild of North America. The authors wish to thank Larraine Feldman and Deborah Lotus, Guild Certified Feldenkrais Practitioners, for their helpful feedback.

## References

1. Nagi S: Disability concepts revisited: implications for prevention. In Pope AM, Tarlov AR (eds): *Disability in America: toward a national agenda for prevention,* Washington, DC, 1991, National Academy Press.
2. Alexander FM: *Constructive conscious control of the individual,* New York, 1923, EP Dutton.
3. Alexander FM: *The use of self,* New York, 1992, EP Dutton.
4. Johnson DH: *Bone, breath, gesture: practices of embodiment,* Berkeley, Calif, 1995, North Atlantic Books.
5. Rolf IP: *Rolfing: the integration of human structures,* New York, 1977, Harper & Row.
6. Feldenkrais M: *Awareness through movement: health exercises for personal growth,* New York, 1972, HarperCollins.
7. Feldenkrais M: *Body awareness as healing therapy: the case of Nora,* Berkeley, Calif, 1993, Frog Ltd.
8. Feldenkrais M: *Awareness through movement lessons with Moshe Feldenkrais* (audiotapes), 1980 (see www.feldenkrais. com).
9. Feldenkrais M: *The elusive obvious or basic Feldenkrais,* Capitola, Calif, 1981, Meta Publications.
10. Feldenkrais M: *The potent self: a guide to spontaneity,* San Francisco, Calif, 1985, HarperCollins.
11. Hanna T: Three elements of somatology: preface to a holistic medicine and to a humanistic psychology, *Main Currents* 31(3):82-87, 1975.
12. Hanna T: *The body of life: creating new pathways for sensory awareness and fluid movement,* New York, 1980, Alfred A Knopf.
13. Hanna T: *Bodies in revolt: a primer in somatic thinking,* ed 2, Novato, Calif, 1985, Freeperson Press.
14. Hanna T: What is somatics? *Somatics* I:4-8, Spring/Summer, 1986.
15. Hanna T: *Somatics: reawakening the body's control of movement,* Cambridge, Mass, 1988, Perseus Books.
16. Aston J: *Aston postural assessment workbook: skills for observing and evaluating body patterns,* San Antonio, Tex, 1998, Therapy Skill Builders.
16a. Cohen BB: Sensing, feeling, and action: the experimental anatomy of body mind centering, Northampton, Mass, 1993, Contact Editions.
17. Rubenfeld I: *Listening hand: self healing through the Rubenfeld Synergy Method of Talk and Touch,* New York, 2000, Bantam Books.
18. Knaster M: *Discovering the body's wisdom,* New York, 1996, Bantam Books.
19. Varela FJ, Thompson E, Rosch E: *The embodied mind: cognitive science and human experience,* Cambridge, 1993, MIT Press.
20. Thelen E, Smith LB: *A dynamic systems approach to the development of cognition and action,* Cambridge, 1994, MIT Press.
21. Edelman G: *Bright air, brilliant fire: on the matter of the mind,* New York, 1992, Basic Books.
22. Damasio AR: *Descartes' error: emotion, reason, and the human brain,* New York, 1994, Avon Books.
23. van der Kolk BA: The body keeps the score: memory and the evolving psychobiology of posttraumatic stress, *Harv Rev Psychiatry* 1(5):253-265, 1994.
24. Borysenko J: *Minding the body, mending the mind,* Reading, Mass, 1987, Addison Wesley.
25. Pert C: *Molecules of emotion: the science of mind-body medicine,* New York, 1997, Simon & Schuster.
26. Cardinali DP, Cutrera RA, Esquifino AI: Psychoimmune neuroendocrine integrative mechanisms revisited, *Biol Signals Recept* 9(5):215-230, 2000.
27. Antoni MH et al: Cognitive-behavioral stress management intervention effects on anxiety, 24-hr urinary norepinephrine output, and T-cytotoxic/suppressor cells over time among symptomatic HIV-infected gay men, *J Consult Clin Psychol* 68(1):31-45, 2000.
28. Goleman D: *Emotional intelligence,* New York, 1995, Bantam Books.
29. Cheever O: *Education as transformation in American psychiatry. From Voices of control to voices of connection* (EdD dissertation), Harvard Graduate School of Education UMI, 1995.
30. Cheever O: Somatic education and somatic empathy in somatic educators and students of somatic education, *ReVision* pp 15-23, spring 2000.

31. Gardner H: *Intelligence reframed: multiple intelligences for the 21st century,* 1999, New York.
32. Moore T: *Care of the soul,* New York, 1992, HarperCollins.
33. Piaget J: *The psychology of intelligence,* London, 1950, Routledge and Kegan Paul. (translated by M Piercy and DE Berlyne).
34. Piaget J: *The origins of intelligence in children,* New York, 1952, International Universities Press.
35. Alon R: *Mindful spontaneity: moving in tune with nature,* New York, 1999, Avery.
36. Alon R: *Mindful spontaneity: returning to natural movement,* Berkeley, Calif, 1996, North Atlantic Books.
37. Ryerant Y: *The Feldenkrais Method: teaching by handling,* San Francisco, 1983, Harper & Row.
38. Zemach-Bersin D, Zemach-Bersin K, Reese M: *Relaxercize: the easy new way to health & fitness,* San Francisco, 1990, HarperSan Francisco.
39. Sharfarman S: *Awareness heals: the Feldenkrais Method of dynamic health,* New York, 1997, Addison Wesley.
40. Jones FP: *Body awareness in action: a study of the Alexander Technique,* New York, 1979, Schocken Books.
41. Myers TW: "Kinesthetic Dystonia": what bodywork can offer a new physical education, *J Bodywork Movement Ther* 2(2):101-114, 1998.
42. Cheever O: Personal communications, 1998.
43. Siler B: *The Pilates body,* New York, 2000, Broadway Books.
44. Cohen LJ: Personal communications, 1999.
45. Feldenkrais M: *Body and mature behavior: a study of anxiety, sex, gravitation & learning,* New York, 1949, International Universities Press.
46. Winner C: Interview with Esther Thelen, PhD, *In touch* (Journal of the Feldenkrais Guild) p 13, 4th quarter 2000.
47. Stern D: *The interpersonal world of the human infant: a view from psychoanalysis and developmental psychology,* New York, 1985, Basic Books.
48. Corcoran KJ: Experiential empathy: a theory of a felt-level experience, *J Humanistic Psychol* 21(1):29-38, 1981.
49. Squire LR, Zola SM: Structure and function of declarative and nondeclarative memory systems, *Proc Natl Acad Sci USA* 93:13515-13522, Nov 1996 (colloquium paper).
50. Reber PJ, Squire LR: Parallel brain systems for learning with and without awareness, *Learn Mem* 1(4):217-229, 1994.
51. Leri D: Learning how to learn, *Gnosis* 29:49-53, 1993.
52. Maturana U, Varela FJ: *The tree of knowledge: the biological roots of understanding,* Boston, 1987, Shambhala Publications.
53. Pribram K: *Languages of the brain: experimental paradoxes and principles in neuropsychology,* Monterey, Calif, 1977, Wadsworth Publishing.
54. Pribram K: *Brain and perception: holonomy and structure in figural processing,* Hillsdale, NJ, 1991, Lawrence Erlbaum Associates.
55. Schmidt R, Wrisberg C: *Motor learning and performance,* ed 2, Champaign, Ill, 2000, Human Kinetics.
56. Georgopoulos AP: Neural aspects of cognitive motor control, *Curr Opin Neurobiol* 10:238-241, 2000.
57. Bizzi E, Mussa-Ivaldi F: Neural basis of motor control and its cognitive implications, *Trends Cogn Sci* 2(3): 97-102, 1998.
58. Sieve AN, King T, Ferguson AR, et al: Pain and negative affect: evidence the inverse benzodiazepine agonist DMCM inhibits pain and learning in rats, *Psychopharmacology* 153:180-190, 2001.
59. Johnson SK, Frederick J, Kaufman M, et al: A controlled investigation of bodywork in multiple sclerosis, *J Altern Complement Med* 5(3):237-243, 1999.
60. Bearman D, Shafarman S: The Feldenkrais Method in the treatment of chronic pain: a study of efficacy and cost effectiveness, *Am J Pain Management* 9(1):22-27, 1999.
61. Lunblad I, Elert J, Gerdle B: Randomized controlled trial of physiotherapy and Feldenkrais interventions in female workers with neck-shoulder complaints, *J Occup Rehabil* 9(3):179-194, 1999.
62. Gutman GM, Herbert CP, Brown SR: Feldenkrais versus conventional exercise for the elderly, *J Gerontol* 32(5): 562-572, 1977.
63. Ofir R: The Feldenkrais Method: on the importance and potency of small and slow movements, *Phys Ther Forum* IX 42:1-5, 1990.
64. Johnson DH (ed): *Groundworks: narratives of embodiment,* Berkeley, Calif, 1997, North Atlantic Books.

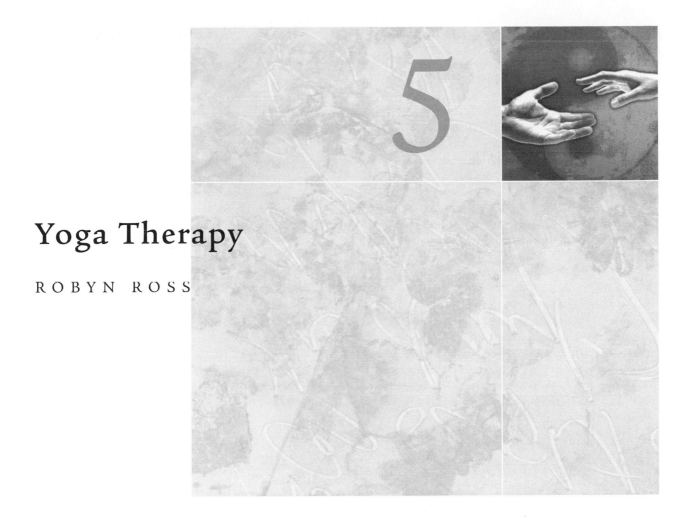

# Yoga Therapy

ROBYN ROSS

$\mathcal{Y}$oga is emerging as a valuable holistic health program for the next millennium. People from all walks of life, including many celebrities, have publicly touted the benefits of yoga in their life. As a result of the increasing popularity of yoga, its influences can be seen in today's fashions, advertising, television programs, movies, and even on the cover of *Time* magazine. In view of this exposure, many patients may be interested in learning how yoga can be incorporated into their current treatment plan.

Yoga is a philosophy of life, a powerful system of self-improvement. It is not a religion. Therefore such diverse groups as local YMCA's, universities, corporations, community centers, churches and synagogues, and major medical institutions sponsor yoga classes.

Yoga is a low-impact activity; therefore people of all ages, shapes, sizes, and conditions can practice it with relative ease and comfort.

Because the culture of this country is pragmatic, it makes sense that a major attraction of yoga in the United States is its documented capacity to support good health and well-being. There is mounting scientific and clinical evidence to support the medical benefits of yoga.[1,2] This chapter illustrates how yoga can be applied as an effective form of therapy for certain neurological disorders.

In the future, mind-body programs such as yoga will play a complementary role in disease management models that focus on self-care.[3] Because of the growing interest in alternative medicine, this is the time to approach healthcare with an integrative perspective.

## WHAT IS YOGA?

In Sanskrit, the word *yoga* translates literally as *yuj,* meaning to yoke together, to make whole. Most commonly, however, yoga is translated as *union*—union of the mind, body, and soul and union of the self to the divine. In the West, yoga has taken many different forms. The most recognizable form today is called *Hatha Yoga,* the physical postures. The Sanskrit root, *ha,* means sun or positive aspect, and *tha* means moon or negative aspect. *Hatha* represents the relationship of opposites, such as dark to light, male to female, and yin to yang. Hatha Yoga seeks to unite polarities and resolve conflicts into a state of balance, harmony, and union. According to ancient yogis, disease occurs when the body is out of balance. Yoga then comes to mean a way to bring the body into a state of balance, homeostasis, and optimal health.

There are many other paths of yoga, including *Raja Yoga,* which is the way to balance and union through meditation and control of the mind; *Jnana Yoga* is knowledge or study; *Bhakti Yoga* is about devotion and selfless love; *Karma Yoga* is union through service, work, and action; and *Mantra Yoga* is union through sound, vibration, and speech.

This chapter focuses on classic Hatha Yoga. This path provides a unique form of physical therapy to help students on their journey toward a broadening knowledge of self and the needs of the mind and body. This therapy helps the student achieve and maintain good physical and mental health and spiritual harmony.

The practice of yoga includes a combination of techniques, including physical postures, breathing exercises, relaxation methodologies, and meditation, to help practitioners reach optimal levels of physical and mental health. Following is a brief overview of the components and benefits that make up a classic yoga session.

*Centering and meditation* begins the session to bring the student into the present. The student begins to connect inward, to develop concentration, and to focus the mind for the session ahead.

*Breath control (pranayama)* is a voluntary regulation of breathing to oxygenate the blood and release carbon dioxide buildup. A series of techniques is used to stimulate, balance, or relax the entire system.

*Warm-ups and stretching* lubricate the joints and start to release muscle tension and increase circulation throughout the body. Warming up increases the range of motion (ROM) and begins to cultivate body awareness.

*Postures (asanas)* strengthen the musculoskeletal system and increase flexibility. Yoga postures reeducate the alignment of the bones, ligaments, and tendons. Each posture series is designed to move the body in all planes of motion, which causes an increase of blood to a specific target organ or gland. Increasing the mobility of the spine can ensure a clear pathway of nerves out to the body.

*Relaxation (yoga nidra or shavasana)* integrates the system into a state of balance, or homeostasis, giving the student time to let go of physical and emotional tension and to rest deeply.

*Affirmation* and *visualization* are sometimes included to recondition the subconscious mind away from negative habitual thoughts. Visualizing health in a certain area brings *prana* (life energy) to that area.

*Meditation* ends each session to create stillness, a sense of non-doing, and a reconnection to the essential self. Meditation helps create clarity and peace of mind and is a major component of a full yoga practice.

When all of these components are synthesized, a consistent practice of yoga can create a powerful state of vitality and rejuvenation and is a formula for health and healing. Yoga refers to the disease process as *dis-ease,* which means a disturbance in the natural ease or balance of the body. Also contributing to this dis-ease is any form of constriction in the flow of prana. Therefore one of the key purposes of yoga is to increase and/or regulate the flow of prana and maintain an environment of organic stability.

Hatha Yoga and meditation, as adjunctive therapies for promoting and maintaining wellness, offer an excellent example of the mind-body connection at work. Hatha Yoga creates balance, both physically and emotionally, as it opens the door to self-actualization to create the perfect union of mind, body, and spirit.[4]

## HISTORY AND PHILOSOPHY

Yoga, which began about 5,000 years ago in India, may be the oldest mind-body health system known today. According to an article in *YogaWorld,* "It is that the great sages spontaneously practiced yoga, evolving out of their relationship and harmony with nature. Using their deepest intuition, intelligence, and experience, they became familiar and instinctual about the energy flowing throughout all life forms. They developed natural ways to access, build, nurture and direct the energy for greater health and awareness."[5]

There is no one historical reference to the beginning of yoga; therefore there is no one manuscript to explicate yoga. Several ancient texts contribute to the body of knowledge of yoga and its history. Among these are the *Vedas,* the *Upanishads,* the *Bhagavad Gita,* and the *Yoga Sutras.*

The Hindu scriptures, the *Vedas* (meaning knowledge), which are the oldest written tradition in India (second century AD), explore the possibilities of the human spirit and discuss the purpose and meaning of life. The *Ayur Vedas* contain early writings about health and medical treatments; *Ayurveda* is the Vedic science of healing that uses yoga as one of its modalities.

The *Upanishads,* possibly dating as far back as the middle of the second millennium BC, are philosophical poems that explore the nature of the universal soul; that is, they are a collection of metaphysical speculations. The *Upanishads* (meaning to sit down close to one's teacher) are a reference to the mode in which esoteric knowledge is transmitted by word of mouth from teacher (guru) to student (disciple).[6] The *Maitri Upanishad* in particular outlines the essential practices of yoga.

The *Bhagavad Gita* (Lord's Song) from the third or fourth century BC is one of the core sacred texts of yoga. Written as a dialog between Lord Krishna and his devotee, Arjuna, it is a story of the battle between the good and evil within us. It also discusses the various yogic paths toward liberation, such as Jnana Yoga, Karma Yoga, Bhakti Yoga, and Hatha Yoga.

The *Yoga Sutras of Pantanjali* (aphorisms on yoga) from the second century BC presents yoga in a coherent and systematized format. Most modern yogis regard it as an authoritative text on yoga, and all the different schools of yoga recognize it. The *Yoga Sutras* are a philosophical compilation with direct techniques for spiritual advancement. Included is the eight-fold path of yoga, or eight limbs.

1. *Yama:* social ethics, restraints
2. *Niyama:* personal ethics, observances
3. *Asana:* discipline of the body
4. *Pranayama:* discipline of the breath
5. *Pratyahara:* withdrawal of the senses
6. *Dharana:* mental concentration
7. *Dhyana:* contemplation, meditation
8. *Samadhi:* bliss, union with the supreme

Various schools of yoga emphasize different techniques, but the goal of *union* is always the same. Hatha Yoga uses practices mentioned in the Yoga Sutras, such as breath control, meditation, and physical postures, as the path to awaken spiritual awareness. This awakening ultimately leads to self-realization and vital health.

Georg Feuerstein wrote, "Yoga is comprised of so many different approaches and schools that one is justified in calling it the most versatile spiritual tradition in the world."[7] Classic yoga as we know it emerged as a tradition around 500 BC. A strong influence of yoga can also be seen in Buddhism, and although yoga originated within the Hindu culture, today Christians, Jews, Muslims, and Hindus all practice yoga while maintaining devotion to their traditional religious beliefs. It cannot be emphasized enough that yoga is not a religion but instead a practical science of self-improvement.

Guided by the texts, various paths, and accomplished teachers, the aim of the yogi is to eventually experience liberation; that is, self-realization and self-knowledge. Liberation or freedom comes when the yogi breaks the bond of old mental habits, destructive patterns, and physical disease, thereby achieving the ability to live in harmony with vitality and peace of mind. Yoga is a valuable philosophy to apply to everyday life. One of the primary reasons that yoga is so effective as a healing tool is that it is not just a dynamic system of physical exercise and health promotion. Rather, yoga is about a deeper understanding of the self.

Yoga can then be described as a true holistic concept, one involving the whole person and affecting the mind, body, and spirit. The yoga teacher simply helps students take control of their body, breath, and mind and thereby begin to take control of their life.

## THERAPEUTIC YOGA FOR REHABILITATION

The power of yoga to affect healing should not be underestimated because its efficacy is well documented in the scientific literature. Yoga techniques are increasingly used as an adjunct to medical management. Many major medical institutions and physicians in private practice now refer their patients to qualified yoga teachers who use yoga as a restorative modality. Yoga techniques have become extremely adaptable and effective for aiding the process of healing and can easily be executed in a chair, in bed, or even in a wheelchair. The ancient postures can be modified in many creative ways, and the results have been very encouraging.

The various components that make up a yoga session can be useful for patients with particular neurological aliments. Using yoga for rehabilitation has diverse applications. Studies show that many physically handicapped subjects had restorations of some degree of functional ability after practicing yoga.[8]

As discussed, breathing techniques, postures, meditation, and relaxation are specifically designed to bring the student into a profound understanding of the self. This understanding leads to *a deeper awareness and understanding of the body,* which will eventually be the ultimate teacher for the student. Patients who practice yoga will be better suited to communicate their symptoms in specific and clear terms, which means that they can be better partner physicians for a more integrative approach to their recovery. Studies reveal that patients are motivated to pursue complementary approaches to become active participants in their own healing process, which can also help patients cope with their disease.[9]

The objective is to use yoga as a therapeutic technique. Yoga therapists (YT's) evaluate the best way to help clients with their particular difficulties and disabilities and adapt the yoga postures accordingly. The YT takes a personal and medical history and then draws on available resources and personal experience, knowledge, and intuition to help the client. Various yogic techniques are incorporated along with props and/or hands-on assistance when necessary. Sessions in restorative yoga can be very nurturing and can heal the effects of chronic stress.[10] Each session is specifically designed to include breathing techniques, gentle movements, and relaxation and meditation routines that accurately address the patient's problems and provide support on the path toward health and wholeness.

Patients should be encouraged to approach the exercises with compassion and to listen deeply to the messages of their body. What makes yoga different from traditional physical therapy is the intense one-pointed concentration on the task at hand and the deep yogic breathing that is incorporated into every movement. The patient learns never to strive or to push the body past its limitations. The postures are all executed with steadiness and ease (*sthria* and *sukha*) and without strain or struggle. Yoga is eventually performed with "effortless effort." A nonjudgmental attitude is also key and should be encouraged throughout the session. Patients should begin to practice accepting the body as it is in the present, from one moment to the next. Movements must be slow and gentle, completely conscious, and always coordinated with the breath. An inner awareness develops; therefore patients learn where the joints and muscles feel restricted and where they feel more flexible. From there patients begin their healing journey.

## REHABILITATION LEVELS

The Yoga Therapist can intervene in any phase of rehabilitation (see box on p 55) to facilitate recovery. Most importantly, the therapist can support the patient by teaching simple yogic techniques to integrate into their daily routine to create a healthy lifestyle. This assimilation may help prevent further illness or disease progression.

## YOGA FOR STRESS REDUCTION

In our society, which is addicted to stress and has a tendency to overactivate the sympathetic high-arousal system, many serious stress-related illnesses have developed. According to medical statistics, 70% of all diseases are stress related. Because its purpose is to relax, rejuvenate, and restore the body, mind, and spirit, yoga is one of the most powerful tools to counteract the stress response. Yoga postures, combined with meditation and pranayama (breath control), can neutralize this overarousal by using clinically proven techniques to help elicit the parasympathetic functions and decrease sympathetic discharges. Postures and breathwork can begin to equalize and alter autonomic responses; thus yoga can create a time for the body to recover from the imbalance stress can place on it and mind.

Numerous studies have shown a statistically significant fall in both systolic and diastolic blood pressure[11] and a reduction of the heart rate with the practice of yoga.[12] Moreover, significant clinical differences

## Rehabilitation Phases

If a patient is hospitalized due to surgery or treatment:

### Phase 1: Inpatient
Yogic techniques can be effectively tailored to the patient's condition and, as a result, be performed in a hospital bed, wheelchair, or any chair available to the practitioner. A yoga session may simply consist of gentle movements and/or yoga breathing exercises. The therapist must be competent and fully informed as to the specific physical limitations and the medical contraindications.

### Phase 2: Immediately after Hospital Discharge
Conservative ambulatory programs are created during early convalescence. After a detailed assessment of the patient's range of motion and physical capabilities, the practitioner can gradually increase the patient's routine with the goal of improving their yoga practice accordingly. This phase is best executed with private yoga therapy sessions.

### Phase 3: Maintenance
Group or individual yoga sessions are provided on a weekly basis. A conventional yoga instructor in the patient's community can lead these classes. The teacher should be fully informed of the details of the patient's condition and should continue to modify the yoga practice accordingly. A special group class for students with similar conditions led by a yoga therapist is optimal. Group support is essential in the overall rehabilitation process.

Before the patient needs aggressive treatment or surgery:

### Pre-Surgery Phase
Whenever possible, a yoga therapist can prepare a patient for surgery by teaching basic breathing and relaxation techniques that can support the patient in managing the procedure ahead. Yogic techniques can be a powerful ally to help soothe the fear and anxiety inherent before surgery.

### Prevention Phase
It is advantageous to enroll a patient in a community-based stress reduction program such as yoga as soon as the patient is informed of a condition. Working with a qualified teacher, the patient can then begin a consistent practice of yoga to provide immediate support. Establishing a course of self-care will empower the patient to incorporate yoga as a part of an ongoing stress reduction routine and, as a result, a healthy lifestyle.

---

can be observed with regard to coping with stress and mood elevation at the end of experiments that use yoga.[13] Pranayama, for example, appears to alter autonomic responses by increasing vagal tone[14] (see "Breathing Techniques"). A regular practice of yoga can therefore be used as an essential recuperative tool for dealing with the effects of stress. According to I.S. Chohan, "Yoga is known to induce beneficial effects on physiological, biochemical, and mental functions in man."[15] It is also important to note that yoga may be used to stimulate sympathetic activity when it is therapeutically indicated.

To maintain health and well-being, the challenges of life must be balanced with periods of rest and relaxation. Sleep disturbances, headaches, and muscle spasms, to name only a few conditions, are often symptomatic of a person's inability to fully relax. Brownstein and Dembert wrote, "Relaxation training, of which yoga is one type, has been reported in the medical literature to have wide clinical application. It should be considered as a nonpharmacological therapy adjunct or alternative for medical disorders."[16]

Jamiel[17] described yoga as follows.

In day to day life, the mindful awareness that yoga cultivates can allow a patient to become more readily aware of any quickened respiration, muscular tension and other physical symptoms of stress. This awareness gives one the ability to consciously interrupt the habitual stress response by doing something as simple as taking a breath or moving the body. Hence the integration of the yogic breathwork, focused awareness and relaxation during day to day life may afford the greatest opportunity for stress reduction. Like traditional Chinese and Tibetan medicine, the Indian system views health as a state of balance sustained by diet, lifestyle and mental attitudes. The traditional view maintains that when this delicate balance is disturbed, various disorders may arise. Yoga is not a medicine, per se, but a system of practices that can restore and maintain this balance.

## POTENTIAL BENEFITS OF YOGA

Following are some of the beneficial clinical outcomes of the practice of yoga.

- Decreased blood pressure
- Reduced heart rate
- Decreased sympathetic stimulation
- Increased parasympathetic tone
- Increased joint ROM
- Increased body strength, stamina, and flexibility
- Improved balance
- Decreased symptoms of carpal tunnel syndrome
- Enhanced mental alertness, memory, concentration, and focus
- Better circulation and oxygenation of the blood
- More efficient breathing
- Decreased muscle stiffness

Beneficial anecdotal outcomes of the practice of yoga include the following.

- Relief of constipation and stimulation of digestion
- Improved body awareness of physical posture
- Decreased muscular fatigue
- Relief of back pain and joint pain
- Reduced pain
- Stress reduction and relaxation
- Improved posture and muscle tone
- Decreased emotional tension
- Decreased premenstrual and menopausal symptoms
- A more positive outlook on life

## POTENTIAL RISKS

Because of the demand for yoga and the many yoga classes that are appearing, it is more important than ever to find a qualified YT. Because yoga uses the body in ways that are perhaps new to most patients, there is always a chance for injury. Depending on the pa-

tient's condition, it may be advantageous for him or her to have private yoga sessions with a certified YT or qualified teacher. For those who are new to yoga, it is advisable to start with a class designed specifically for beginners, regardless of athletic background. The postures must be taught clearly and safely. The teacher must be attentive and involved in each student's participation. The student should not simply be expected to follow along. Just as in the selection of a physician, care must be taken to determine the training and experience of the teacher (see "Finding a Yoga Teacher"). Presently, YTs are not licensed in this country, and the length of training necessary to be certified varies from several years to as little as 1 weekend. Inadequately supervised yoga practice has resulted in injuries ranging from simple strains to a case of sciatic neuropathy in the thigh, resulting from prolonged sitting in the lotus posture.[18]

There are general precautions and contraindications that can be followed to prevent undue injury. Certain inverted postures, those that bring the head below the heart, are contraindicated for people with untreated or malignant hypertension, heart conditions, some nervous disorders, and pregnancy. Recent surgeries and certain chronic conditions or severe inflammation may prohibit specific movements. During acute sciatica or with a herniated disk, certain movements should be prohibited. When balance is impaired from multiple sclerosis (MS) or Parkinson's disease, special modifications are used for balancing postures. When necessary, yoga can even be performed in a wheelchair or in bed.

As mentioned, the advantage of yoga is that it can be modified to meet the needs of even high-risk individuals. Because of its gentle nature, yoga can be applied even when a patient is recovering from a serious injury. I was on staff as a yoga therapist at Columbia-Presbyterian Medical Center in New York City for 3 years developing a yoga program for cardiac patients 3 days postoperative. I worked with these patients bedside or they came to a group chair yoga class. Even with the inherent risks involved, I was able to devise a protocol to guide them through a complete experience of simple yoga postures, breathing techniques, meditation, and relaxation. Patients were able to move their bodies in a safe and gentle way after this invasive major surgery. Many patients reported that following the yoga session they felt a decrease in postoperative pain, mood elevation, increased energy, and a reconnection to the body. They also found that the yoga session had a relaxing and calming effect. D. MacArthur, a heart transplant patient, gratefully reported that "the yogic breathing and stretching was an adaptable tool that I was able to draw on whenever I needed it during my recuperation. I was also able to incorporate the breathing tools into my life, especially within stressful situations." MacArthur race walked the last two New York City marathons and used his yogic breathing as an important addition to his training, as well as during the races. Looking back at the experience at the hospital, I am once again amazed at the adaptability and efficacy of yoga practice for high-risk individuals.

## CLINICAL APPLICATIONS

Yogis have always used themselves as empirical research laboratories. In fact, the brilliance of yoga is that it integrates the spiritual with the empirical. Spiritual practices that lead to desired outcomes are integrated into the discipline, and those that do not are eliminated. The result is a system designed over thousands of years to promote the outcome of good health. In clinical applications, we take much the same empirical approach that is used by yogis. Postures are suggested based on past successes, the yogic literature, and the growing body of evidence-based research; however, client outcome always determines the efficacy of the treatment plan. Because the essence of yoga is developing awareness, beginning to incorporate it can be as straightforward as paying attention to one's breath for a few minutes each day.[17]

## Nadis and the Nervous System

It is fascinating to note that a system in yoga called the *nadis* bears a remarkable resemblance to modern anatomic descriptions of nerves and plexus. The ancient manuals of yoga anatomy describe a network of several thousand *nadis* that are considered to be energy channels, tubes, or pathways throughout the gross and subtle body.[19] They have been compared with the nerve plexus, which controls the autonomic nervous system.

One of the many ways that prana (life energy) passes through the physical body is via the nadis (nerve plexus). To accomplish this, the prana is absorbed and then flows via the nerve plexus throughout the nervous system to the rest of the body. According to Hindu scriptures, there are 350,000 energy channels in the system (Figure 5-1).[20] Of these channels, the *sushumna, ida,* and *pingala* are the most important. The main channel is the sushumna, or line of energy, which stems from the root of the tailbone and goes up the spine. The ida and the pingala are two major energy channels that intertwine up the spine. They are usually pictured as two snakes coiling up a centerline. The coils meet and cross at seven spinning energy centers called the *chakras.* Illustrations of the sushumna with the ida and pingala are an identical representation of the caduceus, which is used as a symbol of the medical model today (Figure 5-2).

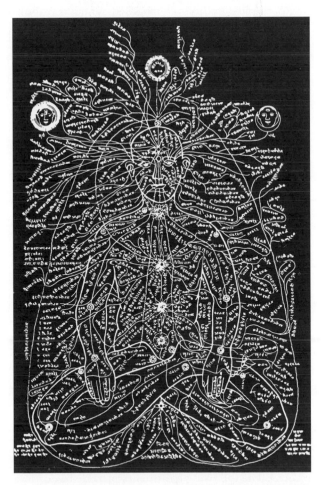

*Figure 5-1* Ancient Hindu drawing of the nadis and chakras. (From Hills C (ed): *Energy, matter & form,* Boulder Creek, Calif, 1975, University of the Trees Press, p 238.)

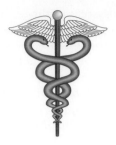

*Figure 5-2* The caduceus, our modern symbol for healing, traces the path of the nadis and chakras, emanating from the base to the two winged petals at the top.

It is easy to see how these ancient texts parallel the modern. For example, the pingala represents the sympathetic nervous system (SNS), which is responsible for the left brain functions, the right nostril breathing,[21,22] the solar energy, and the fight-or-flight reaction. The ida, representing the parasympathetic nervous system (PNS), is responsible for the right brain functions, the left nostril breathing,[21] the lunar energy, and the relaxation response. Various yoga postures, sounds, and pranayama techniques are used to open and balance the vital flow of energy through these nadis. This is a complicated and subtle practice.

## Treatments

There can be no standard treatment plan for yoga. Any program that is prescribed is a synthesis of what a client is able and willing to do and what is appropriate for the client at that moment. The ability to modify traditional postures whenever it is necessary to fit the client's need is vital. It is also important that each program be designed to move all joints within a pain-free ROM. The YT assesses the patient and prescribes the appropriate treatments specific to the problem.

Whenever feasible, it would be helpful for the YT to maintain a working relationship with the student's physician during the yoga treatment. This integrative form of healthcare can lead to strong support for the patient. The following treatments provide basic ideas that can be used to treat certain disorders. Please note that for clarity, the classic Sanskrit terminology is not used when referring to the yoga postures in this sec-

tion. Illustrations of certain yoga postures are provided later in this chapter.

## Breathing Techniques

Proper breathing is the foundation of yoga and may be used by itself as treatment for many disorders. Life force is called *prana,* to master or control is *ayama.* Therefore to master the life force through breath control is translated as *pranayama.* The system of Hatha Yoga asanas (postures) and breathing is based on balancing and increasing the flow of prana in the body. The key to understanding prana and energy is breath. Yoga postures without the awareness of breath are just movement, not yoga.

There are many pranayama techniques that can be incorporated into a yoga practice. The following are recommended.

The way one breathes has a profound effect on health. Many people breathe short, shallow, rapid breaths that actually elicit the SNS. The *three-part yogic breath (dirgha)* is full deep breathing that allows the abdominal area to expand, then opens the rib cage area and brings the breath all the way up to the clavicular region. The breath then releases from the chest, or rib cage area, and finally the abdominal muscles are contracted to promote full exhalation.

This type of breathing encourages the diaphragm, the lower ribs, and the muscles in the back to expand, thereby opening up more space and massaging the abdominal organs. Barbara Phillips, MD, a professor of pulmonary and critical care medicine at the University of Kentucky College of Medicine in Lexington, notes, "As you breathe more slowly and fully with awareness, that brings more oxygen to the body, slowing the heart rate and triggering the PNS, creating a feeling of relaxation and calm." Breathing is clinically shown to influence the PNS and the SNS.

The control of prana is the regulation of inhalation and exhalation. By adjusting the ratio of inhalation to exhalation we can adjust and influence the relative emphasis given to each activity. John Clark, MD, of Harvard Medical School and board certified in cardiology, family practice, and internal medicine, writes, "The technique of 2-to-1 breathing for instance, where the exhalation is twice as long as the inhalation, will indicate a drop in the arousal level of the SNS and increase the influence of the PNS."[23] One can also count the number of breaths to provide a focus for the mind, simply doubling the number of exhalations to inhalations.

Another technique involves *alternate nostril breathing* (ANB), or *nadi shodhanam* and *anuloma viloma.* There are many variations of ANB, each with a particular purpose, yet they all have the common theme of alternating the flow of breath between two nostrils.[24] This is done by simply closing off one nostril with the thumb or ring finger of the right hand, inhaling through one nostril and exhaling through the alternate nostril, back and forth. This is a continuous, long, silent relaxed flow of air. Studies suggest that ANB has a balancing effect on the functional activity of the left and right hemispheres of the brain.[25] Left nostril breathing showed a reduction of the SNS; right nostril breathing showed an increase in metabolism due to increased sympathetic discharge to the adrenal medulla. These results indicate that breathing selectively through either nostril could have a marked activating effect or relaxing effect on the SNS.[21] Therapeutic implications to alter metabolism by changing the breathing pattern may also be hypothesized.[26]

*Kapalabhati pranayama,* referred to as the *breath of fire,* is a technique of rapid respiration. The technique demonstrates a unique unilateral effect on sympathetic stimulation of the heart that may have therapeutic value.[27] This form of pranayama employs quick abdominal contractions and expulsion of air through both nostrils upon exhalation. Using this technique will increase physical and mental energy. According to Dharma Singh Khalsa, MD, in his book *Brain Longevity,* "It is believed to be effective because it stimulates the splanchnic nerves in the abdominal cavity. Stimulation of these nerves causes the release of epinephrine and norepinephrine."[28]

The *ujjayi* breath, also known as the *ocean-sounding breath,* is another pranayama technique used to relax the nervous system. This is done by constricting the epiglottis slightly and creating a hissing sound at the back of the throat. Ujjayi pranayama is deeply soothing and centering. The mind becomes absorbed and focused by the sound, which induces meditation. This technique can be applied to all of the treatments listed.

Thoughts and feelings influence breath; therefore in yoga breath is thought to influence attitudes and emotions. These basic breathing techniques are the simplest and most effective of the stress-management techniques. They can be done anytime, anywhere. Learning how to breathe effectively has a profound balancing effect on the nervous system. Scientific evidence indicates that a yoga therapy program can result in a significant increase in pulmonary function and greater exercise tolerance as well.[29] The adequate flow of breath constantly supports good physical health.[30-32]

## MULTIPLE SCLEROSIS

Stress and tension play a part in an attack of MS. When muscle tension increases spasticity, spasms and clumsiness also increase. Problems with balance and movement tend to make the body compensate by using other muscles, which can also add to chronic muscle tension. Yoga can aid in relaxing the entire body to help reduce this stress and mental stress as well. This awareness is the hallmark of yoga, representing centuries of wisdom. The patient should begin with very slow movements and deep awareness to help locate the muscles that are weak or inflexible and therefore inhibiting movement. The patient can then begin to increase the number of movements, expending the least effort. Through that awareness the patient can work to bring strong and weak muscle groups into balance. The body then becomes less awkward and strain is alleviated.

Yoga asanas (postures) tone the neuromuscular system and may help to correct postural abnormalities, a crucial aspect of proper walking. Yoga postures can also help return joints to their proper alignment. Yogic stretching and strengthening postures can return a degree of usefulness to a limb that has lost its ability to function. Howard Kent, director of the Yoga for Health Foundation in Bedfordshire, England, states, "We have evidence that where people are effectively maintaining a yoga practice both mentally and physically, it is rare for us to find deterioration in patients with MS. By the correct use of breathing, mental relaxation and postures, I have seen people move legs with control, which have not moved in years."[33] In addition, studies have shown improvement in the degree of plasticity in motor control systems with the practice of yoga.[34] Certain stretching exercises may also be useful for temporarily relieving pain.

Because MS brings on inefficient breathing patterns, it is important to incorporate deep rhythmic breathing into the following routine for oxygenation of the cells, relaxation, and energy. The postures can be practiced on the floor, seated in a chair, or standing with support.

## Postures

Cat/dog (Box 5-1)
Supine butterfly
Half locust
Leg lifts
Cobra (modified), sphinx (see Box 5-1)
Bridge (modified)
Boat (modified)
Seated mountain, seated half moon (see Box 5-1)
Hug both knees in chest
Mountain with wall support
Wind reliever and circle knees
Legs on wall
Seated spinal twist (see Box 5-1)
Warrior with chair
Forward bend on floor/chair
Triangle with wall

BOX 5-1

*Yoga Postures*

The following photographs illustrate various yoga postures discussed in this chapter.

Seated mountain, seated half moon with fingers interlaced.

Modifications of the tree posture.

BOX 5-1

*Yoga Postures—cont'd*

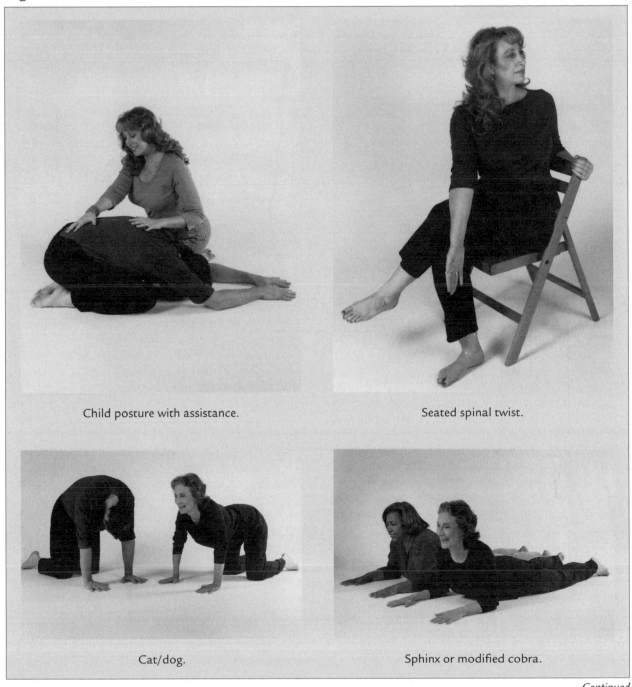

Child posture with assistance.

Seated spinal twist.

Cat/dog.

Sphinx or modified cobra.

*Continued*

BOX 5-1

*Yoga Postures—cont'd*

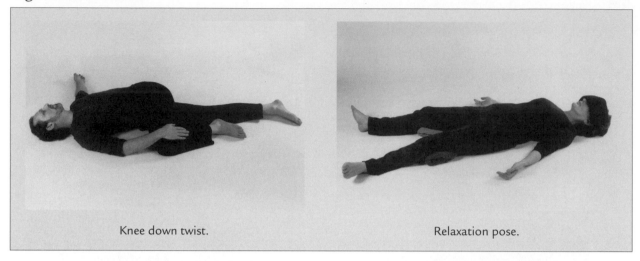

Knee down twist.

Relaxation pose.

## Breathing

Three-part yogic breath
Alternate nostril breathing
Meditation on breath

To what extent these postures can be practiced depends on the individual and the degree of disability. At first patients may find certain movements difficult, but with steady practice they may accomplish actions they would not have thought possible. The routine is very simple and adaptable. Props can be used to aid in safety and stability and to prevent added stress or fatigue. Because people dealing with MS are often advised not to get overheated, yoga can also be done in a pool, where props, such as blocks and ropes, can help the patient hold poses longer. A student with MS, Eric Small, later became a YT. He claimed to feel stronger and less fatigued, his digestion improved, he could walk farther, and he felt more centered after beginning yoga. His depression, which is often associated with MS, lifted. It has been 25 years since he has had a serious attack.[35]

## CARPAL TUNNEL SYNDROME

With the growing use of computer keyboards, there has been a high incidence of carpal tunnel syndrome (CTS) during the past 10 years. Repetitive stress injuries (RSIs) can also affect persons in many other occupations, from musicians and athletes to construction workers. To prevent RSI and CTS the individual must take awareness breaks throughout the day. One of the most beneficial aspects of yoga is the cultivation of body and breath awareness. Patients should be encouraged to apply the awareness they have developed during the yoga session to their body alignment, breath, and repetitive movements.

The easiest way to prevent CTS and RSI is with simple yoga postures concentrating on hand, arm, and body movements coordinated with breath. It is important to establish a routine and to execute it on a regular basis throughout the workday. Exercising the wrists and fingers eases stiffness and tenderness. It is important to focus on upper body yoga postures to improve flexibility and decrease muscle tension. Frequent yoga breaks are crucial because prolonged repetitive physical actions cause CTS. It is also important to get up from the desk intermittently, move around, and do some yoga stretches for the entire body. Proper working posture and correct positioning of everything on the desk also aid in the prevention of CTS because poor posture creates added stress on arms and wrists. Yoga emphasizes correct posture and teaches students techniques for sitting, standing, and moving in proper alignment. Correcting alignment of hands, wrists, arms, and shoulders; stretching; and increasing awareness of optimal joint position during use are all preventive measures for CTS.[36]

A recent study published in *JAMA* shows how yoga and relaxation techniques can alleviate pain and tenderness and increase the ROM for patients with CTS. In this randomized trial, subjects were assigned 11 yoga postures designed for strengthening, stretching, and balancing each joint of the upper body. They were also given relaxation techniques. Patients in the control group were offered a wrist splint to supplement their current treatment. Patients in the yoga group had significant improvement in grip strength and pain reduction. Changes in grip strength and pain were not significant in the control group.[36]

A study conducted at Cedars-Sinai Medical Center in Los Angeles also found yoga to be helpful for persons with CTS and RSI.[37] Yoga stretches and strengthens muscles, nerves, and tendons, which may help untangle spasms and prevent other spasms from developing. Stretching the muscles and tendons seems to stave off more spasms, thus relieving pain.

Proper posture, correct positioning, body awareness, office yoga stretch breaks, and breathing techniques can help prevent and perhaps alleviate CTS symptoms. The following postures and breathing should be practiced regularly.[38-41]

## Postures

Rotate wrists in both directions
Press hand forward and back, stretching wrists and forearms
Spider pushups with fingers spread
Make prayer hands, turning front and back
Shake out hands and arms to increase circulation
Massage palm side of each hand
Move joints in fingers and wrists
Clench hands in a fist, then open; repeat opening and closing
Eye movements (additional)
Reach arms overhead, interlace fingers, and stretch upward and side to side (seated mountain and half moon)
Interlace hands behind body to stretch shoulders and open chest
Chair twists
Dog pose with chair
Standing mountain
Half moon
Shoulder stretch on wall
Rag doll

Child
Relaxation pose

## Breathing

Three-part yogic breath
Kapalabhati breath
2-to-1 breath
Alternate nostril breath

## BACK PAIN

There are many causes of low back pain, ranging from spinal disk injury, nerve damage, and impingement to muscle sprain and tension. Many yoga postures relieve back pain by relaxing muscle tension while releasing pressure on affected nerve centers.[42] For treatment, certain yoga postures can be used to strengthen the muscles that support the back and increase abdominal strength and the surrounding hip flexibility. Yoga practice can include a series of gentle and safe stretches that also stretch the paraspinal muscles. These stretches may increase the intervertebral space, improving the ROM of the spinal column. Yoga practice contributes to reeducating and restructuring the postural alignment. As mentioned, the practice of yoga can increase the patient's body awareness and the structural understanding of how to stand, sit, and lift correctly to avoid possible strain.

In the case of sciatic pain from intervertebral disk syndrome, the YT must be very careful not to exacerbate the injury. Anterior or posterior stretches may be contraindicated. However, if the sciatica is due to piriformis syndrome, certain yoga postures can offer great relief by relaxing and gently stretching the overcontracted muscle that may be impinging on the sciatic nerve root.[18]

The use of gentle yoga postures for back pain may offer the patient a safe and natural alternative to back surgery.

## Postures

Cat/dog (see Box 5-1)
Child (see Box 5-1)
Easy forward bend
Sphinx or modified cobra (see Box 5-1)
Half locust

Bridge
Knees to chest and wind reliever
Knee down twist or seated twist (see Box 5-1)
Pigeon and hero (piriformis stretches)
Mountain
Half moon
Relaxation pose (see Box 5-1)

## Breathing

Three-part yogic breath
Alternate nostril breathing
2-to-1 breath
Ocean-sounding breath
Meditation/visualization

## NECK PAIN

Stretching and relaxing the neck muscles allows for better circulation and improved posture. Again, gentle movements coordinated with the breath performed slowly and with awareness can begin to reduce stiffness and promote mobility of the cervical spine. Special emphasis should be placed on lengthening the neck to temporarily increase the space between the vertebrae, thereby causing less stress on the cervical disks and facet joints and freeing nerve compression. Movements that exacerbate or create pain, numbness, or radicular pain are contraindicated. Special care must be taken to perform movements in a pain-free ROM. These movements can be practiced anywhere to help prevent and relieve neck pain. Following are gentle neck and shoulder movements to relieve neck pain. Isolated cervical movements that do not roll the neck are recommended.

## Postures

Chin to chest
Ear to shoulders (lateral movements)
Head forward and slightly back (posterior, anterior movements)
Trace outline of circle with nose and/or figure 8s
Shoulder squeeze
Rotate shoulders
Facial movements (especially to release tension in jaw)
Cow's head
Eagle arms

Lying down in relaxation pose: turn head from side to side; unclench teeth and relax jaw
Relaxation pose (see Box 5-1)

## Breathing

Three-part yogic breath
Alternate nostril breathing
2-to-1 breath
Ocean-sounding breath
Meditation/visualization

## ANXIETY AND PANIC ATTACK

Anxiety disorders can vary greatly in their severity; they may be mild or completely immobilizing. The yogic three-part breath is an extremely effective tool for reducing panic reactions and a useful and valuable tactic for anyone who finds himself or herself in a frightening or anxiety-producing situation. During most panic reactions the person has the sensation of hyperventilation or loss of breath. Therefore incorporating slow, long, deep yogic breath at the time of an attack can be very beneficial in easing the fear. Visualization, affirmation, and meditation can counteract intruding negative thoughts that add to the attack and can help the person return his or her focus to healthy thoughts.

Inducing deep relaxation of nerves and muscles can help to eliminate the buildup of tension in both mind and body. Studies have shown that practicing yoga postures followed by a period of deep relaxation can help normalize the blood pressure, calm the mind, and relax the symptoms of the fight-or-flight reaction. Clinical evidence indicates that yoga practice has proven most effective with a wide range of psychosomatic and psychiatric disorders.[43] In psychiatric patients, decreases in both self-reported anxiety and anxious behavior and a decrease in cortisol levels were noted after the practice of yoga.[44] Yoga groups showed markedly higher scores in life satisfaction and high spirits and lower scores in excitability, aggressiveness, and somatic complaints.[13]

## Postures

Mountain posture (standing, seated)
Tree (see Box 5-1)
Spinal twist (see Box 5-1)

Sphinx (see Box 5-1)
Easy forward bend
Child
Legs up on wall or chair
Relaxation pose (see Box 5-1)
Progressive relaxation technique (relaxing body parts head to toe, using body scanning)

## Breathing

Three-part yogic breath
Alternate nostril breathing
Counting breath
Ocean-sounding breath
Meditation on breath/visualization

 *A Case Study*

*Anxiety*
A YT is currently working with a 70-year-old woman who has been housebound for 2 years. Through the teacher's work with this woman, she was able to shift her attention away from fear of falling down the stairs to a primary focus on her breath. This allowed her to take her first steps. Within 6 months she had walked down the flight of stairs and outside for the first time in 2 years. This is a good example of the relationship between anxiety and breath. In this work, the goal is not to deny the fear or to change the fear in any way. The focus is shifted to the breath and to the observation of the experience. ∾

## TENSION HEADACHE

Yoga can offer a holistic form of treatment for pain associated with tension headache caused by an overcontraction of the head, neck, and shoulder muscles. Gentle stretching (see "Neck Pain"), relaxation pose and alternate nostril breathing (see "Breathing Techniques"), and meditation can calm emotional and physical tension, providing an alternative to painkillers.

## MIGRAINE HEADACHE

Migraine headaches are more deeply rooted than tension headaches, involving the flow of blood to the brain. Treatments that have been mentioned for neck pain and tension headache may be helpful for the migraine headache sufferer, but sometimes even the slightest movement can be too painful or cause nausea and visual disturbances. Instead, a period of relaxation using yoga nidra and the corpse pose (shavasana) may be beneficial. The corpse pose is the relaxation pose (see Box 5-1) that is done by lying on the floor or bed, giving the full weight of the body to the earth. The arms are spread so that they are 18 inches out from the body with palms open. The feet are 8 to 12 inches apart with the ankles relaxed. Placing a pillow under the knees will reduce the gap between the floor and the lower back. Also recommended is a dark room or a soft dark cloth placed over the eyes, and rest. The goal of the shavasana is for the body and mind to be still and fully relaxed. With the eyes closed, a technique of autogenic relaxation can be used (see "Insomnia"). "Deep breathing and progressive relaxation can help stave off stress," according to Joseph Kandel, MD, and David B. Sudder, MD, in their book, *Migraine: What Works!*[45-48] Watching the gentle flow of breath such as the 2-to-1 breath (see "Breathing Techniques") may also help soothe and relax tension.

## INSOMNIA

Yoga can provide a natural solution to the problem of insomnia caused by excessive tension and anxiety. Here again, the use of simple yogic techniques can calm the body, slow the mind, and reduce anxiety.

A gentle routine of stretching and breathing before retiring to bed will increase the PNS tone and relax muscle tension. While in bed the patient may also try deep yogic-related relaxation techniques, such as autogenic self-suggestive phrases to help induce sleep naturally. The patient concentrates on the different parts of the body from the toes to the head. Using phrases such as "relax the toes, allow them to get warm and heavy" relaxes every region of the body systematically. Each time the mind wanders, it should be brought back to the task at hand. A regular practice of yoga will help eliminate the muscle tension buildup that prevents relaxation at bedtime. It is also important to take breathing breaks periodically throughout the day to release stress buildup. Yoga helps the patient train the wandering mind to reduce the internal mental stimulation that often creates anxiety and tension and keeps the patient from "switching off" the brain at night.

## Postures

Neck stretches
Knees to chest, circle knees
Knee down twist, seated twist (see Box 5-1)
Wind reliever
Cat/dog (see Box 5-1)
Child (see Box 5-1)
Relaxation pose (see Box 5-1)

## Breathing

Three-part yogic breath
Counting breath
Ocean-sounding breath
Meditation on breath/visualization

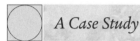 *A Case Study*

### Vertigo and Disequilibrium Syndrome

A YT recently worked with an 83-year-old woman who had fallen repeatedly during the previous year and wanted to increase her strength. During the initial screening, marked ataxia was discovered, and the client was immediately referred to a neurologist for assessment. The physician suspected that the woman had myelin sheath degeneration, but the client's daughter did not want her mother to be subjected to the medical testing required to confirm the diagnosis. The neurologist suggested that the woman continue gentle yoga without restrictions, but he did not express much hope for improvement. In working with the client the neurologist noticed that in addition to the unbalanced gait, the client became easily distracted while walking. While she worked on basic yoga postures and strength-building practices, the major focus was on the breath and concentration. The primary yoga practice consisted of walking meditation in which the client focused on her breath and the sensation on the sole of each foot as it touched down. This created a dramatic change in her ability to even out her erratic gait. She then purchased a treadmill, which she used daily for 5 to 10 minutes to practice her meditative walking. These treadmill meditations increased her focus and strength, and helped reduce her number of falls. After 6 months the client asked her daughter to watch as she walked briskly in a straight line across the length of her lobby. Her daughter wanted to know what new drug she was taking that had finally cured her terrible gait. However, it was a combination of increased strength along with improved mental focus that supported her change. ❧

## MUSCLE WEAKNESS, MYOPATHY, AND MUSCULAR DYSTROPHY

As discussed previously, yoga asanas (postures) may be used therapeutically for most neuromuscular disorders. Using clinically proven techniques to relax the mind and body while strengthening the muscular system can be very effective. The YT should first assess the patient's weaknesses and strengths, then check the ROM and, finally, design a routine that can address the affected areas. Again, yoga is a profound way for the patient to become aware of and therefore understand the strengths and weaknesses of his or her body and begin the process of integration and healing.

## PAIN SYNDROMES

Because many pain medications can cause unhealthy side effects and even addiction, yoga can be used as a potent natural pain control method. The effective use of yoga and yoga-related techniques in pain management have been documented.[49]

One method of pain relief is to influence the "spinal gate" mechanism. The input of stimuli is prevented from reaching the brain by using mental concentration (meditation) and relaxation techniques.

Breathing techniques can also be used to manage pain because the breath is directly linked to the pain stimulus. For example, when one is in great pain, the breath tends to be tense, shallow, and irregular. When one is at ease the breath is relaxed, slow, and rhythmic. Therefore the use of slow, regulated yogic breathing can manage pain by bringing it under the patient's own willful control. Moreover, breathing helps to relax the system. Whenever there is pain in a certain area of the body, the muscles surrounding that area can tense and go into contraction, which further exacerbates the pain. Simple yogic stretching and postures can help relax the muscles in the entire area, decreasing the spasms and thereby decreasing the pain. In addition, Julius Richmond, MD, professor emeritus of health policy at the Department of Social Medicine, Harvard Medical School, supports information previously given in this chapter by saying that "many relaxation techniques can help slow heart rate, lower blood pressure, and relax large muscle groups—all of which can diminish the perception of pain."

## Postures

Balancing postures, such as the tree, to increase
concentration
Stretching to discourage tension buildup
Relaxation postures, such as child and the relaxation
pose

## Breathing

Three-part yogic breath
2-to-1 breath
Alternate nostril breathing
Ocean-sounding breath
Meditation on the breath/visualization

## SUMMARY

With the increasing emphasis on preventive medicine
and the greater awareness of the effects of lifestyle
on health, yoga could be an important adjunctive
complementary treatment for patients. Stephen
Sinatra, MD, author of *Optimal Health* said, "The doctors who are willing to incorporate the disciplines of
nutritional, emotional, and spiritual healing will become our most effective healers as we move into the
next millennium." The future of healthcare will be
the integration of standard allopathic treatments
with ancient therapies such as yoga. Numerous scientific studies have shown that yoga shows great potential for modifying certain neurological impairments and disorders. Yoga techniques merit further
study under controlled situations that could help
lead to new approaches for treating a variety of
disabilities.

B.K.S. Iyengar, one of the founding fathers who
brought yoga to this country, put it this way, "Words
fail to convey the total value of yoga; it has to be
experienced."

## ACKNOWLEDGMENTS

I would like to thank the photographer, Joan Tedeschi,
and models, Jason Frome, Ellen Wallach, and Mar-
garetta (Maji) Richards, for joining me in demonstrating the postures depicted in this chapter. I would also
like to thank Dr. Jeff Migdow, a holistic physician in
private practice in Lenox, Massachusetts, for reviewing this chapter.

## References

1. Upupa KN, Singh RH: The scientific basis of yoga, *JAMA* 220(10):1365, 1972.
2. Hoenig J: Medical research of yoga, *Confin Psychiatr* 11(2):69-89, 1968.
3. La Forge R: Mind-body fitness: encouraging prospects for primary and secondary prevention, *J Cardiovasc Nurs* 11(3):53-65, 1997.
4. Gimbel MA: Yoga, meditation and imagery: clinical ap- plication, *Nurs Pract Forum* 9(4):243-255, 1998.
5. www.yogaworld.org.
6. Feuerstein G: *The Shambhala encyclopedia of yoga,* Boston, 1997, Shambhala Publications.
7. Feuerstein G: *The yoga sutra of Pantanjali,* Rochester, Vt, 1979, Inner Traditions.
8. Telles S, Naveen KV: Yoga for rehabilitation: an overview, *Indian J Med Sci* 51(4):123-127, 1997.
9. Winterholler M, Erbguth F, Neundorfer B: The use of alternative medicine by multiple sclerosis patients— patient characteristics and patterns of use, *Fortschr Neu- rol Psychiatr* 65(12):555-561, 1997.
10. Lasatar J: *Relax and renew: restful yoga for stressful times,* Berkeley, Calif, 1995, Rodmell Press.
11. Sundar S et al: Role of yoga in management of essential hypertension, *Acta Cardiol* 39(3):203-208, 1984.
12. Raju PS et al: Influence of intensive yoga training on physiological changes in 6 adult women: a case report, *J Altern Complement Med* 3(3):291, 1997.
13. Schell FJ, Allolio B, Schonecke OW: Physiological and psychological effects of Hatha-Yoga exercise on healthy women, *Int J Psychosom* 41(1-4):46-52, 1994.
14. Bhargava R, Gogate MG, Mascarenhas JF: Autonomic responses to breath holding and its variations follow- ing pranayama, *Indian J Physiol Pharmacol* 32(4):257- 264, 1988.
15. Chohan IS et al: Influence of yoga on blood coagulation, *Thromb Haemost* 30:51(2):196-197, 1984.
16. Brownstein AH, Dembert ML: Treatment of essential hypertension with yoga relaxation therapy in a USAF aviator: a case report, *Aviat Space Environ Med* 60(7):684- 687, 1989.
17. Jamiel A: *Exercise physiologist and yoga teacher,* unpublished manuscript, 1999.
18. Vogel CM et al: Lotus footdrop: sciatic neuropathy in the thigh, *Neurology* 41(4):605-606, 1991.
19. Rama S, Ballentine R, Hymes A: *Science of breath,* Hones- dale, Penn, 1979, Himalayan Institute.
20. Judith A: *Wheels of life,* St Paul, Minn, 1987, Llewellyn.
21. Mohan SM: Svara (nostril dominance) and bilateral volar GSR, *Indian J Physiol Pharmacol* 40(1):58-64, 1996.

22. Telles S, Nagarathna R, Nagendra HR: Physiological measures of right nostril breathing, *J Altern Complement Med* 2(4):479-484, 1996.

23. Clark J: Slowing down: the practice of 2-to-1 breathing, *Yoga Int* pp 8-10, 1994 (reprint series: Breathing lessons).

24. Davis S: Breathing, *Am Health* 16(9):54-57, 1997.

25. Stancak A Jr, Kuna M: EEG changes during forced alternate nostril breathing, *Int J Psychophysiol* 18(1):75-79, 1994.

26. Telles S, Nagarathna R, Nagendra HR: Breathing through a particular nostril can alter metabolism and autonomic activities, *Indian J Physiol Pharmacol* 38(2):133-137, 1994.

27. Shannahoff-Khalsa DS, Kennedy B: The effects of unilateral forced nostril breathing on the heart, *Int J Neurosci* 73(1-2):47-60, 1993.

28. Khalsa DS: *Brain longevity,* New York, 1997, Warner Books.

29. Jain SC, Talukdar B: Evaluation of yoga therapy programme for patients of bronchial asthma, *Singapore Med J* 34(4):306-308, 1993.

30. Migdow J, Loehr JE: *Breath in, breath out,* New York, 1999, Time Life.

31. Ornish D: *Dr. Dean Ornish's program for reversing heart disease,* New York, 1996, Ballantine.

32. Benson H: *The relaxation response,* New York, 1975, Avon Books.

33. Telles S et al: Plasticity of motor control system demonstrated by yoga training, *Indian J Pharmacol* 38(2):143-144, 1994.

34. Graham J: *MS: a self-help guide to its management,* Rochester, Vt, 1989, Healing Arts Press.

35. Despres L: Yoga and MS, *Yoga J* 135:94-103 July/Aug, 1997.

36. Garfinkel MS et al: Yoga-based intervention for carpal tunnel syndrome, *JAMA* 280(18):1601-1603, 1998.

37. Brody JE: Carpal tunnel syndrome: some new treatment, *New York Times* Feb 28, 1996.

38. Freedman M, Hankes J: *Yoga at work,* Rockport, Mass, 1996, Element.

39. Anderson B: *Stretching at your computer or desk,* Bolinas, Calif, 1997, Shelter.

40. Lusk JT: *Desk top yoga,* New York, 1998, Berkley Books.

41. Schatz MP: *Back care basics,* Berkeley, Calif, 1992, Rodmell Press.

42. Weller S: *The yoga back book,* Hammersmith, London, 1993, HarperCollins.

43. Goyeche JR: Yoga as therapy in psychosomatic medicine, *Psychother Psychosom* 31(1-4):373-381, 1979.

44. Platania-Solazzo A et al: Relaxation therapy reduces anxiety in child and adolescent psychiatric patients, *Acta Paedopsychiatr* 55(2):115-120, 1992.

45. Weller S: *Yoga therapy,* Hammersmith, London, 1995, HarperCollins.

46. Munro R, Nagendra HR, Nagarathna R: *Yoga for common ailments,* New York, 1990, Fireside.

47. Kandel J, Suddert DB: *Migraine: what works!* Roseville, Calif, 1996, Prima.

48. Reilly R: Acute and prophylactic treatment of migraine, *Nurs Times* 90(29):20-26, 35-36, 1994.

49. Nespor K: Pain management and yoga, *Int J Psychosom* 38(1-4):76-81, 1991.

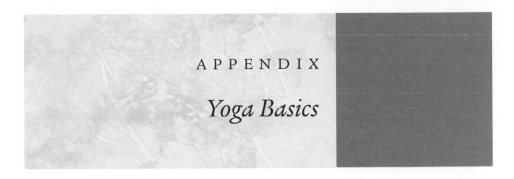

## COSTS

Costs for group classes range from $5 per class in hospital- or school-sponsored programs to $15 per class in a small private yoga studio in New York City. Private session costs range from $30 to more than $100, depending on the location and the training and expertise of the practitioner.

A number of safe videotapes and audiotapes are available for a reasonable price. Although it is possible to learn yoga from books and/or tapes, the safest way to begin yoga is with a qualified teacher.

## FINDING A YOGA TEACHER

Hatha Yoga in its basic form is a series of postures, breath, and meditation. It is important to understand that the approach to Hatha Yoga comes in various styles, levels, and systems.

The type of yoga discussed in this chapter is therapeutic. Neither all schools of yoga nor all YT's are equipped to handle vulnerable patients. Therefore it is imperative to research teachers and their credentials to make sure they have skill, experience, and knowledge about the illness being treated. It is best to make an appointment with the YT and experience his or her teaching personally.

Standards of yoga teaching can vary greatly. The recent rise in popularity of yoga has created a need for a national organization for yoga. The National Yoga Alliance was formed and is creating standards for yoga certification and eligibility requirements for the National Registry of Yoga Therapists. It is important to make sure that the YT's qualifications meet these standards because there are no state licensers at this time. Clients should ask teachers about their qualifications, their philosophy of yoga, their certification, and their teaching style. Their teacher training should include a strong background in anatomy and physiology, teaching methodology, philosophy, ethics, yogic lifestyle, and training in the various yoga techniques and practices.

The following yoga associations may provide names of teachers in your area.

Kripalu Yoga Teachers Association:
(413) 448-3202
Integral Yoga Teachers Association:
(804) 969-3121 ext. 137
Integrative Yoga Therapy: (800) 750-9642
International Association of Yoga Therapists:
(707) 928-9898
B.K.S. Iyengar Yoga National Association of the
United States: (800) 889-9642
Himalayan Institute Teachers Association:
(570) 253-5551 ext. 1305
Prana Yoga Teachers: (413) 448-3446
Yoga International's Guide to Yoga Teachers:
(800) 253-6243
Yoga Journal's Yoga Teacher Directory:
(800) 436-9642

Hatha Yoga is the most familiar type of yoga in the United States. There are many different approaches or schools to the classic Hatha Yoga, based on the work or traditions of particular teachers. Following are but a few of the different approaches: *Kripalu Yoga* is a gentle flowing style that focuses on improving awareness of mind, body, and spirit. *Integral Yoga* focuses mainly on breathing and meditation, with a standard routine of postures. *Iyengar Yoga* focuses primarily on alignment of the body, using props to aid the postures. *Kundalini Yoga* aims to release dormant bodily energy and focuses on purification. *Ashtanga Yoga,* or "power yoga," is more strenuous, involving *vinyasa,* a connection of every asana. *Sivananda Yoga* focuses on proper lifestyle with a vigorous form of yoga. *Viniyoga Yoga* also emphasizes the flow of the movements while coordinating breathing; it is a gentler form of Ashtanga Yoga.

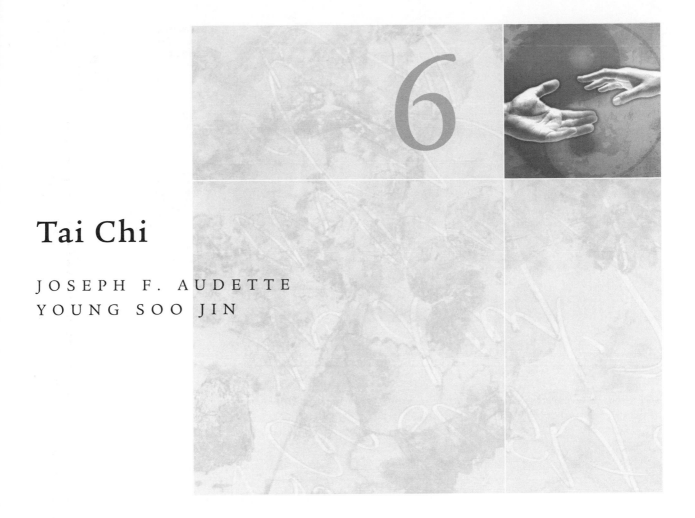

# Tai Chi

## JOSEPH F. AUDETTE
## YOUNG SOO JIN

There is growing recognition that, despite continued technological advancements in medicine, the modern biomedical healthcare model is not equally effective for all types and stages of illness. As a result, many in the healthcare community have looked to the medical wisdom of our historical past to find alternative solutions to modern problems, especially in the area of health promotion and disease prevention. A particularly rich area of ancient knowledge lay in the health value of movement therapies. These exercises offer great potential for informing new therapies in the Rehabilitation arena for the treatment of a variety of chronic conditions.

There are a number of Eastern movement practices that have gained popularity in the West, including Tai Chi, Qigong, and Yoga. Although each of these practices has a distinct origin, the current focus of research and general use is to apply these movements to the development of physical, mental, emotional, and spiritual well-being, as well as disease prevention and treatment. Unique among these, Tai Chi Chuan (TCC) has clear martial beginnings and is considered an effective means of self-defense. In the last 50 to 70 years, however, the development has focused far more on the health and mind-body effects of this discipline.

Taoist theories of health and longevity are based in part on exercise practices such as TCC that can enhance the flow and balance of *Qi,* or *vital energy.* Disease is believed to occur when the Qi is out of balance or blocked, and TCC is one of a number of techniques used to help restore this dynamic, energetic equilibrium in the body. Even today the practice of TCC is an important feature of the Chinese approach to health

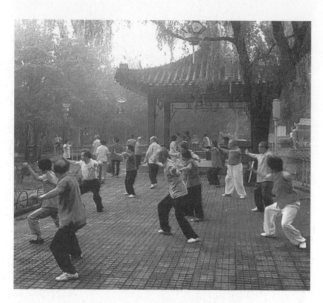

*Figure 6-1* Practice of TCC in China.

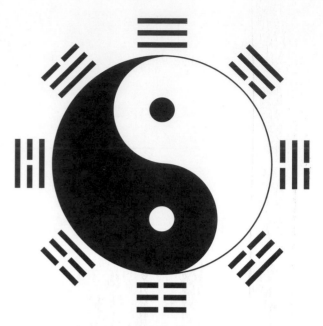

*Figure 6-2  The Great Ultimate.*

and disease prevention, and the practice continues to be taught to students in Traditional Chinese Medical Schools.

As anyone who has visited China knows, TCC has also become popular among Chinese elders, who practice in large numbers in the streets and parks of China primarily for the health benefits (Figure 6-1).

In this chapter, TCC is introduced as a therapeutic exercise rather than a martial art. Information about the history and philosophy of TCC is also provided, along with a detailed review of the scientific literature. At the end of the chapter, two case examples of the practical application of TCC are given.

## HISTORY AND PHILOSOPHY

Tai Chi Chuan (TCC) (also written as Tai Chi, Tai Chi Quan, Taijiquan, or T'ai Chi) developed many centuries ago as one of many different styles of Chinese martial arts, and it continues to be enjoyed in a form true to its beginnings throughout the world. The name is derived from the Chinese characters that mean *The Great Ultimate* (Figure 6-2), which refers to the dynamic and fundamental balance between oppo-

sites in the universe (*Yin,* or unity, balanced with *Yang,* or change).

The historical origins of TCC are controversial and steeped in legend. Douglas Wile has sorted the various historical accounts into different categories to help with the scholarly endeavor of tracing back the true beginnings of this unusual form of exercise. Conceptually, TCC can be traced back to its philosophical origins, the origins of various training techniques and combat strategies, and the origins of the modern postures and forms.[1]

On a philosophical level, the principles of TCC are founded on the teachings of Taoism and the writings of Lao Tzu. The central vehicle of achieving tranquility is to align oneself with the Tao, a term which has been translated as *the way* or *the path.* The Tao is the central mystical underpinning of Lao Tzu's philosophy and is characterized as the formless, unfathomable source of all things. Historically, the writings of Lao Tzu have provided ample inspiration for the movements and theory of TCC. Lao Tzu writes, "Yield and overcome. Bend and be straight." "Returning is the motion of the Tao. Yielding is the way of the Tao." "Stiff and unbending is the principle of death. Gentle and yielding is the principle of life."[2]

Legend has it that the synthesis between Taoist thought and TCC movements occurred some eight centuries ago with Chang San-feng. The available historical data suggests that Chang San-feng may have lived as long ago as the Sung period (960-1279) or as late as the Ming (1368-1644). A legendary Taoist priest, he is said to have developed TCC-like movements based on the inspiration he received while observing a fight between a crane and a snake. In this skirmish, he saw how the soft and yielding could overcome the hard and inflexible. The fundamental wisdom of self-defense lay in the knowledge of softness in the face of strength. The principles of yielding, softness, slowness, balance, suppleness, and remaining rooted and centered are essential tenets of Taoist philosophy that TCC has drawn on in its understanding of movement, both in relation to health and also in its martial applications.

The legend of Chang Sang-feng is tied to the present with the publication of *Epitaph for Wang Cheng-nan,* written by Huang Tsung-hi (1610-1695), and *Methods of the Internal School of Pugilism,* written by his son, Pai-chia.[3] These writings organize various systems of martial arts into internal (soft) and external (hard) styles. The underlying principle of an internal school is illustrated by the aphorism of "stillness overcoming movement." Internal styles of martial arts reversed the principles of the older Shaolin styles, where only superior force could win. Pai-chia traces the transmission of this philosophy of pugilism back to Chang Sang-feng. TCC was subsequently labeled as an internal style and, as a result, identified with the Chang San-feng legend, without there being direct evidence of more than a philosophical connection to modern styles.

In subsequent years foreign invasions and domestic peasant uprisings stimulated the diffusion of martial arts among the people. With the destruction of the Shaolin temple, a new form of boxing evolved and developed with the Chen family that closely resembles styles of TCC practiced today (Chen Family Boxing [1771-1853]). The Yang family then inherited and transformed the Chen TCC movements (Yang Lu-ch'an [1799-1872]), then later the Wu family (Wu Chien-ch'üan [1870-1942]) and the Sun family (Sun Lu-t'ang [1861-1932]) created distinct styles.[1]

Based on these early family traditions, there are several styles of TCC currently practiced. The five main schools (with numerous subdivisions under each) are Chen (quick with large movements), Yang (slow with large movements), Wu (midpaced with compact movements), Sun (quick with compact movements), and Hao (related to Wu). Among these schools, Chen is the oldest and Yang is the most popular.

There are 108 movements in the traditional long form of the Yang style. Yang Ch'eng-fu (1883-1936), grandson of Yang Lu-ch'an, is credited with establishing the Yang style of TCC as the dominant internal marshal art system in China. His period of greatest influence was in the 1920s and 1930s. The Yang style subsequently became the basis for a new, simplified version of TCC adopted in the Peoples Republic of China in 1956. Perhaps Yang Ch'eng-fu's most famous student in the United States was Professor Cheng Man-ch'ing (1900-1975), who subsequently taught in New York for many years and published a number of books on TCC.[4] Professor Cheng Man-ch'ing created a shortened version of the Yang style consisting of 37 movements that has many adherents in the United States, including T.T. Liang. Another accomplished student of Yang Ch'eng-fu was Harn Ch'in-tang, whose son-in-law, Leung Kai-chi, and daughter, Harn Lin, teach in the Boston area today and continue the tradition of teaching the long form of the Yang style.

In the 1950s a national physical fitness program incorporating TCC was first instituted in China. A simplified set of TCC exercises based on the most popular sequences of the Yang school was issued in 1956 by the Chinese National Athletic Committee. This form consists of 24 movements that progress logically from the easy to the difficult and take 5 minutes to complete. In 1990 TCC was included for the first time in the martial arts division of the eleventh Asian games.

## PHYSIOLOGICAL EFFECTS

In China a great deal of anecdotal and survey literature on TCC exists. This literature suggests that significant health benefits are gained by older persons who practice TCC. A summary of these significant health benefits are presented in Table 6-1, and a systematic review of the English language literature follows.

TABLE 6-1

*Survey Data From the Chinese Literature Comparing TCC Practitioners With Sedentary Controls*

| Measure | TCC practice (age >60 yr) | Sedentary (age >60 yr) |
|---|---|---|
| Occurrence of spondylitis | 23.8% | 47.2% |
| Occurrence of osteoarthritis | 14.3% | 79.4% |
| Occurrence of deconditioning | 25.8% | 47.2% |
| Ability to toe touch with hand | 85.7% | 20.6% |
| Average resting systolic BP | 134 mm Hg | 154 mm Hg |
| Occurrence of atherosclerosis | 37.5% | 46.4% |
| Cardiac response to physical stress (sit to stand 20 times in 30 sec) | Without arrhythmia | 35 extra beats |

Modified from Wolf SL, Coogler C, Xu T: *Arch Phys Med Rehab* 78:886-892, 1997.
*TCC*, Tai Chi Chuan; *BP*, blood pressure.

## BALANCE AND STRENGTH

The risk for falls in older persons is a serious health problem in the United States, costing upward of $10 billion annually in direct medical care. Approximately one out of three older persons will sustain a fall this year, and half of those will go on to fall again.[5] A number of studies have reported the positive effects of TCC on balance and lower extremity muscle strength in this population, suggesting that the long-term practice of TCC may help prevent accidental falls.[6,7,8,9,10]

Lan noted significant improvement in thoracolumbar range of motion (ROM) and knee flexion and extension strength among men and women after a 6-month daily training period using the 108-movement Yang style.[11] Judge randomized 21 older women to a control group vs. an intervention group enrolled in a combined training program of leg strengthening; brisk walking; and postural control exercise, including a simplified form of TCC. Compared with the control group, the intervention group exhibited a trend toward less postural sway during single support.[12] Jacobson reported increased lateral stability on tilt board testing after training 24 men and women in TCC for 12 weeks.[13] In addition, TCC practice in older persons has been shown to maintain the improvement in balance made after a non-TCC intensive balance training intervention is given.[9]

There are also a number of studies to support that community TCC practitioners have improved balance when compared with nonpractitioners.[14,15] In 1990, a prospective trial was funded under the acronym of FICSIT (Frailty and Injuries: Cooperative Study of Intervention Techniques) by the National Institute on Aging and the National Center on Nursing Research of the National Institutes of Health (NIH). This was a multicenter trial applying a number of different interventions at the various centers. In the Atlanta trial center, 200 subjects were randomized to 15 weeks of TCC, computerized balance training classes, or education control groups. Across all centers, TCC was the only group exercise intervention that reduced the occurrence of falls after 4 months of follow-up. Also, a reduction in fear of falling in both the TCC and balance training groups occurred. There continued to be significantly fewer falls in the Atlanta TCC group compared with the control group after 1 to 2 years of follow-up. A significant trend toward a decrease in incidence of injurious falls also was reported.[16]

In the older, often arthritic population, the issue of tolerability must be raised, especially with TCC movements, which demand sequential, alternate weight bearing on a single leg with a bent knee (single weighting) (Figure 6-3).[17] This question has been addressed in a population of rheumatoid arthritis (RA) patients by Kirsteins. The findings suggest that TCC appears to be safe for patients with RA and may serve as an alternative form of exercise therapy in rehabilitation programs without risk for causing increased pain.[18] In addition, there is some suggestion in the literature that RA patients demonstrate improved joint ROM after a TCC intervention.[19] TCC, as a weight-bearing exercise, also has the potential advantage of

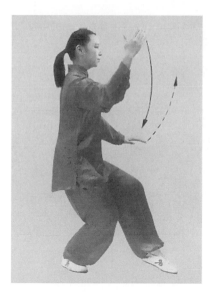

*Figure 6-3* Single weighting in TCC.

stimulating bone growth and strengthening connective tissues, as evidenced by some recent pilot data.[20]

In summary, TCC practice has a positive biological and psychosocial influence on older persons with regard to balance and falls.[21] On a biomechanical level, practicing TCC can improve lower extremity strength and spinal flexibility, and it can lessen sway velocity. Outcomes research has confirmed that TCC can reduce the risk for falls and increase postural stability and balance in older persons. Presumably, some of these effects are mediated by the effect of single weighting during TCC practice. However, the cognitive effect of TCC may also be involved in the psychosocial effects of TCC, including reduced fear of falling, increased confidence in balance and movement, and increased overall well-being. These findings were found in samples of frail elders, community-dwelling elders, and well elders. None of the studies reviewed reported any problems resulting in increased pain from TCC practice, even in the case of RA.

## CARDIOVASCULAR SYSTEM

Exercise training has been shown to have a positive effect on the cardiovascular system. Regular physical activity is associated with multiple health benefits, including a reduced incidence of coronary artery disease and stroke.

### A Case Study

*Cerebral Palsy*
Eve is a 31-year-old woman with spastic paraparesis secondary to cerebral palsy. Although functional and independent in ambulation with bilateral loft-strand crutches, movement can often be seriously impaired by periods of excessive spasticity in her lower extremities that is accompanied by hip pain. Eve is generally intolerant of oral antispasticity agents because of cognitive clouding and fatigue. Standard Physical Therapy techniques such as stretching, proprioceptive neuromuscular facilitation (PNF), and progressive muscle relaxation were only partially beneficial for relieving the episodes of excessive lower extremity tone. Eventually, Eve had the opportunity to attempt practice of a simplified form of Tai Chi Ch'ih. The form had to be even further modified because of Eve's inability to stand without using her crutches. This was accomplished by having Eve perform the practice sitting but still motivating her arm movement from the area of her center of mass below the umbilicus. Her breathing pattern was diaphragmatic and timed with her movements. Practice 2 to 3 times per week had a profound effect on her normal ambulation and movements, dramatically reducing the episodes of incapacitating spasticity. ∽

The metabolic demand of TCC has been shown in a number of studies to be equivalent to light to moderate aerobic activity, depending on the TCC form practiced and the age group studied. In one study of men and women 58 to 70 years of age using the 108-movement Yang style of TCC, the exercise intensity was 52% to 63% of the predicted target heart rate.[11] In a study of experienced TCC practitioners (estimated age range 26 to 48 years), changes in heart rate, blood pressure, and urinary catecholamine levels after a long form of Yang TCC practice were compared with those changes experienced during meditation, brisk walking (6 km/h or 3 mph), and neutral reading. Equivalent cardiovascular changes were found between TCC and brisk walking groups.[22]

In a comparison of the metabolic energy equivalents (METs) of the TCC short form (24 movements) with that of the long form (108 movements), the short form was estimated to cost about 2.9 METs, compared with 4.1 METs for the long form.[23] In another study of a modified short form of TCC called T'ai Chi Ch'ih, the METs for sitting TCC movements were estimated to be 1.5; for slow standing movements, 2.3;

TABLE 6-2

## Comparison of the Metabolic Demands and Changes in Heart Rate Seen in TCC

| Study author | Tai Chi style | METs | HR (% of max) | Equivalent activity |
|---|---|---|---|---|
| Zhuo | Yang long form | 4.1 | | Brisk walking (3.5 mph) |
| | Yang short form | 2.9 | | Walking (3.0 mph) |
| Fontana | TC Ch'ih sitting | 1.5 | | Sewing or eating |
| | TC Ch'ih slowly | 2.3 | 43.0% | Slow walking (2.0-2.5 mph) |
| | TC Ch'ih fast | 2.6 | 49.0% | Walking (2.5 mph) |
| Lan | Yang Long Form | — | 52.0%-63.0% | — |
| Lai | Yang Long Form | — | 70.0% | — |
| Jin | Yang Long Form | — | 58.0% | Brisk walking (4.0 mph) |
| Schneider | Yang Long Form | 4.6 | 59.8% | Brisk walking (4.0 mph) |

TCC, Tai Chi Chuan; METs, metabolic energy equivalents; HR, heart rate.

and for slow standing movements performed at a faster pace, 2.6. In this group, mean maximum heart rates ranged from 43% to 49% of the predicted maximum heart rate for age. An 8% increase in mean systolic and diastolic blood pressures was observed during TCC. There was no difference in response to the movements by gender or experience with TCC exercise. [24] (See Table 6-2 for a comparison of TCC with other activities.)

These studies confirm that a gentle style of TCC requires an energy expenditure comparable to a moderate walking pace and would be safe for persons with low exercise tolerance. Therefore TCC may be an alternative approach to health promotion in a population with chronic disease.

Detailed cardiopulmonary assessments have been made on a group of experienced TCC practitioners and compared to age- and body weight–matched sedentary controls. A total of 90 participants, aged 50 to 64 years, were assessed (21 males and 20 females in the TCC group; 23 males and 26 females in the control group). TCC participants showed significantly higher $VO_2$ max (maximal oxygen consumption in L/min) and work capacity compared with the sedentary controls. In this age group, the mean heart rate exceeded 70% of the predicted maximum during practice of the Yang style long form of TCC.[25] These results have been confirmed by others and demonstrate that TCC practice has a significant cardiorespiratory effect.[10] The exercise intensity of TCC (Yang style, long form) is moderate for older people, and it is aerobic in nature.

On 2-year follow-up of this same group, the rate of decline in $VO_2$ max was significantly less in the TCC subjects than in the control subjects. Collectively, these data reinforce the belief that cardiorespiratory benefits for both younger and older persons can be achieved with TCC training. In summary, practicing TCC regularly may delay the decline of cardiorespiratory function in older persons, and it may be prescribed as a suitable aerobic exercise for that population.[26]

The American Heart Association has endorsed moderate intensity and low impact exercise for cardiac rehabilitation programs to improve functional capacity and reduce cardiac-related morbidity and mortality.[27] For cardiac patients, exercise intensity in the range of 50% to 70% of the calculated target heart rate for age has been shown to improve functional and aerobic capacity.[28]

Regular physical activity is also thought to reduce blood pressure. In 1999, Young presented the result of a pilot study at the American Heart Association's epidemiology and prevention conference. She studied 62 sedentary adults with mild hypertension, 60 years of age and over, who were not taking blood pressure medication. They practiced either moderately intense aerobic exercises or TCC. After 12 weeks, both the TCC and aerobic exercise groups showed significant reduction from baseline in mean systolic (7.0 mm Hg in the TCC group vs. 8.4 mm Hg in the aerobic group) and diastolic (2.4 mm Hg in the TCC group vs. 3.3 mm Hg in the aerobic group) blood pressures.[29]

TCC practice has been shown to safely enhance cardiopulmonary function for low-risk patients following coronary artery bypass graft surgery (CABG). In one study the TCC group included nine men who practiced classical Yang style TCC for 1 year following heart surgery. Exercise intensity during TCC was low to moderate, with heart rates ranging from 48% to 57% of predicted maximum for age. The TCC group showed an increase of 10.3% in $VO_2$ peak compared with the control group, which showed a slight decline in $VO_2$ peak following participation in a home-based phase II cardiac rehabilitation program.[30]

TCC also has been found to be beneficial for patients who have suffered acute myocardial infarction. A sample of 126 patients who were capable of exercising following acute myocardial infarction and who were without severe arthritis or heart failure were randomly assigned to either a TCC (Wu style) group (n = 38), aerobic exercising group (n = 41), or a non-exercise group (n = 47). The TCC and exercise groups met twice weekly for 3 weeks, then once weekly for an additional 5 weeks. Despite the fact that the groups participated in only 11 exercise sessions, trends were shown for decreasing systolic blood pressure in both exercise groups and decreasing diastolic blood pressure in the TCC group. These results suggest that regular TCC or aerobic exercise in the recovery period from acute myocardial infarction may help decrease blood pressure. The researchers suggested that TCC might be a useful alternative to formal aerobic exercise as part of a cardiac rehabilitation program.[31]

The difference between TCC and other forms of aerobic exercise has also been evaluated. Brown examined the ventilatory and cardiovascular response to TCC practice when compared with bicycle ergometry at an equivalent level of oxygen consumption ($VO_2$). The study population included six experienced long-form Yang-style TCC practitioners. Three measures of ventilatory efficiency were studied and showed significant changes during TCC compared with similar measures made on the group during cycle ergometry: lower ventilatory frequency (Vf) (11.3 vs. 15.7 breaths/min-1), ventilatory equivalent ($VE/VO_2$) (23.47 vs. 27.41), and the ratio of dead space ventilation to tidal volume (VD/VT) (20% vs. 27%). This study suggests that the respiratory response to TCC in experienced practitioners is more efficient than the respiratory response to standard forms of aerobic exercise.[32]

Similar findings were obtained by Schneider and Leung when studying 20 male martial arts experts from both TCC and a hard style called Wing Chun. No significant differences in $VO_2$ max or HR (heart rate) max obtained during treadmill exercise were found between the practitioners of the two styles, despite the fact that Wing Chun practice is much more demanding than TCC (6.6 vs. 4.6 METs). The ventilatory equivalent for oxygen ($VE/VO_2$) obtained during TCC exercise (21.7) was significantly lower than that for Wing Chun exercise (24.2), suggesting that TCC practitioners use efficient breathing patterns during exercise.[33] The improved respiratory efficiency found in TCC practice may be due to the slow, deep diaphragmatic breathing required during TCC practice. More intriguing is the question of whether the findings in these studies reflect the physiological benefits of the cognitive aspects of TCC, which are similar to those found in the relaxation response. For example, the state of mindfulness attained during the relaxation response has been shown to have a regulating effect on the autonomic nervous system, and this factor may influence the physiological responses to TCC practice.[34,35]

## COGNITIVE FUNCTION

A mind-body therapy is any treatment method in which the mind is used to alter physiology to promote health and recovery from illness. This is a very broad definition and can include many treatment modalities. Examples include relaxation exercises, meditation, guided imagery, support groups, psychotherapy, Yoga, art and music therapy, TCC, and hypnosis.[36] TCC requires a state of mind that is similar to that found with meditation-based stress reduction techniques. Relaxed breathing and mental attention are essential during the practice of TCC to achieve balance between body and mind. Qigong breathing exercises, which are often incorporated in TCC practice, have been recognized to have a similar physiological effect as mind-body relaxation techniques.[37]

Our knowledge of the influence of cognitive states and the relaxation response on health and disease has greatly increased over the last 10 years. However, little attention has been given to the physiological relationship between exercise and the relaxation response, and no work has been done to compare their relative health benefits. Clearly the potential health benefits of cognitive and physical practices are not the same, as has been illustrated in a recent study in which a 4-month stress management intervention was found to be superior to an exercise intervention in reducing ischemic events in patients with coronary artery disease.[28] In addition, there has not been a great deal of research on whether there is an additive effect on physiological outcomes when combining the relaxation response with exercise.

In an attempt to better understand this relationship, low- and moderate-intensity walking groups were compared with a mindful exercise group performing TCC to determine if the cognitive effect of TCC provided a therapeutic benefit over and above its exercise effect. Subjects were sedentary adults (69 women and 66 men) randomized to various groups that included light to moderate walking exercise and TCC. Outcome measures included self-assessment questionnaires measuring different domains of mood and general health. The most significant finding was that women in the TCC group experienced significant improvements in depression scores and other measures of mood disturbance when compared with the walking groups.[38] The men in this study did not show the same response to TCC. This difference between the male and female response may reflect interesting differences in the willingness to learn the cognitive aspects of TCC.

A study by Jin compared 33 experienced TCC practitioners with 33 beginners (total group age range 16 to 75 years).[22] The experienced practitioners exhibited increased heart rate and noradrenaline excretion in urine but decreased salivary cortisol concentration when compared with the beginners. It was noted in the study that the more experienced group had lower, more strenuous postures during the movements, thus inducing a higher heart rate response and a stronger catecholamine activation. However, the greater physical stress of the practice was not accompanied by an increase in cortisol levels as would normally be expected.[13] These data are compatible with the notion that experienced TCC practitioners are less stress reactive because of the induction of the relaxation response during exercise.

Chen has reviewed the effects of TCC when it is used as a technique to reduce stress-related illnesses such as pain, mood disorders, and nightmares. In one study reviewed, the effectiveness of mind-body interventions in reducing chronic low back pain was assessed. The mind-body interventions included education, relaxation response training, and movement therapy (TCC or Qigong) and were administered in combination. All groups were matched relative to gender, age, and pain scores on visual analog scales. Findings confirmed that this combination of mind-body interventions produced an improvement in affective mood state, pain perception, and functional state.[39] However, because of the combined therapies, the specific outcome effect of TCC is not known.

Jin reported that mood states became more positive during TCC, and they remained positive even 1 hour following exercise. Relative to baseline levels, subjects reported less tension, depression, anger, fatigue, confusion, and state anxiety; felt more vigorous; and, in general, had less total mood disturbance during and after TCC.[40] Similar findings have been found in a population of patients with multiple sclerosis following TCC practice.[41]

## PSYCHONEUROIMMUNOLOGY

The central nervous system and immune system are linked by many important neurohumoral connections. The best described of these is the immunosuppressive action of glucocorticoids that is released in response to stress. These hormones are secreted secondary to activation of the hypothalamic-pituitary adrenal axis (HPA axis), and they act directly on specific receptors in various immune cells. Other neurohumoral systems are also involved in this regulation. At least 20 such neuromodulating peptides have been described that also have been shown to have an immunomodulating effect, including norephinephrine, endogenous opiates, vasopressin, growth hormone, and thyroxine.[42]

Psychological and physical stresses are crucial modifiers of the immune system.[43] It is well documented that various forms of stress influence the balance of the HPA axis.[44,45] Many studies on the modulation of the HPA axis by moderate and intense training have been investigated. The psychoneurological effect of aerobic exercise may participate in the regulation of immune function via the HPA axis and through neurohormones. As previously mentioned, at least one study has shown a decrease in salivary cortisol levels after TCC practice despite physiological evidence of the TCC providing a substantial physical stress, as measured by a significant rise in heart rate and increased noradrenaline excretion in urine.[13] Normally, the physical stress of an exercise intervention will raise cortisol levels, suggesting that TCC practice has unique physiological effects. The lowered cortisol levels correlated with the subjects' reports of less tension and less total mood disturbance. This finding has been partially confirmed in a study of the related practice of Qigong. During Qigong training, the plasma level of beta-endorphin significantly increased at the midpoint of the exercise session, while the level of adrenocorticotropic hormone (ACTH) declined by the mid-point and during the postexercise period, again suggesting a down regulation of the hormonal response of the HPA axis during a movement-based exercise that includes mindfulness.[46]

Acute physical stress can alter the number and function of circulating immune cells. Typical alterations include increased numbers of circulating lymphocytes, natural killer cells, CD8+ T cells, and a decrease in the ratio of CD4+ to CD8+ T cells.[47,48] Acute physical stress has also been found to increase natural killer cell activity (NKCA), and the lymphocyte proliferative response to mitogens has been found to either decrease or remain unchanged.[49,50] There is now some evidence to show that in addition to its central effect on reducing the stress response, TCC practice can enhance immunity. Sun used the sheep erythrocyte rosette method to estimate the number of T lymphocytes and active T lymphocytes and found increased numbers of both parameters in experienced TCC practitioners compared with sedentary controls. Furthermore, immediately following TCC exercise, a marked increase in active T lymphocytes was reported.[51] Similar findings of enhanced measures of immune reactivity have been found using mucosal analysis of antibodies following TCC practice. Such changes were not found in the walking exercise control group.[52] Qigong training has been shown to produce marked increases in the ratio of CD4+/CD8+ T lymphocytes.[53,54] However, little is known about the long-term effects of TCC on the immune system in comparison with other forms of exercise and mind-body interventions.

## FUTURE RESEARCH

Most of the TCC studies reviewed had a relatively small sample size, which limits our ability to generalize the results. Another factor that must be considered when reviewing the effects of TCC is the influence of the practice parameters and style on the outcome. This is a problem that is found in other Complementary and Alternative interventions, where the skill of the practitioner has a great deal to do with the treatment effect.

Because TCC has many different styles and diverse movement protocols and teaching methods, researchers should have a solid understanding of the key elements of a particular TCC technique before implementing it in a study. When learning TCC, a novice should be periodically evaluated on the progress and program adherence with regard to cognitive response, muscular tension, balance, and flexibility to ensure optimal results.[55] Furthermore, longitudinal studies are essential to substantiate the long-term training effects of TCC. This is particularly important with a practice like TCC, which requires learning to integrate a state of deep cognitive relaxation with specific breathing and movement techniques and cannot be learned quickly. Because this mind and body integration is essential for optimal benefit from the practice of TCC, the physiological effects are likely to be more pronounced with sustained practice.

## PRACTICAL CONSIDERATIONS

TCC takes between 5 and 25 minutes to perform. When practicing TCC, the lower body moves within a square, based on the four cardinal directions and their diagonals, while the upper body moves in multi-planed circles. The original intent of the circular movement was to allow the interception of aggression in a fluid motion and deflect it away. Today the circular movements of the hips and waist promote flexibility and central balance. TCC training also teaches one to have an open, quiet mind. Training must emphasize complete relaxation and effortless movement to achieve the intended results. A sense of grounded buoyancy must be achieved, which Cheng Man-ch'ing related to the sensation of swimming or floating in air. From a martial point of view, this was felt to improve reaction time and enhance sensitivity to the actions of the opponent. Today, with the focus on the health benefits of TCC, the importance of this sense of floating is still primary because it allows integration of mindfulness and the relaxation response with conscious movement.

Despite the fact that the individual styles of TCC appear distinct, they share common properties. From a Taoist point of view, all TCC styles seek to balance and strengthen Qi (vital energy) in the body's meridians, consequently reducing the potential for developing serious illness. Originally, the *correct* practice of the styles was motivated to enhance this balance. From a more pragmatic view, even today there are certain essential elements of the modern practice of TCC that provide health benefits.

The first thing a beginner of TCC has to learn is to completely relax. This can be surprisingly difficult for many people. Progressive muscle relaxation techniques to first relax the facial muscles, then the neck and shoulder muscles, and so on down the body, can be used to facilitate complete relaxation. Second, the pattern of movements must be accompanied by a sense of lightness or a floating sensation. To accomplish this, the body should be extended and relaxed, the elbows should always hang to the floor and not point out to the sides, and the body is kept erect, as if there were a string pulling lightly on the crown of the head. Movements should not be exaggerated or forced but should flow from the center of mass below the umbilicus. Third, all movements require the well-coordinated sequencing of body segments. Awareness of this sequencing originates with the center of mass and involves rotation at the waist and upper hips. The movement then flows outward from this center balance point to propel the arms in circular movements. The movements progress in the semi-squat position and use the principle of single weighting, where the weight of the body continuously shifts from one leg to the other and back again without jerky or bobbing movements of the head and shoulders. Finally, breathing should be deep and regular. By using the diaphragm, practitioners should expand the lower abdomen with each breath. With practice, the breath frequency should match the pace of the movements with each weight shift accompanied by the alternation of inhalation and expiration. Wolf has published a sequence of 10 TCC movements that he believes distills these essential elements for practice in the older population without being overly complex or physically demanding (Figure 6-4).

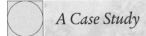 *A Case Study*

### Peripheral Neuropathy

Aida is a 53-year-old woman with a painful 5-year history of an idiopathic peripheral sensory polyneuropathy affecting her hands and feet. She experienced balance problems and pain related to the abnormal sensations in her extremities. She had become increasingly isolated and depressed as a result of the discomfort and was unable to exercise because use of her arms or legs would increase her pain. TCC was started, initially focusing on gentle movements of her upper extremities in a standing position without moving her feet. Initially this actually made her hand pain worse, with increased stinging sensation in her hands, and she wanted to stop after the first few sessions. However, with individual counseling in which she focused her mind onto her center of mass below the umbilicus, Aida was able to completely eliminate the stinging sensations. Eventually, her exercise tolerance increased and she regained normal function for most activities. ∽

## SUMMARY

Tai Chi Chuan (TCC) is known as a slow, smooth, and graceful form of Chinese exercise that includes a form of mindfulness meditation that is reputed for its health benefits. TCC practice has been shown to improve balance, strength, and coordination of body movements and can reduce the risk for falls in older persons. In addition, TCC has been shown to be a safe method of exercise for older persons from a cardiovascular point of view.

TCC requires a state of mind that is similar to that found with meditation-based stress reduction techniques. Qigong breathing exercises, which are often incorporated in TCC practice, have been recognized to have a similar physiological effect as mind-body relaxation techniques. This state of mindfulness has been shown to have a regulating effect on the autonomic nervous system and immune function.

TCC, Qigong, and Yoga represent a class of exercise that differs from the routine strengthening and stretching programs currently employed in physical medicine. Practicing TCC appropriately has various benefits (e.g., balance improvement, fall prevention, cardiovascular enhancement, stress reduction), and it is highly recommended for the appropriate patients.

This class of exercise incorporates a mind-body approach to the rehabilitation of disorders commonly seen by clinicians. Methods such as TCC and Qigong serve to add valuable options to the continuity of care of ambulatory and nonambulatory patients with various chronic illnesses. There is a clear challenge to practitioners of Western medicine to continue to explore the basis of the beneficial effects seen from the practice of the time-honored exercise method of TCC.

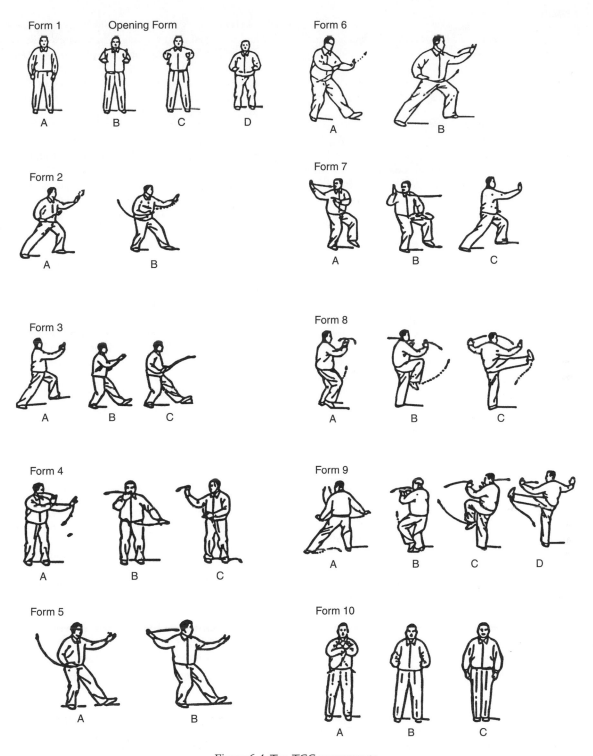

Form 1
Opening Form

Form 6

Form 2

Form 7

Form 3

Form 8

Form 4

Form 9

Form 5

Form 10

*Figure 6-4*  Ten TCC movements.

## References

1. Wile D: *Lost Tai Chi classics from the late Ch'ing Dynasty*, New York, SUNY Press, 1996.
2. Liang TT: *T'ai Chi Ch'uan for health and self-defense: philosophy and practice*, New York, Vintage Books, 1977.
3. Goodrich LC: *The literary inquisition of Ch'ien Lnug*, New York, Paragon Books Reprint, 1966, pp 65, 247.
4. Cheng M: *Tai Chi Ch'uan: a simplified method of calisthenics for health and self defense*, Berkeley, Calif, North Atlantic Books, 1981.
5. Province MA, Hardley EC, Homebrook MC, et al: The effects of exercise on falls in elderly patients: a pre-planned meta-analysis of the FICSIT trials—frailty and injuries: cooperative studies of intervention techniques, *JAMA* 273(17):1341-1347, 1995.
6. Hain TC et al: Effects of Tai Chi on balance, *Arch Otolaryngol* 125(11):1191-1195, 1999.
7. Lan C, Lai JS, Chen S-Y, et al: Tai Chi Chuan to improve muscular strength and endurance in elderly individuals: a pilot study, *Arch Phys Med Rehabil* 81:604-607, 2000.
8. Wolf SL, Coogler C, Xu T: Exploring the basis for Tai Chi Chuan as a therapeutic exercise approach, *Arch Phys Med Rehab* 78:886-892, 1997.
9. Wolfson L, Whipple R, Derby C, et al: Balance and strength training in older adults: intervention gains and Tai Chi maintenance, *J Am Geriatr Soc* 44(5):498-506, 1996.
10. Lan C, Lai JS, Wong MK, et al: Cardiorespiratory function, flexibility, and body composition among geriatric Tai Chi Chuan practitioners, *Arch Phys Med Rehabil* 77(6):612-616, 1996.
11. Lan C, Lai JS, Chen SY, et al: 12-month Tai Chi training in the elderly: its effect on health fitness, *Med Sci Sports Exerc* 30(3):345-351, 1998.
12. Judge JO, Lindsey C, Underwood M, et al: Balance improvements in older women: effects of exercise training, *Phys Ther* 73(4):254-262, 1993.
13. Jacobson BH, Chen HC, Cashel C, et al: The effect of T'ai Chi Chuan training on balance, kinesthetic sense, and strength, *Percept Mot Skills* 84(1):27-33, 1997.
14. Schaller KJ: Tai Chi Chih: an exercise option for older adults, *J Gerontol Nurs* 22(10):12-17, 1996.
15. Tse SK, Bailey DM: T'ai chi and postural control in the well elderly, *Am J Occup Ther* 46(4):295-300, 1992.
16. Wolf SL, Barnhart HX, Kutner NG, et al: Reducing frailty and falls in older persons: an investigation of Tai Chi and computerized balance training: Atlanta FICSIT group—frailty and injuries: cooperative studies of intervention techniques, *J Am Geriatr Soc* 44(5):489-497, 1996.
17. Hartman CA, Mano TM, Winter C, et al: Effects of Tai Chi training on function and quality of life indicators in older adults with osteoarthritis, *J Am Geriatr Soc* 48(12):1553-1559, 2000.
18. Kirsteins AE, Dietz F, Hwang SM: Evaluating the safety and potential use of a weight-bearing exercise, Tai-Chi Chuan, for rheumatoid arthritis patients, *Am J Phys Med Rehabil* 70(3):136-141, 1991.
19. Van Deusen J, Harlowe D: The efficacy of the ROM Dance Program for adults with rheumatoid arthritis, *Am J Occup Ther* 41(2):90-95, 1987.
20. Chan KM, Au SK, Choy WY, et al: Beneficial effect of one-year Tai Chi in retardation of bone loss in post-menopausal women, *J Bone Miner Res* 15:S444, 2000 (abstract).
21. Kessenich CR: Tai Chi as a method of fall prevention in the elderly, *Orthop Nurs* 17(4):27-29, 1998.
22. Jin P: Efficacy of Tai Chi, brisk walking, meditation, and reading in reducing mental and emotional stress, *J Psychosom Res* 36(4):361-370, 1992.
23. Zhou DH: Preventive geriatrics: an overview from traditional Chinese medicine, *Am J Chin Med* 10(1-4):32-39, 1982.
24. Frontana JA: The energy costs of a modified form of Tai Chi exercise, *Nurs Res* 49(2):91-96, 2000.
25. Lai JS, Wong MK, Lan C, et al: Cardiorespiratory responses of Tai Chi Chuan practitioners and sedentary subjects during cycle ergometry, *J Formos Med Assoc* 92(10):894-899, 1993.
26. Lai JS, Lan C, Wong MK, et al: Two-year trends in cardiorespiratory function among older Tai Chi Chuan practitioners and sedentary subjects, *J Am Geriatr Soc* 43(11):1222-1227, 1995.
27. Fletcher GF, Balady G, Blair SN, et al: Statement on exercise: benefits and recommendations for physical activity programs for all Americans—a statement for health professionals by the Committee on Exercise and Cardiac Rehabilitation of the Council on Clinical Cardiology, American Heart Association, *Circulation* 94(4):857-862, 1996.
28. Blumenthal JA, Jiang W, Babyak MA, et al: Stress management and exercise training in cardiac patients with myocardial ischemia: effects on prognosis and evaluation of mechanisms, *Arch Intern Med* 157(19):2213-2223, 1997.
29. Young DR, Appeal LJ, Jee SH, et al: The effects of aerobic exercise and Tai Chi on blood pressure in older people: result of randomized trial, *J Am Geriatr Soc* 47:277-284, 1999.
30. Lan C, Chen SY, Lai JS, et al: The effects of Tai Chi on cardiorespiratory function in patients with coronary artery bypass surgery, *Med Sci Sports Exerc* 31(5):634-638, 1999.
31. Channer KS, Barrow D, Barrow R, et al: Changes in haemodynamic parameters following Tai Chi Chuan and aerobic exercise in patients recovering from acute myocardial infarction, *Postgrad Med* 72(848):349-351, 1996.

32. Brown DD, Mucci WG, Hetzler RK, et al: Cardiovascular and ventilatory responses during formalized T'ai Chi Chuan exercise, *Res Q Exerc Sport* 60(3):246-450, 1989.

33. Schneider D, Leung R: Metabolic and cardiorespiratory responses to the performance of Wing Chun and T'ai Chi Chuan exercise, *Int J Sports Med* 12(3):319-323, 1991.

34. Goldenberg DL, Felson DT, Dinernan H: A randomized controlled trial of amitriptyline and naproxen in the treatment of patients with fibromyalgia, *Arthritis Rheum* 29:1371-1377, 1986.

35. Koh TC: Qigong-Chinese breathing exercise, *Am J Chin Med* 10(1-4):86-91, 1982.

36. Chiaramonte DR: Complementary and alternative therapies in primary care, *Prim Care* 24(4):788-807, 1997.

37. Luskin FM, Newell KA, Griffith M, et al: A review of mind/body therapies in the treatment of musculoskeletal disorders with implications for the elderly, *Altern Ther Health Med* 6(2):46-56, 2000.

38. Brown DR, Wang Y, Ward A, et al: Chronic psychological effects of exercise and exercise plus cognitive strategies, *Med Sci Sports Exerc* 27(5):765-775, 1995.

39. Chen KM, Snyder M: A research-based use of Tai Chi/movement therapy as a nursing intervention, *J Holist Nurs* 17(3):267-279, 1999.

40. Jin P: Changes in heart rate, noradrenaline, cortisol and mood during Tai Chi, *J Psychosom Res* 33(2):197-201, 1989.

41. Mills N, Allen J: Mindfulness of movement as a coping strategy in multiple sclerosis: a pilot study, *Gen Hosp Psych* 22(6):425-431, 2000.

42. Maier SF, Watkins LR. Cytokines for psychologists: implications of bidirectional immune-to-brain communication for understanding behavior, mood, and cognition, *Psychol Rev* 105(1):83-107, 1998.

43. Khansari DN, Murgo A, Faith RE: Effects of stress on the immune system, *Immunol Today* 11:170-174, 1990.

44. Besedovsky H, Sorkin E: Network of immune-neuroendocrine interactions, *Clin Exp Immunol* 27:1-12, 1977.

45. Vanoli E, Cerati D, Pedretti RF: Autonomic control of heart rate: pharmacological and nonpharmacological modulation, *Basic Res Cardiol* 93(Suppl 1):133-142, 1998.

46. Ryu H, Lee HS, Shin YS, et al: Acute effect of Qigong training on stress hormonal levels in man, *Am J Chin Med* 24(2):193-198, 1996.

47. Nieman DC, Henson DA, Gusewitch G, et al: Physical activity and immune function in elderly women, *Med Sci Sports Exerc* 25(7):823-831, 1993.

48. Van Titts LJ, Michel MC, Grosse-Wilde H, et al: Catecholamines increase lymphocyte beta 2-adrenergic receptors via 2-adrenergic, spleen-dependent process, *Am J Physiol* 258(1 Pt 1):E91-202, 1990.

49. Jin YS, Park JY, Kim MH, et al: The effects of exercise pattern on acute response of T lymphocyte and Nk cell, *Med Sci Sports Exerc* 31(5; Suppl):S61, 1999.

50. Shinkai S, Konishi M, Shephard RJ: Aging and immune response to exercise, *Can J Physiol Pharmacol* 76(5):562-572, 1998.

51. Sun X, Xu Y, Xia Y: Determination of E-rosette-forming lymphocytes in aged subjects with Taichiquan exercise, *Int J Sports Med* 10(3):217-219, 1989.

52. Verity LS, Czubryt P, Hamilton L, et al: Effects of Taichi, meditation and walking on stress and immune responses, *Med Sci Sports Exerc* 31(5; Suppl):S346, 1999.

53. Ryu H, Mo HY, Mo GD, et al: Delayed cutaneous hypersensitivity reaction in Qigong (Chun Do Sun Bup) trainees by multi-test cell mediated immunity, *Am J Chin Med* 23:139-144, 1995.

54. Ryu H, Jun CD, Lee BS, et al: Effect of Qigong training on proportion of lymphocyte subsets in human peripheral blood, *Am J Chin Med* 23:27-36, 1995.

55. La Forge R: Mind-body fitness: encouraging prospects for primary and secondary prevention, *J Cardiovasc Nurs* 11(3):53-65, 1997.

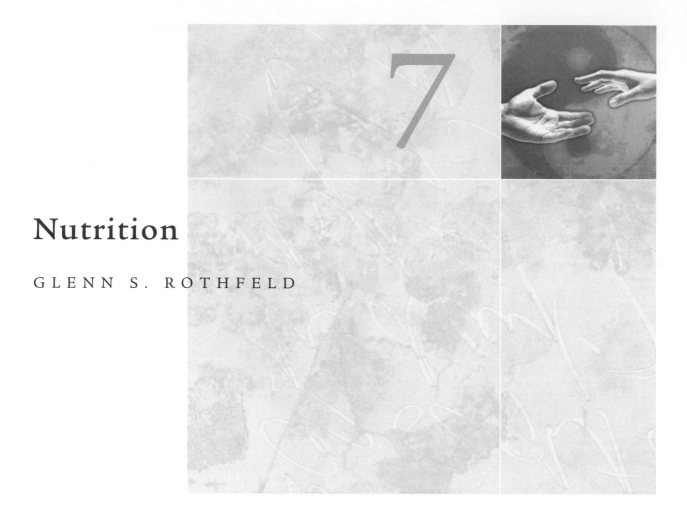

# Nutrition

GLENN S. ROTHFELD

The importance of wound healing in the recovery from injury, surgery, and chronic illness is classically underrepresented in the medical literature. In fact, one could argue that there is no recovery without the complex interplay of cellular and biochemical reactions that lead to tissue inflammation, repair, and then the remodeling and anatomical restructuring that complete the repair process. As with other physiological and biochemical processes, the proper delivery of nutrients and other natural factors to the tissues has a profound influence on the rate and completeness of healing.

Recovery from illness and injury can be vague in its description. In the conventional medical paradigm, it involves the circulatory, neurological, hematological, immunological, dermatological, musculoskeletal, and clotting systems, in addition to the various end-

organ functions. Therefore in order to look at natural factors in recovery, it is necessary to limit the scope of the effects somewhat. This chapter looks at nutritional and herbal influences on recovery or, more specifically, on inflammation, pain, and the complex biochemical and cellular changes involved in wound healing.

Wound healing starts with the triggering of the inflammatory process. This tissue response is automatically activated by any injury that affects or destroys cellular elements such as epithelial or endothelial cells, muscle cells, or blood cells (leukocytes, erythrocytes, platelets). In acute inflammation, the blood vessel wall is compromised and blood components leach out, entering the site of the injury. These cells have specific roles, including the control of infection (lymphocytes, neutrophils), phagocytosis and the removal of debris (macrophages, monocytes), and the walling off of the injured site to prevent further spread and bleeding (platelets, fibroblasts).

Various biochemical mediators are released, including cytokinins, histamine, complement moieties, and eicosanoids of various sorts (including leukotrienes and prostaglandins). Some of these modify and control the inflammatory process while others initiate the beginning of the next phase, involving the formation of fibrin, the laying down of collagen and granulation tissue, and the modeling of scar tissue. All mediators are produced from nutritional raw materials in the body, and all reactions involve nutritional cofactors. Therefore a natural medicine plan to improve the inflammatory process and wound healing involves attention to proper general nutriture and the delivery of specific nutritional substances.

## GENERAL NUTRITION

Even general nutritional status is difficult to evaluate. However, some studies look at the simple measurement of common laboratory tests as indicators or nutritional status. In one study, patients with abnormally low total lymphocyte counts and low serum albumin, two measures of general nutritional status, had significantly greater mortality and less recovery after hip fracture surgery.[1] Other studies measured specific nutrients and charted their effects on healing.[2,3] It is difficult to look at this data reliably because changes in micronutrient status are not easily measured. In fact, most biochemical tests are notoriously insensitive in measuring variability in micronutrient tissue levels.

## SPECIFIC NUTRIENTS

Some specific nutrients illustrate this problem. For example, magnesium is an intracellular mineral that is critical to almost every level of the healing process. In its action at the calcium channels, it is responsible for the proper relaxation of muscle tissue and for nerve relaxation. Magnesium is a cofactor in the production of steroid hormones and of neurotransmitters such as serotonin, is used at several places in the energy-producing Krebs Cycle, and is necessary for over 50 common biochemical reactions. Nevertheless, it is difficult to assess true magnesium status in the body. Because the mineral is buffered in the blood, serum

levels are fairly useless. Erythrocyte magnesium levels are somewhat more useful than serum levels. Leukocyte magnesium levels are more useful than either serum or erythrocyte magnesium levels, but they are not readily available. The gold standard test of magnesium deficiency in the body is a magnesium load assay in which a standardized dose of magnesium is given before and after a 24-hour urine collection and whole body retention of magnesium is calculated, giving an indirect measurement of magnesium deficiency. However, this test is cumbersome, and the amount of magnesium and threshold for deficiency are debated in the literature.

Other nutrients are similarly difficult to measure effectively. For example, pyridoxine, or vitamin $B_6$, is best assayed in an uncommonly performed and largely unavailable laboratory test, an erythrocyte glutamate-oxalate transferase challenge, and even this test only measures pyridoxine availability for this one enzyme. Vitamin C is best measured in the leukocyte, as is zinc. However, these nutrients also are best measured functionally under certain conditions. Vitamin C can be measured by a capillary fragility test, and zinc by an oral zinc sulfate taste test, using the necessity of good zinc nutrition for proper taste to occur.

It should be remembered that all studies of nutrient effects on rehabilitation (or anything else for that matter) are flawed by the limitations in the state of the art of nutrient testing. Therefore the preponderance of studies are either laboratory studies of isolated effects of nutrients or outcome studies looking at specific doses of a substance or substances in a specific clinical situation. In the case of nutrients, there is usually no attempt to answer the question of whether that nutrient dose is optimal for the situation.

## BOTANICALS

Herbal studies pose a different problem. As opposed to a pharmaceutical medication, an herbal formula or preparation uses multiple parts of a plant and therefore has a number of different ingredients. These ingredients can come from roots, leaves, stems, seeds, or fruit and contain aromatic hydrocarbons, saponins, glycosides, and other diverse chemical structures. It is difficult or impossible to isolate the active ingredient(s). Sometimes it is the confluence of ingredients that result in the unique properties of herbs. For example, white willow has natural salicylates, but it also contains other active substances that protect the stomach lining from the harmful erosion that aspirin can cause.

To get around this problem, many herbal studies have identified a single ingredient and standardized the extract to that ingredient. Most published trials of St. John's wort *(Hypericum perforatum)* have standardized the extract to 0.3% hypericin, an alkaloid thought to be responsible for the antidepressant activity. However, more recent research has suggested that other components of St. John's wort are just as psychoactive, if not more so.

## INFLAMMATION

### Essential Fatty Acids

The actions and proper quantities of both omega-6 and omega-3 fatty acids are required for proper inflammatory response. Through the action of delta-6-desaturase, linoleic acid is converted to gamma linolenic acid (GLA). This is the rate-limiting step, and a number of factors affect the delta-6-desaturase enzyme, including magnesium, zinc, vitamin $B_6$, alcohol, aging, elevated cholesterol, and trans fatty acids. If GLA is not produced in the body, then there is a deficiency of substrate for the production of dihomo-gamma-linolenic acid (DGLA). This intermediate fatty acid is converted by delta-5-desaturase into arachidonic acid (AA). AA is then converted into proinflammatory prostaglandin PGE2 by the action of cyclooxygenase. Aspirin and most common nonsteroidal antiinflammatory drugs (NSAIDs) act by inhibiting cyclooxygenase, thereby limiting PGE2-mediated inflammation. Arachidonic acid can also by altered by lipoxygenase enzyme to become the leukotriene LTB4, another proinflammatory messenger.

AA is released in response to tissue injury, and it is the main fatty acid responsible for triggering the inflammatory process. AA also is obtained through the diet, mostly from meat. Eggs and peanuts also have high AA content and therefore can be proinflammatory foods under certain conditions.

Some DGLA is diverted to become the antiinflammatory prostaglandin PGE1. Thus omega-6 fatty acids can act both as proinflammatory and antiinflammatory precursors. However, omega-3 fatty acids have more profound antiinflammatory effects (Figure 7-1). This essential fatty acid (EFA) can be obtained by eat-

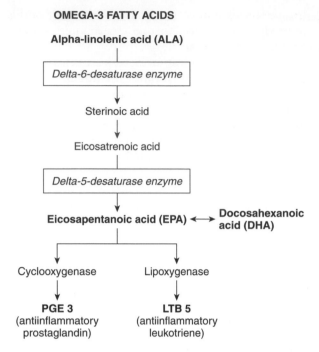

*Figure 7-1* Omega-3 fatty acids and inflammation.

ing fish, primarily of the cold water variety. Flaxseed oil and canola oil also have high omega-3 content. The primary omega-3 oil is alpha-linolenic acid, which is converted by the same delta-6-desaturase enzyme into an intermediate fatty acid that is then converted by the delta-5-desaturase into eicosapentaenoic acid (EPA). EPA can also interconvert with docosahexanoic acid (DHA). EPA is the precursor for the antiinflammatory prostaglandin PGE3 and the antiinflammatory leukotriene LTB5.

Thus a nutritional strategy for lowering inflammation involves an increase in omega-3–containing foods accompanied by a drastic reduction in foods high in arachidonic acid and a relative decrease in omega-6–containing foods. This creates a fatty acid balance favoring the formation of PGE3 and LTB5. In addition, the mineral cofactors magnesium, zinc, and $B_6$ can be used, along with the restriction of alcohol and trans fatty acids.

Several articles support the supplementation of omega-3 fatty acids as antiinflammatory agents.[4,5,6] In a randomized study,[7] 85 patients who underwent abdominal surgery for gastrointestinal malignancies were given either a standard diet or a diet supplemented with omega-3 fatty acids, along with the amino acid arginine and oral RNA.[7] The patients on the supplemented diet developed 70% fewer infections, left the hospital an average of 4 days earlier, and had fewer episodes of postsurgical wound dehiscence and fewer pneumonias than the patients on the standard diet.

Inflammatory conditions as diverse as ulcerative colitis and Crohn's disease,[8] rheumatoid arthritis (RA),[9,10,11] systemic lupus erythematosus (SLE),[12] psoriasis,[13] asthma,[14] and eczema[15,16] have been found in studies to respond to omega-3 fatty acid supplementation. There is some evidence that supplementing GLA has antiinflammatory effects, probably by its encouragement of PGE1 production.[17] In studies, eczema,[18] Sjögren's syndrome,[19] and RA,[20] among other inflammatory illnesses, have been treated successfully with oral GLA.

## Zinc

Zinc does not have specific antiinflammatory properties, but it is a required cofactor for almost 200 enzymes, including the critical antioxidant enzyme superoxide dismutase (SOD). SOD is the most important enzyme used by the cells to convert superoxide free radicals (generated as part of the inflammatory process) into hydrogen peroxide and then, through the action of another enzyme, catalase, into oxygen and water. SOD comes in two forms, the mitochondrial form, which is manganese dependent, and the cytoplasmic form, which is dependent on both zinc and copper.

Zinc is necessary for proper immune system function.[21] Some studies have suggested that this might be more of a factor in older persons, who are prone to zinc deficiency.[22]

## Vitamin C

Ascorbic acid, or vitamin C, is particularly critical to the collagen production phase of healing. However, there are few aspects of physiology that do not involve this ubiquitous nutrient in some form. Vitamin C does not possess antiinflammatory activity directly, but it has antihistamine activity, is an antiviral agent,[23] and can both prevent and treat infection.

One of the most important roles of vitamin C is as an antioxidant, and its most important antioxidant function may be to protect the body from harmful low-density lipoprotein (LDL) cholesterol. However, it also prevents harmful oxidation damage to tissues in the event of injury, and it prevents the breakdown of vitamin E, another antioxidant. In addition, vitamin C seems to improve nitric oxide activity, thus providing for the dilation of blood vessels and improved capillary flow into an injured area.

## Bromelain

Several mechanisms have been proposed for the wound-healing and antiinflammatory properties of proteolytic enzymes. Part of the inflammatory process involves the deposition of fibrin, which loculates the area of inflammation and promotes swelling and localized destruction of tissue. Proteolytic enzymes have fibrinolytic activity. This allows better circulation into the area of inflammation, improved removal of necrotic and inflammatory tissue, and increased tissue levels of medications such as antibiotics.

In one experimental double-blind study[24] of 80 patients undergoing tooth extraction, the group taking oral enzymes maintained statistically significantly better health and experienced less swelling and pain than a similar placebo group. Other studies have demonstrated reduced swelling, bruising, and pain in women receiving episiotomies.[25,26] The antiinflammatory effects of bromelain have been suggested in preliminary studies of its effect on RA.[27] A double-blind study of urinary tract infections treated by antibiotics plus either placebo or proteolytic enzymes showed that the enzyme-treated group reduced symptoms more than twice as successfully as those treated by antibiotics alone.[28] Double-blind studies of sinusitis patients showed similar success in the bromelain-treated patients vs. placebo, particularly when combined with antibiotics.[29] In an animal study, the combination of proteolytic enzymes, flavonoids, and vitamin C were superior to seven NSAIDs in experimentally induced inflammation.[30]

The use of bromelain and other proteolytic enzymes in trauma has been well documented. In one experimental double-blind study[31] following blunt wounds to the soft tissue with distortion of the ankle joint from sports injuries, ice and tape were applied to all study participants, but one group received hydrolytic enzymes while the other received placebo.

Recovery was better in the enzyme-treated group. The time during which the patients were unable to work or train was reduced by about 50%, a statistically significant difference, by enzyme therapy (see Case Study). Other double-blind and observational studies have yielded similar results,[32] including studies of injury healing in boxers, karate fighters,[33] and other athletes.[34]

 *A Case Study*

### Multiple Sclerosis

A 48-year-old patient is wheelchair bound with multiple sclerosis and has a variety of medical problems, including gastrointestinal reflux disease (GERD). She is generally unable to take NSAIDs of any kind. She suffers a hip fracture.

Postoperatively the patient is placed on a proprietary combination of nutrients and bromelain. Her medication includes bromelain 200 mg in a time-released formula; the enzymes trypsin, chymotrypsin, papain, and pepsin; vitamin C 500 mg; manganese 150 mg; calcium aspartate 150 mg; magnesium aspartate 75 mg; zinc aspartate 75 mg; B complex 50 mg; bioflavonoids 350 mg; glucosamine sulfate 125 mg; and a base of herbs (valerian, passionflower) that are known for their relaxing properties.

Despite her inability to easily move and exercise, she heals well from her surgery, and there is little pain and no inflammation. Her orthopedist comments on the rapidity with which she heals from this potentially serious injury and surgical repair.

Some clinical trials have looked directly at the ability of bromelain to decrease platelet stickiness, which may account for its suggested positive effects in angina and in thrombophlebitis.[35] This blood-thinning activity also mandates that bromelain and similar enzymes not be given presurgically and that they be used with caution when combined with other blood thinners. Proteolytic enzymes also have a mucolytic effect, suggesting a positive effect in chronic bronchitis. ❧

## Flavonoids

Bioflavonoids are polyphenols, aromatic compounds in plants that give them their rich variety of colors, smells, and tastes. Among their many functions are antioxidant activity and protection of collagen and hyaluronan in connective tissue. Bioflavonoids have antiinflammatory activity, probably through their in-

hibition of enzymes involved in arachidonic acid metabolism. Certain bioflavonoids can slow leukocyte infiltration into the site of inflammation. Lipoxygenases are inhibited by quercetin, a flavonoid that has been well studied for its profound range of activities.

In an experimental double-blind study,[36] 48 football players randomly received either 600 mg citrus bioflavonoids before lunch and 300 mg before suit-up time or placebo. In the treated group, there was significant improvement in recovery time and a decrease in the number of sprains and injuries overall. Similar studies have been performed on baseball players and other athletes. Flavonoids will be discussed later in greater detail with regard to their varied effects on capillary and wound strengthening and their antioxidant properties.

## Capsaicin

Capsaicin is the main ingredient in several herbs with antiinflammatory properties, including cayenne pepper *(Capsicum annum)*, ginger *(Zingiber officinale)*, and turmeric *(Curcuma longa)*. Capsaicin has been demonstrated in vitro to block cyclooxygenase activity, thereby inhibiting prostaglandin synthesis. It lowers histamine levels and possibly stimulates the natural production of cortisol by the adrenal gland, thus enhancing the body's stress response. It has also been studied for its pain control uses because it selectively depletes the neuropeptide substance P in superficial nerves that transmit pain. Because substance P is one of the primary neurotransmitters of the pain mechanism, capsaicin-containing substances are currently being used in postherpetic neuralgia and other pain syndromes.

In one double-blind controlled study of 252 patients with diabetic neuropathy,[37,38] pain intensity and pain relief were both statistically improved with topical capsaicin over a placebo cream. A meta-analysis of capsaicin cream studies showed statistically significant improvement in osteoarthritis[39] and psoriasis,[40] among other inflammatory conditions. In a Phase-III placebo-controlled study of 99 postsurgical cancer patients with neuropathic pain,[41] capsaicin cream decreased pain and was preferred by patients.

## Turmeric/Curcumin

Ginger and turmeric have other antiinflammatory activity, separate from their content of capsaicin. Both inhibit lipoxygenase and cyclooxygenase, presumably decreasing the release of proinflammatory leukotrienes. Turmeric in particular has a long folk history of use in inflammatory conditions, particularly in the indigenous form of Indian medicine known as Ayurveda. This substance, also known as curcumin, interferes with the incorporation of arachidonic acid into platelet phospholipids, thereby reducing its availability for the production of proinflammatory messengers. Unlike NSAIDs, curcumin-containing substances are not known to cause gastritis or ulcerations.

One double-blind study of curcumin vs. the antiinflammatory agent phenylbutazone[42] showed significantly less pain and tenderness after hernia and hydrocele surgery, but another similar study was not as definitive. While clinical studies of turmeric/curcumin are generally lacking in the literature, laboratory studies are supportive of its antiinflammatory activity, and the historical uses are well documented.

## Echinacea

Echinacea is not known to have antiinflammatory activity, but its use as an antimicrobial agent and immunomodulator has been well documented. In vitro, echinacea has been shown to stimulate natural killer cell activity, and it may increase antibody-dependent cell cytotoxicity as well.

While studies of the effects of echinacea on viruses, including the common cold, have varied in reliability and efficacy, the preponderance of evidence supports its use in viral illnesses. One recent meta-analysis of studies on the prevention and treatment of the common cold, encompassing 16 good clinical trials and 3,396 patients, concluded that, based on available evidence, echinacea preparations generally show more positive effects than placebo and may be more effective.

## Boswellia

Another herb used commonly in Indian medicine is boswellia, derived from the *Boswellia serrata* tree. The boswellic acids, which are the active ingredients of this resin, inhibit 5-lipoxygenase, thereby interfering with leukotriene synthesis. These acids also have been shown in vitro to interfere with the complement system, thereby slowing an important step in the inflammatory process.

Controlled, double-blind studies have suggested an antiinflammatory role for boswellia extracts in ulcerative colitis[43] and in both RA[44] and degenerative arthritis.

## White Willow, Meadowsweet, and Nettle

Several herbs are known to have natural antiinflammatory activity similar to aspirin. In fact, aspirin was first synthesized from white willow bark *(Salix alba),* which contains high levels of the glycoside salicin. Salicin is converted into the antiinflammatory salicylic acid, which is pharmacologically close to aspirin (acetylsalicylic acid). The actions of white willow are similar to aspirin, though milder and more long lasting. Clinical studies support the use of white willow in osteoarthritis. In one double-blind study of 82 arthritic subjects,[45] a proprietary herbal combination with white willow as the chief ingredient was significantly more effective than placebo in lowering pain. Another herb with similar constituents is meadowsweet *(Filipendula ulmaria).* The effects of meadowsweet are reported to be similar to those of white willow, although milder. There are no reliable clinical studies of meadowsweet, however.

Nettle, or stinging nettles *(Urtica dioica),* is another herb that seems to have antiinflammatory activity. This appears to be due to a direct effect on prostaglandin synthesis from one or more components of the nettle leaf. Clinically, nettle has been studied in double-blind studies for its antiinflammatory effect in allergic rhinitis[46] and in prostate problems.[47]

# CONNECTIVE TISSUE REPAIR

## Amino Acids

Collagen consists of long chains of amino acids, particularly glycine, proline, hydroxyproline, and hydroxylysine. The latter two are produced by a process called hydroxylation in the presence of a reducing agent such as ascorbic acid (vitamin C) that requires alpha-ketoglutarate or another substrate.[48] Because research suggests that hydroxyproline and hydroxylysine are incorporated into collagen through this hydroxylation reaction, it has been suggested that providing the necessary amino acids, alpha-ketoglutarate, and vitamin

C would improve collagen synthesis. There is some clinical evidence of this. Other evidence demonstrates that wound healing is impaired in protein-deficient patients.

In a study that evaluated three groups undergoing total hip replacement,[49] 13 postsurgical subjects were given either intravenous glucose, glucose and L-glutamine, or glucose plus a combination of L-glutamine and alpha-ketoglutarate during and after surgery. Protein synthesis was greater and there was less wasting of muscle tissue in the groups with L-glutamine, particularly the group which also included alpha ketoglutarate.

L-Glutamine has been particularly studied for its effects on healing. It is the most abundant free amino acid in skeletal muscle, a component of glutathione production and the prime source of nutritional fuel for the small intestinal mucosa, thus conserving glucose in the body for its use in energy production elsewhere.

After surgery, sepsis, and trauma, circulating concentrations of glutamine are reduced despite the release of this amino acid from skeletal muscle and other tissues and the increased kidney uptake. Among the other positive effects of L-glutamine supplementation after injury or surgery is the protection of the intestinal mucosa from peptic ulcers and a protective effect against aspirin-induced gastric ulceration. Studies have demonstrated the safety and potential benefits of glutamine supplementation in nutritional support of surgical patients. Glutamine supplementation in total parenteral nutrition solutions improves nitrogen balance and reduces skeletal muscle glutamine loss in patients undergoing elective cholecystectomy or colon or rectum resection for cancer.

L-Arginine is another *conditionally essential* component of the diet of healthy individuals, but there is evidence that the stresses of rehabilitation create an increased need for this amino acid.[50] L-Arginine seems to stimulate pituitary release of growth hormone and prolactin and the pancreatic release of insulin. Supplemental arginine has been shown to improve weight gain, nitrogen retention, and wound healing in various situations.[51] In animal models, supplementary arginine caused an increase in thymic weight and reduction of postinjury thymic shrinking. Supplementing the diet with arginine has led to enhanced T lymphocyte activity, less host skin graft rejection, improved survival and immune response after severe burn injury, and improved survival after experimentally induced peritonitis. In addition, it has resulted in better postoperative lymphocyte responses to mitogens than seen with unsupplemented diets in cancer patients undergoing major surgery.

Other amino acids that have been shown to impact wound healing include the sulfur-containing amino acids methionine and cystine, as well as carnosine and histidine.

## Zinc

Zinc is commonly used topically on the body. One familiar available form is calamine lotion, a topical antiinflammatory. The use of topical zinc is as common today as it was over 4,000 years ago in ancient Egypt. Many studies have looked at the effects of topical zinc compounds on wound healing, pressure ulcers, and vascular sores.

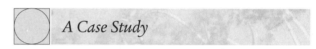

*A Case Study*

*Stasis Ulcers*

A 78-year-old nursing home patient had a 1-inch venous stasis ulcer that had persisted for 3 months. The ulcer had been treated with topical and systemic antibiotics and with an Unna boot but still had not formed good granulation tissue. An assessment of the patient's diet revealed that it consisted largely of white bread, rice, cereal, soda, and an occasional cheese sandwich. Because it is known that zinc is deficient in over 33% of older persons, zinc deficiency was determined to be a factor in the lack of healing.

The patient was placed on zinc picolinate, a particularly absorbable form of zinc, at 30 mg twice daily. The patient was also given vitamin C 500 mg daily, and a multivitamin that contained an additional 10 mg of zinc. The ulcer was debrided, cleaned, and covered with zinc oxide ointment daily. Within 10 days, granulation tissue began to appear, and the wound was totally closed within 6 weeks. ❧

In several studies, topical zinc oxide has resulted in reduced inflammation and infection, as well as improvement in the growth of new epithelial cells in leg ulcers.[52,53] Interestingly, this response has not been duplicated when zinc sulfate is used. There is some evidence that zinc levels are decreased in patients with chronic vascular ulcers.[54] In those patients with documented zinc deficiency, supplementation seems to improve healing. Zinc nutrition has profound implications for wound healing, skin integrity, and proper immune function.[55]

## Copper, Manganese, and Other Minerals

Copper is a cofactor for the action of lysyl amine oxidase in the aldehyde reactions, which generate strong covalent bonds in collagen, creating the cross-linking of connective tissue. Along with zinc, it also is a necessary factor for the proper function of the antioxidant enzyme SOD in the cytoplasm.

Copper is commonly used in folk medicine to improve joint function and lessen pain in arthritis and to increase flexibility. Copper bracelets have been widely used for centuries. There is little clinical evidence, however, that copper supplementation leads to these specific effects.

Manganese is necessary for the glycosylation of hydroxyproline during the formation of collagen. It is the cofactor for the mitochondrial form of the antioxidant enzyme superoxide dismutase and is commonly used empirically to assist in the repair of wounds and injuries, although to date this has not been investigated in controlled studies.

Iron is also required for proper hydroxylation of proline and lysine in the production of collagen. However, this mineral may be more important for its oxygen-carrying role in the formation of erythrocytes and its resultant effects on the proper function of the immune system. Molybdenum and silicon are also involved in connective tissue metabolism.

## Vitamin C (Ascorbic Acid)

The ascorbic acid (AA) relationship to healing is based on the old concept of asymptomatic scurvy. Adequate tissue levels of AA would seem to be required for collagen fiber production, and deficiency of AA will both delay wound healing and produce a weaker collagen matrix. This is because, along with iron and alpha-ketoglutarate, AA is necessary for the hydroxylation of proline and lysine to form hydroxyproline, thus enhancing the cross-linking structure of connective tissue. AA also is necessary for adequate angiogenesis of

healing tissue, and its deficiency leads to weakened capillaries.

A number of studies have looked at specific effects of AA on collagen and elastin formation. In one laboratory study,[56] collagen formation increased by a factor of 8 when vitamin C was introduced. In another, vitamin C was decreased in the diet, leading to deficiency and to delayed wound healing.[57]

Studies of AA on pressure sore healing have shown mixed results, and its effects in these situations may be related to the preexisting concentration of vitamin C in the tissues because measurably lower AA tissue levels lead to decreased healing of skin ulcers.

There is also a suggestion that concurrent nutrients are important in the success of AA in treating wound healing. For example, pantothenic acid and vitamin C together increased tensile strength of wounds in patients healing from tattoo removal, and the results were dose dependent.[58]

AA levels decrease sharply in response to stress, as demonstrated in a number of studies. There is some evidence that AA in levels significantly greater than the RDA can support adrenal function and decrease high cortisol levels. In one study, vitamin C prevented adrenocorticotropic hormone (ACTH)-stimulated increases in cortisol, while in another, AA with vitamins $B_1$ and $B_6$ intravenously improved the glucocorticoid function of the adrenal gland.

## Vitamin A

Vitamin A seems to increase collagen synthesis, thereby strengthening scar tissue. Several animal studies have supported the use of vitamin A in wound healing, particularly in vitamin A–deficient conditions. In one experimental animal study,[59] rats were fed a vitamin A–deficient diet for 2 weeks, then divided into two groups. One group received a diet containing basal amounts of vitamin A while the other received additional vitamin A, both as beta carotene and retinyl acetate. Within 5 days there was demonstrably increased wound tensile strength in the vitamin A group, especially those given beta carotene.

Corticosteroids have a well-known inhibitory effect on the healing of wounds. It appears from a published case report that vitamin A may reverse this effect.[60] Reports have been for both animals and humans.

## Vitamin E

Several animal studies have supported the use of vitamin E in the strengthening of surgical wounds and the lessening of adhesions. In one study,[61] three groups of rats received varying amounts of vitamin E injected into the abdominal cavity, followed by radiation and surgical incision. Increasing levels of vitamin E increased the breaking strength of wounds exposed to preoperative radiation. Other studies have focused on the ability of vitamin E to prevent postsurgical scarring.[62]

There is at least one study in which very high doses of vitamin E inhibited wound healing,[63] a finding that was reversed with the concurrent addition of vitamin A. Although vitamin E is traditionally used both topically and internally for burns and topically for wound healing and scar reduction, there is currently no clinical study that has looked at this convincingly.

## Glucosamine/Chondroitin

Glycosaminoglycans (GAG) are mucopolysaccharides, long chain polymers of repeating disaccharide units. These GAGs form proteoglycans (PGs), which are major constituents of cartilage. They allow circulation of nutrients and fluids through the tissue while providing its structure. GAGs, in turn, are made up of smaller mucopolysaccharides called glucosamine sulfate (GS) and larger mucopolysaccharides called chondroitin sulfate (CS).

There is considerable research support for the use of glucosamine sulfate in osteoarthritis[64,65] and some support for the use of chondroitin sulfate as well,[66] although the absorption of this large molecule may be difficult. Injectable chondroitin, on the other hand, has been used worldwide to treat athletic injuries and joint degeneration.

Wound healing seems to be accelerated by the use of cartilage preparations that contain GS and CS, or treatment by these supplements directly. Many experimental and animal studies support this finding, and several controlled human studies are currently underway. Cartilage preparations are usually extracted from bovine sources, although shark and poultry are also used.

There is also some support for cartilage powder used topically on open wounds. In one experimental controlled study,[67] 15 volunteers had two skin incisions, one treated with a finely ground acid-pepsin digested calf tracheal cartilage powder, the other left alone. After the wounds were healed, tensile strength was measured and found to be increased in the treated wounds an average of 45% over the control group. There is some suggestion that polymers of *N*-acetylglucosamine, a type of GS, are contained in the cartilage preparations and promote wound healing.

## Arnica/Traumeel

Homeopathy is a 200-year-old system of medicine that uses minute doses of natural substances to deliver an "energy" message to tissue, encouraging healing and balance. One of the most common homeopathic medications is *Arnica montana,* which is used in both acute and chronic injuries.

There are a number of interesting studies recently that have looked at the efficacy of homeopathic medicines. Two recent meta-analyses of these studies have found positive results in over 70% of the studies.[68,69]

Preparations containing homeopathic arnica have been tested in a variety of circumstances related to injuries. While the definitive study has by no means been conceived as yet, there are some intriguing findings in existing studies. In one controlled double-blind study involving 69 subjects with acute ankle injuries, the group using the arnica preparation Traumeel had a reduction of pain in 28 of 33 participants, vs. 13 of 36 participants in the placebo group.[70]

## Aloe Vera

The gel of this long-leaf plant has been used in many cultures for sunburns and other minor injuries. Latex is gotten from the aloe plant by allowing the cut leaves to dry. This latex contains glycosides that have been shown to have antiinflammatory and wound healing effects. There is also some indication that aloe latex might be antibacterial.

In rat studies, aloe vera has shown uses both topically and orally to lessen inflammation and accelerate wound healing.[71] This finding has not been repeated in humans, however. There have been positive findings in double-blind placebo controlled studies of aloe topically in psoriasis,[72] but there were negative findings in a similar study of radiation burns,[73] although earlier case reports suggested that aloe could be helpful with burns.

## Other Topical Herbs

Several other studies have suggested uses for various herbal creams and ointments. One German study of sea buckthorn ointment (Olei Hippopheae) suggested a positive effect on wound healing.[74] Another, employing an ointment of the herb echinacea, demonstrated an increased healing of skin lesions.

A double-blind study employing the herb gotu kola (Centella asiatica)[75] both topically and orally concluded this treatment to be "of clinical value in stopping the inflammatory phase of hypertrophic scars and keloids . . . a preventive effect on burns and postoperative hypertrophic scars" and that it gave "more lasting results than intralesional cortisone or radiation therapy." Gotu kola has uses in rehabilitation medicine as well. The triterpenoids, or saponins, contained in this Asian herb have specific effects on collagen, including the promotion of GAG formation and the inhibition of hyperactive scar tissue. One uncontrolled study suggested that gotu kola promotes the healing of infected wounds, while other double-blind studies support its use in chronic venous insufficiency.

## Sugar/Honey

Several studies of wound healing support the use of a natural substance that may not be an herb, or even a food, at all. Granulated sugar has been used successfully to debride infected wounds and to promote granulation of tissue.[76,77] Honey, as well, has its proponents in wound healing. Raw honey has been used for centuries to prevent infection in open burn wounds and to enable healing in stasis ulcers.

## PAIN CONTROL

It should be noted that much information exists about the use of natural medicines and nutrients in pain relief, although it is beyond the scope of this chapter to cover this topic in depth. Magnesium is necessary for both muscle and nerve relaxation, and its deficiency has been associated with both chronic and acute pain,[78] as well as muscle spasm. Likewise, calcium supplementation can be useful in chronic pain conditions.

The amino acid, DL-phenylalanine, while not strictly a natural medicine (the D-forms of amino acids are not found in nature), has been studied for its uses in chronic pain.[79] Other treatments for pain, previously mentioned, include topical capsaicin, ginger, bromelain, EFAs, and white willow.

## RELAXATION AND ENERGY ENHANCEMENT

Several herbs are used for their relaxing and hypnotic properties. Passionflower (Passiflora incarnata), hops (Humulus lupulus), melissa (Melissa officinalis), and valerian (Valeriana officinalis) are all used as sedatives in natural medicine, either alone or in combination. Kava (Piper methysticum) is useful in anxiety states and has been found to be superior to placebo in some studies.[80] Magnesium and several amino acids, including tyrosine, taurine and tryptophan, are also useful in relaxation.

Natural energy enhancement is a lengthy topic, and many uses involve a group of botanicals that have adaptogenic activity. In other words, they enable the adrenal gland and stress-response organs to adapt to stresses without exhausting reserves to the same extent. The herbs that have been studied for this activity include ginseng, both Korean ginseng (Panax ginseng) and Siberian ginseng (Eleutherococcus sinensis), licorice (Glycyrrhiza glabra), gotu kola (Centella asiatica), astragalus (Astragalus membranaceus), and schisandra (Schisandra chinensis). Mushrooms, including reishi, shiitake, and maitake, also seem to have this effect, and ginkgo biloba has been studied extensively for its positive effects on circulation and respiration.

Finally, it is critical not to discount the beneficial effects of a healthy diet on both energy and the healing process. Although there are many popular diets with radically different principles, general recommendations include eating a diet free of additives and preservatives. A healthy diet is rich in fruits, vegetables, lean protein, and whole grains. In addition, it is best to avoid a diet with saturated fats, fried foods, sugar, and white flour.

## References

1. Koval KJ, Maurer SG, Su ET, et al: The effects of nutritional status on outcome after hip fracture, *J Orthop Trauma* 13(3):164-169, 1999.
2. Thomas DR: Specific nutritional factors in wound healing, *Adv Wound Care* 10(4):40-43, 1997.
3. Shenkin A: Micronutrients and outcome, *Nutrition* 13(9):825-828, 1997.
4. Meydani SN: Effect of (n-3) polyunsaturated fatty acids on cytokine production and their biologic function, *Nutrition* 12:S8-S14, 1996.
5. Kremer JM, Lawrence DA, Petrillo GF, et al: Effects of high dose fish oil on rheumatoid arthritis after stopping non-steroidal anti-inflammatory drugs, *Arthritis Rheum* 38(8):1107-1114, 1995.
6. Meydani M, Natiello F, Goldin B, et al: Effect of long-term fish oil supplementation on vitamin E status and lipid peroxidation in women, *J Nutr* 121:484-491, 1991.
7. Daly JM: Enteral nutrition with supplemental arginine, RNA, and omega-3 fatty acids in patients after operation: immunologic, metabolic and clinical outcome, *Surgery* 112(1):56-57, 1992.
8. Mate J, Castanos R, Garcia-Samaniego J, et al: Does dietary fish oil maintain the remission of Crohn's disease: a case control study, *Gastroenterology* 100:A228, 1991 (abstract).
9. Geusens P, Wouters C, Nijs J, et al: Long-term effect of omega-3 fatty acid supplementation in active rheumatoid arthritis, *Arthritis Rheum* 37:824-829, 1994.
10. van der Tempel H, Tulleken JE, Limburg PC, et al: Effects of fish oil supplementation in rheumatoid arthritis, *Ann Rheum Dis* 49:76-80, 1990.
11. Kremer JM, Lawrence DA, Petrillo GF, et al: Effects of high-dose fish oil on rheumatoid arthritis after stopping nonsteroidal anti-inflammatory drugs, *Arthritis Rheum* 38:1107-1114, 1995.
12. Westberg G, Tarkowski A: Effect of MaxEPA in patients with SLE: a double-blind, crossover study, *Scand J Rheumatol* 19(2):137-143, 1990.
13. Kojima T, Ternao T, Tanabe E, et al: Long-term administration of highly purified eicosapentaenoic acid provides improvement of psoriasis, *Dermatologica* 182:225-230, 1991.
14. Arm JP, Horton CE, Eiser NM, et al: The effects of dietary supplementation with fish oil on asthmatic responses to antigen, *Allerg Clin Immunol* 81:183, 1988 (abstract #57).
15. Bjornboe A, Soyland E, Bjorneboe GE, et al: Effect of dietary supplementation with eicosapentaenoic acid in the treatment of atopic dermatitis, *Br J Dermatol* 117(4):463-469, 1987.
16. Bjornboe A, Soyland E, Bjornboe GE, et al: Effect of n-3 fatty acid supplement to patients with atopic dermatitis, *J Intern Med Suppl* 225(731):233-236, 1989.
17. Horrobin DF: The importance of gamma-linolenic acid and prostaglandin E1 in human nutrition and medicine, *J Holistic Med* 3:118-139, 1981.
18. Schalin-Karrila M, Mattila L, Jansen CT, et al: Evening primrose oil in the treatment of atopic eczema: effect on clinical status, plasma phospholipid fatty acids and circulating blood prostaglandins, *Br J Dermatol* 117:11-19, 1987.
19. Horrobin DF: Essential fatty acid metabolism in diseases of connective tissue with special reference to scleroderma and to Sjögren's syndrome, *Med Hypotheses* 14(3):233-247, 1984.
20. Joe LA, Hart LL: Evening primrose oil in rheumatoid arthritis, *Ann Pharmacother* 27:1475-1477, 1993 (review).
21. Fraker PJ, Gershwin ME, Good RA, et al: Interrelationships between zinc and immune function, *Fed Proc* 4:1474-1479, 1986.
22. Girodon F, Lombard M, Galan P, et al: Effect of micronutrient supplementation on infection in institutionalized elderly subjects: a controlled trial, *Ann Nutr Metab* 41:98-107, 1997.
23. Gerber WF et al: Effect of ascorbic acid, sodium salicylate, and caffeine on the serum interferon level in response to viral infection, *Pharmacology* 13:228, 1975.
24. Vinzenz K: Edema therapy in dental interventions with hydrolytic enzymes, *Quintessenz* 42(7):1053-1064, 1991 (German).
25. Howat RCL, Lewis GD: The effect of bromelain therapy on episiotomy wounds: a double blind controlled clinical trial, *J Obstet Gynaecol Br Commonwealth* 79:951-953, 1972.
26. Zatuchni GI, Colombi DJ: Bromelain therapy for the prevention of episiotomy pain, *Obstet Gynecol* 29:275-278, 1967.
27. Cohen A, Goldman J: Bromelain therapy in rheumatoid arthritis, *Pa Med* 67:27-30, 1964.
28. Mori S, Ojima Y, Hirose T, et al: The clinical effect of proteolytic enzyme containing bromelain and trypsin on urinary tract infection evaluated by double blind method, *Acta Obstet Gynaecol Jpn* 19(3):147-153, 1972.
29. Ryan RE: A double-blind clinical evaluation of bromelain in the treatment of acute sinusitis, *Headache* 7:13-17, 1967.
30. Tarayre JP, Lauresserguess H: Advantages of a combination of proteolytic enzymes and ascorbic acid in comparison with non-steroid anti-inflammatory agents, *Drug Res* 27(6):1144-1449, 1977.
31. Baumuller M: Therapy of ankle joint distortions with hydrolytic enzymes: results of double-blind clinical trials. In Hermans GPH, Mosterd WL (eds): *Sports, medicine and health,* Amsterdam, Excerpta Medica, 1990, p 1137.
32. Rathgeber WF: The use of proteolytic enzymes (Chymoral) in sporting injuries, *S Afr Med J* 45(7):181-183, 1971.

33. Zuschlag JM: *Double-blind clinical study using certain proteolytic enzyme mixtures in karate fighters,* Geretsried, Germany, Mucos Pharma 1988, pp 1-5 (working paper).

34. Masson M: Bromelain in the treatment of blunt injuries to the musculoskeletal system: a case observation study by an orthopedic surgeon in private practice, *Fortschr Med* 113(19):303-306, 1995.

35. Seligman B: Oral bromelains as adjuncts in the treatment of acute thrombophlebitis, *Angiology* 20:22-26, 1969.

36. Broussard MU: Evaluation of citrus bioflavonoids in contact sports, *Citrus in Med* 2(2), 1963.

37. Capsaicin study group: Treatment of painful diabetic neuropathy with topical capsaicin: a multicenter, double-blind, vehicle-controlled study, *Arch Int Med* 151: 2225-2229, 1991.

38. Capsaicin study group: Effect of treatment with capsaicin on daily activities of patients with painful diabetic neuropathy, *Diabet Care* 15:159-165, 1992.

39. McCarthy GM, McCarty DJ: Effect of topical capsaicin in the therapy of painful osteoarthritis of the hands, *J Rheumatol* 19:604-607, 1992.

40. Bernstein JE, Parish LC, Rapaport M, et al: Effects on topically applied capsaicin on moderate and severe psoriasis vulgaris, *J Am Acad Dermatol* 15:504-507, 1986.

41. Ellison N, Loprinzi CL, Kugler J, et al: Phase III placebo-controlled trial of capsaicin cream in the management of surgical neuropathic pain in cancer patients, *J Clin Oncol* 15:2974-2980, 1997.

42. Satoskar RR, Shah SJ, Shenoy SG: Evaluation of anti-inflammatory property of curcumin (diferuloyl methane) in patients with postoperative inflammation, *Int J Clin Pharmacol Ther Toxicol* 24:651-654, 1986.

43. Gupta I, Parihar A, Malhotra P, et al: Effects of *Boswellia serrata* gum resin in patients with ulcerative colitis, *Eur J Med Res* 2:37-43, 1997.

44. Etzel R: Special extract of *Boswellia serrata* (H15) in the treatment of rheumatoid arthritis, *Phytomedicine* 3:91-94, 1996.

45. Mills SY, Jacoby RK, Chacksfield M, et al: Effect of a proprietary herbal medicine on the relief of chronic arthritic pain: a double-blind study, *Br J Rheumatol* 35:874-878, 1996.

46. Vontobel H, Herzog R, Rutishauser G, et al: Results of a double-blind study on the effectiveness of ERU *(extractum radicis Urticae)* capsules in conservative treatment of benign prostatic hyperplasia, *Urologe* 24(1):49-51, 1985 (German).

47. Mittman P: Randomized, double-blind study of freeze-dried *Urtica dioica* in the treatment of allergic rhinitis, *Planta Med* 56:44-47, 1990.

48. Percival M: Treating injury and supporting musculoskeletal healing, *Appl Nutr Sci Res* 2000.

49. Blomqvist B et al: Glutamine and ketoglutarate prevent the decrease in muscle free glutamine concentration and influence protein synthesis after total hip replacement, *Metabolism* 44(9):1215-1222, 1995.

50. Dudrick PS, Souba WW: Amino acids and surgical nutrition: principles and practice *Surg Clin North Am* 71(3):459-476, 1991.

51. Kirk SJ, Hurson M, Regan MC, et al: Arginine stimulates wound healing and immune function in elderly human beings, *Surgery* 114:155-160, 1993.

52. Agren MS: Studies on zinc in wound healing, *Acta Derm Venereol Suppl* 154:1-36, 1990 (review).

53. Liszewski RF: The effect of zinc on wound healing: a collective review, *J Am Osteopath Assoc* 81:104-106, 1981 (review).

54. Hallböök T, Lanner E: Serum-zinc and healing of venous leg ulcers, *Lancet* 2(7781):780-782, 1972.

55. Young B, Ott L, Kasarskis E, et al: Zinc supplementation is associated with improved neurologic recovery rate and visceral protein levels of patients with severe closed head injury, *J Neurotrauma* 13:25-34, 1996.

56. Murad S et al: Regulation of collagen synthesis by ascorbic acid, *Proc Natl Acad Sci USA* 78(5):2879-2882, 1981.

57. Schwartz PL: Ascorbic acid in wound healing: a review, *J Am Diet Assoc* 56(6):497-503, 1970.

58. Vaxman F, Olender S, Lambert A, et al: Effect of pantothenic acid and ascorbic acid supplementation on human skin wound healing process: a double-blind, prospective and randomized trial, *Eur Surg Res* 27:158-166, 1995.

59. Gerber LE, Erdman JW Jr: Wound healing in rats fed small supplements of retinyl acetate, beta-carotene or retinoic acid, *Fed Proc* 3453:838, 1981.

60. Hunt TK et al: Effect of vitamin A on reversing the inhibitory effect of cortisone on healing of open wounds in animals and man, *Ann Surg* 170(2):203-206, 1969.

61. Taren DL et al: Increasing the breaking strength of wounds exposed to pre-operative irradiation using vitamin E supplementation, *Int J Vitam Nutr Res* 57:133-137, 1987.

62. Ehrlich H, Tarver H, Hunt T: Inhibitory effects of vitamin E on collagen synthesis and wound repair, *Ann Surg* 175:235-240, 1972.

63. Rucker RB, Kosonen T, Clegg MS, et al: Copper lysyl oxidase, and extracellular matrix protein cross-linking, *Am J Clin Nutr* 67(5 Suppl):996s-1002s, 1998.

64. Drovanti A: Therapeutic activity of oral glucosamine sulfate in osteoarthritis: a placebo-controlled double-blind investigation, *Clin Ther* 3:260, 1980.

65. Noack W, Fischer M, Forster KK, et al: Glucosamine sulfate in osteoarthritis of the knee, *Osteoarthritis Cartilage* 2:51-59, 1994.

66. Bourgeois P: Efficacy and tolerability of chondroitin sulfate 1200 mg/day vs chondrolitin sulfate 3 × 400 mg per day vs placebo, *Osteoarthritis Cartilage* 6:25, 1998.

67. Prudden JF, Allen J: The clinical acceleration of healing with a cartilage preparation: a controlled study, *JAMA* 192:352-356, 1965.

68. Linde K, Clausius N, Ramirez G, et al: Are the clinical effects of homeopathy placebo effects? A meta-analysis of placebo-controlled trials, *Lancet* 250:834-843, 1997.

69. Kleijnen J, Knipschild P, ter Riet G: Clinical trials of homeopathy, *Br Med J* 302:316-323, 1991.

70. Zell J, Connert WD, Mau J, et al: Treatment of acute sprains of the ankle joint: double-blind study assessing the effectiveness of a homeopathic ointment preparation, *Biol Ther* 7(1):1-6, 1989.

71. Davis RH, Leitner MG, Russo JM, et al: Wound healing: oral and topical activity of aloe vera, *J Am Podiatr Med Assoc* 79(11):559-562, 1989.

72. Syed TA, Ahmad SA, Holt AH, et al: Management of psoriasis with aloe vera extract in a hydrophilic cream: a placebo-controlled double blind study, *Trop Med Int Health* 1:505-509, 1996.

73. Williams MS, Burk M, Loprinzi CL, et al: Phase III double blind evaluation of an aloe vera gel as a prophylactic agent for radiation-induced skin toxicity, *Int J Radiat Oncol Biol Phys* 36:345-349, 1996.

74. Ianev E, Radev S, Balutsov M, et al: The effect of an extract of sea buckthorn (*Hippophae rhamnoides* L.) on the healing of experimental skin wounds in rats, *Khirurgiia* 48(3):30-33, 1995 (Bulgarian).

75. Bosse JP, Papillon J, Frenette G, et al: Clinical study of a new antikeloid drug, *Ann Plas Surg* 3:13-21, 1979.

76. Trouillet JL et al: Use of granulated sugar in treatment of open mediastinitis after cardiac surgery, *Lancet* 2(8448):180-184, 1985.

77. Chirife J, Scarmatto G, Herszage L: Scientific basis for the use of granulated sugar in the treatment of infected wounds, *Lancet* 1(8271):560-561, 1982.

78. Bilbey DL, Prabhakaran VM: Muscle cramps and magnesium deficiency: case reports, *Can Fam Phys* 42:1348-1351, 1996.

79. Budd K: Use of D-phenylalanine, an enkephalinase inhibitor, in the treatment of intractable pain, *Adv Pain Res Ther* 5:305-308, 1983.

80. Volz HP, Kieser M: Kava-kava extract WS 1490 versus placebo in anxiety disorder in a randomized placebo controlled 25-week outpatient trial, *Pharmacopsychiatry* 30:1-5, 1997.

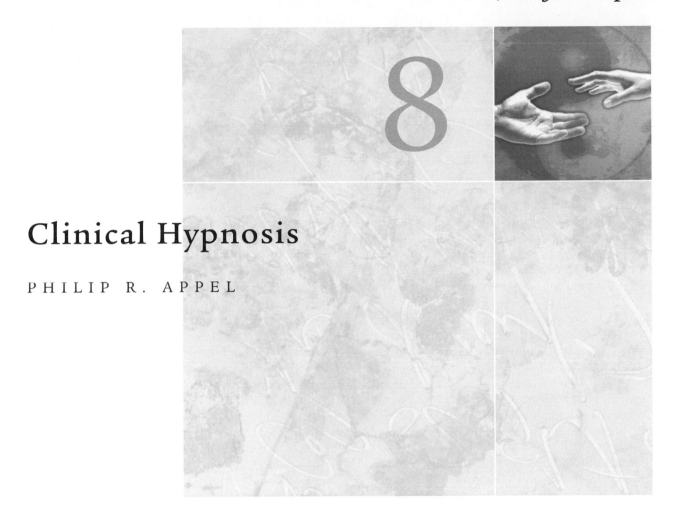

# Clinical Hypnosis

PHILIP R. APPEL

In the late 1960s and early 1970s a revolution was taking place in healthcare. Many healthcare practitioners who had been frustrated with the Newtonian-Cartesian model of medicine and healthcare in the West over the last several hundred years began to embrace what was then called a Holistic Health model. This philosophical approach to healthcare embodied a biopsychosocial perspective and drew on the changes in physics from the classical model to a quantum mechanics perspective in which the body was the densest part of the mind. No longer was there the perception that the mind and body were separate. Instead there was an emphasis on treating the whole person and addressing all the different factors that might facilitate wellness. In many ways, the alternative and complementary medicine movement grew out of this philosophical revolution as healthcare providers looked for ways and modalities to treat their patients instead of just treating their patients' diseases. Understanding patients from a perspective that included looking at their stressors (both internal and external), diet, and health behaviors, as well as seeing how illness was a reflection of an organism's life expression gone awry, became the hallmark of the new revolution in healthcare. James Gordon, author of *Manifesto for a New Medicine,* points out the intimate connection between mind and body and states that humans are fundamentally unique beings along multiple parameters and that every person is really quite different from another.[1]

## MIND-BODY MEDICINE

Mind-body medicine is considered to be one of the five complementary and alternative healthcare domains by

97

the National Center for Complementary and Alternative Medicine. The holistic health revolution had argued for looking at how the mind through cognitive and affective activity could affect the body. Dossey[2] stated that it is clear that human factors can no longer be regarded as peripheral to the causation of disease. Mind-body medicine interventions essentially are interventions designed to facilitate the mind's capacity and ability to affect body functions and symptomatology.

Pelletier wrote about how states of mind affect the health and homeostasis of the body. He stated that mind and body are inextricably linked, and their second-by-second interaction exerts a profound influence on health and illness, life and death.[3] Attitudes, beliefs, and emotional states ranging from love and compassion to fear and anger can trigger chain reactions that affect blood chemistry, heart rate, and the activity of every cell and organ system in the body from the stomach and gastrointestinal tract to the immune system. Physiatrist John Sarno[4] has written extensively how from his point of view that much of illness and chronic pain is the result of a mind-body disorder in which repressed unconscious emotions generate abnormal autonomic activity and spawn neuropeptide activity that then influence the way the body functions.

Many mind-body medicine interventions are about changing consciousness and awareness of self to promote a different way of being, not only mentally and emotionally but physically and even spiritually. Hypnosis, which this chapter is about, has been an important modality for centuries in altering consciousness. Tart[5] defined an altered state of consciousness as follows: "An altered state of consciousness for a given individual is one in which he clearly feels a qualitative shift in his pattern of mental functioning; that is, he feels not just a quantitative shift (more or less alert, more or less visual imagery, shaper or duller, etc.) but

*To change the printout of the body, you must learn to rewrite the software of the mind.* ∾

DEEPAK CHOPRA

also that some quality or qualities of his mental processes are different. Mental functions operate that do not operate at all ordinarily, perceptual qualities appear that have no normal counterparts, and so forth." Clinical hypnosis has allowed individuals to express and experience themselves in different ways in the pursuit of some health goal.

## HYPNOSIS

To date there is little agreement among researchers or clinicians with regard to the nature of hypnosis. The major controversy is whether hypnosis creates an altered state of consciousness or whether suggestion and variables related to social interaction are responsible for the elicited social behavior. One of the more comprehensive theoretical texts on hypnosis presents seven different theoretical models, and it is fascinating how little agreement there is among these models.[6] A possible explanation for the differences in the theoretical frames of reference may be the difference in what is being studied by each of the proponents of the various theories. In general, it appears that the theoretical disagreements are between academic researchers studying hypnotic phenomena unrelated to a clinical situation in a lab with research subjects and clinicians studying the phenomena in clinical situations with patients who by their nature have emotional or physical problems or both. Obviously the groups are studying different phenomena and subjects.

State theorists view hypnosis as an altered state of consciousness and that such cognitive-perceptual states are different from the ordinary waking state. They further believe that there is permeability between those realms of the mind known as conscious and unconscious in a manner that allows for unconscious material to be easily accessible. Barber[7] states that hypnosis is an altered condition or state of consciousness characterized by a markedly increased receptivity to suggestion, the capacity for modification of perception and memory, and the potential for systematic control of a variety of usually involuntary physiological functions (e.g., glandular activity, vasomotor activity).

When we talk about hypnosis and hypnotic behavior it is important to realize that in reality any behavior that can be elicited in a hypnotic trance can also be elicited outside of the trance state as well. Individuals cannot transcend their human condition and initiate behaviors that are not part of the human experience. Thus what makes the hypnotic state different is not the behavior per se, but the experience of the behavior. Often it is the meaning that the behavior has at the time that it is expressed that contributes to the individual experiencing it as unusual. Tart[5] pointed out that individuals have a particular phenomenological experience of a state of mind that is familiar and identified as self. When an individual is in this familiar conditioned state of awareness and processing, the individual thinks of himself or herself in his or her usual state of mind. From my own experience with being hypnotized, and through my observations of hypnotized patients, it appears to me that a hypnotized individual is in an altered state of consciousness. It seems that the hypnotized individual is in a state of mind where there is a high degree of absorption, dissociated cognitive control, a general fading of a reality orientation, a willingness to follow suggestion, and an expectancy of experiencing the suggested goal.

## Some Basic Assumptions

Clinical hypnosis is very much an interpersonal process and a context with demand characteristics that facilitates a change in consciousness of the subject. It is a process and context in which a healthcare provider proffers suggestions designed to alter the attention, concentration, and perception of experience of a patient for the purpose of achieving a change in functioning. As stated earlier in this chapter, from a holistic perspective, each individual is seen as a unique being. As such the clinical task is to find a way of communicating and offering suggestions that will be readily acceptable to the patient given the life experiences that he or she has had and the expectations that he or she may hold. Barber[8] points out that to use hypnosis effectively one must be like a locksmith in that the task is to find the communication strategy and personal suggestions that would help alter the person's consciousness so that a trance state could be created. An example of some beginning suggestions for a hypnotic induction would be the following:

Go ahead right now, and close your eyes . . . allow yourself to become aware of the air going through your nostrils, feel the gentle sensation that the air makes as it goes in and out . . . feel the gentle friction made by the air as it goes through your nasal passages and with each exhalation allow your self to relax into the furniture. Even now as you become aware of the sound of my voice, the sounds both within the office and coming from outside the office . . . you can become more aware of how quiet and still you are, and how with each exhalation you are relaxing more and more. . . . As you feel your body relaxing in the chair, you can become aware of mother earth's gentle pull and you can relax in her gravitational field and allow your body to become heavy and warm. . . . With each exhalation relaxing more and more. . . .

A hypnotic induction is capturing someone's attention, pacing their experience, and leading their concentrated attention in particular ways.

Similar to many practitioners of CAM who believe that healing is integral to the body, most clinicians who use hypnosis to facilitate their treatment regimen believe that their patients have sufficient resources within themselves to accomplish their goals. The clinical task is to help the patient acquire access to those inner resources that will then help the patient achieve his or her goals. An inner resource could be a quality such as wisdom, insight, or courage or a skill such as triggering a relaxation response. The trance state makes it possible for an individual to not only access various cognitive resources and skills but also to behave in a manner that personifies those accessed resources. The hypnotic state can facilitate a state in which the individual acts as if he or she were really thinking and behaving in the suggested manner. The trance state can facilitate the individual's ability to access a state of awareness in which he or she can influence body systems such as the sympathetic nervous system or the cardiovascular system. The behavior of any of the body systems can be potentially influenced by hypnosis. Hypnosis promotes awareness of the process of experiencing and can facilitate internal communication that leads to a change in consciousness. This change in consciousness can in turn lead to a different set of psychophysiological responses.

## The Agent of Change

Promoting changes in microbehaviors (body systems) or macrobehaviors (complex patterns of behaviors involving movements and intended actions) can be accomplished by enhancing awareness of the targeted behavior. Hypnosis is a useful tool for promoting awareness by using suggestion to focus attention and concentration. In many ways hypnosis could be described as an exquisite state of highly concentrated attention, attention so concentrated that nothing else seems to exist except that which is being attended to. In addition, the hypnotic state allows for an individual to become so absorbed and identified with the object of attention that he or she can mentally become like that object. Hypnosis has many uses clinically, whether it is promoting identification with a certain mood state or a particular pattern of macrobehavior or manifesting a certain psychophysiological state.

To accomplish their goals with hypnosis, clinicians will direct the patient's attention and pattern of awareness by giving suggestions that shape and direct the patient's experience. Such suggestions usually consist of directing the patient's attention to aspects of experience such as sensations, imaginings, thoughts, emotions, intuitions, or impulses. Patients usually have conditioned patterns of awareness in which they operate, and typically they don't consciously attend to all of the elements of their experience. For example, a patient experiencing chronic pain might be very focused on the nociceptive signals and be unaware of other sensory feedback from the rest of the body. Or a patient with a prosthesis may be very focused on thoughts of being unable to ambulate, so much so that the patient is not really attending to sensory experiences that might guide him or her to successfully accomplishing ambulation. Increasing awareness of what one is actually experiencing allows for greater insight and choice in response. The clinician will seek to promote greater awareness of the ongoing flow of experience by giving the patient suggestions to attend to more aspects of experience (sensations, imaginings, thoughts, emotions, intuitions, or impulses) than the patient usually attends to in his or her everyday discrete pattern of awareness and consciousness.

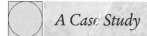

*A Case Study*

*Anxiety*

Susan, a young woman with a spinal cord injury, was learning to brace walk and was extremely anxious. Both the physical therapist and patient surmised that her anxiety had to do with falling. Therefore she was referred to me to alter her symptoms so that therapeutic goals could be achieved. During hypnosis, when the cognitive aspects of the experience were brought into awareness, it became apparent that Susan's anxiety was in response to the fear of her own rage at her physical therapist, whom she depended on. When Susan was able to recognize that her anxiety was based on the interpersonal aspects of the experience and not on the personal performance aspects, she was able to perform significantly better in physical therapy.

In this case, by using hypnosis, I was able within one session to get to the issue and bring about a change in Susan's performance. Once she realized that her anxiety was not about brace walking, her performance improved. The task had been to connect Susan with an important element of her experience that was out of her awareness yet was influencing her performance. Several sessions were spent with Susan examining her dependency needs and how she could be more assertive in her life. ∾

A way of thinking about the importance of increasing awareness is to realize that often the patient's inability to find a solution to his or her problem is a result of the conditioned pattern of awareness out of which the patient is operating.

## Research

In reviewing the research one would find that there is a consensus about the reality of hypnotic phenomena. Furthermore, hypnotic responsivity appears to be more or less normally distributed in the population and is as stable and enduring as personality traits. The controversy that exists has been about the best way to conceptualize the phenomena. Hypnosis has been difficult to study because until recently there have been few ways to understand what may be happening from a neuropsychophysiological perspective. As such, researchers have tended to focus on that which has been most readily observable: the subjects' behaviors and verbal reports of their subjective experiences. One of the most powerful subjective experiences to be had in the hypnotic state is the experience that what is happening is out of one's volitional control. It is this key effect of the experience of dissociated control that has given rise to the different theoretical interpretations of hypnosis. Much of the hypnotic research has been of a comparative nature, looking at differences between subjects at either end of the hypnotic responsiveness continuum. The effects of the hypnotic state on memory, problem solving, creativity, personality correlates, and even neuropsychological differences have been examined and reported in the literature.

Highly hypnotic subjects have been characterized as having the ability to shift attention and cognitive set easily. They have been found to be capable of vivid imagery; to engage in holistic thinking; to have extremely focused and sustained attention; and to be easily absorbed in imaginative activities, even outside of the hypnotic context.[9] It appears that hypnotic ability lies along a continuum and that, as has been measured, hypnotic ability is not a unitary construct or a phenomenon. There are several different types of hypnotic phenomena in which an individual may excel, and little is known about the differences between individuals who excel in demonstrating the different phenomena. Hypnotic capacity and responsiveness have been assessed by tests of hypnotic susceptibility. These tests ascertain the individual's ability to demonstrate certain types of hypnotic phenomena and the degree to which the individual can demonstrate. The various tests of hypnotizability essentially measure a subject's ability to perform a proffered suggestion. Some tests also seek to determine the degree to which the subject then experienced his or her response to the suggestion as nonvolitional, as well as the degree of absorption that the subject experienced while performing the suggestion. Tests of hypnotizability focus on that which is observable, the objective behavioral response to the hypnotic suggestion. Tests of hypnotic susceptibility employ suggestions for behaviors that can be found in the following clusters.[10]

1. Ideomotor phenomena
2. Cognitive abilities (imagery, dreams, age regression, hypermnesia)
3. Sensory denial or negation (analgesia, negative hallucinations)
4. Cognitive-perceptual distortion of reality (positive hallucinations, hyperesthesias, alteration in meaning)
5. Posthypnotic effects (amnesia, response to posthypnotic suggestions)

## Physiological Correlates

Finally, with the ever-advancing progression of technology, diagnostic tools have been invented that at long last allow us to see correlates of brain-mind behavior. With the advent of such diagnostic tools as electroencephalographic (EEG) frequency analysis, EEG topographic brain mapping, somatosensory event-related potential (SERP), topographic brain mapping, positron emission tomography (PET), regional cerebral blood flow (rCBF) and functional magnetic resonance imaging (fMRI), researchers have been learning about the brain-mind functions of highly hypnotizable individuals when they are in a hypnotic state. Unfortunately this research has not yet resolved the fundamental question of what hypnosis is or why or how it works. The research seems to suggest that the consciousness of highly hypnotizable individuals shows some unique patterns that are held in common. In comparing highly hypnotizable individuals to low-hypnotizable individuals, it is evident that the more highly hypnotizable subjects have greater cognitive flexibility, an easier ability to shift perceptual set (shift from a detail-oriented to holistic perspective), and a greater ability to shift from left to right anterior brain functioning as demonstrated by neuropsychological tests.[9,11] Several authors in review of various imaging studies (rCBF, PET, and SPECT) found strong evidence for neurophysiological changes in subjects during hypnosis.[11-13] Gruzelier[11,13] found positive correlations between shifts in cognitive strategy and neurophysiological hemispheric specificity or dominance across cognitive tasks. Kuzendorf and Boisvert[14] demonstrated that when highly hypnotizable individuals were engaged in auditory imaging tasks with instructions to image auditory deafening stimuli, they actually succeeded in physiologically masking their brainstem auditory evoked potentials (BSAEPs) and thus muffled their actual perceptual sensations. Barabasz and associates,[15] looking at differences between high- and low-hypnotizable individuals who were given the task to positively hallucinate sensory stimuli while being monitored by EEG cortical event-related potentials (ERPs) (visual and auditory P300 ERPs), found that individuals who were highly hypnotizable showed greater ERP amplitudes while experiencing positive hallucinations, in contrast to individuals who had low hypnotic capacity. De Pascalis[16] found that individuals who were highly hypnotizable and were experiencing hypnotic analgesia showed significantly smaller total, delta, and beta amplitudes in the right hemisphere across all frontal, central, and posterior recordings so that a significantly more pronounced hemispheric asymmetry in favor of the left hemisphere was displayed.

## The Use of Hypnosis in Healthcare

Much of the hypnotic research literature is experimental rather than clinical in nature. In recent years, given new ways of measuring mind-body interactions, more attempts have been made to study the effects of how mind-body modulations can be facilitated. Holroyd[17] reviewed the research of the influence of suggestion on mind-body interactions and found that there is clear evidence that both hypnosis and waking suggestion can influence vasoconstriction and dilation, enhance the immune system (beta-endorphin–like immunoreactive material in the blood; B-cells and white blood cells), and limit the pathological response of burns. Ruzyla-Smith, et al,[18] studied the effects of hypnosis on the immune system, specifically looking at B-cells, T-cells, helper, and suppressor cells when subjects were hypnotized. They found that there was a significant alteration of the immune response as measured by increased B-cell and helper T-cell activity in the high-hypnotizable subjects but not in low-hypnotizable subjects.

Over the last several decades there has been much discussion about the use of hypnosis in medicine. Since the beginning the primary use for hypnosis in medicine has been pain control, and that is still a major use today. The anesthesiologist, William Kroger,[19] who wrote one of the first comprehensive modern clinical texts about the use of hypnosis, described its use in the various specialties of medicine, such as internal medicine, surgery, anesthesiology, obstetrics, gynecology, dermatology, physical medicine and rehabilitation, urology, oncology, orthopedics, pediatrics, and psychiatry. Hypnosis has been very useful in the management of symptoms of various medical conditions.[20-22] The clinical hypnosis literature is extensive.

One of the classic texts in behavioral medicine that discusses the use of hypnosis is by Brown and Fromm.[22] In this text the authors discuss the hypnobehavioral treatment of various psychophysiological disorders such as pain, hypertension, asthma, various gastrointestinal diseases (e.g., peptic ulcer disease, irritable bowel syndrome, inflammatory bowel disease), various skin diseases, and immune-related diseases. They discuss the various clinical interventions ranging from symptom alleviation (as in pain control), retraining of physiological functioning (as in irritable bowel syndrome), stress reduction, and modification of lifestyle to enhancement of health behaviors and wellness. Brown[23] has stated that the main contributions of hypnosis to clinical outcome lie in positive subjective effects (e.g., decreased distress and increased well-being) and in behavioral changes (e.g., symptom reduction, a decrease in the use of medication, and the frequency of medical visits).

The majority of clinical interventions have been directed at symptom relief or restoration of homeostasis. Holroyd[17] points out that for much of recorded human history and across cultures there has been a belief in the ability of the mind to cure illness. It appears that the hypnotic state fosters a change in the everyday discrete state of consciousness that even relaxation by itself does not engender. Rossi,[24] more than other writer of hypnosis, stands out for his work in exploring the mind-body connection. He has attempted to describe how hypnosis functions as a mind-body therapy by using state-dependent memory, learning, and behavior and seeing the limbic-hypothalamic system of the brain as a vehicle for information transduction between the mind and body.

## The Use of Hypnosis in Physical Medicine and Rehabilitation

Wright[25] has portrayed the rehabilitation process as an educational process in which patients learn new motor skills and how to adapt to modified sensory organizational patterns and changes in cognitive activity. He has stated that as part of that educational process, patients have to develop new values and a new sense of self to be able to live in a cultural and societal milieu that often has negative attitudes about disabled individuals. Given that rehabilitation is a biopsychosocial endeavor, mind-body medicine consultations and interventions can be an integral part of the treatment regimen.

The majority of written work pertaining to the use of hypnosis in physical medicine and rehabilitation is similar in nature to that of the use of hypnosis in other medical specialties in that it tends to be all clinical report and anecdotal evidence. There is very little clinical research that has been performed, outside of the use of hypnosis for pain. The history of the use of hypnosis in rehabilitation to facilitate psychological and physical change began some 40 years ago. Alexander[26] pointed out that the psychological sequelae of illness and/or injury often intensified the experience of disability and loss of functional capacity and that hypnosis was an effective modality for promoting motivation and for facilitating better goal attainment. Becker[27] also pointed out that hypnosis, when used to reduce the effects of pain, fear, and anxiety associated with disability, could help patients achieve greater concentration, thus enabling them to participate more fully in their rehabilitation regimen.

Crasilneck and Hall[21] wrote that hypnotic interventions could be used with rehabilitation patients to enhance functional ability, to decrease both the sensory and affective components of pain, and to increase the patients' ability to tolerate the emotional sequelae and dysphoria in response to illness or disability. They also found that hypnosis was useful for increasing the patients' motivation to participate in the rehabilitation regimen. Hypnotically mediated psychotherapy interventions have been quite effective for reducing negative emotional reactions to the rehabilitation treatment regimen itself and for increasing motivation.[21,28] With lengths of stay becoming shorter in acute rehabilitation settings, it can be critical that dysphoric mental states be treated so that rehabilitation efforts can proceed and patients can attain their goals.

Hypnotic interventions have been used to deal with motor impairment associated with various illnesses and injuries in such ways as reducing muscle tone and decreasing spasticity,[29-31] increasing range of motion (ROM),[28,32,33] reeducating movement,[32,34,37] and increasing bowel and bladder control.[38] Hypnosis has also been used to facilitate speech therapy[39] and to reduce dysphagia.[40] Thompson, et al,[39] in a pilot study investigating whether naming behavior could be positively enhanced in patients with Brocca's aphasia by using hypnosis, showed that all subjects improved over baseline measurements. The study also showed that hypnosis can be effective with patients who have sustained brain impairment, particularly impairment in language-related areas of the brain. Hypnosis has been found to be useful for improving movement in hemiparetics[41] and for assisting in the voluntary movement of muscles that were weakly innervated because of peripheral nerve lesions.[42]

Eisenberg and Jansen[43] have reviewed the use of clinical hypnosis as an adjunctive tool for the rehabilitation psychologist in the treatment of neuromuscular disorders and have found that it was an effective modality. Hypnosis has been used as an adjunctive modality for enhancing functional outcomes and dealing with the emotional sequelae that can often diminish performance in conjunction with the treatment of such illnesses as Parkinson's disease,[44] Huntington's disease,[45] multiple sclerosis,[46] cerebral palsy,[29,30] and juvenile rheumatoid arthritis.[28] Hypnotic interventions with patients who have had cerebrovascular accidents* or traumatic brain injury[48,49] have been used for increasing motivation for treatment, facilitating attainment of goals, improving memory, and reducing headaches. Holroyd and Hill[32] used hypnosis with patients who had cerebrovascular accidents for pain management, mental practice, reframing of experience and attitude, and increasing sensitivity to somatic sensations. Moore and Wiesner[50] used hypnosis to induce vasodilatation in patients with repetitive strain injuries to reduce discomfort and pain.

Domangue et al[51] studied the effects of hypnotic treatments with arthritic patients and found that there were clinically and statistically significant decreases in the phenomenological experiences of pain, anxiety, and levels of depression and that there were increases in the beta-endorphin–like immunoreactive material. In a study comparing physical therapy and hypnotherapy with 40 fibromyalgia patients refractory to treatment, Haanen et al[52] found that the hypnotherapy group experienced a significant decrease in somatic and psychological discomfort as measured by the Hopkins Symptom Checklist, less fatigue on awakening, and better sleep patterns. Hypnosis has also been used as an adjunctive treatment for chronic fatigue syndrome and with post-polio syndrome for pain management and for dealing with the various aspects of the emotional sequelae of the illness.

Finally, hypnosis has been used in vocational rehabilitation with disabled individuals in preparing them for work by assisting them with handling the preperformance anxiety of job interviews and engaging in covert rehearsal of various job tasks.

# MIND-BODY INTERVENTIONS IN REHABILITATION

From a simplistic point of view, behavioral medicine interventions in the rehabilitation setting have been directed at (1) enhancing the patient's attainment of rehabilitation goals, (2) facilitating the psychological adjustment and adaptation to disability; and (3) treating existing psychological conditions exacerbated by the disability. Hypnotic interventions have been successfully used in all three areas. Because we are focusing on mind-body interventions, we shall focus only on the first two areas.

---

*References 21, 28, 32, 39-41, 47.

## Goal Attainment

Rehabilitation is unique in that, as compared with acute care, the main clinical activities are directed at attainment of functional goals and mastery of expression of self. With goal attainment so crucial, particularly in today's outcome-driven healthcare economic environment, healthcare providers often seek behavioral medicine consultation to facilitate compliance with treatment or enhance patient performance.

Management of pain and suffering is of paramount importance in assisting patients to derive the maximum benefit from their rehabilitation regimen. Many of the injuries or illnesses for which rehabilitation patients are treated are accompanied by pain, and at times even the treatment interventions themselves, such as ROM exercises in a patient who has had a knee or hip arthroplasty, can be painful. Hypnosis for pain control and management has a long history and has been well documented by several authors over the years.* Hypnosis has been used to treat a variety of pain syndromes ranging from malignant and phantom pain to chronic pain. In rehabilitation, hypnosis has been used for pain management with amputees for both stump and phantom pain,[53] as well as for management of phantom pain in paralyzed limbs[54] and for central pain in individuals with acute spinal cord injury.[55] I have used hypnosis extensively for self-regulation training of unwanted sensations such as pain, paresthesias, muscle stiffness, itching, nausea, and other unpleasant sensory experiences.

Related to pain is suffering, and hypnotically mediated interventions have been used quite successfully to help patients regulate their affect and negative emotional states, whether it be in response to pain, illness, accident, or disability. The goals of such interventions are to reduce stress, promote well-being, and foster a sense of self that transcends identification with the body. Changing the way patients think about their situations, themselves, and their outcomes can be critical to promote a sense of well-being and the ability to respond to their existential situations.

Many rehabilitation goals are physical in nature, involving the learning of motor skills and tasks. Hypnosis has been used to facilitate the learning of new motor patterns in such diverse approaches as neuromuscular reeducation, neuromotor facilitation, hypnotically hallucinated physical therapy, and mental practice.[33] All intentional movements are part of behavioral repertoires,

*References 7, 17, 19, 21, 22, 33.

and even the bracing and guarding that are often expressed in reaction to pain (pain behavior) can be modified and regulated. Hypnosis can be used to teach the patient how to have influence over conditioned or ineffective movement patterns (e.g., kinesophobia and compensatory but maladaptive behavioral patterns that actually interfere with optimum movement). I have written about the use of hypnosis to enhance performance through increasing ROM, to decrease muscle tone to reduce stiffness, to teach sequencing and coordination of movements for self-dressing tasks, and to enhance ambulation skills in individuals using prostheses through promotion of mental practice of balance and sequencing and coordination of movements.[33] I have also used hypnosis for enhancing patient performance in maintaining balance, posture, coordination, and sequencing of movements for fine motor tasks such as writing or playing a musical instrument.

Many times the ability to execute what can be seen as a challenging physical demand can be interfered with by negative mentation and attributions about one's ability to perform the task. As such it becomes critical to change preperformance mental set, beliefs, and internal dialogue. I have used hypnotically mediated cognitive interventions to change a patient's mental set and attitude and thus facilitate the patient's attempting the perceived difficult motor challenges and tasks with a "can do" attitude. Examples of using hypnosis to enhance physical performance can be seen in the Case Studies.

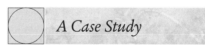

## A Case Study

*Performance Enhancement with Musculoskeletal Dysfunction*
A young woodwind musician who developed left scapular dysfunction, bilateral upper extremity aches in joints and muscles, and right wrist and hand pain was referred for depression as the pain and musculoskeletal problems severely impacted his ability to play his instrument. He had been suffering with these problems for several years. Because the young man's depression was in response to his loss of ability and identity, one of the ways to reduce the depression was to help him to be able to play for longer periods without pain, thereby engendering hope that through rehabilitation he could once again pursue his passion. All of the following strategies were performed within a hypnotic context. He was first taught self-regulation exercises for muscle relaxation and pain control. The relaxation exercises consisted of (1) a hypnosuggestive progressive sensory muscle

relaxation exercise coupled with elements of autogenic training and visual imagery, (2) auditory imagery of relaxing music coupled with suggestions to imagine feeling the music he heard as physical sensations in his body, and (3) a variation of a mindfulness technique in which he was helped to achieve a state of diffuse awareness that enabled him to be aware of everything and no particular thing at the same time and able to just witness his experience. The pain management techniques consisted of (1) guided imagery techniques in which the images were direct suggestions to transform the experience of the pain and (2) a variation of a mindfulness technique. He was then taught self-regulation techniques for affect control, which consisted of ego-state work via visual imagery and disidentification.

Next we worked on improving physical function and performance by (1) increasing ROM through mental practice exercises (consisting of internal and external imagery[33]), (2) relearning how to maintain neutral relaxed postures while holding his instrument (he had a tendency to tighten and elevate left shoulder as he played) through mental practice, and (3) learning how to stay relaxed while blowing the instrument through mental practice and focusing exercises. After observing his behavior, I gave him the following suggestions: (1) maintain awareness of the left elbow while playing (by focusing awareness on where the elbow should be, paradoxically he was able to relax his shoulder); (2) experience the movement of the hands—the dance of the hands across the keys (By focusing on the hands, the arms and shoulders would do what they needed to do to facilitate the hand movement. Given his previous attention on his shoulders, he was more aware of the discomfort and inadvertently was tightening up in response to the pain.); and (3) experience the tension of the body in the breath when blowing the instrument, feeling the body moving around the breath. The aforementioned strategies, which were done within a hypnotic context, allowed the patient to extinguish conditioned motor patterns in response to pain that were actually interfering with his performance. He was able to regain more natural movement patterns, allowing him to play without pain and thus offering him a sense of mastery and hope, which also brought about a reduction in his depression. ∾

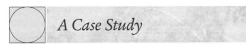

## A Case Study

*Performance Enhancement with Bilateral Amputation*
A 65-year-old female patient with bilateral below-the-knee amputation secondary to peripheral vascular disease and insulin-dependent diabetes mellitus was helped to improve her ambulation skills through hypnotically mediated mental practice. Mental practice was used in a hierarchical fashion, having her first perform the mental

practice of standing on both her prostheses in a balanced manner with good posture incorporating all of the suggestions and instructions that her physical therapist had been giving her. As the patient was being instructed in the mental practice of being on her prostheses with good balance, she was also given suggestions for mastery, skill, competence, and self-appreciation.

Follow-up mental practice sessions concentrated on using external imagery, with which she would see herself in the physical therapy gym, walking between the parallel bars in the manner in which her physical therapist had been instructing her. While she was imaging herself ambulating, she was given the suggestion that she could correct the images of her movement patterns until they looked perfect to her. She was instructed to signal me when she had achieved a level of satisfaction with the images of how she was walking, at which point I began giving her suggestions for internal imagery. The internal imagery consisted of suggestions to merge with the external image of herself and experience herself kinesthetically walking in just the way she had pictured herself (so that she could feel her prostheses, could lightly feel the parallel bars beneath her palms, see the gym, etc.).

Once the patient became proficient with her mental practice skills, cotreatment with her physical therapist was initiated. During a physical therapy session, before actual physical practice of her ambulation skills, she was asked to go into a hypnotic trance and mentally rehearse what she was about to do. (This was a "psyching up" strategy.) The hypnosis relaxed her and concentrated her attention on the task at hand so that any anticipatory anxiety about her physical therapy would be diminished.

Further hypnotic sessions for performance enhancement then focused on her ambulating in the following hierarchical situations: at the physical therapy gym outside of the parallel bars, at the nursing unit, in her home, at a friend's house, in her favorite store, and in a supermarket. Her physical therapist was instructed to create time for the patient in future therapy sessions to practice her self-hypnosis as a prelude to the therapy and to ensure that the patient rehearsed what they were doing through mental practice. After 1 week the patient's mood and actual physical performance increased significantly. At the end of 2 weeks the patient was ambulating more skillfully with her prostheses and was experiencing more confidence. By the time of discharge she had learned to control her pain, had significantly increased her sense of self-esteem and self-efficacy, and had acquired the skills necessary for ambulation with bilateral prostheses. ∾

Disability, when it is the result of an accident or a sudden biological event such as a stroke or heart attack, is often experienced as traumatic. The trauma is usually experienced as an assault on one's sense of self and how the world works. The individual's notions of invulnerability and assumptions that the world is an orderly and safe place are confronted and sometimes shattered by the injury or illness. Rehabilitation must encompass helping the individual to develop the cognitive schemes and a model of the world that include not only adapting and accommodating to the disability but also having emerged from victimhood. Treatment often must focus on the patient's depression or anxiety over the loss and rejection of that which is perceived as self, not being able to make his or her way in the world independently, and feeling impotent and dependent. The emotional sequelae of traumatic injury or illness can be quite varied. Premorbid personality, emotional temperament, and biological disposition, as well as prior life experiences, all combine synergistically to influence whether the response to the disability will be one of depression, anxiety, or posttraumatic stress, or something altogether different.

How an individual reacts to his or her disability also has much to do with the meaning that the individual ascribes to his or her injury. A physicist may have a very different reaction to being a paraplegic than will a professional dancer as both individuals begin to ponder what comes next after rehabilitation. In a similar fashion, the meaning of a body part that is lost may have much to do with the significance and attributions made to that body part. Another crucial hurdle that needs to be overcome along the path to adjustment is the ability to see beyond the trauma and foresee beginning a new life. Hypnotically mediated psychotherapeutic interventions have been useful in helping patients develop a new sense of self and cognitive schemes of the world in which they must live.

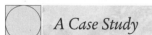

### A Case Study

*Adjustment to Disability: Scoliosis with Chronic Pain*
An example of how hypnosis can be used to facilitate adjustment to disability can be seen in the case of a 43-year-old female with a history of thoracic scoliosis that had required four different surgeries to correct the curvature and resulting pain. The patient was referred for treatment of anxiety and depression related to her medical condition. She had actually begun to feel phobic over the possibility of having another episode of pain. Her medical condition had led her to feel vulnerable and as a victim of changes in her own body. She was overwhelmed with the thoughts

and feelings about the foreign objects (instrumentation) within her that were stabilizing her spine. Treatment was performed within a hypnotic context and began with teaching her self-regulation strategies of sensory experience similar to the relaxation strategies mentioned in the previous case so that she could relax and soothe herself. The relaxation and mindfulness exercises allowed her to feel more able to influence her experience and realize that she could begin to have mastery over her experience. Although the patient was taught imagery techniques for hypnoanalgesia, she responded best to mindfulness-type strategies in which she was allowed to go into a diffuse state of awareness and experience the body in pain rather than the back in pain. Paradoxically, as she learned to experience the pain without emotion, she became less afraid of being in pain. Treatment then focused on the meaning of having a crooked back and bringing into conscious awareness her beliefs and reactions to the various surgeries she had endured. Through the use of an "affect bridge" she was helped to process the emotions that she had never expressed and reconceptualize her experiences from the vantage point of hindsight and an adult perspective. This is a technique in which a patient is helped to develop awareness and insight into an emotional state through directed free association of the particular emotion being explored. She was helped to make conscious some state-dependent learned memory behaviors and change the cognitive stimulus consequence chain that was driving her emotions. She was further helped to symbolize herself through the visual image of a professional, capable woman who had accomplished much in spite of her medical condition rather than the image of a young teenager with a crooked back. After five sessions (hypnotically mediated psychotherapy typically reduces the time needed to achieve change) the patient was no longer feeling depressed and anxious about her situation and she was able to take steps to make some vocational changes that had been on hold because of her mood. ∞

## SUMMARY

At the heart of rehabilitation is the restoration of the physical and psychological capacities and abilities of individuals who have suffered functional losses because of traumatic injury or illness. The rehabilitation process as stated previously is at once a biopsychosocial endeavor and a true model of a holistic health interventional approach. The primary contribution of hypnosis to rehabilitation lies with its potential for facilitating learning and accelerating change.[56] In this chapter the phenomenon of hypnosis has been introduced and a rudimentary discourse on its nature presented. I have suggested that there is a neuropsychophysiological understanding of the phenomenon of hypnosis and further suggest to you that there are unique brain processes peculiar to the hypnotic state that allow for what sometimes seem to be remarkable results to be obtained. While hypnotic responsivity is randomly distributed in the population at large, even low- to moderately hypnotizable patients can gain some benefit from learning to focus their attention and act on self-suggestion. The various ways that hypnosis has been used in rehabilitation also have been presented in this chapter.

Alexander[26] pointed out many years ago that the psychological sequelae of neurological illnesses often intensify the disability and that hypnosis is an effective tool to foster motivation; change attitudes about illness and situation; and facilitate better accommodation, adjustment, and rehabilitation outcomes. Hypnosis helps patients to gain cognitive mastery over the emotional sequelae of disability through teaching them how to alter their perception, reframe their perspective, access internal cognitive and emotional resources, and provide covert experiences of mastery and achievement. Hypnosis can promote a situation for the patient in which the patient can become so absorbed with his or her phenomenological experience that nothing else may seem to exist in that moment except that which is being attended to. In that moment, free from extraneous sensory, emotional, or cognitive information, new experiences can be had that can alter the patient's perception of self and sense of what is possible to experience. Self-hypnosis, when used with a variety of self-administered cognitive-behavioral–based interventions, allows patients to develop an experience of self that reflects mastery and competence.

When one considers the variety of rehabilitation populations and functional problems for which hypnosis has been used, a persuasive argument can be made for teaching more patients how to apply their cognitive skills and direct their will on their own behalf. Martin,[57] an ardent advocate of the use of hypnosis in rehabilitation, suggested that healthcare providers should use every adjunctive treatment in the clinical realm that they can to achieve better outcomes and that hypnosis should be an indispensable part of treatment. For the better half of a century now, hypnosis has been used in rehabilitation with great success to facilitate outcomes and promote greater mastery in physical medicine patients.

## References

1. Gordon JS: *Manifesto for a new medicine,* Reading, Mass, Addison-Wesley, 1996, p 57.
2. Dossey L: *Space, time medicine,* Boston, Shambhala, 1982, p 61.
3. Pelletier KR: *Towards a science of consciousness,* New York, Delta, 1978, p 19.
4. Sarno JE: *The mindbody prescription: healing the body, healing the pain,* New York, Warner Books, 1998.
5. Tart CT: *Altered states of consciousness,* Garden City, NJ, Doubleday Anchor, 1972, pp 1-2.
6. Lynn SJ, Rhue JW (eds): *Theories of hypnosis: current models and perspectives,* New York, Guilford Press, 1991, pp 241-274.
7. Barber J: *Hypnosis and suggestion in the treatment of pain,* New York, Norton, 1996, p 5.
8. Barber J: The locksmith model: accessing hypnotic responsiveness. In Lynn SJ, Rhue JW (eds): *Theories of hypnosis: current models and perspectives,* New York, Guilford Press, 1991, pp 241-274.
9. Crawford HJ, Gruzelier JH: A midstream view of the neuropsychophysiology of hypnosis: recent research and future directions. In Fromm E, Nash MR (eds): *Contemporary hypnosis research,* New York, Guilford Press, 1992, pp 227-266.
10. Hammond DC: *Learning clinical hypnosis: an educational resource compendium,* Chicago, American Society of Clinical Hypnosis, 1988.
11. Gruzelier JH, Warren K: Neuropsychological evidence of reductions on left frontal tests with hypnosis, *Psychol Med* 23:93-101, 1993.
12. Crawford HJ: Brain dynamics and hypnosis, *Int J Clin Exp Hyp* 42(3):204-232, 1994.
13. Gruzelier JH: Neuropsychological investigations of hypnosis: cerebral laterality and beyond. In Van Dyck R, Spinhoven PH, Van Der Does AJW (eds): *Hypnosis: theory, research and clinical practice,* Amsterdam, Free University Press, 1990, pp 37-51.
14. Kuzendorf RG, Boisvert P: Presence vs. absence of a "hidden observer" during total deafness: the hypnotic illusion of subconsciousness vs. the imaginal attenuation of brainstem evoked potentials. In Kunzendorf RG, Spanos NP, Wallace B (eds): *Hypnosis and imagination,* Amityville, NY, Baywood, 1996.
15. Barabasz A, Barabasz M, Jensen S, et al: Cortical event-related potentials show the structure of hypnotic suggestions is crucial, *Int J Clin Exp Hyp* 47:5-22, 1999.
16. De Pascalis V: Psychophysiological correlates of hypnosis and hypnotic susceptibility, *Int J Clin Exp Hyp* 47:117-143, 1999.
17. Holroyd J: Hypnosis as a methodology in psychological research. In Fromm E, Nash MR (eds): *Contemporary hypnosis research,* New York, Guilford Press, 1992, pp 201-226.

18. Ruzyla-Smith P, Barabasz A, Barabasz M, et al: Effects of hypnosis on the immune response: B-cells, T-cells, helper and suppressor cells, *Am J Clin Hypn* 38:71-79, 1995.

19. Kroger WS: Clinical and experimental hypnosis in medicine, dentistry, and psychology, Philadelphia, Lippincott, 1963.

20. Spiegel D: Uses of hypnosis in managing medical symptoms, *Psychiatr Med* 9:521-533, 1991.

21. Crasilneck HB, Hall JA: *Clinical hypnosis principles and applications,* ed 2, Orlando, Grune & Stratton, 1985.

22. Brown DP, Fromm E: *Hypnosis and behavioral medicine,* Hillsdale, NJ, Lawrence Earlbaum Assoc, 1987.

23. Brown DP: Clinical hypnosis research since 1986. In Fromm E, Nash MR (eds): *Contemporary hypnosis research,* New York, Guilford, 1992, pp 427-458.

24. Rossi EL: *The psychobiology of mind-body healing: new concepts of therapeutic hypnosis,* ed 2, New York, WW Norton, 1993.

25. Wright ME: Hypnosis and rehabilitation, *Rehabil Literature* 21:(1)2-12, 1960.

26. Alexander L: Hypnosis in primarily organic illness, *Am J Clin Hypn* 4:250-253, 1966.

27. Becker F: Modification of anxiety through the use of hypnosis in physical medicine, *J Am Geriatr Soc* 11:235-237, 1963.

28. Appel PR: Clinical applications of hypnosis in the physical medicine and rehabilitation setting: three case reports, *Am J Clin Hypn* 33:85-93, 1990.

29. Secter IL, Gilberd MB: Hypnosis as a relaxant for the cerebral palsied patient, *Am J Clin Hypn* 6:363-364, 1964.

30. Spankus WH, Freeman LG: Hypnosis in cerebral palsy, *Int J Clin Exp Hyp* 10:135-139, 1962.

31. Feher TL: Hypnosis in clinical neurology. In Wester W (ed): *Clinical hypnosis: a case management approach,* Cincinnati, Behavioral Science Center, 1987.

32. Holroyd J, Hill A: Pushing the limits of recovery: hypnotherapy with a stroke patient, *Int J Clin Exp Hyp* 37: 189-191, 1989.

33. Appel PR: Performance enhancement in physical medicine and rehabilitation, *Am J Clin Hypn* 35:11-19, 1992.

34. Yensen R: Hypnosis and movement re-education in partially paralyzed subjects, *Percept Mot Skills* 17:211-222, 1963.

35. McCord H: Hypnotically hallucinated physical therapy with a multiple sclerosis patient, *Am J Clin Hypn* 5:168, 1963.

36. Garver RB: The enhancement of human performance with hypnosis through neuromotor facilitation and control arousal level, *Am J Clin Hypn* 19:177-181, 1977.

37. Warner L, McNeil ME: Mental imagery and its potential for physical therapy, *Phys Ther* 68(4):516-521, 1988.

38. Baer RF: Hypnosis applied to bowel and bladder control in multiple sclerosis, syringomelia and traumatic transverse myelitis, *Am J Clin Hypn* 4:22-23, 1961.

39. Thompson CK, Hall HR, Sison CE: Effects of hypnosis and imagery training on naming behavior in aphasia, *Brain Lang* 28:141-153, 1986.

40. Kopel KF, Quinn M: Hypnotherapy treatment for dysphagia, *Int J Clin Exp Hyp* 44:101-105, 1996.

41. Radil T, Snydrova I, Hacik L, et al: Attempts to influence movement disorders in hemiparetics, *Scand J Rehabil Med Suppl* 17:157-161, 1988.

42. Pajntar M, Jeglic A, Stefancic M, et al: Improvements of motor response by means of hypnosis in patients with peripheral nerve lesions, *Int J Clin Exp Hyp* 28:16-26, 1980.

43. Eisenberg MG, Jansen MA: Rehabilitation psychology: state of the art, *Ann Rev Rehabil* 3:1-31, 1983.

44. Wain HJ, Amen D, Jabbari B: The effects of hypnosis on a parkinsonian tremor: case report with polygraph/EEG recordings, *Am J Clin Hypn* 33:94-98, 1990.

45. Witz M, Kahn S: Hypnosis and the treatment of Huntington's disease, *Am J Clin Hypn* 34:79-90, 1991.

46. Dane JR: Hypnosis for pain and neuromuscular rehabilitation with multiple sclerosis: case summary, literature review, and analysis of outcomes, *Int J Clin Exp Hyp* 44:208-231, 1996.

47. Halama P: Hypnotherapy for stroke patients, *Hypnosis* 20(3):154-162, 1993.

48. Spellacy F: Hypnotherapy following traumatic brain injuries, *Hypnosis* 19(1):34-39, 1992.

49. Laidlaw T: Hypnosis and attention deficits after closed head injury, *Int J Clin Exp Hyp* 41:97-111, 1993.

50. More LE, Wiesner SL: Hypnotically-induced vasodilatation in the treatment of repetitive strain injuries, *Am J Clin Hypn* 39:97-104, 1996.

51. Domangue BB, Margolis C, Lieberman D, et al: Biochemical correlates of hypnoanalgesia in arthritic pain patients, *J Clin Psychiatry* 46:235-238, 1985.

52. Haanen HCM, Hoenderdos HTW, Van Romunde LKJ, et al: Controlled trial of hypnotherapy in the treatment of refractory fibromyalgia, *J Rheum* 18(1):72-75, 1991.

53. McGarry J: Hypnotic interventions in psychological and physiological aspects of amputation, *Aust J Clin Hypnother Hypn* 14:7-12, 1993.

54. Sthalekar H: Hypnosis for relief of chronic phantom pain in a paralyzed limb: a case study, *Austral J Clin Hypnother Hypnosis* 14:75-80, 1993.

55. Alden P: The use of hypnosis in the management of pain on a spinal injuries unit, *Hypnosis* 20(2):106-116, 1993.

56. Wright ME: Hypnosis and rehabilitation, *Rehabil Literature* 21(1):2-12, 1960.

57. Martin J: Hypnosis is also useful in rehabilitation therapy, *JAMA* 249:153-168, 1983.

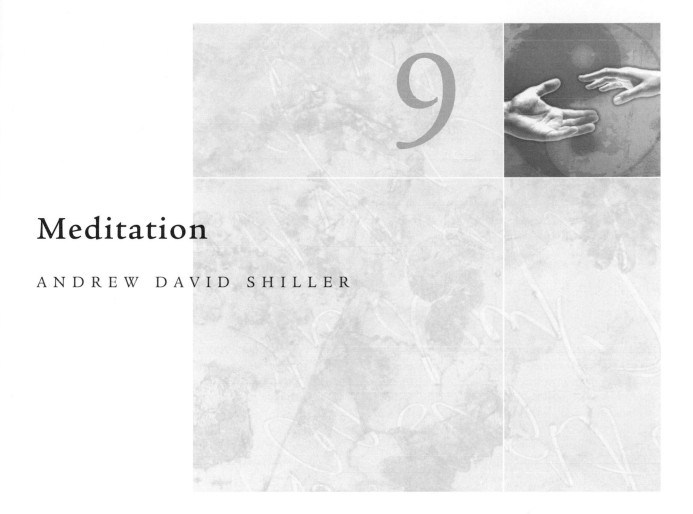

# Meditation

ANDREW DAVID SHILLER

Meditation complements the traditional rehabilitation process via three potential pathways. First, abundant data demonstrate the deleterious physiological effects of chronic mental and physical stress. Meditation and related stress reduction techniques have been shown to oppose the physiological correlates of stress. Also, regular meditation practice speeds the return to the resting state after stress-induced physiological change. Second, meditation facilitates psychological changes that can enhance learning, improve health-related behavior, and facilitate enhanced psychological adaptation to illness and disability. Finally, regular meditation practice empowers practitioners to play an active role in enhancing their health and sense of well-being. In so doing, it enhances the self-efficacy and sense of control that are so often compromised with persons with disability and chronic illness.

This chapter asserts that meditation and meditation-based behavioral interventions are useful adjuncts to traditional rehabilitation interventions for people with disability and chronic illness. The important messages in this chapter are the following.

- *Meditation* is a general term that refers to a wide variety of techniques for regulation of the mind-body-spirit system. There is significant overlap among the effects of different types of meditation. Many techniques do not require any particular belief system or spiritual orientation and are widely practiced in modern society.
- Meditation has important physiological effects. The best documented is a restful state of hypoarousal that differs from sleep and opposes the physiological "fight-or-flight" response.
- Research supports the efficacy of meditation and cognitive-behavioral stress management interven-

tions in improving chronic disease outcomes, reducing psychological distress, and reducing healthcare usage.

- There is a rationale for the efficacy of meditation that is based on the current science of mind-body interactions and the effects of chronic psychophysiological stress.
- Existing data suggest that meditation has important implications for patients in rehabilitation settings.
- Meditation can have a positive impact on healthcare providers. It may improve empathy and communication, as well as diagnostic accuracy and clinical decision making.

# OVERVIEW

## History

The meditation techniques that are practiced today have their roots in ancient spiritual and religious traditions. In many traditional cultures, the functional systems that modern medical science currently divides into *mind* and *body* were seen as inseparable parts of a seamless whole. Meditation was part of a system of practices intended to integrate the emotional, physical, mental, and spiritual realms of being.

While many modern meditators practice as part of spiritual discipline, meditation is often practiced in a context that is not explicitly spiritual. Rather, meditation is used as means to facilitate higher functioning of mind-body processes. Meditation has been used to improve athletic and job performance, facilitate learning, reduce stress, and ease suffering for people with a broad variety of symptoms and illnesses.

## Demographics

Meditation is a prevalent mode of self-care. In Eisenberg's 1997 random telephone survey of roughly 2,000 residents of the United States, 16.3% reported regular practice of some sort of relaxation technique. Of the "relaxers," 75% said they used meditation, and 15% of them saw practitioners for the therapy, with an average of 21 visits per user over the previous year. Based on these data and a U.S. population of 198 million, the authors estimated that in 1997 there were 103 million visits to practitioners for relaxation or meditation

therapies. The authors found that many of the visits were for the treatment of conditions (e.g., back pain, arthritis, fatigue, headaches, insomnia, anxiety) that are often treated by rehabilitation professionals.[1] A smaller survey focused on persons with disabilities to determine their patterns of complementary care use. Of 401 patients interviewed, 31.7% (127) had used a relaxation technique in the previous 12 months.[2]

# Meditation Techniques

Meditation could be broadly defined as the intentional control or manipulation of attention to cultivate particular qualities of mind and body. This is an intentionally vague definition because there are many kinds of meditation practice. To get a clearer sense of the possibilities, it is helpful to consider three parameters of meditation practice that illustrate the variability in approaches. It should be kept in mind that there is considerable overlap among the different possibilities within these three categories.

1. *What is done with the body?* Meditation can be done with eyes closed or open, while lying down, sitting, standing, walking, or in the choreographed movements of yoga and tai chi. (See chapters 5 and 6.) Some traditions bring meditative awareness to daily activities such as washing dishes, serving food, painting, and archery, among others.
2. *Where is the attention directed?* Some meditation traditions involve an "open focus" of attention that develops nonreactive awareness of the flow of thoughts, bodily sensations, emotions, and environmental stimuli. Other traditions involve a "closed focus" of attention that is fixed on a word, sound, idea, candle flame, etc. Some traditions use visualizations of colors or complex images that are intended to bring about particular transcendental mind states. Visual imagery relevant to desired health outcomes might be considered a type of meditation.
3. *What quality or skill is cultivated?* Some techniques focus on accessing a state of mental and physical relaxation. Body-centered meditation such as tai chi or yoga can also develop a heightened sense of body awareness and coordination of body, mind, and breathing. Mantra and closed-focus meditations tend to develop focused concentration. Open-focus techniques develop nonjudgmental awareness and a more accepting relationship with

life experiences. Other techniques are meant to elicit feelings of lovingkindness, connection with other living beings, or the sense of a transcendent Self, consciousness, or deity. There is typically a great deal of overlap of effects among practices.

An entire book could be devoted to a discussion of the types of meditation practiced today. This section describes mindfulness meditation, the relaxation response, and Transcendental Meditation, which are commonly practiced in healthcare settings and used in clinical research. The relative emphasis on mindfulness meditation reflects the author's greater experience with the technique. There are a variety of other "relaxation techniques" that are used in healthcare settings that meet the broad definition of meditation previously described.

It is important for healthcare providers and meditation practitioners to acknowledge the subtle and subjective nature of meditation practice. Meditation should not be learned from a book. As the practitioner relaxes, difficult sensations or mind states can arise. Most beginning practitioners need help in such situations. In the appropriate setting, this can pave the way for healing of emotional, psychological, and physical pain. An individual who is interested in practicing meditation should do so under the supervision of an experienced teacher. See the box on p. 112 for further sources of information.

## Mindfulness-Based Stress Reduction

*Mindfulness* is an approach to meditation that has its roots in the Theravada Buddhist teachings and has been practiced for at least 2,500 years. Mindfulness is often described as nonjudgmental awareness of the flow of experience. Mindfulness meditation can involve formal and informal practice. During formal practice, the practitioner sets aside time for cultivating mindfulness. This is typically done in various meditation postures or during walking meditation. Informal practice brings nonreactive awareness to daily activities such as household chores, eating, and traveling, among others.

Mindfulness-Based Stress Reduction (MBSR) is a clinical regimen that has been popularized by the work of Jon Kabat-Zinn and colleagues at the University of Massachusetts (UMass) (see box on p. 112). There are many clinical sites around the United States that offer MBSR based on the program developed at UMass. MBSR trains participants to develop mindfulness through sitting meditation, walking meditation, a supine body scan, hatha yoga, observation and discussion of habits of perception and communication, and other behaviors.

MBSR participants meet for approximately 2½ hours each week for 8 weeks. There is typically a 7-hour intensive practice session toward the end of the program. The sessions provide meditation training and practice with the support of an instructor who has significant experience with mindfulness meditation. Group discussion and exercises encourage awareness of habitual patterns of perception, communication, behavior, and emotional coping during daily life. Homework assignments involve daily practice of sitting meditation, walking meditation, body scan or gentle yoga, informal meditation practice, and written exercises meant to integrate the lessons learned in class.

As part of daily life, mindfulness meditation is typically practiced for 30 to 45 minutes. Some prefer walking, while others prefer sitting meditation or yoga. Many teachers recommend practicing twice daily, once in the morning and once in the evening. Some practitioners pursue prolonged retreats, which can last from 1 to 14 days or longer. Informal practice is encouraged as a way of bringing mindful awareness into daily activities.

During both formal and informal practice, the practitioner anchors his or her attention to a present moment sensation such as the breath moving through the nostrils, shifting pressure on the feet during walking, environmental sounds, or the details of a household chore. The practitioner learns to notice when the attention wanders to thoughts about the future or past, emotions, bodily sensations, or other "objects of attention." The basic practice is to *gently* bring the attention back to the present moment sensation.

Most beginning practitioners find that their attention is unstable and incessantly drawn to commentary or judgments about their experience, thoughts about the future or past, feelings, or various body sensations. With practice, however, the mind settles down and is less likely to be pulled away from present moment awareness. As the mind becomes steady, one sees directly that most thoughts, feelings, and sensations are transient and insubstantial. There is less attachment to pleasant objects of mind, and less aversion to unpleasant ones. Practitioners develop enhanced freedom from habitual patterns of thought, emotional reactions, and

## Resources

Stress Reduction Clinic University of Massachusetts
    Memorial Medical Center Shaw Building
55 Lake Avenue North
Worcester, MA 01655
mindfulness@umassmed.edu
www.umassmed.edu/cfm

The UMASS stress reduction clinic pioneered the use of mindfulness meditation in mainstream healthcare. It has grown into the Center for Mindfulness in Medicine, Health Care, and Society (CFM), which continues to provide clinical and research programs and to offer mindfulness training to businesses, teachers, the prison system, and other groups. Professional training resources include an 8-week professional internship program for healthcare providers and intensive mindfulness teacher development programs. The ongoing clinic program is covered by some insurance programs and provides services in response to many different kinds of referrals. The website contains a nationwide list of sites that offer mindfulness-based stress reduction, a bibliography of relevant references, and information to facilitate referral of patients.

Mind/Body Medical Institute at Beth Israel
    Deaconess Medical Center
110 Francis Street
Boston, MA 02215
(617) 632-9530
mbmi@caregroup.harvard.edu
www.mbmi.org

The Institute offers mind-body programs for patients and training courses for healthcare providers. It maintains a list of affiliated programs in many cities around the United States. The website includes links to references of relevant research. Professional training courses are offered directly through the MBMI and through Harvard Medical School.

Mind/Body Medical Institute Center for Training
Shirley Selhub
Director, Center for Training
(617) 632-9542
sselhub@caregroup.harvard.edu

Transcendental Meditation (TM) Information
The official website for TM is www.tm.org. It contains links to resources for learning the TM techniques, as well as links to research documenting the physiological, psychological, and social effects of TM practice. The research is heterogeneous in quality.

The Center for Natural Medicine and Prevention at Maharishi University of Management studies TM and natural medicine approaches to cardiovascular disease and other chronic illness. Visit www.mum.edu/CNMP/index.html.

Multiple links to organizations that promote Mindfulness Meditation: www.dharma.org/other resources.htm. ∾

---

behavioral responses. The steadiness and nonattachment to thoughts, feelings, and body sensations allows greater insight into the dynamics of mind-body processes. It should be mentioned that the nonattachment and acceptance that are developed do not imply passivity or resignation. Rather, acceptance and awareness are typically important aspects of transforming difficult circumstances. Most practitioners report an enhanced ability to manage potentially difficult situations with skill and grace. Mindfulness empowers them to make more conscious and effective choices about the allocation of psychological, emotional, spiritual, and physical energy.

## Transcendental Meditation

Transcendental Meditation (TM) was introduced to the United States in 1959 by Maharishi Mahesh Yogi and draws from ancient Hindu and Vedic traditions. The Maharishi's organization has been successful in promoting the practice and creating an infrastructure to support extensive research and practical application. As a result, TM is probably the most widely practiced form of meditation in the United States. Most meditation research has been carried out with practitioners of TM. The TM research and clinical program are unusual in that they focus on TM alone without additional cognitive or behavioral strategies. This is in contrast to most meditation and stress management research, which often incorporates cognitive behavioral techniques. The box on p. 112 contains links to more information about TM.

The TM technique is typically practiced for 20 minutes twice daily. It is stated that the technique does not require any particular belief system. The practitioner sits comfortably with eyes closed and effortlessly pays attention to the sound of a simple mantra. The mantra is a sound/syllable that is chosen for the individual by an experienced teacher. When thoughts or distractions arise, attention is brought back to the mantra.

According to the Maharishi, the TM technique allows the mind to settle into a quiet state of restful alertness that is characterized by "unbounded awareness." Practitioners of TM report a deep state of relaxation and clear awareness that is associated with a greater sense of energy and well-being and improved relationships with others. Proponents of TM hold that the practice enlivens the natural intelligence of the mind-body system and enhances creativity and innate mechanisms of self-repair and healing.[3]

### Relaxation Response

*Relaxation response* is a term coined by Herbert Benson, MD, to describe a set of physiological changes that often accompany meditation practice.[4] Based on research over the past 4 decades, the relaxation response appears to oppose the physiological changes of the fight-or-flight response. It is a state of hypoarousal that includes decreased respiration, decreased oxygen consumption, cardiovascular relaxation, reduced muscle tension, and other physiological changes.[5] Most types of meditation have the potential to elicit the relaxation response. Drawing on meditation practices that are often embedded in religious traditions, Dr. Benson devised a simple, secular approach to meditation that consistently brings on the relaxation response. The easy-to-learn technique involves (1) repeating a word, sound, phrase, prayer, or simple movement; (2) passively disregarding thoughts that inevitably come to mind; and (3) returning to the repetition.

The clinical programs developed by Dr. Benson and colleagues at the Mind-Body Medical Institute (see box on p. 112) employ the relaxation response as a foundation for a number of mind-body interventions. Participants learn to identify and adapt to stressors and inaccurate or unproductive cognitive patterns. They practice techniques to improve emotional self-management, communication skills, and social support. Information is provided relevant to diet, exercise, and other health behaviors. The groups typically meet for several hours once weekly for 8 to 10 weeks.

### Overlap Among Techniques

Experience suggests that there is overlap in the effects of the different techniques previously described. For example, subjects who go through programs based on the relaxation response often report effects ascribed to TM such as improvement in concentration, sense of connection to others, and sense of coherence in life. Practitioners of mindfulness typically experience the relaxation response. TM practitioners often develop the nonreactive, heightened sense of awareness that is typical of mindfulness.

Nevertheless, some have argued that there are differences in effects among the techniques. For example, TM has been shown to be more effective than other techniques in some clinical situations.[6] Also, simple elicitation of the relaxation response is not always practical in daily circumstances. In contrast, advocates of mindfulness meditation assert that mindful attention can be brought to bear in even the most stressful situations and can enable a more skillful, and sometimes less stressful, handling of difficult circumstances. However, the relaxation response is often taught along with cognitive-behavioral skills that encourage students to develop coping skills for real-time stressful situations. Further research is needed to determine the differential effects of the techniques.

### Other Clinical Approaches

Numerous other techniques of stress reduction incorporate attention control and breathing techniques to elicit the relaxation response. Clinical and research settings have employed progressive muscle relaxation, autogenic training, and visualization techniques. A few of the clinical studies cited later in this chapter were carried out with such techniques.

### Combined Interventions

Many mind-body meditation programs offered in clinical settings today combine meditation with cognitive-behavioral strategies that address a variety of psychological and behavioral variables. Many names are used for this type of program, including *behavioral medicine* and *cognitive-behavioral stress management (CBSM)*.

Such combined interventions offer several approaches to mind-body health. Programs are typically delivered in a group setting, which probably affords important benefits in terms of social support. Participants learn to identify stressors and to self-regulate with meditation or another form of stress reduction. Information is provided about health behaviors such as diet, exercise, and smoking. Practical exercises develop skills in problem solving, emotional self-management, and interpersonal communication. It seems likely that these approaches are synergistic in reducing psychophysiological arousal and the resulting deleterious effects of chronic stress.

It is difficult to distinguish the effects of the various components of combined interventions. The reductionist approach that has dominated biomedical science suggests that we can and should determine the detailed mechanisms and contributions of the various components. However, with the exception of the TM program, much of the clinical and investigative work in mind-body medicine involves combined interventions. The individual interventions probably operate via multiple pathways that we are just beginning to understand. Further, the deleterious effects of chronic stress and other mind-states are likely to be multifactorial. Because of the complexity of mind-body relationships, the reductionist approach may be insufficient to guide rational development of clinical programs. It may be more fruitful to look at global health outcomes to determine whether combined interventions are reliable and cost effective.[7]

# EFFECTS OF MEDITATION

## Physiological Effects

Accumulating data have demonstrated significant physiological changes during various types of meditation. It is important to distinguish between acute effects (those that occur during or shortly after meditation practice) and chronic effects (those that occur after weeks to months of practice). There is also evidence that acute physiological effects differ between experienced (those practicing for more than 6 months) and inexperienced practitioners.

Jevning et al[8] summarized some of the early studies of the acute and chronic effects of TM. The authors noted that acute effects typically occurred after TM periods of 15 to 30 minutes. Consistent findings included decreased oxygen consumption and respiratory rate with stable plasma pH. These were associated with decreased muscle and red blood cell metabolism and decreased serum lactate. Increased cardiac output was associated with stable blood pressure, suggesting a decrease in systemic vascular resistance. Autonomic effects included increased galvanic skin resistance (GSR) and decreased heart rate. Treadmill studies have demonstrated decreased oxygen consumption at constant workload while eliciting the relaxation response.[9]

In long-term meditators, acute neuroendocrine changes include decreased adrenocorticotropic hormone (ACTH) and urinary cortisol excretion. In contrast, short-term practitioners did not demonstrate decreased adrenocortical activity based on plasma cortisol levels. Two studies showed increases in the urinary metabolite of serotonin. Consistent acute electroencephalographic (EEG) findings in meditation included increased hemispheric coherence and increased theta-wave activity. In deeper states of meditation, disappearance of tonic electromyography (EMG) activity has been reported.

Jevning also reports chronic effects of TM. Several studies showed decreased urinary cortisol after 4 to 6 months of practice. Three studies suggested increased autonomic stability in experienced meditators. In these studies, meditators and controls were subject to noxious stimuli, resulting in increased heart rate and decreased GSR. In the meditators, these values returned to baseline more quickly and plasma cortisol levels rose less significantly than in controls.

Some of the effects described may be related to reduced end-organ responsivity to catecholamines. A number of small studies support this hypothesis. In a study of 30 subjects, practitioners of the relaxation response (20 minutes twice daily for 30 days) were compared with controls (ordinary rest for similar period). In response to postural challenge, subjects practicing the relaxation response demonstrated increased plasma catecholamine responses without changes in blood pressure or heart rate.[10] Similar results were found with subjects who were stressed by isometric exercise and painful stimuli.[11] Another study found that 4 to 6 weeks of meditation led to reduced pupillary dilatation in response to topical phenylephrine (alpha-adrenergic agonist).[12] Long-term meditators demonstrate blunting of the lymphocyte redistribution that normally occurs in response to physical stress.[13] Other evidence suggests that meditation brings about a downregulation of the adrenergic receptors that mediate the action of catecholamines.[14]

Meditation has also been shown to increase heart rate variability.[15] Robust heart rate variability suggests balance between the parasympathetic and sympathetic nervous systems and is consistent with earlier findings demonstrating increased autonomic stability. Decreased heart rate variability has been associated with increased cardiac death, chronic pain, fibromyalgia, and other pathological states. As of yet it is unknown whether meditation-induced increases in heart rate variability are associated with improvements in these conditions.

# Psychological Effects of Meditation

The psychological effects of meditation are more difficult to measure than the physiological effects. Research has suggested improvements in concentration, memory, alertness, empathy, and learning ability,[16] as well as reduction in psychological symptoms and increased sense of control over stressful experiences.[17] Furthermore, many meditation traditions report states of mind that may have important implications for health. For example, "mindfulness" and a "sense of interconnection" are often described. These psychological states may be helpful in the setting of the loss, grief, anger, social isolation, and chronic stress that often accompany chronic illness or disability. These mind states are described briefly.

## Mindfulness

Mindfulness might also be called *non-neurotic awareness* or *equanimity*. According to most authorities, mindfulness is not a mystical or spiritual concept. It is a natural quality of mind that everyone possesses to some degree. It develops further by many meditation techniques, including mindfulness meditation. Mindfulness could be described as a state of steady, open awareness that enables one to see things clearly, with minimal distortion by habits of perception, thought, feeling, or action. A thorough discussion of the topic is beyond the scope of this text. Numerous authors from religious and nonreligious backgrounds have discussed the topic in depth.[18,19]

By developing mindfulness, patients can enhance their conscious awareness of mind-body processes. This can allow them to interpret their experience more clearly, and to make more effective, conscious choices

in how they relate to symptoms or functional limitations. In the case of chronic pain, for instance, a patient might learn to notice the quality of persistent pain, its location, quality, associated muscle tension, the flow of emotions that arise and fall in relation to the pain, and so on. The patient begins to notice that pain unconsciously leads to an increase in muscle tension and anxious feelings. There is often a habitual *story line* or commentary, perhaps attributing blame for the pain, concerns about pain-induced inability to work or fulfill family roles, or need for medication. Patients typically notice that the thoughts, feelings, and story line are part of a vicious cycle that worsens pain and leads to a sense of disempowerment. Mindfulness is empowering because it brings awareness to the cascade of thoughts, feelings, physiological responses, and interpretations that arise automatically and habitually in response to the pain sensation. Mindful, conscious awareness of these previously-unconscious mind-body processes enable the patient to stop feeding the vicious cycle of pain, tension, anxiety, and more pain, by making a conscious choice to let go of the muscle tension or disengage from the anxious thoughts and commentary. With time, the tension, anxiety, and story line may not even arise in response to the pain.

Mindfulness also facilitates acceptance of the naturally occurring inner conflict and confusion that go along with being human in a complex world. Meditation practitioners often describe relating to themselves and to the challenges of life with greater gentleness and compassion. This often translates into greater understanding and acceptance of the complexities and behavioral inconsistencies in others and improved interpersonal relationships.

## Interconnectedness

Practitioners of various types of meditation often describe an enhanced sense of interconnectedness with others. There is a feeling of joy and profound well-being and a sense of coherence in otherwise challenging and confusing circumstances. Some people report momentary experiences or steady development of unconditional love for others.

Epidemiological data suggest that psychosocial constructs such as social connectedness and sense of coherence have implications for health. Other data suggest that hostility and cynicism predict negative outcomes. The subjective descriptions of expanded consciousness associated with meditation practice suggest a role for meditation in enhancing a sense of coherence and social connectedness while reducing hostility. Research might further define these constructs, evaluating whether they are changed with meditation practice and whether this correlates with improved health outcomes.

# CLINICAL EFFECTS OF MEDITATION

## Overview

The outcome that is typically most important to rehabilitation professionals is functional status. Unfortunately, minimal research has evaluated whether meditation can improve functional outcomes. However, research has demonstrated that meditation can have positive effects on some of the disease processes, symptoms, and psychosocial challenges faced by patients treated in rehabilitation settings.

The methodological quality of meditation research is quite variable. A critical review is beyond the scope of this text. This chapter cites studies that suggest a role for meditation and cognitive-behavioral stress management (CBSM) in rehabilitation. The development of clinical programs in specific populations would benefit from critical reviews of the relevant research. Further research is needed to assess the safety and efficacy of meditation and behavioral medicine as an adjunct to rehabilitation.

## Arthritis

Self-management courses consisting of relaxation training and cognitive-behavioral training for patients with arthritis have been shown to reduce pain, reduce depressive symptoms, and facilitate increased physical activity. Data suggests that they also reduce healthcare costs by decreasing demand for physician care.[20] Similar interventions have been shown to reduce pain and helplessness and improve self-efficacy.[21]

## Cardiovascular Disease

### Hypertension

Many studies have evaluated meditation and stress management in the treatment of hypertension. Most of the early studies had methodological problems and conflicting results.[22] Since then, a few trials have suggested that meditation can reliably reduce blood pressure. In a randomized controlled trial (RCT) of 213 hypertensive African Americans, 3 months of TM led to significant reductions in systolic and diastolic blood pressure compared with controls.[23] In that study, progressive muscle relaxation also lowered blood pressure, but significantly less than TM. Another RCT showed that relaxation exercise plus education was superior to education alone in allowing reduction of blood pressure medication while maintaining normal pressures.[24] A recent Canadian Medical Association review of the topic led to the conclusion that stress reduction strategies are likely to be helpful in the treatment of hypertension in patients for whom psychosocial stress is an issue.[25]

### Atherosclerosis and Myocardial Ischemia

Studies of stress reduction–based interventions in atherosclerotic heart disease have produced conflicting results. A controlled study evaluated the effects of counseling and stress reduction in 2,328 patients discharged home after myocardial infarction.[26] The patients in the intervention group had a lower frequency of angina, but clinical complications, clinical sequelae, and mortality did not differ between groups at 12 months.

A randomized controlled trial of 60 hypertensive African Americans showed that 6 months of TM reduced carotid artery wall thickness, suggesting regression of atherosclerotic disease.[27]

In a 5-year study of 107 patients with mental stress– or treadmill-induced myocardial ischemia, subjects were randomized to usual care; usual care and exercise; or usual care, stress reduction, and exercise. Endpoints included bypass surgery, angioplasty, and myocardial infarction. At least one of these adverse outcomes occurred in 10% of patients in the stress management group, 21% of patients in the exercise group, and 30% of patients in the usual care group.[28]

In another RCT of 21 middle-aged men with chronic stable angina who were awaiting bypass surgery, 8 months of TM increased exercise tolerance and improved hemodynamic parameters during exercise[29] in meditators, but not in controls.

### Cardiovascular Risk Reduction

A small trial randomized subjects to a program of either education and exercise or stress management plus education and exercise and followed cardiovascular risk factors. The stress management group (progressive muscle relaxation was the self-regulation technique used) demonstrated more significant improvements in blood pressure, obesity indices, cholesterol profile, and cardiovascular conditioning.[30] Similar results have been found with the TM program.

## Chronic Pain

A recent systematic review failed to find convincing evidence that relaxation-type therapies provided more pain relief than various control interventions.[31] However, the review did not include trials that involved multifactorial treatment (i.e., relaxation plus cognitive-behavioral therapy or other interventions in addition to medical treatment). This is unfortunate because multifactorial treatment has become the accepted method of treating chronic pain, which typically develops and is perpetuated by a complex interaction among behavioral, socioeconomic, psychological, and biological factors. At a recent National Institutes of Health (NIH) technology assessment conference, it was concluded that there is strong evidence to support the efficacy of relaxation therapies as adjunctive treatments in the multidisciplinary management of chronic pain.[32] Evidence shows that multifactorial interventions incorporating relaxation or meditation can also reduce the use of healthcare services among people with chronic pain.[33]

## Affective Disorders

Ernst et al[34] reported on three randomized controlled trials of meditation in depressed patients. All three were small trials, and two did not control for the effects of additional attention from providers in the meditation groups. Two of the studies showed that the meditation intervention provided greater relief from depressive symptoms than no intervention. The third found relaxation therapy superior to tricyclic antidepressants.

Patients with anxiety and panic disorder who participated in an 8-week mindfulness-oriented stress reduction program had fewer panic attacks and anxiety symptoms 3 years later.[35]

## Psychological Distress Associated With Chronic Illness

A number of studies have demonstrated that CBSM can reduce psychological distress and stress hormone levels in HIV-positive men. For example, an

RCT of CBSM in symptomatic HIV-positive men demonstrated significant reductions in self-reported anger, anxiety, depressed mood, and confusion compared with controls. The treatment group also had reduced 24-hour urine cortisol levels compared to controls.[36]

In an RCT of 68 patients with malignant melanoma, 6 weeks of multifactorial stress reduction reduced standardized measures of confusion, depression, and fatigue and improved sense of vigor, use of active coping methods, and quality of life. The effects persisted at 6 months. At 6-year follow-up there was a trend for recurrence in the control group, and there was a significantly higher rate of death in the control group (10 of 34 participants) compared with the experimental group (3 of 34 participants).[37]

Another RCT of 90 patients with various cancers found that mindfulness meditation led to similar reductions in emotional distress, as well as reduced somatic symptomatology.[38]

## Insomnia

At a recent NIH technology assessment conference, it was concluded that there is strong evidence for the use of relaxation therapies in appropriate patients with insomnia. The evidence suggests that cognitive therapies such as meditation are more effective than bodily therapies such as progressive muscle relaxation. While the improvements in sleep onset and total sleep time were statistically significant, the report acknowledged that the clinical significance was uncertain. It suggested that patient-by-patient analysis might demonstrate clinical benefit in selected patients.[32]

## Self-Management for People with Chronic Disease

The Chronic Disease Self-Management Program is a CBSM program designed for a mixed population of patients with various chronic illnesses. In an RCT of 952 patients with congestive heart failure, chronic pulmonary disease, osteoarthritis, or stroke, participants demonstrated significant improvements in health behaviors, self-reported health, health distress, and disability when compared with controls. They also spent fewer nights in the hospital than wait-listed controls.[39]

## Somatization

Somatization is the expression of physical symptoms that likely represent psychological distress. It is commonly known that the majority of symptoms presented in primary care offices are ultimately not associated with organic disease. In a retrospective study of 1,000 patients over 3 years, it was found that 84% of the most common presenting symptoms were not found to have an organic basis despite diagnostic evaluation.[40] Compared with controls, people with somatization disorder exhibit increased levels of physiological arousal (heart rate, serum cortisol) and subjective feelings of tension in response to laboratory stressors. Further, the control subjects demonstrated blunting of stress responses (habituation) in response to repeated stress. In contrast, the subjects who were somatizing demonstrated a lack of habituation in heart rate and a subjective sense of tension.[41] This suggests that people with somatization have an impaired ability to tolerate acute stress and fail to adapt to recurrent stress. In an RCT of 68 outpatients with multiple somatic symptoms and high clinic usage, the meditation-based CBSM program reduced physical and psychological symptoms and decreased clinic usage. The education-only control group demonstrated minimal or no improvement in these measures.[42]

## WHY SHOULD MEDITATION IMPROVE HEALTH?

## Assumptions

Data show that chronic psychological stress has important biological and clinical effects that can contribute to the development and progression of a variety of illnesses. The general assumption is that the health impact of psychological stress is mediated by the physiological stress response. The physiological stress response consists of an increased ratio of sympathetic to parasympathetic outflow from the autonomic nervous system and increases in neuroendocrine stress modulators such as catecholamines and cortisol. Chronic psychological stress has been associated with impaired memory; hippocampal neuronal atrophy and death; impaired immune function and wound healing; increased infection rates; increased adverse events related to atherosclerotic heart disease; increased gastrointestinal and somatic symptoms; increased musculoskeletal pain;[43] and impaired ability to control unhealthy behaviors such as smoking, overeating, and substance abuse.[44]

Box 9-1 summarizes some of the mechanisms by which meditation and CBSM might reduce chronic or excessive stress and its potentially damaging effects. Items marked with an asterisk (*) are supported by scientific study. Others extrapolate from clinical experience and indirect research.

Reduction of chronic stress is likely to be part of the mechanism by which meditation and CBSM can be therapeutic. It is generally understood that stress is harmful when the physiological stress response is excessive and/or prolonged. McEwen[45] discusses four factors that seem to determine whether a given stimulus will contribute to dangerous chronic elevation of stress mediators. These factors vary among individuals depending on genetic, environmental, and behavioral variables.

1.  Does the person's mind-body perceive the stimulus as stressful? For example, an academic examination or a parking ticket may be stressful to one person but not another.

---

BOX 9-1

*Physiological and Psychological Changes by Which Meditation May Reduce Stress*

- Decreased cortisol levels*
- Decreased end-organ responsivity to stress hormones*
- Decreased magnitude of stress response*
- Reduced duration of stress response (faster return to baseline after arousal resulting from stressor)*
- Enhanced awareness of stressors and development of coping strategies
- Cognitive restructuring and reinterpretation of stimuli as less stressful*
- Improved communication skills and interpersonal relationships
- Enhanced self-efficacy in health behaviors (i.e., exercise, diet, medication use)
- Decreased stress-induced practice of unhealthy behaviors (i.e., smoking, substance abuse)

*Changes that have been demonstrated in scientific studies of meditators.

2.  What is the magnitude of the physiological stress response to the stimulus?
3.  After the stimulus is removed, does the stress response shut off or persist? Some people seem to hold onto a persistent state of psychophysiological arousal after a stressor, while others quickly return to baseline. Posttraumatic stress disorder is an extreme example of this.
4.  How does the person respond to recurrent stimuli? Is there a behavioral, psychological, or physiological process that reduces the stress response to recurrent stimuli (habituation)? Or does the stress response get larger with recurrent stimuli (sensitization)?

Meditation may reduce stress by modulating one or more of these factors. Therefore these four factors have implications for referral of patients to clinical programs and for the design and interpretation of meditation research. For example, strategies directed at reducing the effects of stress are unlikely to be helpful for individuals who mount stress responses that are small or short in duration. On the other hand, greater benefit might be expected for individuals who respond to daily circumstances with a large or prolonged stress response. Further research is needed to guide thinking in this area.

## Physical Attributes

The autonomic nervous system and hypothalamic-pituitary adrenal axis (HPA axis) are well-established mechanisms by which chronic or excessive psychological stress can influence disease processes. There is evidence for other mechanisms of mind-body interaction. Emotional and psychological experiences are associated with nearly instantaneous communication of information to the immune system via neuropeptides. In turn, immune cells produce neuropeptides that can modulate thoughts and emotion.[46] Similar pathways connect the mind and other organ systems.[47] The emerging picture suggests that information is constantly being shared among the organ systems that are responsible for psychological, emotional, and biological processes.

These pathways suggest a mechanistic substrate by which mental states can have important positive or negative effects on health. Besides reducing stress, meditation brings about psychological states such as increased empathy and joy and a sense of well-being, interconnection with others, and coherence. There are also measurable changes in brain activity, including enhanced hemispheric coherence and increased slow-wave activity. It seems possible that these changes in brain activity and psychological states are associated with clinically important effects on endogenous systems of self-repair and self-healing. Further research is needed to evaluate the mechanisms by which this might occur.

## IMPLICATIONS FOR REHABILITATION

It is unfortunate that more research has not yet evaluated the effects of meditation and CBSM in rehabilitation populations. Nonetheless, data from other patient populations suggest that meditation can have several possible benefits in the rehabilitation setting. The breadth of these findings suggests that widespread application of meditation and CBSM in the rehabilitation setting could reduce morbidity, improve psychological coping, facilitate more effective rehabilitation, and reduce costs. There are four primary ways in which meditation and CBSM might improve rehabilitation outcomes.

1.  As discussed, meditation and CBSM can improve outcomes of chronic illnesses such as cardiovascular disease, lung disease, arthritis, and diabetes that underlie or accompany many rehabilitation diagnoses.
2.  Chronic illness is associated with psychological distress that is correlated with degree of disability.[48] Meditation can directly reduce psychological distress. CBSM provides skills for dealing with the psychosocial challenges that are present in daily life and often exacerbated by chronic illness and disability. Further, as Kabat-Zinn discusses in the foreword to this book and as described in the box on p. 118, mindfulness can help rehabilitation patients accept the changes that accompany disablement and access inner resources that are so important to the process of becoming reenabled.
3.  A reduction in nonorganic somatic symptoms may facilitate more successful rehabilitation. Clinical experience suggests that selected patients in both outpatient and inpatient rehabilitation settings present symptoms that resolve when psychological, emotional, and spiritual concerns are addressed. A previous section of this chapter referred to studies demonstrating that meditation-based interventions reduce symptoms and healthcare

usage in high-use medical outpatients with multiple symptoms and in cancer patients. It is likely that similar reductions in symptoms would be enjoyed by somatizing patients in rehabilitation settings. A reduction in somatic symptoms could improve participation in therapy and reduce unnecessary diagnostic and therapeutic interventions.

4. Reduction in psychological stress could have a variety of clinically important short-term effects. Research demonstrates that psychological stress impairs immune function and wound healing,[49] increases viral infection rate,[50] and impairs learning and memory.[51] Psychological stress can also contribute to increased pain, anxiety, and insomnia. Further research could evaluate whether effective stress reduction through meditation can improve wound-healing rates in postoperative patients and amputees. Other possible effects include reduced viral infection rates among inpatients (and perhaps staff) if carrier rates decrease within a hospital. Finally, meditation can reduce pain, anxiety, and insomnia. The associated reduction in the use of narcotics, benzodiazepines, and other sedatives might afford improvements in mental status and facilitate more effective rehabilitation efforts (see Case Study).

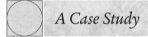

## A Case Study

### Spinal Cord Injury

JB is a 53-year-old man who sustained a T9 burst fracture at 19 years of age in 1967. He has no voluntary motor or sensation below the level of his injury.

*How did you begin practicing meditation?* I had been seeing a massage therapist who introduced me to his meditation teacher. I began to practice Zen meditation in my late 20's. Later I switched to vipassana, or mindfulness meditation.

*Has it been helpful? How so?* Yes, in a few ways. First, it has helped me develop more clarity in my thinking and I'm better at calming down when I become anxious. The vipassana teachings and practice also have helped me to see how much I was a prisoner of my emotional states, especially aversion.

*What do you mean by "prisoner of aversion"?* I was having lots of problems with my bowels, difficulty integrating into society, and financial problems. When something unpleasant came up, I would get incredibly frustrated and aggravated. The recurrent frustration led to discouragement,

despair, and fatigue. I think that contributed to the depression that I often experienced.

*How has the meditation practice helped?* I saw pretty quickly that I was making matters worse by reacting to the unpleasant stuff with frustration leading to anger leading to discouragement and so on. The practice let me see that the unpleasant thought, no matter how intense, is a transient phenomenon. It may be related to a circumstance that is real and important and needs attention and effort. But the thought that is generated, be it frustration or anger or confusion, is just a thought. When mindfulness isn't present, it's easy for me to identify with the unpleasant thoughts and get into a negative spiral. Mindfulness practice has provided a lifeline that helps me pull myself out of the spiral. When discouraging thoughts come, they are less overwhelming. I have learned to notice the difficult stuff without trying to push it away so much. The difficult situations haven't gone away, of course, but there is less anger and frustration and discouragement. Because I'm not consuming mental and physical energy by churning with anger and frustration, I have more resources to deal effectively with reality.

*Has meditation helped you in other ways?* Yes. The body awareness practice has been very helpful. I'm less likely to overreach or overstress myself. And it seems like I'm able to tune in better to what is happening in my body, again without so much aversion, and do what is needed. You know, to take care of business without making a drama out of it. Also, I find that many doctors don't know how to take care of people with spinal cord injuries, especially in the rural area where live. I have to really be in charge of my care. This has been especially helpful in dealing with my neurogenic bowel.

*Did you have any adverse effects?* Yes. In the beginning, I wanted to do things just right, so I would sit on one of those hard cushions at the meditation center. I developed coccygeal pressure sores that took awhile to heal. Now I use my wheelchair cushion and don't have problems.  ❧

# MEDITATION AND HEALTHCARE PROVIDERS

## Relationship

The quality of relationship between provider and patient can have a powerful influence on clinical outcomes and the satisfaction of patients and providers.[52] This relationship can be affected by a caregiver's personality, values, attitudes, and emotional needs. When these highly personal variables are unrecognized, they can interfere with discussions about difficult topics such as end-of-life care and emotional despair. Unconscious biases can also prevent the experience or clear communication of empathy. A variety of approaches have been developed to improve physicians' self-awareness and ability to process information and communicate clearly on mental and emotional levels.[53] Epstein[54] and Connelly[55] eloquently discuss mindfulness, or present moment awareness, as a way of being that facilitates a provider's ability to self-monitor, be aware of deeply held values and biases, use implicit knowledge and experience, and empathize with others. Meditation can facilitate the development of mindfulness, thereby improving reflective self-awareness and empathy.[56]

Further, most physicians and healthcare providers are tightly scheduled and overwhelmed with urgent demands and interruptions. These stressful and distracting conditions can impair diagnostic accuracy and decision making. By reducing stress and developing concentration, meditation can reduce the likelihood of burnout and improve decision making (see Case Study).

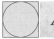 *A Case Study*

*Physician Stress*
DJ is a 33-year-old physician.

*What kind of meditation do you do, and why did you start?* I've been practicing mindfulness meditation on and off for about 8 years. I was drawn to it as a way of reducing stress during medical school.

*How has it affected you?* Possibly the most important effect of the practice is that I have a smoother relationship with the ups and downs of life and medical practice. To use a surfing metaphor, I feel that when the waves come in, I'm more able to ride them instead of having them crash over my head. It's not that I don't have any stress, but I have less than I used to, and I know when it's building up so I can let it go a bit. I also feel that I've learned to see more clearly what is going on inside of me when difficult situations arise, and it lets me make more conscious choices about my responses, instead of being pushed along by knee-jerk reactions. It is as if there is an extra voice inside of me that lets me know when I'm reacting unconsciously. My meditation teacher used to call it "observer consciousness."

*Can you give an example?* Sure. I was trying to finish rounds and get to a meeting last week. Mrs. J. was complaining about everything, it seemed. (Lots of things bother her.) I was standing at the foot of the bed getting increasingly impatient and frustrated with her, trying to quickly fix her complaints so I could go on with my day. It seemed as though the more I responded to her complaints, the more complaints she presented. I was getting really annoyed. Then that observer voice came in and said, "Relax and breathe." I took a mindful breath, relaxed and let go a bit, and sat down at the bedside at eye level and listened to her complaints for about 3 minutes with all of my attention, letting myself be open to what she might be feeling. As I listened, I remembered that her son was supposed to come visit her that weekend and asked her about that. She said he wasn't coming because of his job and she was angry about it. Her anger turned to sadness and she started sobbing. I just listened and gave her hand a squeeze. I asked her if anything else was troubling her. She said she felt much better and thanked me profusely for listening to her. The whole thing took less than 10 minutes and really seemed to help her.

*Anything else you want to say?* Yes. The "observer consciousness" seems like the long-term benefit of meditation practice that goes with me even when I'm not practicing. But the actual practice still has immediate benefits. When I'm having a particularly stressful day, I sit down for about 10 minutes before lunch, close my eyes, tune into my breathing, and let go of the physical and mental tension I've been carrying around. I get a boost of energy, I think more clearly, and my lunch tastes better. ❧

## ECONOMIC CONSIDERATIONS

Most efforts to reduce healthcare costs have focused on reducing the supply of services. In such a framework, it is difficult to imagine adding interventions such as meditation or other mind-body therapies. However, mind-body interventions affect many of the determinants of demand for healthcare services. By reducing symptoms and psychological distress and possibly improving disease outcomes, these interventions reduce demand for care, thus reducing costs. This has been borne out in controlled studies that have estimated significant cost savings and improved outcomes with behavioral programs.[57] For example, the Chronic Disease Self-Management Program that was discussed earlier led to reduced hospital stays for the subjects compared with waitlist controls. Assuming that a day in the hospital costs $1,000, the healthcare expenditure savings (savings in hospital visits minus program costs) approximated $750 per participant—more than 10 times the cost of the program.

Mind-body programs can yield a cost offset that will benefit forward-looking managed care companies. Some third-party payers have taken note and begun to reimburse for such programs. In the future, more payers may reimburse for meditation-based mind-body programs.[58]

## SUMMARY

In conclusion, the term *meditation* applies to a variety of attentional techniques that share clinically important physiological and psychological effects. There is a rational foundation and evidence to support the assertion that meditation and CBSM can reduce psychological distress and have meaningful impacts on some chronic illnesses. Further evidence suggests that the initial cost of meditation-based programs can be offset by reduced usage of healthcare services. The sense of interconnectedness and mindfulness that develop with meditation practice may have important implications for functional status and chronic illness outcomes. Further research is needed to design meditation-based interventions that can reliably improve rehabilitation outcomes.

In closing, it is notable that part of the therapeutic power of meditation may be rooted in its encouragement of "non-effort." This is in strong contrast to most rehabilitation interventions. Most of what we do in rehabilitation is goal oriented. Whether it is enhanced cardiovascular conditioning, improved upper extremity coordination, or independent mobility or self-care skills, rehabilitation patients and providers alike conceptualize what is important and create plans for how to achieve goals. In contrast, most approaches to meditation cultivate acceptance of things as they are. The emphasis is on allowing one's experience to "be" just as it is without judgment or manipulation. "Successful" meditation involves dropping the goal, dropping the agenda, and noticing what is happening. This passive, receptive state of mind is not seen as superior or as an alternative to a goal orientation. Rather, it is complementary to the goal orientation that one needs to regain function after illness or injury.

Why would a passive state of mind be complementary to a goal orientation? From a purely mechanistic point of view, the mind-body system needs to cycle between rest and activity for optimal functioning. Meditation can provide deep mind-body rest at any time, in any place, without special equipment. As the practitioner shifts from "doing" to "being," there is enhancement of homeostatic mechanisms associated with increased activity of the parasympathetic nervous system. This is in contrast to the increased sympathetic tone associated with exercise.

From another view, this "letting go" often puts practitioners in contact with important inner sources of emotional and psychological strength. Most of the world's spiritual and healing traditions acknowledge the innate healing intelligence that inhabits our mind-body system. Likewise, healers of many kinds discuss the importance of listening deeply and nonjudgmentally to the whole person, making room for expression of the natural intelligence that moves through every individual. Thoughtful practitioners of modern scientifically based healing arts such as medicine and psychotherapy typically agree that deep empathetic listening can itself be a therapeutic intervention. Meditation helps its practitioners listen deeply and unconditionally to their own mind-body processes. In so doing, it empowers patients and practitioners to heal themselves.

## References

1. Eisenberg D et al: Trends in alternative medicine use in the United States, 1990-1997: results of a follow-up national survey, *JAMA* 280(18):1569-1575, 1998.
2. Krauss HH et al: Alternative health care: its use by individuals with physical disabilities, *Arch Phys Med Rehabil* 79:1440-1446, 1998.
3. Schneider RJL, Maharishi International University of Management, Fairfield, Iowa. Personal communication, 2001.
4. Benson H: *The relaxation response,* New York, Morrow, 1975.
5. Wallace RK, Benson H, Wilson AF: A wakeful hypometabolic physiologic state, *Am J Physiol* 221(3):795-799, 1971.
6. Orme-Johnson DW, Walton KG: All approaches to preventing or reversing the effects of stress are not the same, *Am J Health Promot* 2(5):297-299, 1998.
7. Myers SS, Benson H: Psychological factors in healing: a new perspective on an old debate, *Behav Med* 18(1):5-11, 1992.
8. Jevning R, Wallace R, Beidebach M: The physiology of meditation: a review—a wakeful hypometabolic integrated response, *Neurosci Biobehav Rev* 16:415-424, 1992.
9. Benson H, Dryer T, Hartley L: Decreased VO2 consumption during exercise with elicitation of the relaxation response, *J Human Stress* 4(2):38-42, 1978.
10. Hoffman JW et al: Reduced sympathetic nervous system responsivity associated with the relaxation response, *Science* 215(4529):190-192, 1982.
11. Morrell EM, Hollandsworth JG Jr: Norepinephrine alterations under stress conditions following the regular practice of meditation, *Psychosom Med* 48:270-277, 1986.

12. Lehmann JW, Goodale IL, Benson H: Reduced pupillary sensitivity to topical phenylephrine associated with the relaxation response, *J Human Stress* 12:101-104, 1986.

13. Solber EE, Halvorsen R, et al: Meditation: a modulator of the immune response to physical stress? *Br J Sports Med* 29(4):255-257, 1995.

14. Mills P et al: Beta-adrenergic receptor sensitivity in subjects practicing transcendental meditation, *J Psychosom Res* 34(1):29-33, 1990.

15. Sakakibara M, Satoshi R, et al: Effect relaxation training on cardiac parasympathetic tone, *Psychophysiology* 31:223-228, 1994.

16. Murphy M, Donovan S: *The physical and psychological effects of meditation: a review of contemporary research with a comprehensive bibliography, 1931-1996,* ed 2, Sausalito, Calif, Institute of Noetic Sciences, 1999.

17. Astin J: Stress reduction through mindfulness meditation: effects on psychological symptomatology, sense of control, and spiritual experiences, *Pscyhother Psychosom Med Psychol* 66(2):97-106, 1997.

18. Nhat Hahn T: *Peace is every step: the path of mindfulness in daily life,* New York, Bantam Books, 1992.

19. Santorelli S: *Heal thy self: lessons on mindfulness in medicine* Bell Tower, 1999.

20. Lorig K, Holman HR: Evidence suggesting that health education for self-management in patient with chronic arthritis has sustained health benefits while reducing health care costs, *Arthritis Rheum* 36:439-446, 1993.

21. Parker JC, Buckelew SP, Stucky-Ropp RC, et al: Effects of stress management on clinical outcomes in rheumatoid arthritis, *Arthritis Rheum* 38(12):1807-1818, 1995.

22. Eisenberg DM, Delbanco TL, Berkey CS, et al: Cognitive behavioral techniques for hypertension: are they effective? *Ann Intern Med* 118:964-972, 1993.

23. Schneider RH et al: A randomized controlled trial of stress reduction for hypertension in older African Americans, *Hypertension* 26(5):820-827, 1995.

24. Shapiro D, Hui KK, Oakley ME, et al: Reduction in drug requirements by means of a cognitive-behavioral intervention, *Am J Hypertens* 10:9-17, 1997.

25. Spence JD et al: Recommendations on stress management: lifestyle modifications to prevent and control hypertension, *CMAJ* 160(9 Suppl):S46-50, 1999.

26. Jones DA, West RR: Psychological rehabilitation after myocardial infarction: multicentre randomised controlled trial, *BMJ* 313:1517-1521, 1996.

27. Castillo-Richmond A et al: Effects of stress reduction on carotid atherosclerosis in hypertensive African Americans, *Stroke* 31(3):568-573, 2000.

28. Blumenthal JA et al: Stress management and exercise training in cardiac patients with myocardial ischemia: effects on prognosis and evaluation of mechanisms, *Arch Intern Med* 157(19):2213-2223, 1997.

29. Zamarra JW et al: Usefulness of the transcendental meditation program in the treatment of patients with coronary artery disease, *Am J Cardiol* 77(10):867-870, 1996.

30. McCrone SH, Brendle D, Barton KM: A multibehavioral intervention to decrease cardiovascular disease risk factors in older men, *AACN Clin Issues* 12(1):5-16, 2001.

31. Carroll D et al: Relaxation for the relief of chronic pain: a systematic review, *J Adv Nurs* 27(3):476-487, 1998.

32. Integration of Behavioral and Relaxation Approaches into the Treatment of Chronic Pain and Insomnia. NIH Technology Assessment Statement, 1995.

33. Caudill M et al: Decreased clinic utilization by chronic pain patients after behavioral medicine intervention, *Pain* 45(3):334-335, 1991 (letter).

34. Ernst E, Rand JI, Stevinson C: Complementary therapies for depression: an overview, *Arch Gen Psychiatry* 55(11):1026-1032, 1998.

35. Miller J et al: Three-year follow-up and clinical implications of a mindfulness meditation-based stress reduction intervention in the treatment of anxiety disorders, *Gen Hosp Psychiatry* 17:192-200, 1995.

36. Antoni MH et al: Cognitive-behavioral stress management reduces distress and 24-hour urinary free cortisol output among symptomatic HIV-infected gay men, *Ann Behav Med* 22(1):29-37, 2000.

37. Fawzy FI, Fawzy NW, et al: Malignant melanoma: effects of an early structured psychiatric intervention, coping, and affective state on recurrence and survival 6 years later, *Arch Gen Psychiatry* 50:681-689, 1993.

38. Speca MP et al: A randomized, wait-list controlled clinical trial: the effect of a mindfulness meditation-based stress reduction program on mood and symptoms of stress in cancer outpatients, *Psychosom Med* 62(5):613-622, 2000.

39. Lorig KR et al: Evidence suggesting that a chronic disease self-management program can improve health status while reducing hospitalization: a randomized trial, *Med Care* 37(1):5-14, 1999.

40. Kroenke K, Mangelsdorff AD, et al: Common symptoms in ambulatory care: incidence evaluation, therapy, and outcome, *Am J Med* 86(3):262-266, 1989.

41. Rief WP, Shaw RP, Fichter MM: Elevated levels of psychophysiological arousal and cortisol in patients with somatization syndrome, *Psychosom Med* 60(2):198-203, 1998.

42. Hellman CJC, Budd M, Borysenko J, et al: A study of the effectiveness of two group behavioral medicine interventions for patients with psychosomatic complaints, *Behav Med* 16:165-173, 1990.

43. Hubbard J, Workman E: *Handbook of stress medicine: an organ system approach,* New York, CRC Press, 1998.

44. Heatherton TF, Renn RJ: Stress and the disinhibition of behavior, *Mind/Body Med* 1:72-81, 1995.

45. McEwen BS: Protective and damaging effects of stress mediators: central role of the brain, *Prog Brain Res* 122:25-42, 2000.

46. Pert C: *Molecules of emotion,* New York, Scribner, 1997.

47. Mayer E, Naliboff B, Munakata J: The evolving neurobiology of gut feelings, *Prog Brain Res* 122:195-206, 2000.

48. Ormel J et al: Chronic medical conditions and mental health in older people: disability and psychosocial resources mediate specific mental health effects, *Psychol Med* 27(5):1065-1077, 1997.

49. Rozlog LA et al: Stress and immunity: implications for viral disease and wound healing (review), *J Periodontol* 70(7):786-792, 1999.

50. Cohen S, Tyrrell DAJ, Smith AP: Psychological stress and susceptibility to the common cold, *New Engl J Med* 325:606-612, 1991.

51. McEwen BS, Sapolsky RM: Stress and cognitive function, *Curr Opin Neurobiol* 5(2):205-216, 1995.

52. Tresolini CP, Pew-Fetzer Task Force: *Health professions education and relationship-centered care,* San Francisco, Pew Health Professions Commission, 1994.

53. Novack D et al: Calibrating the physician: personal awareness and effective patient care, *JAMA* 278(6):502-509, 1997.

54. Epstein RM: Mindful practice, *JAMA* 282(9):833-839, 1999.

55. Connelly J: Being in the present moment: developing the capacity for mindfulness in medicine, *Acad Med* 74(4):420-424, 1999.

56. Shapiro SL, Schwartz GE, Bonner G: Effects of mindfulness-based stress reduction on medical and premedical students, *J Behav Med* 21(6):581-599, 1998.

57. Sobel D: The cost-effectiveness of mind-body medicine interventions, *Prog Brain Res* 122:393-412, 2000. In Mayer EA, Saber CB (eds): *The biological basis for mind body interactions, vol 122,* New York, Elsevier Science, 2000.

58. Marwick C: Managed care may feature behavioral medicine, *JAMA* 275(15):1144-1146, 1996.

## Suggested Readings

Ader R, Felten DL, Cohen N (eds): *Psychoneuroimmunology,* ed 3, San Diego, Academic Press, 2001.

The definitive textbook in the field. The research that is summarized demonstrates the indivisibility of somatic and psychological processes and the inseparability of immunological and neuroendocrine processes. The book also discusses the clinical implications of psychoneuroimmunology, covering neurological and psychiatric diseases, infection, surgical trauma, cardiovascular disease, periodontal disease, alcoholism, and aging. It also addresses the influence of emotions on immune responsiveness and the ways in which personal and social support can help in the recovery from an immune-mediated disease.

Mayer EA, Saper CB (eds): *The biological basis for mind body interactions, vol 122,* Elsevier Science, New York, 2000.

A collection of state-of-the-art reviews of different aspects of brain-mind-body interactions in health and disease. Main sections include I. The relationship between mind, brain, and emotions; II. Neurobiology of the stress response; III. Early life experiences and the developing brain; IV. Influences of the internal environment on the brain; V. Influences of the body on the brain; VI. Influences of the brain and mind on the body; and VII. Practical use of mind-body interactions in medicine.

Hubbard J, Workman E (eds): *Handbook of Stress Medicine: an organ system approach,* New York, CRC Press, 1998.

Discusses the implications of stress for health and disease in all the organ systems. Most chapters contain detailed reviews of the relevant literature.

Murphy M, Donovan S: *The physical and psychological effects of meditation: a review of contemporary research with a comprehensive bibliography, 1931-1996,* ed 2, Sausalito, Calif, Institute of Noetic Sciences, 1999.

Provides a thoughtful overview of various meditation traditions and their potential implications. The bibliography is extensive, though it does not rate the methodological quality of cited research.

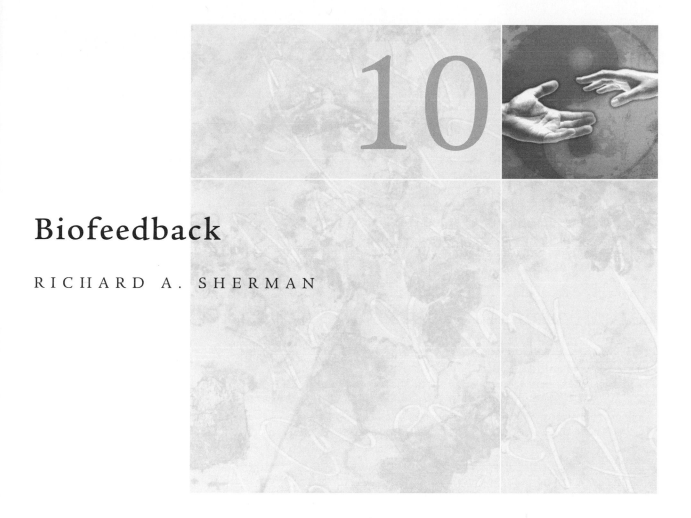

# Biofeedback

RICHARD A. SHERMAN

In this chapter,* you will learn about biofeedback, including a bit of its history, some of its typical uses, psychophysiological recording and biofeedback techniques used in the evaluative and interventional processes, and typical clinical interventions that incorporate biofeedback into the rehabilitation process.

Biofeedback is the act of showing someone real-time recordings of one or more physiological systems (e.g., muscle tension in the jaw) as they are made. This permits both the person being recorded and any coach or therapist who may be present to be instantly aware of (1) the level at which the physiological system is functioning and (2) changes in the level of functioning.

This information can be used to increase the person's awareness of the functioning of the particular physiological system and/or to correct the level of functioning if it is not optimal for the given circumstances. The true strength of biofeedback is that it can be used to objectively demonstrate to both the patient and therapist the underlying physiological dysfunctions (e.g., elevated muscle tension) causing the disorder. Both the patient and the therapist can actually see the changes in physiology as the training progresses through the rehabilitation process. Thus this chapter is about how to help people learn self-regulation skills to control a clinical problem by enhancing their ability to perform in physiologically optimal ways.

---

*This chapter is adapted from Sherman RA: *Psychophysiology in Pain Assessment and Control,* which was accepted for publication by the Association for Applied Psychophysiology in 1999.

People do not function in physiologically optimal ways for innumerable reasons. One of the most common is not realizing when a physiological system is not functioning at the best level for the particular situation. For example, many runners do not use optimal breathing patterns for sustained running. Many people get headaches because they keep muscles in their jaws too tense for too long either because they do not realize their jaw muscles are tense or because they do not habitually relax their muscles after the need for them to be tense has passed. Techniques such as biofeedback help people (1) recognize how a physiological system is functioning and (2) learn to form a habit of controlling the system so that it works optimally. Biofeedback can be used in the realms of sports, education, medicine, and many more.

## THE BIOFEEDBACK PROCESS

*Psychophysiology* is the study of interrelationships between the mind and the body. Therefore *applied psychophysiology* is the use of knowledge about these interactions to develop and apply techniques for altering the relationships to correct clinical problems. Applied psychophysiological techniques include biofeedback, progressive muscle relaxation training, and autogenic training, among others. These techniques are used in conjunction with techniques as diverse as muscle balance training, cognitive therapy, classical conditioning, and urodynamics drawn from virtually every healthcare field.

Within the context of applied psychophysiology, when biofeedback instruments are discussed, we usually mean an electronic device that can record one or more physiological parameters and can show the information to the patient as it happens. However, mirrors and similar simple devices are equally valid and often very useful biofeedback devices. Each physiological parameter recorded normally has a shorthand description. For example, *sEMG* stands for a surface electromyogram. This is an electrical signal moderately correlated with a person's muscle contraction, which is recorded from the surface of the skin. *Biofeedback* is a dynamic combination of learning processes and procedures in which the patient and therapist receive information about the immediate status of a physiological parameter. This information is usually provided by instrumented biofeedback using physiological recording instruments (e.g., surface muscle tension monitors or

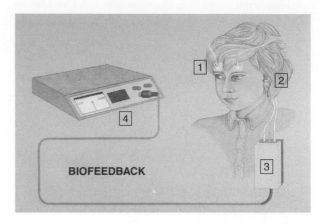

*Figure 10-1* Simplified biofeedback system. Sensors *(1)* for picking up tiny signals from muscles are taped to the forehead and compared with signals from a reference sensor *(2)* to minimize noise from the body. The signals are then amplified *(3)* to minimize contamination by noise from the environment and sent to a biofeedback device *(4)* which displays the signals.

mirrors) with displays designed to optimize the subject's ability to recognize information of interest. The information is used to (1) recognize abnormalities in the parameter's functioning and (2) correct the abnormalities. Home practice of awareness and control exercises (e.g., progressive muscle relaxation exercises) are usually used to heighten the subject's own perceptions of the functioning of the parameter both at home and in the workplace. Patients learn to be very aware of changes in the parameter of interest while they are in their normal environments so that they can learn what causes changes that lead to problems. The feedback from the biofeedback device is used to help relate various intensities of sensations to the actual level at which the parameter is functioning that second. Once the patient can tell that a parameter is functioning abnormally, he or she can correct the function with skills learned during biofeedback and home practice sessions. Biofeedback devices are thought to shorten the time required to learn to control physiological parameters because (1) patients can see the results of their control strategies instantly by monitoring the biofeedback signal and (2) comparing the signal showing actual levels of a parameter with sensations coming from the body permits accurate calibration of the meaning of sensations to what the body is actually doing. If patients do not learn these skills, they are not likely to get better. Figure 10-1 shows a sim-

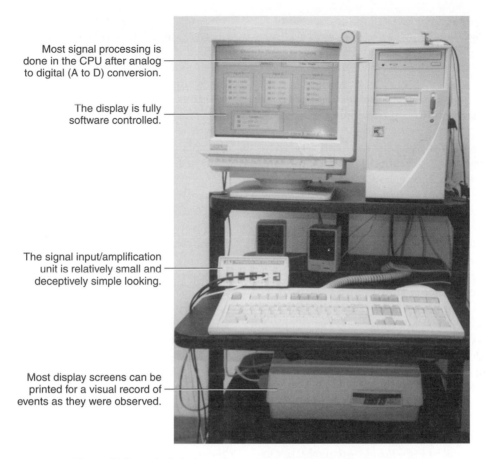

Most signal processing is done in the CPU after analog to digital (A to D) conversion.

The display is fully software controlled.

The signal input/amplification unit is relatively small and deceptively simple looking.

Most display screens can be printed for a visual record of events as they were observed.

*Figure 10-2* Typical desktop computer-based biofeedback system.

plified biofeedback system, and Figure 10-2 is a typical desktop computer-based biofeedback system.

Tiny biofeedback devices capable of fitting into a pocket are sometimes used to record relationships between change in the intensity of the disorder and change in related physiological parameters. These battery-powered ambulatory units can go anywhere dry that a patient goes. For example, a patient may wear the unit for several days and use the keypad to enter changes in back pain and types of activities engaged in while sensors taped to the low back muscles record changes in muscle tension. Figure 10-3 shows such a device set to record two channels of muscle tension and motion. Feedback can be from headphones, a vibrator, the digital display window near the top of the unit, or the analog light bars that run along the bottom of the unit. Small biofeedback devices are commonly used as home trainers, as are fingertip-size thermometers and

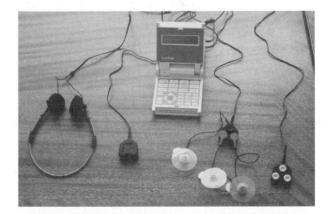

*Figure 10-3* Typical ambulatory recorder/biofeedback device, which can be used to record patterns of muscle tension, motion, and keyboard representations of pain intensity in the patient's normal environment. The device can go anywhere the patient goes and can provide both auditory and visual feedback.

other simple devices, to cue patients to the status of their physiology.

An example of the logic behind a typical intervention will help clarify the issues. When a patient comes to the orthopedic clinic where I practice, complaining of pain in the upper back and shoulders that often radiates to the neck and head, he or she gets a traditional workup. Most patients have already been evaluated by a physical medicine healthcare provider; therefore trigger points (TrPs) and postural problems such as forward head thrust have already been ruled out, and conservative modalities provided by physical therapy have failed. If the physical examination and the usual array of imaging tests have not shown any particular results other than potential muscle tension problems, the patient is likely to have an opportunity to talk with me.

When patients report that their pain is exacerbated by physical and psychological stresses and that the pain tends to begin with tightness in the back and shoulders before it extends to the neck and head, I know that this person is probably a reasonable candidate for psychophysiological intervention. Of course, such "clean," obvious patients with a decent workup are rare. Most are a complex maze of problems.

The usual first step is to conduct a stress profile, during which several physiological systems reactive to stress (e.g., muscle tension in the forehead and shoulders, heart rate, respiration, and fingertip temperature) are recorded while the patient is somewhat relaxed, imagining stressful and relaxing situations. The typical evaluation will be discussed later in this chapter. However, this step might well be skipped for our sample patient because we already know from his history that he tenses up his shoulder and facial muscles when he is tense. By the same logic, he is probably appropriate for muscle tension awareness—relaxation training including feedback of surface electromyographic (EMG) representations of muscle tension and home use of relaxation exercises. This combination is chosen because muscles become painful when kept too tense for too long as a result of spasms, stress, incorrect posture, and guarding due to pain. Typical examples include tension-type headaches, pain due to spasms following a stroke, and cramping phantom limb pain due to spikes in muscles of the residual limb. As you might expect, the relationship between muscle tension and pain is not simple for any of these problems.

After an appropriate assessment, the patient is taught a simple muscle tension awareness and control exercise to use at home several times per day in conjunction with a tape recording of the exercise. During succeeding sessions, tension in the forehead and trapezius muscles is shown to the patient and therapist. The patient learns to relate sensations from the muscle to actual levels of tension (calibration) and to habitually control them when they are incorrect. The therapist uses the information provided by the biofeedback device to coach the patient toward better strategies of control and to track progress throughout the treatment.

The patient learns to recognize incorrect tension in the normal environment through home practice emphasizing muscle tension awareness/control/relaxation exercises. No attempt is made to teach patients not to tense their muscles in response to a physically or psychologically stressful situation because responses to stress are part of our basic wiring. Rather, the idea is for patients to learn not to become tenser than necessary in any given situation or to remain tense longer than necessary. Patients tend to progress through various stages of training as they get better at recognizing their muscle tension levels, recognizing what affects those levels, and controlling them.

Figure 10-4 illustrates a typical biofeedback display of "raw" muscle tension recorded from the biceps and triceps as the arm is sequentially bent and straightened at the elbow several times. The raw signal is a digitized representation of the electricity produced by motor units in the muscle firing virtually at the same time. This summation of electricity from many motor units creates the envelope of power, which is proportional to signal strength. Thus the larger the envelope (vertically) the greater the signal strength (and, in this case, the greater the muscle tension).

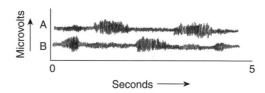

*Figure 10-4* "Raw" signals changing over time from the bicep and tricep muscles as the arm is consecutively bent and straightened at the elbow.

These raw signals can be averaged so that each signal appears as a moving line on the screen. The dot at the end of each line goes up as signal strength increases (and, in this case, as muscles tense) and goes down as the signal gets smaller. By observing the relationship of the lines, both the therapist and patient can watch what the muscles are doing in relation to each other at any moment and compare the relationship with what it was moments ago. Instead of showing a moving dot going across the screen, each signal can be represented as a bar going up and down or across the screen. Typical line and bar displays are illustrated in Figure 10-5.

Physiological parameters commonly recorded to aid in assessing a patient's problems include skin conductance (to pick up changes in sweating, which occur with changes in the autonomic nervous system), respiration from both the chest and abdomen (to evaluate breathing habits that cause feelings of anxiety and to assess breathing patterns), heart rate, skin temperature (to measure the near surface blood flow, which causes heat at the skin's surface), muscle tension, and the electroencephalogram (EEG).

## BIOFEEDBACK IN THE ASSESSMENT AND TRACKING PROCESSES

Psychophysiological recordings made on biofeedback machines can be very helpful adjuncts to the evaluation of a patient. Preintervention baselines can give an excellent idea of underlying physiological dysfunctions causing the patient's problem. Brief psychophysiological assessments can be repeated both before and after a treatment to assess progress and at the end of the intervention to assess learning and changes that have occurred during therapy. For example, patients with headaches and upper back pain are commonly not convinced that their posture at a computer terminal causes the problem. Simply showing patients their own muscle tension levels in the shoulders, arms, and head while in good and poor postures is highly convincing. Patients are quickly motivated to correct the problem and can use the feedback display both to work toward correcting their postures and to know when they have achieved their goal. Figure 10-6 shows typical trapezius muscle

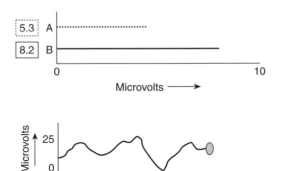

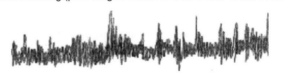

Before training (pain ranged from 2 to 3 on a zero to ten scale)

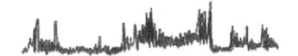

After training (pain ranged from 0 to 1 on a zero to ten scale)

*Figure 10-5* Biofeedback of tension from several muscles provided in the form of bars and digits (*upper* graph). The relative magnitudes of averaged or slow-changing signals are frequently shown as bars moving across a graph as the signals get stronger and weaker. Actual magnitudes are shown by digital displays. A moving line (*lower* graph) is used to display changes in signal strength over time. Vertical height is proportionate to strength. The dot at the right end of the line is the current strength; the tail shows what the signal's strength has been in the past few moments.

*Figure 10-6* Relationships between bilateral upper trapezius sEMG and tension headache recorded in a subject's normal environment before and after muscle tension awareness and control training (a combination of sEMG biofeedback and progressive relaxation muscle training). Pen tracing of an actual recording for clarity. Activity types and levels during two 4-hour periods were similar. Height of vertical deflection is indicative of amount of muscle tension. Note that after training sEMG is not only lower but quiet periods of exceedingly low tension appear in the recording.

tension patterns recorded in an upper-back-pain/ tension-headache patient's normal environment before and after biofeedback training. This type of objective data shows that biofeedback has actually had an effect. Patients with tension-related upper back pain and headache who do not show changes in their muscle tension patterns typically do not show significant improvements with treatment.

Patients with urge and stress urinary incontinence typically have weak pelvic floor muscles that easily go into spasm and cannot sustain a contraction. When these patients are evaluated, patterns of relative muscle tension in the lower abdomen and the pelvic floor are recorded. Figure 10-7 shows the typical relationship between these two muscle groups when the patient attempts to contract the pelvic floor muscles while keeping the lower abdominal muscles relaxed. The abdominal muscles show the pattern the pelvic muscles should show—a sharp increase at the start of contraction, then a relatively level, powerful, smoothly maintained contraction until rapid relaxation at the end of the required period of contraction. The pelvic floor muscle usually takes a while to contract and does not contract very much; the muscle tension fluctuates widely, and tension drops off gradually long before the required time is up. Because the abdominal muscles are much larger and stronger than the pelvic floor muscles and because of their strategic location relative to the bladder, this improper pattern of relative tension, combined with the weak pelvic floor, causes much of the inability to hold in urine observed in people with urge and stress urinary incontinence. Teaching these patients to correct the patterns by observing them on a biofeedback display and performing various strengthening exercises is highly effective in reducing urinary incontinence. Both the therapist

and patient can track success of the treatment by observing successive approximations to the correct patterns as illustrated in Figure 10-7.

When assessing a patient's muscular problems, it is crucial to record muscle tension during movements because muscles that can appear perfectly normal when not under a load may be obviously abnormal when under a load. During a motion, each muscle needs to work in conjunction with the rest of the muscle group responsible for getting the job done smoothly and effectively with the minimum of extra effort. However, muscles may work at the wrong point in a motion, not tense sufficiently to play their role in the task, tense too much, spasm when the task is completed (rather than relaxing back to normal baseline immediately), or any of a variety of other abnormalities. Kinesiological profiles can assist in evaluating muscle tension problems during motion.[1] They usually include postural analysis (e.g., forward head thrust for upper back pain and headache), agonist/ antagonist synergistic patterns, functional activity and muscle substitution analysis, active range of motion, isometric and dynamic contractions, and evaluation of kinematic chains (linked joints [for foot, ankle, knee, or hip problems]). It should be remembered that any group of muscles performs multiple functions; therefore the group may behave normally when performing one task but abnormally when performing another. Watching the relative tension of the muscles as they go about their tasks gives unparalleled evidence of where and when the problems occur.

It is often the case that neither the patient nor the therapist can tell from symptoms or history just which physiological systems are most responsive to stress. When working with patients who have stress-related problems, it is crucial to determine which systems are most responsive to stress because these are the systems that can be tracked from session to session to determine the extent to which interventions such as desensitization and cognitive restructuring are working. Patients and therapists can monitor physiological reactions to simulated stressful situations to determine whether they are indeed producing a reaction. Which physiological systems are reactive during simulated stressful and relaxing conditions is evaluated by conducting a psychophysiological profile. The most common systems to record are muscle tension in the forehead and trapezius, heart rate, galvanic skin response, respiration, and fingertip temperature. The procedure typically consists of taking a 5-minute rest-

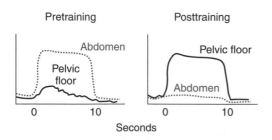

*Figure 10-7* Patterns of relative muscle tension in the lower abdomen and pelvic floor before and after biofeedback training.

ing baseline followed by 3 minutes of guided imagery during which the patient imagines a stressful event in great detail. This is followed by a 5-minute recovery period and then 2 or 3 minutes during which the patient imagines a quietly relaxing situation. The profile ends with a final 5-minute baseline. The tricky part of the profile is to ensure that patients actually imagine stressful and relaxing events in great enough detail to produce physiological responses. When patients cannot think of their own scenarios, therapists guide them through typical scenes such as driving along an ice-covered highway at night during a sleet storm and being cut off by a huge truck.

## EFFICACY

There are several ways to judge the efficacy of a treatment. On a patient-by-patient basis, psychophysiological recordings made before and after treatment can provide conclusive evidence that changes in underlying physiology have occurred. For those disorders in which there is excellent evidence supporting the relationship between the physiological dysfunction and the symptoms, the sustained change in physiology corroborates the change in symptoms and demonstrates that the patient has learned the required skills. This is crucial because the patient will not get better if the required skills are not learned. Examples include the tight relationship between spasms in the residual limb and the occurrence of cramping phantom limb pain and decreased blood flow in the residual limb with intensity of burning phantom limb pain. When patients are trained to stop the spasms or increase blood flow to the residual limb, the pain is relieved to the extent that the spasms are prevented or blood flow is increased respectively. Pretreatment to posttreatment changes in muscle tension are especially evident when prerecordings and postrecordings of pelvic floor and lower abdominal muscle tension patterns are compared among patients with stress and urge urinary incontinence.

Applied psychophysiology is a developing field. Many of its uses are in early stages of evaluation but a number have been proven effective in many controlled studies and regular clinical use. Jacobson[2] published the results of many studies using progressive muscle relaxation training for the control of pain. Linden[3] provided a truly spectacular analysis of the incredibly voluminous German literature on auto-genic training, which differentiates between rare high-quality, controlled studies and the plethora of uncontrolled case reports. Hatch et al[4] reviewed studies on clinical efficacy of biofeedback in their book, which is being updated.

The weaknesses in applied psychophysiological studies—especially the lack of follow-up—greatly influenced the following recommendations on which conditions have been demonstrated to be amenable to these interventions. Thus although psychophysiological techniques have been used to ameliorate such conditions as arthritis, carpel tunnel syndrome, herpes, cancer, sickle-cell anemia, torticollis, reflex sympathetic dystrophy, and causalgia, they are not listed here simply because there is insufficient data to show that they are effective. Their use with such conditions as dysmenorrhea, premenstrual syndrome (PMS), and pelvic area pain are on the borderline and therefore are discussed but presented with reservations.

Two areas, carpel tunnel syndromes related to upper extremity EMG and myofascial pain syndromes related to TrP/EMG complexes, are nearly ready to be included. Donaldson's work[5] relating some carpel tunnel problems to upper extremity EMG activity and the work of Gevirtz,[6] Lewis et al,[7] and Headley[8] that show the relationship between TrP activity and muscle pain are very convincing, although they do not have the treatment studies with follow-ups yet published. As soon as the studies are completed and replicated by a few other groups, these techniques will be ready for standard clinical practice.

The following list is based on my best judgments of the current status of demonstrated effectiveness of biofeedback-augmented interventions.

1. Proven effective in numerous clinical, controlled, comparative, and outcome studies with reasonably large groups and long follow-ups
   - Migraine headache[9]
   - Tension headache[9]
   - Muscle-related orofacial pain[10]
2. Shown to be effective by numerous clinical and some controlled studies but more comparative and outcome studies with larger groups and longer follow-ups are needed
   - Stress and urge (as well as mixed stress and urge) urinary incontinence
   - Muscle tension–related fecal incontinence[11]
   - Cramping and burning phantom limb pain[12]
   - Irritable bowel syndrome[13,14]

- Raynaud's syndrome[15-17]
- Anxiety related to incorrect breathing patterns[18]
- Anxiety and stress responses
- Posture-related pain problems such as forward head thrust[19]
- Stress labile (essential) hypertension[20]
- Attention deficit hyperactivity disorder (ADHD) among children with math concentration problems[21]
- Drug and alcohol addiction[22,23]
- Stroke rehabilitation in conjunction with training to overcome learned nonuse[24]
- Chest pain and other cardiac symptoms related to stress rather than heart problems[18]
- Bruxism[10]
- Epilepsy[25]
- Phobia: Biofeedback recordings used to track progress of desensitization

3. Clinical studies indicate effectiveness but many more studies with larger groups, longer follow-ups, and controls are required[4]
   - PMS and dysmenorrhea[26]
   - Pain from spastic muscles and muscle spasms[1]
   - Subluxation of the patella and patellofemoral pain[27,28]
   - Rheumatoid arthritis pain
   - Magnification of pain by stress and anxiety
   - Pelvic floor pain syndromes[29,30]
   - Pain from carpel tunnel syndromes related to upper arm muscle tension[5]
   - Myofascial pain syndrome/TrP–related pain[6,31]
   - Pain and spasticity due to not taking micro-breaks among sign language translators, musicians, factory workers, computer workers, and others
   - Coordination dysfunctions due to accidents, stroke; actual correction of the problem has enough evidence to warrant a higher category, but there are no studies showing that the results last, and clinical follow-ups are generally negative
   - Balance problems
   - Tics causes by stress-related disorders
   - Asthma[32,33]

4. A variety of studies indicate that applied psychophysiological interventions are usually *not* effective in controlling these problems, but some clinical work shows that they may sometimes be useful
   - Cluster headaches[34]
   - Shocking-shooting phantom limb pain[11]

## BIOFEEDBACK-AUGMENTED INTERVENTIONS OF GENERAL INTEREST

There is not sufficient space in a chapter of this type to go into detail about the evidence supporting the efficacy of biofeedback-augmented interventions for all of the disorders listed previously. Thus a few of the most likely to be applied are reviewed.

## Migraine and Tension Headache

Numerous clinical and controlled studies demonstrate that psychophysiological interventions, including biofeedback,[9,34] autogenic exercises,[3] and progressive muscle relaxation training,[2] are effective for the treatment of both migraine and tension headache among adults and children. The best review of biofeedback interventions for headaches was written by Blanchard in 1992.[9] The outcome criteria for large studies required decreases in intensity, duration, and frequency of at least 50% with changes in use of medication factored in. Long-term follow-up studies show that the treatments are effective for at least 5 years. Comparative studies show that biofeedback is at least as effective as, if not more effective than, standard interventions. Blanchard et al[35] demonstrated that 3-week pretreatment and posttreatment baselines are adequate for evaluating the *initial* effects of any intervention on headache activity. Thus most of the studies in the literature actually have sufficient baseline and follow-up periods to give a reasonable idea of their initial success rate. Follow-ups are for as long as 15 years and demonstrate sustained effectiveness.

Some patients who have headaches have a mainly physical reason for their headaches such as a TrP or poor posture. Some have a mixture of migraine and tension headaches with the pain of one initiating the other. Other patients have predominantly stress responses causing a chain of events leading to migraines, tension headaches, or both. A typical example of the latter is shown in the following case study.

*A Case Study*

*Stress Response Causing Migraines and Tension Headaches*
A 24-year-old active-duty female soldier was referred to a psychotherapist by family practice for treatment of headaches and anxiety. She appeared to be a very anx-

ious young woman who did not make good eye contact and was obviously uncomfortable in the therapy environment. She reported great anxiety as a result of not being able to perform sufficient sit-ups to pass the physical fitness test and general anxiety about stresses in her unit and social life. She was working with a psychotherapist whose initial contacts were oriented toward cognitive restructuring of stressors in her unit and encouraging practicing sit-ups so that she could pass the physical fitness test.

The physiological profile showed that her trapezius muscles and respiration responded to imagined stressors more than any other muscles or other physiological systems recorded. Further evaluation showed that (1) pressure on an obvious TrP on her right shoulder exactly reproduced the headache and (2) she was breathing incorrectly during sit-ups (breathing in with the chest while breathing out with the abdomen) and therefore she became exhausted rapidly. Correction of the bending-related breathing pattern resulted in her being able to perform her sit-ups adequately. A combination of stretching exercises and muscle tension biofeedback from the trapezius eliminated the headaches. Her stress responsive breathing patterns (shallow, rapid breathing using only the chest muscles) indicated a very long history of incorrect breathing, which caused chronic anxiety. Changes in these breathing patterns resulted in decreased feelings of anxiety. In addition, very brief cognitive restructuring helped her deal better with stresses in her unit. ∾

## Muscle Tension–Related Orofacial Pain

Glaros and Glass,[10] Hatch et al,[25] and Gevirtz et al[6] reviewed the literature in this area and provided sufficient convincing details and analyses of numerous clinical and several controlled studies to reach the firm conclusion that the treatment works as long as the problem is due to muscle-related pain rather than pain originating in the temporomandibular (TM) joint. Studies in my lab done in conjunction with oral surgeons confirmed this conclusion. Relatively recent studies included reasonably large sample sizes, control groups, limited follow-ups (6 months to 2 years), and outcome measures that included dental examinations and EMG levels.[36] Several comparative studies showed that biofeedback was as good as or better than splint therapy and that gains were maintained for longer periods with biofeedback.[37,38]

## Muscle Tension–Related (Musculoskeletal) Upper and Lower Back Pain

The use of psychophysiological assessments and treatments for chronic musculoskeletal pain is one of the staples of clinical psychophysiology. The basic idea is that much of the pain people experience is caused by muscles being kept too tense for too long. Muscles may be kept that way as a result of guarding (preventing movement due to pain from some other source), poor posture, stress reactions, or incorrect sequencing of muscles during movement.

Most practitioners who use biofeedback and other psychophysiological interventions to treat chronic back pain mix them relatively randomly with every other intervention available at their sites,[39] and it is usually impossible to determine whether the psychophysiological intervention had any effect or even how it was applied. Both Flor et al[36] and our team[40] reviewed the literature on the use of biofeedback for treatment of low back pain. In 29 clinical studies,[40] as well as several more recent studies, biofeedback was found to help some patients with muscle tension–related low back pain to some extent. But almost all of the studies have serious flaws in design. There have been no large single-group or multi-practitioner studies of applied psychophysiological interventions for back pain similar to those performed with headache patients.

Flor's group[36,41] completed a series of studies with chronic back pain patients. They found an overall improvement rate of about 65% at short-term follow-up relative to about a one-third improvement rate for placebo controls and no improvement for non-treatment controls. The improvement was sustained on 2- to 2½-year follow-up and resulted in a corresponding decrease in use of the healthcare system. Several hundred patients participated in this series of studies; therefore the results are unlikely to be random.

Middaugh and colleagues[19] conducted numerous studies in which correction of abnormal muscle tension was usually assessed as resulting from incorrect posture. Middaugh emphasizes the need for patients to be trained to minimize tension in painful muscles during normal activities involving the muscle and to keep the muscle quiet during activities that do not involve the muscle. This means that tension in the painful muscles is shown to the patients ("fed back") while they are performing a variety of activities associated with pain. Patients are shown the differences in muscle tension when posture is correct vs. incorrect.

Headley,[31,42] Fogel,[43] and Kasman[1] developed specific protocols for physical therapists to use that incorporate surface EMG into pain evaluation and treatment (including biofeedback) programs. Unfortunately, none of these studies conducted or reported on large studies that verify their logical recommendations. Thus numerous case reports and clinical lore form the basis for conducting these evaluations and treatments. These reports are similar to Middaugh's work[19] in that they use surface EMG to assess the function of a muscle or muscle group while normal activities are attempted. EMG biofeedback is incorporated into standard physical therapy to give the therapist and patient an excellent idea of how the muscle is performing. This feedback permits rapid change of activity to desired levels. Although large studies with long-term follow-up that confirms the effectiveness of these techniques have not been performed, the problems with muscle activity are so apparent during multi-channel recordings that viewers have little doubt that an actual problem exists. When the levels of activity are altered to "normal" through the use of biofeedback, the difference is obvious and the patient reports rapid, sustained resolution of the problem.

When biofeedback is incorporated into a treatment of muscle tension–related low back pain, it is usually used in conjunction with the home use of tape recorded muscle tension awareness and control exercises such as Jacobson's progressive muscle training.[44] A typical case is shown in the following case study.

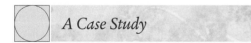

## A Case Study

### Muscle Tension–Related Low Back Pain

A 20-year-old male soldier experienced low back pain and muscle spasms while participating in combat simulation exercises but not while performing similarly demanding tasks of similar duration in his normal work environment. Changes in sleep patterns, loads carried, work-rest cycles, and other obvious possible causes had already been evaluated and found to be insignificant in the problem. A stress profile showed his low back paraspinal muscles to be highly reactive to stress with a particular propensity to remain tense long after either a simulated physical stressor

or an imagined psychological stressor was completed. He was unable to accurately tell how tense his muscles were. Ambulatory recording of paraspinal muscle activity both at the garrison and in the field confirmed that he tensed his muscles more than necessary when under psychological stress and that he kept his muscles tense far longer than usual after both physical and psychological stresses had passed.

The patient was given four sessions of biofeedback from the paraspinal muscles with the aim of teaching him to correctly recognize the actual level of tension in his muscles (calibration). He was also given a tape-recorded progressive muscle tension awareness exercise to listen to twice a day for 2 weeks to increase his ability to relax his paraspinal muscles quickly when appropriate and enhance his awareness of the difference between tense and relaxed muscles. This training significantly reduced his back pain during field exercises. The patient reported being more aware of when he was tense during breaks between physically active periods and that he was able to relax his muscles when he wished. ∾

## Burning and Cramping Phantom Limb Pain

Treatment of phantom pain illustrates the importance of applying the correct treatment to the related underlying physiological problem; in other words, throwing just any behavioral intervention at phantom pain will be as ineffective as throwing any other random treatment at it. Studies from our laboratory[12] and others have shown that burning phantom pain is caused by decreased blood flow to the residual limb while cramping phantom pain is caused by spasms in the residual limb. Treatments that relieve spasms have no effect on burning phantom pain, and vice versa. Our studies[45] and those of Flor[41] show that nearly all amputees with cramping phantom limb pain can learn to recognize the relationship between their pain and spikes in the surface EMG of the residual limb. These patients also can learn to prevent the spikes from occurring and then can prevent their phantom pain to the extent that they can prevent the spikes. If the spikes continue, so will the cramping phantom pain. If the spikes can be voluntarily stopped once an episode of phantom pain begins, the episode can nearly always be almost entirely aborted. Although this method has many qualifiers, it is a clinical reality. Our studies show that the vast majority of people can learn to control nearly all of their cramping phantom pain. (However, *no* learning means *no* control.) Follow-up studies of 1 to 3 years show that the results are sustained.

The same premise holds true for burning as for cramping phantom pain. If patients can learn to increase blood flow to the residual limb, burning phantom pain will decrease to the extent that blood flow is normalized. The burning will remain decreased as long as blood flow remains normal. Unfortunately, about half of our patients have not been able to learn to raise the blood flow in their residual limbs to a significant extent.

## Pelvic Floor Disorders

The major pelvic floor disorders currently treated with biofeedback include muscle tension–related fecal incontinence, urinary incontinence (stress and urge, as well as mixed stress and urge), musculoskeletal pelvic floor pain, pain with intercourse/chronic sensitivity, and constipation. In 1948 Kegel developed biofeedback devices for urinary incontinence, and biofeedback has been in use for pelvic floor disorders at least since that time. Current biofeedback treatments of urinary incontinence are detailed in Tries and Eisman.[29] Although biofeedback for fecal and urinary incontinence is traditionally given to elderly persons whose muscle tone has decreased with age, our studies concentrate on young, athletic adults who leak during physical activity.[12] There is no doubt that feedback of muscle tension from the pelvic floor and abdomen that teaches people to stabilize and strengthen the pelvic floor while relaxing the lower abdomen is effective in controlling stress and urge urinary incontinence.

Schuster and Engle developed similar, highly effective techniques for controlling fecal incontinence. In their technique, sensors are placed under the inner and outer anal sphincters. Patients use the information to contract the sphincters sufficiently and in the correct pattern to avoid incontinence.[46]

Glazer[30] is the major pioneer in using muscle tension feedback from the pelvic floor to relax, strengthen, and stabilize the muscles to control pelvic area pain during intercourse and other situations.

## Alcohol and Drug Addiction

The biofeedback technique for alcohol and drug addiction with the most solid support was developed by Peniston.[22] This technique requires many sessions and uses a combination of temperature biofeedback, EEG biofeedback, and imagery. Good clinical and semi-controlled studies show that the technique works with the most difficult, chronic patients. Ten-year follow-up data are now available that show not only that the technique works for very difficult patients but also that its effects last.[23] Fahrion[46a] treated 360 chronic addicts and followed them for up to several years with excellent results.

## Stroke Rehabilitation and Relearning Balance Control

Muscle tension biofeedback is clearly effective in helping most people with stroke-related loss of muscle control regain considerable control. Unfortunately, the gains commonly are not sufficient to return upper extremity control, especially of the fingers, to useful levels. Thus the vast majority of patients do not make use of their gains and lose their control once again over time.[47-49] Numerous studies now show that most of the gains elicited through any of the standard occupational therapy techniques used with upper extremity stroke patients are lost by the end of the first year as a result. Thus biofeedback is a waste of time unless specific tasks the patient wishes to accomplish can be identified and worked toward successfully. Taub et al[24] recently incorporated techniques for rectifying "learned nonuse" into therapy. Their techniques include tying down the arm not affected by stroke to encourage patients to use the debilitated arm to the fullest extent possible. They found enormous, sustained gains when biofeedback, highly concentrated standard therapy, and learned nonuse training were combined. Brucker[50] used biofeedback based on operant conditioning paradigms with considerable success for people with a wide range of muscular disabilities.

Patients who lose their sense of balance after a stroke or with the general proprioceptive loss that accompanies aging can often be helped with biofeedback. The most common technique in current use is to have the patient stand on a balance platform that records differences in weight distribution.[51,52] The patient then receives visual and/or auditory feedback indicating how far from neutral they are standing.

# EFFECTIVE APPLICATION OF BIOFEEDBACK

A variety of books and journals, as well as meetings of the Association for Applied Psychophysiology and Biofeedback (AAPB),* are available to the clinician seeking more information about biofeedback. This chapter emphasizes what biofeedback is and what it is used for rather than how to do it. Clinical practice courses that detail how the devices work, how to use them, and how to incorporate biofeedback techniques into clinical treatments are widely available. The Biofeedback Certification Institute of America (BCIA)† can be contacted for information on these courses, as well as for listings of local clinicians with experience using biofeedback.

# ACKNOWLEDGMENTS

The drawing of the person receiving biofeedback in Figure 10-1 was finalized from the author's sketch by Karen Wyatt, who was the medical illustrator at Fitzsimons Army Medical Center.

## *References*

1. Kasman G, Cram J, Wolf S: *Clinical applications in EMG,* Gaithersburg, Md, 1998, Aspen.
2. Jacobson E: *Modern treatment of tense patients,* Springfield, Ill, 1970, Charles C Thomas.
3. Linden W: Autogenic training: a narrative and quantitative review of clinical outcome, *Biofeedback Self Regul* 19:227-264, 1994.
4. Hatch J, Fisher J, Rugh J: *Biofeedback: studies in clinical efficacy,* New York, 1987, Plenum Press.
5. Donaldson CCS, Nelson DV, Skubick DL, et al: Potential contributions of neck muscle dysfunctions to initiation and maintenance of carpal tunnel syndrome, *Appl Psychphys Bio* 23:59-72, 1998.
6. Gevirtz R, Glaros A, Hopper D, et al: Temporomandibular disorders. In Schwartz M (ed): *Biofeedback: a practitioner's guide,* New York, 1995, Guilford Press, pp 411-428.
7. Lewis C, Gervirtz R, Hubbard D, et al: Needle trigger point and surface frontal EMG in tension-type headache, *Biofeedback Self Regul* 19:274-275, 1996.
8. Headley B: *Dynamic EMG evaluation: Interpreting postural dysfunction,* St Paul, Minn, 1990, Pain Resources.
9. Blanchard E, Edward B: Psychological treatment of benign headache disorders, *J Consult Clin Psychol* 60:537-551, 1992.
10. Glaros A, Glass E: Temporomandibular disorders. In Gatchel R, Blanchard E (eds): *Psychophysiological disorders: research and clinical application,* Washington, DC, American Psychological Association, pp 299-356, 1993.
11. Whitehead W, Drossman D: Biofeedback for disorders of elimination, *Prof Psychol Res Pract* 27:234-240, 1996.
12. Sherman R, Davis G, Wong M: Behavioral treatment of urinary incontinence among female soldiers, *Mil Med* 162:690-694, 1997.
13. Blanchard EB, Greene B, Scharff L, et al: Relaxation training as a treatment for irritable bowel syndrome, *Biofeedback Self Regul* 18:125-132, 1993.
14. Humphreys PA, Gevirtz RN: Treatment of recurrent abdominal pain: components analysis of four treatment protocols, *J Pediatr Gastroenterol Nutr* 31:47-51, 2000.
15. Freedman R, Lanni P, Wenig P: Behavioral treatment of Raynaud's disease: long-term follow-up, *J Consult Clin Psychol* 5:136, 1985.
16. Freedman R, Morris M, Norton D, et al: Physiological mechanism of digital vasoconstriction training, *Biofeedback Self Regul* 13:299-305, 1988.
17. Freedman R: Physiological mechanisms of temperature biofeedback, *Biofeedback Self Regul* 16:95-115, 1991.
18. DeGuire S, Gevirtz R, Hawkinson D, et al: Breathing retraining: a three-year follow-up study of treatment for hyperventilation syndrome and associated functional cardiac symptoms, *Biofeedback Self Regul* 21:191-198, 1996.
19. Middaugh S, Kee W, Nicholson J: Muscle overuse and posture as factors in the development and maintenance of chronic musculoskeletal pain. In Grzesiak R, Cicconie D (eds): *Psychological vulnerability to chronic pain,* New York, 1994, Springer.
20. McGrady A: Good news—bad press: applied psychophysiology in cardiovascular disorders, *Biofeedback Self Regul* 21:335-346, 1996.
21. Lubar JF, Swartwood MO, Swartwood JN, et al: Evaluation of the effectiveness of EEG neurofeedback training for ADHD in a clinical setting as measured by changes in T.O.V.A. scores, behavioral ratings, and WISC-R performance, *Biofeedback Self Regul* 20:83-99, 1995.
22. Peniston E, Kulkosky P: Alpha-theta brainwave training and beta-endorphin levels in alcoholics, *Alcohol Clin Exp Res* 13(2):271-279, 1989.
23. Walters D: EEG neurofeedback treatment for alcoholism, *Biofeedback* pp 18-33, Spring 1998.

*The AAFB, formerly known as the Biofeedback Research Society and the Biofeedback Society of America, can be contacted at (800) 477-8892 and through their website at www.aapb.org, or e-mail fbutler@resourcenter.org.

†The BCIA can be contacted at (800) 477-8892 or through their website at www.bcia.org.

24. Taub E, Uswatte G, Pidikiti R: Constrain-induced movement therapy: a new family of techniques with broad application to physical rehabilitation, *J Rehabil Res Dev* 36:237-251, 1999.

25. Sterman MB: Basic concepts and clinical findings in the treatment of seizure disorders with EEG operant conditioning, *Clin Electroencephalogr* 31(1):45-55, 2000.

26. Breckenridge R, Gates D, Hall H, et al: EMG biofeedback as a treatment for primary dysmenorrhea, *South Psychol* 1:75-76, 1983.

27. Ingersoll CD, Knight KL: Patellar location changes following EMG biofeedback or progressive resistive exercises, *Med Sci Sports Exerc* 23:1122-1127, 1991.

28. LeVeau B, Rogers C: Selective training of the vastus medialis muscle using EMG biofeedback, *Phys Ther* 60(11):1410-1415, 1980.

29. Tries J, Eisman E: Urinary incontinence: evaluation and biofeedback treatment. In Schwartz M (ed): *Biofeedback: a practitioner's guide,* New York, 1995, Guilford Press, pp 597-632.

30. Glazer H, Rodke G, Swencionis C, et al: Treatment of vulvar vestibulitis syndrome with electromyographic biofeedback of pelvic floor musculature, *J Reprod Med* 40:283-290, 1995.

31. Headley B: Evaluation and treatment of myofascial pain syndrome utilizing biofeedback. In Cram J (ed): *Clinical EMG for surface recordings,* vol 2, Nevada City, Calif, 1990, Clinical Resources, pp 235-254.

32. Lehrer PM: Emotionally triggered asthma: a review of research literature and some hypotheses for self-regulation therapies, *Appl Psychophysiol Biofeedback* 23:13-41, 1998.

33. Lehrer PM, Hochron SM, Mayne TM, et al: Relationship between changes in EMG and respiratory sinus arrhythmia in a study of relaxation therapy for asthma, *Appl Psychophysiol Biofeedback* 22:183-191, 1997.

34. Blanchard E, Andrasik F: *Management of chronic headaches,* New York, 1985, Pergamon Press.

35. Blanchard E, Hillhouse J, Appelbaum K, et al: What is an adequate length of baseline in research and clinical practice with chronic headache? *Biofeedback Self Regul* 12:323-329, 1987.

36. Flor H, Birbaumer N: Comparison of the efficacy of EMG biofeedback, cognitive-behavioral therapy, and conservative medical interventions in the treatment of chronic musculoskeletal pain, *J Consult Clin Psychol* 61:653-658, 1993.

37. Dahlstrom L, Carlsson S: Treatment of mandibular dysfunction: the clinical usefulness of biofeedback in relation to splint therapy, *J Oral Rehabil* 11:277-284, 1984.

38. Hijzen T, Slangen J, Van Houweligen H: Subjective, clinical, and EMG effects of biofeedback and splint treatment, *J Oral Rehabil* 13:529-539, 1986.

39. Roberts D: Physiotherapy exercises and back pain, *BMJ* 303(6797):314, 1991.

40. Sherman R, Arena J: Biofeedback for low back pain. In Basbajian J, Nyberg R (eds): *Rational manual therapies,* Baltimore, 1992, Williams & Wilkins.

41. Flor H, Birbaumer N: Psychophysiological methods in the assessment and treatment of chronic musculoskeletal pain. In Carlson J, Seifert R, Birbaumer N (eds): *Clinical applied psychophysiology,* New York, 1994, Plenum Press.

42. Headley B: The use of biofeedback in pain management, *Phys Ther Pract* 2:29-40, 1993.

43. Fogel E: Biofeedback-assisted musculoskeletal therapy and neuromuscular re-education. In Schwartz M (ed): *Biofeedback: a practitioner's guide,* New York, 1995, Guilford Press, pp 560-593.

44. Jacobson E: *Progressive relaxation,* Chicago, 1938, University of Chicago Press.

45. Sherman RA, Devor M, Jones D, et al: *Phantom pain,* New York, 1996, Plenum.

46. Whitehead WE, Wald A, Norton NJ: Treatment options for fecal incontinence, *Dis Colon Rectum* 44(1):131-142, 2001.

46a. Fahrion SL: Human potential and personal transformation, *Subtle Energies* 6(1):55, 1995.

47. Basmajian JV, Gowland CA, Finlayson MA: Stroke treatment: comparison of integrated behavioral—physical therapy vs. traditional physical therapy programs, *Arch Phys Med Rehabil* 68:267-272, 1987.

48. Inglis J, Donald M, Monga T, et al: EMG biofeedback and physical therapy of the hemiplegic upper limb, *Arch Phys Med Rehabil* 65:755-759, 1984.

49. de Pedro-Cuesta J, Widen-Holmqvist L, Bach-y-Rita P: Evaluation of stroke rehabilitation by randomized controlled studies: a review, *Acta Neurol Scand* 86:422-439, 1992.

50. Brucker BS, Bulaeva NV: Biofeedback effect on electromyography responses in patients with spinal cord injury, *Arch Phys Med Rehabil* 77(2):133-137, 1996.

51. Nichols D: Balance retraining after stroke using platform biofeedback, *Phys Ther* 77:553-558, 1997.

52. Simons R, Smith K, et al: Balance retraining, *Percept Mot Skills* 87:603-609, 1998.

## Suggested Readings

Blanchard E, Andrasik F, Neff D, et al: Sequential comparisons of relaxation training and biofeedback in the treatment of three kinds of chronic headaches or, the machines may be necessary some of the time, *Behav Res Ther* 20:469-481, 1982.

Budzynski T, Stoyva J, Adler C, et al: EMG biofeedback and tension headache: a controlled outcome study, *Psychosom Med* 35(6):484-496, 1973.

Kasman G: Use of integrated EMG for the assessment and treatment of musculoskeletal pain: guidelines for physical medicine practitioners. In Cram J (ed): *Clinical EMG for surface recordings,* vol 2, Nevada City, Calif, 1990, Clinical Resources, pp 255-302.

Luthe W: *Autogenic therapy,* New York, 1969, Grune and Stratton.

Schwartz M: *Biofeedback: a practitioner's guide,* New York, 1995, Guilford Press.

Sherman R: Relationships between jaw pain and jaw muscle contraction level: underlying factors and treatment effectiveness, *J Prosthet Dent* 54(1):114-118, 1985.

Sherman R: Relationships between strength of low back muscle contraction and intensity of chronic low back pain, *Am J Phys Med* 64:190-200, 1985.

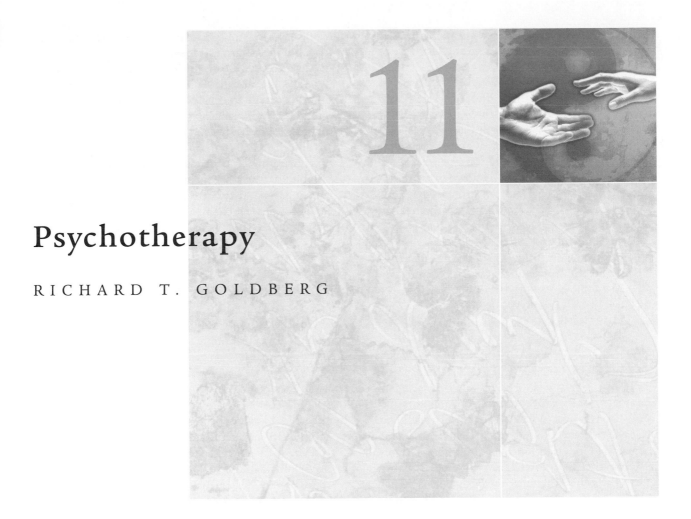

# Psychotherapy

RICHARD T. GOLDBERG

The aim of psychotherapy is to alleviate mental suffering, alter or remove the physical and mental symptoms that interfere or block the person's ability to function in everyday life activities, gain insight into the nature of the person's drives, motives, and behaviors, and enhance positive mental health.

Psychotherapy is the treatment of a psychological problem in which a relationship is established between one person trained as a professional therapist and another person seeking help with a psychological problem. Both persons have equally important, albeit different, perspectives on the problem. The person with the problem approaches the relationship with the unique perspective of one who has experienced the suffering, pain, and mental and physical symptoms resulting from the inability to resolve the problem. The trained professional therapist approaches the relationship with the unique perspective of someone who has helped numerous others who have presented similar problems. Neither the therapist nor the person seeking therapy is superior or inferior to the other. Both must be respected for their unique vantage point.

Persons who consent to engage in psychotherapy with a professionally trained therapist may voluntarily withdraw their consent at any time. A therapist may be called doctor, psychologist, social worker, pastoral counselor, or any other nomenclature as long as appropriate training, licensure, and ethical standards are met. A person engaged in psychotherapy may be called patient, client, or any other name that recognizes the professional relationship involved. The recent trend toward use of the terms *healthcare provider* and *consumer* cheapens the ethical relationship between the two and therefore is not favored by this author.

Psychotherapy may be perceived as a form of alternative medicine because it affects the mind-body relationship. The evidence for the impact of the brain on physical illness is overwhelming. The early works of Menninger,[1] Dunbar,[2] and Horney[3] demonstrate the use of psychotherapy as a form of treatment for psychosomatic illnesses such as allergies, warts, ulcers, and histrionic or conversion disorders. As applied to patients with chronic pain disorders, psychotherapy may be used to uncover the underlying reasons for perpetuation of pain past the period of initial tissue damage, disease, or injury. Insight into the meaning of pain and the conversion of mental conflicts into pain sensation is a major goal of psychotherapy. Distorted thoughts and unexpressed feelings are the raw material for psychotherapy with chronic pain patients.

## PSYCHOTHERAPY AS ART

The influence of psychotherapy on popular culture cannot be ignored. With the advent of psychoanalysis at the beginning of the twentieth century, the influence of Freud, Jung, and Adler permeated all of the arts, first in Europe and later in America.[4] During the 1930's the general revulsion against Nazism in central Europe forced psychotherapists of all schools to flee Europe for England and America. These "exiles in paradise" brought their particular ideologies, methods, and procedures to the practice of psychotherapy.[5] In the United States their influence was particularly felt in New York with the founding of the New School for Social Research, and in California they settled and practiced near Los Angeles and Beverly Hills. Postwar practice saw the emergence of the interpersonal school of psychiatry with Erich Fromm,[6] Karen Horney,[3] and Harry Stack Sullivan. Kurt Lewin,[7,8] a psychologist associated with Wolfgang Kohler at the University of Berlin, brought a special view of personality that saw human behavior as a function of forces in the surrounding environment. Although he was not a psychotherapist, his field theory of personality had a major influence on therapists who understood the psychological environment of the person. Lewin's protégé, Tamara Dembo, who followed him from Berlin to the United States, founded the psychology of disability. In 1944 she was asked to study the psychological adjustment to loss after amputation among veterans of World War II.[9] In her interviews with veterans in military hospitals and later in veterans' hospitals, she constructed the basic concepts of adjustment to disability, which we now take for granted. (I was privileged to have known her and to have worked with her.) These concepts include denial, acceptance of loss, devaluation of self by disability, the phenomenon of spread, the inferior status of the disabled vs. the superior position of the nondisabled, and the integration of the former concept of self as able bodied with the new concept of self as a person with a disability. The most difficult adjustment to disability is not physical but mental.

## TYPES OF PSYCHOTHERAPY

Psychotherapy is primarily a relationship between two persons, not a technique or procedure. However, many techniques are recognized as useful for enhancing the relationship and achieving the outcomes of therapy. The types of therapy discussed in this chapter are insight-oriented and psychodynamic therapies, counseling, supportive therapy, nondirective therapy, and cognitive-behavioral therapy. Psychoanalysis is a special form of treatment in which the unconscious drives of the individual are made conscious through transference. The expense and prolonged treatment by psychoanalysis make it impractical for most patients seeking an alternative form of medicine.

## Insight-Oriented and Psychodynamic Therapies

Insight-oriented therapy consists of probing the root causes of human behavior based on childhood development, family dynamics, instinctual drives, and inherited genetic traits. Whereas traditional Freudian psychoanalytic theory subordinates the study of human behavior to the study of unconscious drives, modern psychotherapy makes use of both instinctual drives and conscious, rational thought. Current interests, values, and goals are based on childhood traits and the unfolding of childhood development. These traits are as important as unconscious drives in the making of human personality. A psychotherapist therefore must explore a person's current motives as an end in themselves. Fortunately a therapist can ask a person what he or she wants or plans to do, and what a person of average intelligence tells me is as important as how that person responds on a psychological test.

The social, biological, and psychological material are integrated in the evaluation phase before insight therapy is begun. This synthesis is especially important in a clinical setting such as a hospital or rehabilitation center where a person's medical history and problems are the primary reasons for hospitalization. For example, a person with traumatic brain injury poses unique problems of differential diagnosis. Is a depression consequent to the brain injury or is there a preexistent depression? As another example, a person with chronic low back pain is addicted to narcotics for pain relief. Is the addiction consequent to chronic pain or was the person vulnerable to addiction before the pain began? The relationship between chronic pain and depression is often due to an underlying history of child abuse. Persons who have been sexually or physically abused as children become both depressed and more vulnerable to pain as adults.[10] Some recent research suggests that a traumatic event in childhood may leave a permanent imprint on the visual cortex that may be reawakened by a painful event in childhood or adulthood.[11]

Psychodynamic therapy helps to unearth the earlier repressed material and to make it whole again. Patients who have experienced severe traumas, such as sexual abuse, wars, concentration camps, earthquakes, and bombings, feel disconnected to family and community. In the case of severe natural or manmade disasters, such as the Oklahoma City bombing, the Mexico City earthquake, the World Trade Center attack, or the atomic bombings, the environment has been so obliterated that the patient no longer recognizes it, which causes a sense of *anomie*.[12-14] Patients who have experienced such disasters tell me that they can remember every chronological happening but cannot remember the emotion attached to the happening. For example, a 42-year-old woman who had been repeatedly raped at ages 10 and 11 by her grandfather told me that she could remember lying in her bedroom looking up at the ceiling, pretending that he was not there. Even today she cannot connect the emotions of rage and humiliation to the event. A traumatized patient feels more vulnerable to future stressful events such as illness or accident. The task of the psychotherapist is to attach the emotion to the event and to reconnect the traumatized patient to family and community and to the integrity of his or her own body.

Insight therapy can be especially useful for the treatment of conversion disorders. Often conversion disorders are seen in pain management and trauma clinics. When a person understands the underlying reasons for using the body to convert mental conflicts into somatic disorders, the emotional expression is openly directed toward the therapist in the therapy session and the symptom abates.

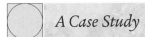

## A Case Study

*Conversion Paralysis*

A 51-year-old woman was suddenly unable to walk while on vacation. She felt weak, dizzy, and was paralyzed in her lower extremities. After her return home, she was taken to the emergency psychiatric service at her local hospital, where she was recommended for acute psychiatric hospitalization. However, she refused to enter the hospital as an inpatient. I was called for consultation because of my experience with conversion disorders. I immediately formed a therapeutic relationship by validating her desire to remain out of a hospital and by contracting with her for safety. She was not suicidal or homicidal, was fully oriented, and was willing to see me again for therapy. I recommended that hospitalization be deferred. On the following day, I saw her for further assessment and began psychotherapy. After a series of therapy sessions, she expressed her basic conflicts: a dying father who doted on her, a family business divided by an internecine struggle for power, a male partner unacceptable to her family, and ambivalence toward independence vs. passivity. As the therapy progressed, her paralytic attacks became infrequent and she gained greater control over her social situation. As she became more assertive and independent of family influence, her conversion attacks subsided. Every now and then she experienced a mild depression when some new family stress reoccurred, but she never again experienced a full-blown conversion disorder. She understood the psychological roots of her conversion disorder and was mindful of the salutary expression of her emotions. Still to be addressed is the relationship with her children and the prevention of the cycle of emotional repression in the next generation. ✍

## Counseling

Counseling is a form of psychotherapy that focuses on specific, everyday issues such as vocational plans, school choices, marital conflicts, and rehabilitation after accidents. The difference between counseling and insight therapy is that the former is concerned with specific, short-term issues that can be resolved within a concrete period and that do not usually spread to deeper emotional conflicts. In contrast, insight therapy does not end with the resolution of a specific problem but continues over a lifetime with or without the help of a therapist. Insight therapy is concerned with basic developmental and inner psychological conflicts that manifest as specific problems.

*Rehabilitation counseling* is a form of counseling that began in 1920 as a specific service offered by the state to help individuals with physical disability return to their former occupation or prepare for a new occupation after experiencing an industrial accident. Counseling and physical restoration were required before vocational training was undertaken. Although rehabilitation counseling was first applied to physical disability, the federal-state program in 1943 expanded the definition of disability to include persons with mental retardation and mental illness. Federal funds became available for surgery and other necessary medical treatments to make the person employable. While counseling is given to prepare a person for work, it is recognized that long-term psychotherapy may be needed to penetrate the emotional block that shrouds the individual with physical or mental disability. Rehabilitation counseling became more inclusive after World War II. The civil rights movement of the 1960s and the consumer movement of the 1970s and 1980s led to the landmark Americans with Disabilities Act in 1990 that has influenced all medical, psychological, social, and vocational services for people with disability.[15]

Psychotherapy now is seen as one of many services that a person with disability could choose. Neither the person with disability nor the therapist is superior or inferior to the other; each has something to give in the relationship. Psychotherapy is not a prescription written by a doctor for a sick individual. In psychotherapy a person begins the process of knowing himself or herself and of changing in the direction most appropriate for him or her. In a rehabilitation hospital or clinic devoted to rehabilitation, counseling may be used to arrest the depression and maladaptive behaviors associated with chronic physical and/or mental disability.

 *A Case Study*

### Traumatic Brain Injury

A 40-year-old married man who had sustained traumatic brain injury 5 years earlier was referred to me for counsel-

ing. He had completed his physical and occupational therapy and was in the last stages of his speech and language therapy. He had full range of motion in upper and lower extremities and had learned to drive in heavy traffic. He complained of posttraumatic headache and neck pain that occurred once or twice monthly with no apparent trigger. Neuropsychological testing indicated mild problems of concentration, attention, and short-term memory. The patient reported that in his home he would forget a task given by his wife when he left one room and went into another. Nevertheless, he could remember directions to the hospital, drove along crowded highways, and unfailingly made it to his appointments.

In counseling, he spent the first half of each hour reporting that he could not function at home the way he did before the injury and that he felt exasperated by the expectations of his therapists and his wife, who did not understand his disability. He was a college graduate who had worked for several years in the insurance industry as a sales manager. He had received several awards for selling the most insurance in his region. Now he could not concentrate enough to return to his former job and he was worried that he would not have enough money to support his wife and children. He was afraid to accept a settlement without having been retrained for another occupation. The industrial accident board was pressuring him to make a settlement.

After 1 year of counseling, the patient had learned to reflect on his assets rather than his liabilities. He made positive statements about his education, religious training, and family support. I had asked him to write down at least five positive self-statements and to refer regularly to those statements, which he kept by his bedside. He became more confident in his abilities and less preoccupied with the limitations imposed by his traumatic brain injury. We looked at all of his options, after which he agreed to try a course in art history with the objective of becoming a museum administrator. He had always been interested in art and hoped that a combination of skills in business management, sales, and art would lead to a remunerative occupation. This is an example of reflecting an individual's choice in counseling while providing him with the trust he needs to make the next step in his rehabilitation without jeopardizing his benefits. The patient settled his case and began his training in art history. ∾

## Supportive Therapy

Supportive therapy is used to help a person faced with extraordinary life stressors that have undermined or broken down that person's usual defenses or adaptive behaviors. Life stressors may include unfavorable change in health; loss of spouse, child, or other family member; loss of occupation and income; ambiguous loss; acts of nature such as earthquakes, fires, and hurricanes; acts of human beings such as wars, bombings, concentration camp internment; and abusive acts, such as verbal, physical, or sexual abuse. A psychotherapist is a neutral figure, "the third ear," as Theodore Reik would say, who listens but does not judge, who accepts a person's anger toward God and nature, and who supports life even in the face of death. It is always easier to succumb to passivity, withdrawal, and death. "Why me, God?" It is more difficult to struggle against losses. Blaming one's own failings on someone else or some past traumatic event interferes with personal growth. Supportive therapy is useful for relieving anxiety, substituting positive for negative thoughts, providing relaxation, teaching coping techniques, and rebuilding defenses.

In my work with terminally ill persons on a complex medical disorders unit, I help to ease the transition between life and death. Some common diagnoses on this unit are end-stage renal disease; chronic respiratory failure; amyotrophic lateral sclerosis; and repeated amputations due to diabetes mellitus, peripheral vascular disease, and cancer. Persons facing death have existential problems that extend beyond the usual specific problems of daily living. They want closure in their life. They want to resolve the issues or at least mend the loosened threads of their family life. They want to feel loved and respected despite their deteriorated physical condition. They do not want to be alone. The most important service I can provide as a psychotherapist is to be *present* for the patient. Long after a patient had died, his family wrote to me to tell me how much my coming into the patient's room meant to him and to them.

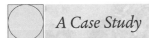

## A Case Study

### End-Stage Renal Failure

A 41-year-old former physician was treated for complex end-stage renal disease and respiratory failure in a rehabilitation hospital. He had been transferred to a rehabilitation setting after having experienced inadequate treatment at a local acute care hospital. I began seeing him for supportive therapy to maintain his interests in medicine, politics, and current events. For the first few months he showed considerable improvement and was hopeful of returning home with a reduced schedule. He even regained hope of doing some editorial work for a medical journal. At the same time, I began seeing his wife, first in conjunction with my visits to him, and later separately. There were

dynamic interactions of guilt, anger, resentment, abandonment, and loneliness expressed by both of them. She took an apartment near the hospital. I encouraged him to become more independent of her and to trust more in the hospital staff. I encouraged her to take more respite time for herself. As his condition declined, he became more dependent and she became guiltier. I spent more time in his room, just listening and talking about current events. His death occurred on his birthday, after a family celebration, at a time of resolution of the family dynamics. ∽

Therapy for terminally ill persons often borders on pastoral counseling. For a patient who has a strong religious faith, I often recommend that a hospital chaplain also see the patient to help resolve the spiritual issues that I feel less equipped to manage. I often work hand in hand with the chaplain to help a patient decide whether to ask for life supports or to withdraw from a respirator or dialysis. The attending physician explains the procedures for resuscitation in case of cardiac arrest or sudden drop in blood pressure. The patient is given information to help him or her decide whether to ask for a DNR (do not resuscitate) order to be placed in the medical record. Whenever there is a doubt or a conflict between the wishes of the patient and the wishes of the family, I help to clarify and to mediate the issues. The wishes of the patient are paramount. I may see the patient alone and more than once to establish reliability.

The questions of whether to prolong life or to prolong the dying process are not strictly medical questions. When alternative medicine is proposed as a treatment for a dying person, we must consider not only the curative or restorative properties of herbal medicine, homeopathy, or magnet therapy but also the healing properties of words, loving gestures, and nonverbal communication. The same healing occurs when a concerned family member is present. Many of us in the health professions have observed that a dying parent, brother, or sister will cling to life until his or her distant child or sibling has flown thousands of miles to be with him or her at the time of death. Then the dying person will let go. I remember a patient with metastatic breast cancer who clung to life with many remissions and reoccurrences until her brother, whom she had not seen for a year, came to visit from California. After 2 weeks all of her body tissues became swollen and she died peacefully.

Words can heal; words can also kill. A fine line exists between telling the truth and killing the hope. While it is true that many physicians are afraid to tell their patients the truth about a fatal illness, it is better to err on the side of life than death. When a patient asks how much longer he or she has to live, the physician can honestly reply that the patient has a fatal illness but that no one can predict with any certainty when the final day will occur. As a psychotherapist, I focus on helping the patient decide how to spend the remaining days. I review with the patient his or her accomplishments in various spheres of life—family, parenting, work, school, hobbies—and I ask whether there is anything more a patient wants to accomplish or look forward to, such as family celebrations, before death. Time is short, and there is a lot of work to be done. I do not divert the patient into miracle cures or faith healing but instead make use of the natural healing ability of the human mind to cope with even the most extreme natural calamities and malevolent human actions. We know that some human beings have recovered emotionally from atomic bombings, concentration camp internment, earthquakes, and typhoons. A psychotherapist uses the natural abilities and energies of the human mind and spirit to cope with traumas.

## Nondirective Therapy

Nondirective therapy is a process in which a helping relationship exists between two persons, a therapist and a client. The main aim of the therapist is to help a client become himself or herself. This definition borrows heavily from Carl Rogers,[16] whose many books and writings have influenced therapists for the past 50 years. Perhaps a good analogy is a gardener who helps each plant develop according to its own unique nature. Nondirective therapy is an important complement to insight therapy. For persons with normal everyday concerns who want to make changes in their life, nondirective therapy can be useful for clarifying, reflecting, and supporting their choices. The therapist is a reflecting mirror that the client uses to understand and accept his or her feelings. The client is the subject of the helping relationship, not the object of dissection. Interpretation of the client's thoughts and feelings are kept to a minimum.

### *A Case Study*

*Chronic Pain and Opiate Abuse*
A 56-year-old man with chronic low back pain and a history of opioid abuse was referred to me to evaluate his po-

tential for successful completion of a pain management program. He was taking opioid medications from multiple sources and was buying illegally several opiates on the street. He was apprehended for drug possession and asked to serve 1 year of probation. Random drug screenings and individual psychotherapy were mandated by the court. He was compliant with both court orders. During the course of psychotherapy, the emphasis shifted from compliance to an exploration of the roots of his substance abuse, chronic pain, and depression. Nondirective therapy permitted the client to dig deeply into his childhood development, which exposed an indifferent father, a powerless mother, an adolescence without parental guidance, and a loveless family. A brief, unsuccessful marriage and a series of sexual partners characterized his adulthood. His career development consisted of fragmentary jobs with no career pattern or advancement.

The client's back pain was a metaphor for the pain in his life. When he recognized the psychological roots of his pain, he stopped buying illicit drugs, participated in random drug screenings, and began an outpatient program for pain management. He continues to consult a physician with pain specialization and sees me regularly for psychotherapy. With the help of nondirective therapy, he identified the deprivation of his childhood and the losses engendered by his back pain. He still needs to plan for the future with an elderly mother, limited friendships, and chronic pain. ✎

## Cognitive-Behavioral Therapy

Cognitive-behavioral therapy applies the principles of operant conditioning to the management of patients with chronic pain, addiction, and chronic physical disability. This form of therapy is especially useful in rehabilitation settings in which behavioral methods can be used not only by individual practitioners but also by the entire staff. Based on the work of B.F. Skinner, cognitive-behavioral therapy is predicated on the theory that human behavior is purposive; influenced by consequences; reinforced by positive rewards; and altered by a structured set of cues, tasks, environmental conditions, and human experiences. Positive reinforcements of any effort or structured activity such as occupational or physical therapy are helpful in encouraging well behaviors and in discouraging ill behaviors. Cognitive-behavioral therapy alters both thoughts and behaviors. By reinforcing positive thoughts through a series of positive self-statements and by converting negative thoughts into positive thoughts, a patient learns to acquire greater control of his or her behavior. Cognitive-behavioral therapy is very useful for managing pain behaviors and the residual sequelae of traumatic brain injury. Negative reinforcement of pain behaviors, such as grimacing, limping, guarding an impaired limb, passivity, or dependency, needs to be replaced by positive reinforcement of structured activities that build a repertoire of skills that involve active and functional behaviors. Cognitive-behavioral therapy was pioneered by Beck[17] and applied to the treatment of persons with disability and chronic pain by Fordyce.[18] In the last 25 years it has become the most commonly used treatment in rehabilitation medicine.

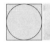

## A Case Study

*Traumatic Brain Injury*

A 28-year-old man with a traumatic brain injury and a history of polysubstance abuse had been acting out aggressively in a residential home for substance abusers and was randomly aggressive on the street. He came to the attention of the Cambridge, Massachusetts, police while they were arresting an unlicensed street vendor in Harvard Square. The patient sympathized with the street vendor and tried to block the arrest. The police warned but did not arrest him. After this incident, I used cognitive-behavioral techniques with him to help him control his anger by (1) compartmentalizing angry thoughts, (2) counting slowly from one to ten and saying "STOP," and (3) using guided imagery (i.e., visualizing a peaceful time and place either from the past, the present, or the future). Whenever he became angry at home, he was to go directly to his room. Whenever he ventured out on the street, he was to use a Walkman to screen out distracting stimuli, such as the police. As a result, the patient has successfully managed to control his anger and has obtained a job as a kitchen worker in a downtown Boston hotel. ◦↞

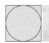

## A Case Study

*Traumatic Brain Injury with Cognitive Impairment*

A 35-year-old man with a traumatic brain injury resulting from a 30-foot fall from scaffolding into Boston Harbor was seen for chronic tension headaches with a migrainous component, attention deficit disorder, and short-term memory disorder. He successfully completed a pain program, with improvement in functional abilities in ambulation, balance, and range of motion in both shoulders. After discharge from the pain program, he was referred to

me for psychotherapy. I used cognitive-behavioral techniques to help him organize his daily schedule. He purchased a microcomputer to schedule daily appointments and to perform simple arithmetic. As his cognitive functions improved, his depression lifted. Although the patient still had intermittent headaches, he was capable of performing his daily activities, which included speech, occupational, and physical therapy. His next goal is to complete the requirements for a driver's license and to return to work.

This patient is a good example of someone who needs the combined approach of behavioral therapy and counseling. Without this combination of therapies and programs, he would still be drifting and adding to the costs of long-term disability benefits. Insurance carriers need to be educated about the cost-benefit ratio of psychological treatment in rehabilitation. ◦↞

## PSYCHOTHERAPY AS SCIENCE

One of the major objections to alternative medicine is that it is not an empirical science. Traditional medicine is held as a model of classical science, with testing of alternative hypotheses; gathering of reliable, valid, and replicable observations; use of randomized experimental and control groups; and testing of statistical significance against probability tables for error. It is not sufficient to demonstrate differences between placebo controls and experimental groups. There must also be the opportunity for falsifiability of a hypothesis by testing its alternative.[19]

In contrast, alternative medicine often relies on case studies without placebo controls. The question facing alternative medicine is whether any effects produced by intervention are greater than a sham intervention expected by placebo controls. However, even placebo control studies have scientific caveats.[20] For starters, such studies are often circumscribed by limited samples, inadequate age and gender criteria, reliability and validity of measures, faulty recruitment, lack of informed consent, and heterogeneous samples that cannot be generalized. For example, in review of studies of low back pain, only a very few qualified as valid placebo-controlled research.[21]

Wait list controls can be an alternative to randomized experimental placebo controlled studies. A patient can be enrolled as a participant in an alternative medicine study without placebo controls with the understanding before starting the study that he or she will eventually be offered a different treatment that has an inactive substance (placebo) that does not affect his or her current treatment after the study is completed. The advantage of wait-list controls is that the participant can be offered either the experimental treatment or the control treatment without jeopardizing his or her health.

Psychotherapy has been compared with faith healing by some critics of psychodynamic methods. As Weil[22] and others have suggested, there is at least a surface similarity between psychotherapy and faith healing. Both methods rely on the belief of the participant and the emotional excitement of participation. Both focus on the charisma of the leader. However, whereas faith healing depends on a spiritual epiphany, psychotherapy depends on a rational understanding of internal and external forces that motivate human behavior. Whereas faith healing depends on human submission to God's will, psychotherapy depends on the ability to master the hidden drives of sex, aggression, power, fear, anger, and jealousy that motivate our behavior and change our equilibrium. Anxiety is a result of disturbed equilibrium, an unpleasant state that propels us to find a method to reduce it. Otherwise, anxiety becomes so salient that everything else in human experience becomes an adaptation to it. Psychotherapy works toward the reduction of anxiety.

## PSYCHOLOGICAL LIFE SPACE

When an individual is perceived as a self-contained organism that can be treated mechanically like an object, then the intervention of medications, the invasion by surgery, and the application of psychiatry in the classical model of medicine follows logically as the commonly accepted best treatment. When an individual is perceived as inhabiting a life space that can be permeated by the outside world, with continuous communication between the two worlds (inner and outer), then the practitioners of medicine must take into account both worlds to provide the best treatment.

For example, the treatment of persons with disability must account for environmental barriers such as architectural barriers, lack of transportation, inaccessible housing, communication barriers for the deaf and hard of hearing, excessive stimuli for the head injured and the mentally ill, and public places without accommodation for handicap. The stigma attached to disabilities such as mental illness, epilepsy, AIDS, heart disease, and cancer can be an obstruction to treatment and rehabilitation. Medicine cannot treat the individual without treating the environment. A combined approach of complementary medicine, classical medicine, and social-psychological intervention works best.

## PSYCHOTHERAPY AS COMPLEMENTARY MEDICINE

Complementary medicine includes homeopathy, herbalism, acupuncture, and osteopathy. The question is whether psychotherapy should be included as complementary medicine. Psychotherapy treats the inner thoughts and feelings of a person, which have a profound effect on a person's health and well-being. Psychotherapy does not treat the "whole person"; no psychological treatment can do that. Psychotherapy may have a placebo effect; so does classical medicine. The nonspecific effects of psychotherapy may be greater than the specific effects of a specific medication. For example, studies of women undergoing psychotherapy following medical treatment for breast cancer indicated that the women improved their quality of life, although their survival time was not extended. The nonspecific effect of an unscientific treatment may be greater than the total effect of a scientific treatment.[23] Whether psychotherapy produces an effect based on classical scientific principles or a sham effect can be tested only by examining the evidence.

## EVIDENCED-BASED MEDICINE

The major argument for classical medicine is that it is evidence based. Delbanco et al[24] have insisted that the methods and procedures of alternative and complementary medicine be tested objectively in the same way other methods are tested. Anecdotal reports and case findings, as well as formal double-blind randomized experimental-placebo control studies, are often reported in the medical literature. The common denominator between alternative and classical medicine must be found in objective evidence. Thus far the majority of studies of alternative medicine has used small numbers of patients and has not been replicated in several centers using the same methods and similar patients.

As an example, Cunningham and associates[25] studied 22 patients with a variety of diagnoses of metastatic cancer who were offered weekly group psychotherapy. Three subgroups of patients with high, medium, and low involvement with psychological therapy were followed for nearly 3 years. Age, severity of disease, quality of life, and attendance at group therapy sessions were similar across the three subgroups. Before group therapy began, a medical panel predicted survival time. Observed survival outcomes were compared with predicted outcomes. Three patients in the high-involvement group were alive 2.8 years and one patient in the medium-involvement group was alive at 1.8 years after intervention, whereas none of the low-involvement group was alive at time of follow-up. Of the seven patients in the low-involvement group, median observed survival time was 1.2 years.

Limitations of the study consisted of the following: (1) it was a correlative study, (2) there were no controls, (3) there were no standard psychological tests, and (4) persons in the high-involvement group may have been psychologically healthier than the others to begin with. The latter limitation is arguably difficult to prove because the medical panel had observed no differences in medical status among the groups. However, psychological health is subtle and more difficult to measure than physical health. The study is illustrative of both the novelty and the pitfalls of small samples, heterogeneous diagnoses, and a consecutive series of clinical patients.

## PSYCHOTHERAPY AND MIND-BODY TECHNIQUES

Meditation, relaxation, yoga, and spiritual contemplation have been used for centuries to manage emotional distress. Because these techniques have not been subjected to classic scientific testing and many derive from complex philosophical and religious systems, it is not useful to compare them with psychotherapy. The use of self-regulation techniques to treat stress and stress-related medical conditions has proven effective and is being studied by several investigations sponsored by the alternative medicine division of the National Institutes of Health.[26] However, self-regulation techniques are not comparable to modern psychotherapy, which derives from studies of psychiatry and psychology. Psychotherapy seeks understanding of motives, feelings, and actions. The outcomes of psychotherapy must be subjected to the same scrutiny to which any other medical treatment is subjected. Outcomes are measured by reliable and valid psychological measures, such as

scales of quality of life, and are reported in experimental-placebo control studies. Mind-body techniques derive from Eastern religious philosophies and are not measurable by Western psychological tests. For example, yoga derives from Indian philosophy and requires intensive training to attain self-regulation of thought. The experience of yoga is internal and cannot be measured by an independent observer trained in Western methods of psychological research.[27] However, many variables of homeostasis, such as blood pressure, heart rate, and galvanic skin reflex, can be measured to determine whether yoga and other mind-body techniques contribute to a sense of well-being.

The work of Rosenman and associates[28] in linking psychosocial factors to coronary artery disease is a good example of the influence of patient actions on health status. In this group study follow-up, patients' compliance with physician orders was more important in calculating 5-year mortality than a specific medicine prescribed for lowering lipids. Other social factors include Type A personality, stressful environment, and psychological dependency.

## PSYCHOTHERAPY AND MILIEU THERAPY

Psychotherapy is most effective when it is combined with milieu therapy. An individual makes important changes when supported by a healthy milieu. The social milieu in which an individual lives may either support or obstruct any changes of feeling or thought in psychotherapy. Family members who do not accept the contribution of psychotherapy may sabotage any effort made in a patient's therapy. For example, a wife or husband may feel threatened by a change in the status quo of the marital relationship. A wife who becomes more assertive is a threat to a dominant husband. Codependent relationships with family members tend to perpetuate substance abuse. To intervene in the cycle of dependency, depression, and inertia, I may recommend an inpatient stay for patients with alcohol or drug dependence or chronic pain. Hospitalization offers the potential for change in a "therapeutic community" in which the milieu itself is a treatment. How else can one explain positive outcomes in patients who previously had undergone months if not years in individual psychotherapy. Individual psychotherapy works well as part of a structured milieu program.

## SUMMARY

Psychotherapy is an alternative form of medicine that complements classical medicine and psychopharmacology. It affects the mind-body relationship by altering the mental and emotional symptoms that express themselves in somatic preoccupation and by liberating a person to function in everyday life activities despite medical illness. Psychodynamic therapy, counseling, supportive therapy, nondirective therapy, and cognitive behavioral therapy are various forms of psychotherapy that can be employed with rehabilitation patients to affect the mind-body relationship. Psychotherapy is both a science and an art in which a relationship is established between two persons who are equal to one another and who seek to alter human thought, feeling, and behavior so that one person, called a patient, client, or consumer, can be liberated to live up to an optimal level of human capacity.

## References

1. Menninger KA: *The vital balance: the life process in mental health and illness,* Magnolia, Mass, 1983, Peter Smith.
2. Dunbar F: *Emotions and bodily changes,* New York, 1954, Columbia University Press.
3. Horney K: *Our inner conflicts,* New York, 1992, Norton.
4. Freud S: *The basic writings of Sigmund Freud* (edited by A.A. Brill), New York, 1995, Random House.
5. Heilbut A: *Exiled in paradise: German refugee artists and intellectuals in America from the 1930s to the present,* Los Angeles, 1997, University of California Press.
6. Fromm E: *Man for himself: an inquiry into the psychology of ethics,* New York, 1990, Holt.
7. Lewin K: *Field theory in social science: selected theoretical papers,* New York, 1951, Harper.
8. Lewin K: *The complete social scientist: a Kurt Lewin reader* (edited by M. Gold), Washington, DC, 1999, American Psychological Association.
9. Dembo T, Leviton GL, Wright BA: Adjustment to misfortune: a problem of social psychological rehabilitation, *Artificial Limbs* 2:4-62, 1956.
10. Goldberg RT, Goldstein R: A comparison of chronic pain patients and controls on traumatic events in childhood, *Disabil Rehabil* 22(17):756-763, 2000.
11. Rauch SL, Van der kolk BA, Fisler RE, et al: A symptom provocation study of post-traumatic stress disorder using positron emission tomography and script driven imagery, *Arch Gen Psychiatry* 53:380-387, 1996.
12. Langer L: *Holocaust testimonies: the ruins of memory,* New Haven, 1993, Yale University Press.
13. Lifton RJ: *Death in life: survivors of Hiroshima,* New York, 1967, Random House (University of North Carolina Press, reprint edition, 1991).
14. Lifton RJ: *The Nazi doctors: medical killing and the psychology of genocide,* New York, 1986, Basic Books.
15. Walker ML: History of rehabilitation. In Dell Orto AE, Marinelli RP (eds): *Encyclopedia of disability and rehabilitation,* New York, 1995, Macmillan Library Reference USA.
16. Rogers C: *On becoming a person,* Boston, 1961, Houghton Mifflin.
17. Beck AT: *Cognitive therapy and the emotional disorders,* New York, 1979, NAL.
18. Fordyce W: *Behavioral methods for chronic pain and illness,* St Louis, 1976, Mosby.
19. Popper K: *The logic of scientific discovery,* London, 1992, Routledge.
20. Kleijnen J, de Craen AJM: The importance of the placebo effect: a proposal for further research. In Ernst E (ed): *Complementary medicine: an objective appraisal,* Oxford, 1996, Butterworth-Heinemann.
21. Goldberg RT, Lox DM: The role of the psyche in low back pain: the mind-body connection. In Lox DM (ed): *Low back pain, physical medicine and rehabilitation: state of the art reviews,* Philadephia, 1999, Hanley & Belfus.
22. Weil A: *Health and healing,* Boston, 1988, Houghton Mifflin.
23. Kaptchuk TJ, Edwards RA, Eisenberg DM: Complementary medicine: efficacy beyond the placebo. In Ernst E (ed): *Complementary medicine: an objective appraisal,* Oxford, 1996, Butterworth-Heinemann.
24. Delbanco T, Ivker R, Relman A, et al: Complementary and alternative therapies and the question of evidence: a panel discussion, *Adv Mind Body Med* 16:244-260, 2000.
25. Cunningham AJ, Phillips C, Lockwood GA, et al: Association of involvement in psychological self-regulation with longer survival in patients with metastatic cancer: an exploratory study, *Adv Mind-Body Med* 16:276-294, 2000.
26. Loizzo J: Meditation and psychotherapy: stress, allostasis, and enriched learning, *Rev Psychiatry* 19(1):141-197, 2000.
27. Becker I: Uses of yoga in psychiatry and medicine. In Muskin PR (ed): *Complementary and alternative medicine and psychiatry,* Washington, DC, 2000, American Psychiatric Press.
28. Rosenman RH, Brand RJ, Jenkins CD, et al: Coronary heart disease in the Western Collaborative Group Study: final follow-up experience of 8½ years, *JAMA* 233(8):872-877, 1975.

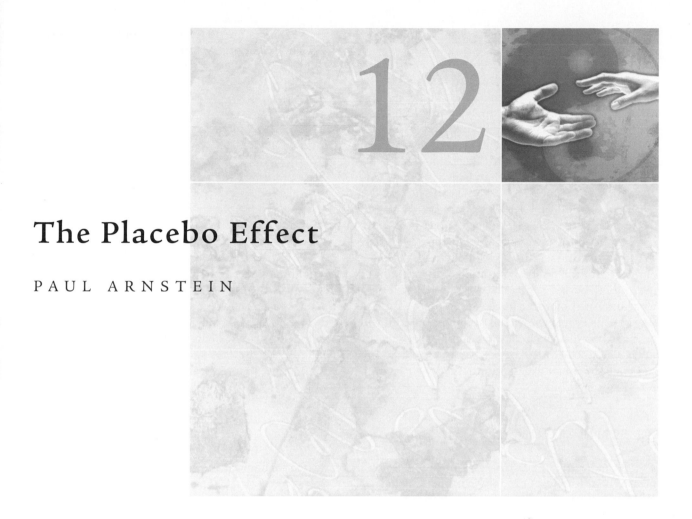

# The Placebo Effect

PAUL ARNSTEIN

We are a drug-obsessed society that waffles between the antidrug mantra of "just say no!" and a media bombardment convincing us that we need Advil, Extra Strength Tylenol, "prescription strength" remedies, or dozens of other drugs. When sick, you are told to stay home and take medications as prescribed. You do not even have to be sick to "need" drugs or nutritional supplements that reportedly provide a source of good health and vitality. Given these mixed messages, it is no mystery why the social ills related to drug use and abuse will not go away.

A powerful and versatile therapeutic tool may help us overcome this obsession. It is called the *placebo effect* because we have learned of its power through the use of placebos. A placebo is an inert substance (e.g., sugar pill or saline injection) or sham physical/electrical manipulation believed to have no chemical, electrical, or physical effect on the patient. Indeed, powerful chemical, electromagnetic, and physical transformations have occurred in patients after exposure to placebos. Placebos have been used to "switch on" and "switch off" serious breathing difficulties associated with asthma. They have demonstrated at times remarkable potency in relieving troublesome symptoms (pain, depression, anxiety, etc.), reducing signs associated with a wide variety of illnesses (involving virtually every part of the body), shortening recovery time, and even reducing mortality. Objective and measurable bodily functions that defy conscious control (concentrations of hormones, immunological markers, neurotransmitters, and the electrical activity of the heart) have been changed following exposure to the placebo arm of research studies.

If these powerful health effects are not the result of a strong drug or precise surgical procedure, what explanation is possible? This chapter provides possible explanations and delineates issues related to the use of placebos and the mobilization of inner healing powers. Clear distinctions must be made between questionable "placebo interventions" and the beneficial placebo effect. When used in modern clinical practice, placebos often represent degrading, deceptive practices that harm rather than benefit patients. Arguments are developed to show that the current use of placebos is not consistent with good science or professional practice. Given the legal and ethical risks, readers are urged to support at least a limited ban on their use. In contrast, the placebo effect is a desirable outgrowth of the skilled application of the art of healing for both patients and rehabilitation professionals, regardless of the professional's discipline or the setting in which care is provided. Recommendations will be made for clinicians to always capitalize on this art form when providing care and on ways to help patients get in touch with and mobilize their healing powers from within.

## DEFINITIONS

The term *placebo* is a Latin word meaning "I shall please," with the implied "false consolation" having roots in colloquial speech dating back to the twelfth century.[1] A placebo is an intervention designed to simulate medical therapy, but is believed by the investigator or clinician not to be therapeutically beneficial. Placebos are believed to produce an effect in patients resulting from their implicit or explicit intent and not from their specific physical or chemical properties. Placebos often take the form of sugar pills, saline injections, miniscule doses of drugs, or a sham procedure (designed to be void of any known therapeutic value).[2]

Placebos have reportedly mimicked the action of a wide variety of drugs, exhibiting measurable drug-like properties.[3] When given intravenously, the placebo begins to work in 15 to 60 minutes, with a peak effect over the next 15 to 45 minutes and a duration of action lasting several hours or days. Pills or injections have an onset, peak, and duration of action the same as the drug they are substituting for.[4] Dose response effects have been demonstrated. For example, two capsules work much better than one and "shots" (injections) are more powerful than pills. Larger (especially brown or purple) pills or capsules typically are stronger than smaller ones, with the exception of very small bright red or yellow pills, which are the most effective.[5]

## Clinical Effects

The literature on the variety of disorders that improve with placebos is quite impressive. Placebos have successfully treated stomach ulcers, hypertension, bedsores, and herpes infections and even have a profound effect on some people with incurable cancer.[6-8] Placebos have been successfully used to control physical symptoms associated with angina pectoris, headache, rheumatoid and degenerative arthritis, temporomandibular (TM) joint disorder, reflex sympathetic dystrophy, asthma, and even the common cold.[9-11] Additionally, placebos have been useful for controlling emotional symptoms such as anxiety, depression, insomnia, and premenstrual tension.[12,13]

## Pain

In 1955, Dr. Beecher of Harvard Medical School conducted a landmark meta-analysis that summarized reports from over 1000 patients with different types of pain. Of these patients, 35% had satisfactory relief from placebos, even with severe postoperative pain.[9] Other investigators administering placebos have reported a reduction in edema, blood pressure, gastric acid, and serum cholesterol levels, as well as improved blood counts and electrolyte and hormonal balances.[12] Even desirable electrocardiographic changes were noted in heart disease patients following a placebo intervention.[14] But before buying some snake oil guaranteed to cure what ails you, remember: it is not the placebo that is causing these changes.

The *placebo effect* (not the placebo itself) is believed responsible for the symptomatic relief and physiological changes reported for a wide variety of conditions.[7,9-14] The placebo effect is a perceptible, measurable, and desirable consequence of the symbolic import of the therapy rather than its ability to change the physical or chemical structure and function of the body. However, physical and chemical changes, beyond those anticipated by the Hawthorne effect, do occur. These may be the result of interpersonal factors such as the presence of a caring person,[15] or what I term the "healer effect." High technology or novel techniques seem to be especially good at eliciting a placebo effect,[4,5,16] to the extent that we are encouraged to use the newest operations, drugs, techniques, and technologies while they still work. When an innovative treatment is introduced, 70% of patients will have a good or excellent effect for several years, until that treatment is discredited and abandoned.[17]

## Surgery

Surgery is considered to have a strong placebo effect, often related to the confidence-instilling attitude of the surgeon. In the 1950's there were two double-blind randomized trials of internal mammary artery ligation surgery (vs. artery exposure without ligation) for the treatment of angina pectoris. These studies demonstrated a marked improvement in angina from skin incision alone, with benefits such as less pain, less medicine required, and improved electrocardiogram tracings lasting at least 6 months.[14] Other sham surgical procedures for TM joint disease and disabling back pain have been shown to be as effective as the standard surgical procedures.[5,8]

In Beecher's 1955 article, he calculated that 50% of the therapeutic benefit of any drug administered is related to the placebo effect, although there were considerable variations noted among the studies regarding the percentage of patients who benefited from the placebo effect. On average, 35% of the patients experience placebo effects; however, response rates ranged from 15% to 80% of the samples in various studies.[9] Beecher noted that more confident, enthusiastic physicians (or researchers) seemed to have better results, accounting for at least some of the discrepancy. This suggests that a majority of the patients do not get the beneficial outcomes associated with the placebo effect, and that even the most confident, enthusiastic provider will not elicit the effect in all patients.

## Nocebos

Despite all the reported potential benefits, placebos can also have a powerful negative "nocebo" effect that increases pain and suffering or worsens disease. The *nocebo effect* is defined as the causation of sickness, symptoms, or even death that results from the belief that these undesired outcomes will occur. We often hear the direct-to-consumer marketing of the pharmaceutical companies state, "The occurrence of side effects is similar to that of sugar pills." What goes unsaid is that mild side effects are experienced by 20% to 30% of patients receiving placebos, including edema, pain, diarrhea, nausea, palpitations, urticaria, and rashes.[18] The rate of nocebo effect responses can also vary considerably, with one sham treatment (a nonexistent electric current applied to the scalp) noted to produce headaches in 70% of healthy subjects.[5]

Some patients experience potential harmful effects from placebos such as dizziness, depression, insomnia, drowsiness, vomiting, numbness, hallucinations, or addiction.[5,13,18,19] Other patients' symptoms get worse because the placebo fails to treat what is wrong with them. Nearly 25% of patients in one study believed that they were permanently disabled and destined to live with greater intensity of pain because of their participation in the placebo arm of a study.[5]

The nocebo effect has been linked to untimely deaths, such as in the case where people seem to "will" themselves to die in certain circumstances. Anecdotes have been widely published about physicians or clergy rendering end-of-life care to the wrong patient, who subsequently dies expediently or unexpectedly, while the intended recipient survives for a prolonged period. Hard data linking the nocebo effect to death comes from the 20-year Framingham Study, which showed a nearly fourfold greater rate of death from heart attacks among women who believed they would die from heart disease, even after controlling for known risk factors (e.g., smoking, cholesterol levels, and high blood pressure).[20]

The nocebo effect may represent a major public health problem, with pain and infectious, stress-related, and autoimmune disorders theoretically linked by related physiological mechanisms.[1] Hahn,[21] an anthropologist and epidemiologist, expresses a concern about the media coverage of health-related problems in that sociogenic illnesses (also called psychogenic illnesses, mass hysteria, or assembly line hysteria) may result from the associated nocebo effect. He postulates that the nocebo phenomenon may account for a significant portion and a substantial variety of pathology suffered around the world. Support of this hypothesis is provided by several case examples detailing outbreaks of disorders more closely aligned with the beliefs of the sufferers than any known medical conditions. Hahn also points out a convincing link between media coverage of suicides and an increase in both suicides and motor vehicle fatality rates.

Hahn concludes that until we know more about the nocebo effect, it may be healthier for society if the media were to err on the side of optimism when reporting messages about health, and to err on the side of caution when reporting suspected causes of disease. Unfortunately, since Hahn's report, we have seen a proliferation of "news magazine" television programs and front page headlines that thrive on pessimism, playing up the catastrophic consequences of exposure to seemingly harmless agents. Indeed, these programs seem to feed into a mass hysteria mindset that is, quite literally, sickening.

## THEORY

### Personal and Interpersonal Characteristics

The comforting and healing power of the placebo effect may be active in all therapies. As a clinician, consider the potential benefits of spending a few minutes during each encounter with a patient to help the patient develop confidence in you and the treatment, to foster a sense of hope, and to develop trust. Research suggests that the quality of the patient-provider interaction can have either a therapeutic or a toxic effect on the patient and that high-quality, caring interactions may be the key that mobilizes the comforting and self-healing potential within individuals.[15] Placebo effects are strongest when the provider is friendly, warm, concerned, sympathetic, empathetic, prestigious, thorough, and competent.[22,23] In addition to the patient's belief in the clinician's abilities, the clinician's explanation of the diagnosis[24] and belief in the treatment being offered[25] are important. Rapport with the patient, confidence in the diagnostic label, and enthusiasm for the treatment are believed to enhance the effectiveness of the interventions provided by activating placebo effects.

Many studies have tried to identify the traits of people who respond to placebos. Certain tendencies have been observed, yet no clearly predictable traits have been confirmed in repeated studies. Spiegel[26] has proposed that a patient's degree of suggestibility is an important factor in placebo responsiveness. The degree of suggestibility is measurable by techniques used to evaluate hypnotizability. In addition, patients who are able to dissociate their thoughts from an awareness of their body and to focus intensely on an idea or instruction are believed to be best suited to experiencing a strong placebo effect. Spiegel concludes, "The placebo effect can occur when conditions are optimal for hope, faith, trust, and love." Supporting this conclusion, research by Lasagna[19] found that good reactors tend to have an affirming, cooperative attitude. Ironically, these are the patients least likely to receive placebos.[27]

## Proposed Mechanism of Action

Even before the patient-clinician interaction, the stage is set for the placebo effect to occur. Patients begin the process by merely seeking, expecting, and accepting help from care providers whom they perceive as competent. The previous interactions between a patient and clinician set the stage for expectations of the impending encounter and have established a prior pattern of conditioned responses that will affect the process and outcome of the encounter. These expectations and conditioned responses appear to be the major factors contributing to the placebo effect.

## Patient Expectations

Patient expectations are one important part of the equation. The role of expectations was demonstrated beautifully in a study of patients with asthma who were to be given two inhalers. Patients were told that one inhaler contained a possible irritant or allergen to aggravate asthma symptoms so that they could test a powerful new form of therapy that was being evaluated in the second inhaler. Inhaling two puffs from the first inhaler resulted in an increase in airway obstruction with more difficulty in breathing and poorer gas volume measures for nearly half of the patients. Then the treatment inhaler was administered, causing the airways to open up, facilitating breathing and improving objective measures of effective breathing. In fact, however, both inhalers contained the same concentration of saltwater.[10]

Further supporting the importance of patient expectation to the magnitude of placebo responses, Evans[28] calculated the pain-relieving potency of placebos to be approximately 5 mg of morphine when the patients thought they received morphine (a standard

10-mg dose), but only 1 mg of morphine when the patients thought they received aspirin (estimated potency of 2 mg of morphine). Many other disease or symptom-related improvements have been linked to patient expectations. Impressively highlighting the role of expectation, one study demonstrated that the use of ipecac syrup (which induces vomiting) can successfully control morning sickness in pregnant women, who were told it would help.

## Provider Expectation

Provider expectations form another key ingredient of the placebo effect. In a multi-center trial of a new antihypertensive agent, researchers at one site were very enthusiastic about the safety and superior efficacy of a new drug. Their patients had indeed demonstrated substantial reductions in their blood pressure. When discussing their results with other researchers, they discovered that the drug was no better than placebos in the other research settings. Thus their enthusiasm for the new drug waned. Despite requests from other researchers to stop the trial of this apparently useless drug, they agreed to complete the study. With less enthusiastic researchers, both the experimental and placebo groups experienced an immediate, marked, and sustained elevation in blood pressure despite earlier reductions.[25]

The way in which clinicians communicate their expectations to patients seems to be another important component of the placebo effect. Thomas[24] randomly selected patients who reported symptoms but displayed no signs of disease. He found that by giving patients a diagnosis and telling them they will get better in a few days, twice as many patients spontaneously recovered than those who were told of the physician's uncertainty.

## Conditioned Responses

In addition to the role of expectations, prior experiences set the stage for conditioned responses to become established and play a part in the placebo effect. It is no secret, for example, that college students have been known to go to social gatherings, consume alcohol, and show signs of intoxication. An annual lesson at one school of pharmacy reportedly involves a Christmas party where word gets out that the punch is "spiked" with a high-potency, colorless, tasteless form of grain alcohol. As reliable as the appearance of Santa at local malls each Christmastime, students attending this party become visibly intoxicated, with some stumbling while others feel woozy and sick. Each year at the end of the party, the students are assured that there was no alcohol in the punch. Invariably the signs of intoxication diminish rapidly; however, students long remember this lesson on the power of suggestion.

Several animal-based research studies have recently been published that point toward operant conditioning as a primary mechanism for explaining the placebo effect. Similar to the college students, rats have demonstrated hyperactive, intoxicated behavior in response to sugar water after first being conditioned with amphetamines. The rats that were not previously conditioned with drugs did not demonstrate these behavioral changes. This conditioned response hypothesis has some support in humans as well. For example, when studying placebo responses in a double-blind crossover study using a potent narcotic agent in one arm of the study, patients who received the active ingredient first had a stronger effect than those who received the placebo first. In a follow-up study, the group that never received an active ingredient was the only group to fail to mount a placebo effect.[29]

## Other Explanations

Although the role of expectations and conditioning has strong support from the research cited, other explanations of the placebo/nocebo effects warrant consideration. The range of possible explanations is vast. At one end of the continuum is the claim that the placebo effect is nothing more than the "tincture of time," explained by natural healing processes for acute illnesses or injuries, or a "regression to the mean" for chronic ailments. On the other end of the continuum is a claim that universal healing energies are tapped and directed to the patient through the healer's compassion and intent to help. Early work by Diers,[15] demonstrating the pain-relieving effect of the presence of a caring person, and more recent research supporting the benefits of energy field manipulation (e.g., Therapeutic Touch) seem to support this latter perspective.

There is also considerable evidence that particular thought patterns are capable of activating psychophysiological self-regulatory mechanisms that mobilize hormones, neurotransmitters, and components of the immune system. For example, volumes of research support a link between self-efficacy belief (the optimistic belief in your own abilities) and health benefits. Bandura and colleagues[30] determined in an elegantly designed study that the pain-relieving placebo effects were mediated by at least two mechanisms. The first is the result of higher self-efficacy beliefs raising pain thresholds and improving the ability to withstand a painful stimulus. Then, as the effects of cognitive control of pain diminish, the body increases production and release of natural pain relievers (endorphins), which accounts for a sustained mediation of pain tolerance.[30]

Further supporting a biobehavioral link between the placebo effect and the body's production of endorphins, investigators from two different studies found that an elevation in endorphin levels correlated to placebo responses and that the morphine antidote naloxone reversed this beneficial placebo effect.[31,32] In separate research studies, people with stronger self-efficacy beliefs were found to have higher levels of endorphins.[30] In contrast, people who had belief patterns associated with learned helplessness had suppressed levels of beta endorphin[33] and reported more pain and depression (perhaps a nocebo response).

Recently, strong physiological links have been made between placebo effects and the relaxation response. Both processes involve an activation of natural (constitutive) antibacterial and antinociceptive peptides, while suppressing potentially harmful (inducible) catecholamines and cytokines.[1] In addition to emerging functional MRI evidence, decades of research have consistently demonstrated that a remarkable number of stress-related conditions can be improved by the placebo effect, thus supporting the notion of this psychoneuroimmunological link.

## IMPLICATIONS FOR PRACTICE

### Use of Placebos in Research

The placebo effect raises some interesting questions for the science and epistemology within the health professions and healing arts. How can we come to know the patient or demonstrate effectiveness of our interventions given the existence of the placebo effect? Does the use of placebos in clinical practice indicate that we value knowing and using the power of drugs more than interpersonal knowledge and power? Is progress in the health sciences being accelerated or stifled by the current methods of inquiry used? Experimental design is considered the only method that can establish cause-effect relationships; however, placebos are not required for this methodology. In fact, the use of placebos may confound the interpretation of findings from studies using this esteemed research design.[34-36] Experiments are often designed to include a control group that receives no intervention; however, it is clear that giving a placebo is not the same as doing nothing.

Soon after the standardization of randomized clinical trial methodology in the late 1940's, it became evident that the large magnitude of placebo effects often encountered (yielding both false-positive and false-negative results) invalidated the findings of even well-designed studies. Investigators were left wondering if the outcomes resulted from the specific treatment effects being studied or the nonspecific placebo effects. Despite these well-established limitations, the randomized clinical trial remains for many the gold standard among research methodologies.

Given that the placebo effect is such a potent confounding variable, are placebos really required to conduct experimental research? The consensus is that randomized clinical trials are best when a double-blind method is used. Double-blind means that neither the investigator nor the patient is aware of whether the patient is receiving the active or placebo treatment. Many randomized clinical trials are not truly double-blind because either the investigator or the patient is aware of which treatment is being used. The more potent the drug being tested, or the stronger the side-effect burden, the more likely it is that the study is not truly blind. Animal and human studies have shown inherent weaknesses with the use of single-blind studies[4,34] that blur the ability to distinguish treatment effects from placebo effects.

Another criticism of randomized clinical trials is that they focus on only a small part of the patient, separate from the whole person and the social/environmental context, and as a result it is easy to overlook the actual cause-effect relationship. Current debates in health sciences support a mixing of research methods to obtain a richer, more insightful perspective. Although the value of evidence-based medicine remains strong, there is a call to look beyond disease-specific outcomes to include Patient Oriented Evidence that Matters (POEMs). Thus including data that describes the subject's perception of the condition and the intervention (e.g., patient satisfaction or improved quality of life) enhances the dialectic process and allows a more comprehensive understanding.[37]

In addition to expanding what we consider to be outcome variables of interest and taking measures to preserve the double-blind nature of the study, researchers can strengthen investigations by ensuring that they are independently evaluated by investigators who are not intervening or collecting the data.[4] When control treatment groups are used, they should be as similar as possible to the active treatment group to create similar expectations. Patients in both groups should have the same frequency of contact and quality of support by the investigator regardless of group assignment.[38] A completely untreated group controls for the effects of the passage of time but not for patients' expectations; therefore many investigations that include a control group also include a standard treatment group, or simply compare the experimental group treatment outcomes with the standard treatments with established efficacy.

Another method of double-blind study that is gaining popularity and is designed to overcome some of the problems inherent in the use of placebos uses patients as their own controls. This method is a randomized clinical trial designed specifically for individual patients. The patients consent to try a random sequence of treatment trials. Some treatments are believed active and others are not (subtherapeutic doses of active medications may be used rather than placebo). Both the patient and the researcher are blinded as to whether a particular treatment is active or not. Measures are made during all treatment periods until there is a clear difference or lack of difference noted between the treatments.[34] This methodology may be flawed, however, because the patient may be unblinded by perceptible (desirable or adverse) effects of the active treatments and because this method does not account for the effects of time during the lengthy trials that require washout periods to prevent the carryover effects of drugs or metabolites.

Amanzio and colleagues[29] recently described a methodology that controls for the placebo effect in multiple ways. First, the use of open vs. hidden administrations controls for patient expectations (hidden administrations are less effective). Second, the use

of reversal agents (e.g., the morphine antidote naloxone) controls for biobehavioral aspects of the placebo response. Last, a completely untreated group is used to control for the nonspecific effects of the passage of time. Although more comprehensive than previous methodologies, factors such as the effects of conditioning and individual and interpersonal features are not controlled for.

In addition to methodological concerns, the use of placebos in research raises some ethical concerns. Tesh[39] discussed the presence of a science-ethics dualism in which researchers may become aware of ethical problems related to their research, but if they break their code of silence they will be discredited as subjective and not scientific. An example of this, and perhaps the greatest misuse of placebos in American history, is the Tuskegee Syphilis Experiment. Primarily poor black men were not told they had syphilis or that they were being treated with placebos. They received a hot meal once a year (so that doctors could perform a physical exam and obtain a blood sample) along with burial money paid to their family on their death in exchange for the opportunity of the U.S. Public Health Service to discover how long it takes untreated syphilis to kill a person. Dozens of nurses, hundreds of researchers, and an estimated 100,000 physicians were aware of the study and did not try to stop it for 40 years until 1972, when the Associated Press broke the story.[40]

## Use of Placebos in Clinical Practice

The use of placebos in the clinical practice of medicine preceded its use as a part of medical research methodology. At about the same time that George Washington was dying from the "heroic" treatment of his sore throat, Hahnemann was developing homeopathic medicines that were more than 99.9% inert,[39] and Thomas Jefferson was reporting the use of bread pills or colored water by the most successful physicians of the day. Jefferson called this a "pious fraud," less harmful than the standard treatment. Heroic treatments of the day included purging; puncturing; cupping; leeching; and the use of poisons (including snake oil), lizard blood, crocodile dung, and fox lungs. Within 50 years, despite the ethical issues raised, 40% of treatments prescribed were placebos.[6] By that time Mary Baker Eddy, who worried about the dangers of available medicine, consciously deceived patients who insisted on drug treatments by administering unmedicated pellets to them.[41]

Similarly, some clinicians today still administer placebos, either to punish patients whose motives are questioned or because of their (perhaps misguided) belief that the benefits of placebos outweigh the harms of available active treatments. Kleinman and associates[42] described the type of patients that are most likely to be prescribed placebos. The patients may be perceived as seeking drugs for abusive rather than therapeutic reasons. Typically the patients have a long and unusual medical diagnosis or get worse instead of better during treatment. Patients who are "treated" with placebos are more likely to have difficulties with interpersonal relationships, especially with the treatment team. Patients are often given placebos for subjective symptoms like pain because they are mistakenly believed to be useful in distinguishing between organic and functional conditions, or to prove that a patient is malingering, exaggerating symptoms for secondary gain, or has some undiagnosed psychiatric disorder. It is ironic that placebos are used by healthcare professionals who do not believe that patients are being honest because it is the integrity of the deceptive healthcare professional who orders or administer placebos that must be questioned.

It is wrong to think that placebo responders had nothing wrong with them to begin with; however, there are still reports in the literature that some professionals interpret the effectiveness of placebos as evidence that discredits a patient's report of discomfort.[43] Those suggestions are the exceptions rather than the rule in the current literature, especially in the area of pain management, where most pain specialists agree that *absence of evidence is not evidence of absence,* meaning that their pain is real, even if the MRI does not reveal an anatomical abnormality. The unconsented use of placebos clinically raises concerns and jeopardizes patient trust; it also damages the reputation of the professional who permits such deception. This weighs heavily against the negligible or even nonexistent benefits of placebos. Some may argue that the beneficial outcomes of placebos justify their use. This justification is misguided and potentially dangerous.[44] Failure to believe patients poses a serious risk of decreased vigilance, missed diagnosis, worsening of symptoms, or perhaps disability or death from a failure to treat a treatable condition.

## Legal and Ethical Issues Pertaining to Placebo Use

Although the concealed administration of placebos occurs in medical practice, the legal and ethical implications are often overlooked. The justification for the current use of placebos in clinical practice seems to be that a physician's right to exercise therapeutic privilege overrides a patient's right to informed consent. However, clinical practice guidelines established by the Agency for Health Care Policy and Research,[45] the American Society of Pain Management Nurses, and the American Pain Society[46] clearly state that the clinical use of placebos is potentially harmful, represents substandard care, and is morally wrong. Similarly, most professional codes of ethics support the notion that placebo use is an unacceptable practice. Professionals are expected to tell the truth and protect patients from substandard care, unethical practices, misrepresentation, or threats to the patients' right to self-determination.

The concealed use of placebos carries the risk of liability for fraud, malpractice, breach of contract, and the violation of informed consent requirements.[47] Attorneys from different parts of the country have concurred that placebos violate informed consent and their use constitutes both medical negligence and deception that no court would excuse.[47] This premise has been tested in the courts, awarding $15 million to the estate of Henry James, a 71-year-old bone cancer patient who was given placebos instead of opiates for pain.[48] Unfortunately it was too late to award anything to Mr. James, who died a horrible, undignified, painful death.

Another issue is the prescribing of a placebo when there is no effective medication available, which reinforces the unhealthy attitude that drugs are the only way to treat illness and human suffering. It raises expectations that relief of disease or pain is as simple as pushing a button or swallowing a pill, shifting the burden of responsibility for healing away from the patient to the clinician. Ironically, by compromising the therapeutic relationship and eroding the necessary environment of trust, the use of placebos reduces the likelihood that benefits of the placebo effect will be realized. There are no win-win situations but there is so much to lose in the tangled web of deception that is weaved by the practice of administering placebos outside of the research context.

## Relationship of Placebos to Complementary and Alternative Medicine

Because it lacked a scientific basis that measures up to today's standards, many claim that the history of medicine before the second half of the nineteenth century is the history of the placebo effect. This period in history is marked by a shift in medicine from the "art" of healing to the "science" of therapeutics. Recently there has been a resurgence of interest in long-abandoned healing techniques. Rather than viewing this as a renaissance of the art of healing, skeptics of alternative forms of therapy (e.g., acupuncture, reiki, nutritional and herbal supplements) revert to the explanation that these techniques are nothing more than the placebo effect. However, given the flaws cited earlier with even well-designed research, it could similarly be argued that a majority of the benefits of modern therapeutics are also derived from the placebo effect.

Without clear objective measures and widely accepted research methods that control for the placebo effect, strong arguments claiming that complementary and alternative therapies derive their benefit solely from the placebo effect are hard to refute. Arguments are particularly difficult with some forms of therapy such as homeopathy and imagery. Medical science could point to the fact that powerful homeopathic agents are 99% inert, just like the placebos used in clinical trials, as evidence of their claim. However, Chapter 14 in this book contains some strong evidence that the benefits of homeopathy are *not* mediated by the placebo effect.

Imagery and the placebo effect can be linked by the fact that placebos are a physical representation of a therapy that is not present, whereas imagery therapeutically uses a mental representation of something that is not present. Imagery, a tool used to promote health by healers throughout history,[49-51] may bring about a placebo effect. Alternatively, the placebo effect may have always derived its benefit from being a form of imagery, which is believed to be the communication bridge between the mind and the body that creates a milieu to promote healing and for the fulfillment of self-fulfilling prophesies. The process of imagery begins with verbal (written, spoken, thought, or mechanically reproduced) instructions, followed by a perceived sensory experience involving one or more of the five senses. This pseudosensory experience makes the image as real as possible, which results in physical, mental, social, and perhaps spiritual change that can be measured and/or reported by the patient.

The described health benefits include improved immune responses that better prevent or fight disease and the promotion of healing, comforting, and biopsychosocial processes. Like placebos, imagery has been found to have a wide variety of benefits, including the reduction of pain and anxiety, accelerated wound healing, and even the reduction in size of cancerous tumors.[51,52] However, potentially harmful effects may result from imagery, such as a suggestion of warmth that may increase peripheral blood flow and worsen conditions associated with shock or bleeding. Indeed, imagery may elicit effects similar to those described as *nocebo* (even to the point of death) if negative images are conjured. Both imagery and placebos seem to rely on cognitive processes to mobilize the comforting and self-healing potential within individuals, the phenomenon Benson calls "remembered wellness."[53]

## A Case Study

### Degenerative Arthritis of the Hip

I volunteered to help Mrs. Mahoney after her daughter heard me speak on a local television program. Within 1 week I obtained the written doctor's order and permission from the nursing home necessary to conduct a pain consultation. Never having been to that nursing home, I was taken aback by the noise level on the third floor, southwest. Nurses were sitting at the nurse's station laughing and shouting over the blaring call lights, discussing their social life. I answered the closest call light and met Mrs. Mahoney.

Mrs. Mahoney was a frail older woman who was struggling to scoot her wheelchair to the bathroom door. "Thank God," she said. "I've been trying to get to the bathroom for a half hour." It was obvious to me while I was helping her to the bathroom that Mrs. Mahoney was severely distressed. Her moans, grimace, body posture, and movements suggested severe, unrelieved hip pain.

When questioned, Mrs. Mahoney reported excruciating left hip pain at the highest intensity on the pain scale. She believed that strong medicine like morphine was responsible for her stroke, so she "would not take any medicine like that." However, there was some medicine that helped in the past, "back when Cathy worked the evening shift," and heat or gentle massage also helped reduce the pain, but her current medicine really did nothing. The distribution of her pain was consistent in location and quality with documented nerve, joint, and bone damage.

The medical record included a CAT scan report of "extreme degenerative changes . . . obliteration of the joint space . . . fracture of the femoral neck . . . and end-stage osteoarthritis requiring surgery." It also detailed her history of cancer, unstable angina, and stroke. Tylenol, Darvocet, or Obecalp were ordered as needed for pain, but nothing had been administered for pain all day. Obecalp was the only pain medicine used for the previous 3 months.

When her nurse, Ms. Conrad, was approached, she agreed to medicate Mrs. Mahoney, stating, "I'll get her Obecalp after I have supper; she's always like this." When I asked what Obecalp was, Nurse Conrad replied, "The red pill, just spell it backward" (i.e., placebo).

Stunned, I sat down and considered how to respond to this appalling situation. There were many clinical, administrative, and ethical issues that needed to be addressed. The pattern of using placebos started when the nurse called "Cathy" still worked there on evenings. Cathy would reportedly come in to Mrs. Mahoney's room in the evening, administer the placebo, and spend some time talking with her and gently massaging her until she fell asleep. When Cathy left the nursing home, the other nurses noted her documentation of the good effect of Obecalp and assumed that they would get the same response merely by administering the "red pill." The Obecalp lost its effectiveness because the staff failed to display Cathy's empathy, sympathy, compassion, or genuine intent to alleviate her pain. They neither had confidence in the treatment nor did they use the power of a caring presence to comfort Mrs. Mahoney.

This represented not only incompetent care but also an egregious breech of professional practice by failing to alleviate Mrs. Mahoney's pain and ensure her human dignity. Nurse Conrad and I spoke privately, and after reviewing my assessment and the CAT scan report, she informed me that placebo was used because of the side effects of strong pain relievers and Mrs. Mahoney's refusal to take them. We discussed the total lack of effectiveness of Obecalp after the comforting interventions of Nurse Cathy were no longer part of the way that the "red pill" was administered. Additionally, we reviewed the legal and ethical liabilities related to continuing with the administration of placebos for severe pain. Nurse Conrad agreed to administer Tylenol and spend some time with Mrs. Mahoney by comforting her at bedtime.

Long-term management of Mrs. Mahoney's pain included discussions with the medical and administrative staff about clinical practice and legal and ethical issues related to this case. Medical orders were changed to discontinue the use of Obecalp and add a routinely administered analgesic with a low side-effect burden. Staff training sessions were carried out to promote characteristics of professional encounters that were more therapeutic than those observed, and information about pharmacological and nonpharmacological methods of pain control were provided. Mrs. Mahoney's daughter became very involved in the care of her mother, and she learned to assist her mother in the use of a variety of pain control methods, including imagery techniques. Pleasant/guided imagery was so effective in controlling pain and promoting functioning that within 1 month Mrs. Mahoney was discharged from the nursing home to the care of her daughter. ∾

## SUMMARY

The use of placebos threatens research investigations and professional integrity in the healthcare sciences. Research methods and clinical protocols need to be modified to control for the placebo effect while minimizing both the false interpretation of data and undesired nocebo responses. The deceptive use of placebos should never be for the convenience of staff, to placate the patient, or in lieu of specialty (e.g., pain specialist or psychiatric) consultation. Healthcare organizations should recognize the potential harm and liability that can result from the uncontrolled use of placebos. Policies should be developed that prohibit, or at least restrict, their use.

Additionally, it should be remembered that the placebo effect is an active, albeit nonspecific, component common to all allopathic, complementary, and alternative therapies. It should be noted that patients vary considerably in the occurrence and magnitude of placebo effects. Because we cannot count on placebo effects to occur all the time, we must use the best therapies available for the patient's specific condition. By using the newest, most effective treatments that we are most confident will help, we enhance the placebo effects in those patients who mount a placebo response.

Definitive evidence of whether the placebo effect is best explained by a "remembered wellness" or "healer effect" model is not currently available. Therefore healthcare providers should recognize that patient, professional, and social interaction factors can be modified to optimize the effect of any and all treatment interventions. Often a simple sentence or two on the part of the healthcare professional can add 15% efficacy to the treatment, which is a substantial return on a modest investment.

Promoting biopsychosocial wellness in a comprehensive fashion helps remove barriers to optimal use of innate self-healing processes. Helping patients to understand their condition and enhancing confidence in the abilities of the professional team in general, and the therapeutic modalities in particular, will help mobilize the beneficial placebo effects. Given the importance of expectations and conditioning, spending time talking with the patient about what he or she thinks will help and what treatments were helpful for similar conditions in the past can facilitate the integration into the treatment plan of interventions likely to elicit placebo effects. Awareness of the patient's misperceptions or unrealistic expectations also helps the professional avoid a common cause of therapeutic failure.

Healthcare is an art, a science, and an ethical obligation that compels professionals to stay abreast of the latest knowledge and skills while honing interpersonal skills and remaining committed to helping the population served. When trust or confidence is undermined, the relationship may take on toxic rather than therapeutic characteristics, with nocebo rather than placebo effects likely to prevail. Striving to develop and maintain high-quality relationships can be the key to enhancing treatment plan effectiveness by activating the placebo effect, which unlocks the natural comfort and healing powers within individuals.

## References

1. Stefano GB, Fricchione GL, Slingsby GD, et al: The placebo effect and relaxation response: neural processes and the coupling to constitutive nitric oxide, *Brain Res Rev* 35(1):1-19, 2001.
2. Bok S: The ethics of giving placebos, *Sci Am* 231(5):17-23, 1974.
3. Fine PG, Roberts WJ, Gillette RG, et al: Slowly developing placebo responses confound tests of intravenous phentolamine to determine mechanisms underlying idiopathic chronic low back pain, *Pain* 56(2):235-242, 1994.
4. Wall PD: The placebo effect: an unpopular topic, *Pain* 51:1-3, 1992.
5. Turner JA, Deyo RA, Loeser JD, et al: The importance of placebo effects in pain treatment and research, *JAMA* 271(20):1609-1614, 1994.
6. Brody H: Placebos and the philosophy of medicine, ed 2, Chicago, 1980, University of Chicago Press.
7. LeVasseur SA, Helme RD: A double-blind study to compare the efficacy of an active based cream against placebo cream for the treatment of pressure ulcers, *J Adv Nurs* 16(8):952-956, 1991.
8. Tsolka P, Morris RW, Preiskel HW: Occlusion therapy for craniomandibular disorders: a clinical assessment by a double blind method, *J Prosthet Dent* 68(6):957-964, 1992.
9. Beecher HK: The powerful placebo, *JAMA* 159(17):1602-1606, 1955.
10. Benson H, Epstein MD: The placebo effect: a neglected asset in the care of patients, *JAMA* 232(12):1225-1227, 1975.
11. Blanchard J, Ramamurthy S, Walsh N, et al: Intravenous regional sympatholysis: a double-blind comparison of guanethidine, reserpine and normal saline, *J Pain Symptom Manage* 5(6):357-361, 1990.
12. Gowdy CW: A guide to the pharmacology of placebos, *CMAJ* 128:921-925, 1983.
13. Lavin MR: Placebo effects on the mind and body, *JAMA* 265:1753-1754, 1991.
14. Cobb LA, Thomas GI, Dillard DH, et al: An evaluation of internal-mammary-artery-ligation by a double-blind technique, *N Engl J Med* 260:1115-1118, 1959.
15. Diers D: The effect of nursing interaction on patients in pain, *Nurs Res* 21(5):419-428, 1972.
16. Meehan TC: Therapeutic Touch and postoperative pain, *Nurs Sci Q* 6(2):69-78, 1993.
17. Murray TH: Medical ethics, moral philosophy and moral tradition, *Soc Sci Med* 25(6):637-644, 1987.
18. Wolf S, Pinsky RH: Effect of placebo administration and occurrence of toxic reactions, *JAMA* 155:339-341, 1954.
19. Lasagna L: The placebo effect, *J Allerg Clin Immunol* 78:161-165, 1986.
20. Eaker E, Pinsky L, Castelli WP: Myocardial infarction and coronary death among women: psychosocial predictors from a 20-year follow-up of women in the Framingham Study, *Am J Epidemiol* 135:854-864, 1992.
21. Hahn RA: The nocebo phenomenon: scope and foundations. In Harrington A (ed): *The placebo effect: an interdisciplinary exploration,* Cambridge, 1997, Harvard University Press, pp 56-76.
22. Alagaratnam WJ: Pain and the nature of the placebo effect, *Nurs Times* 28:1883-1884, 1981.
23. Seeley D: Selected nonpharmacologic therapies for chronic pain: the therapeutic use of the placebo effect, *J Am Acad Nurse Pract* 2(1):10-16, 1990.
24. Thomas KB: General practice consultations: is there any point to being positive? *BMJ* 294:1200-1202, 1987.
25. Graceley RH, Dubner R, Deeter WR, et al: Clinicians' expectations influence placebo analgesia, *Lancet* 331(1):43, 1985.
26. Spiegel H: Nocebo: the power of suggestibility, *Prev Med* 26(5 pt 1):616-621, 1997.
27. Goodwin JS, Goodwin JM, Vogel AA: Knowledge and use of placebos by house officers and nurses, *Ann Int Med* 91:106-110, 1979.

28. Evans FJ: The power of the sugar pill, *Psychol Today* 7:55-61, 1974.

29. Amanzio M, Pollo A, Maggi G, et al: Response variability to analgesics: a role for non-specific activation of endogenous opioids, *Pain* 90(3):205-215, 2001.

30. Bandura A, O'Leary A, Taylor CB, et al: Perceived self-efficacy and pain control: opioid and non-opioid mechanisms, *J Personal Soc Psychol* 53(3):563-571, 1987.

31. Lipmann JJ, Miller BE, Mays KS, et al: Peak β-endorphin concentration in cerebrospinal fluid: reduced in chronic pain patients & increased during the placebo response, *Psychopharmacology* 102(1):112-116, 1990.

32. Levine JD, Gordon NC, Fields HL: The mechanism of placebo analgesia, *Lancet* 2:654-657, 1978.

33. Tejedor-Real P, Mico JA, Malsonado R, et al: Implications of endogenous opioid system in the learned helplessness model of depression, *Pharmacol Biochem Behav* 52(1):145-152, 1995.

34. Enserink M: Psychiatry: are placebo-controlled drug trials ethical? *Science* 288(5465):416, 2000.

35. Chiodo GT, Tolle SW, Bevan L: Placebo-controlled trials: good science or medical neglect? *West J Med* 172(4): 271-273, 2000.

36. Krishnan KR: Efficient trial designs to reduce placebo requirements, *Biol Psychiatry* 47(8):724-726, 2000.

37. Ganiats TG: What to do until the POEMS arrive, *J Fam Pract* 49(4):362-368, 2000.

38. Geden EA: A perspective on the proper use of placebos in research and therapy, *AORN J* 40(6):912-916, 1984.

39. Tesh SN: *Hidden arguments: political ideologies and disease prevention,* New Brunswick, 1983, Rutgers University Press, pp 154-177.

40. Jones JH: *Bad blood: the Tuskegee Syphilis Experiment,* ed 2, New York, 1993, The Free Press.

41. Kaufman M: *Homeopathy in America: the rise and fall of medical heresy,* Baltimore, 1971, The Johns Hopkins Press.

42. Kleinman I, Brown P, Librach L: Placebo pain medications: ethical and practical considerations, *Arch Fam Med* 3(5):453-457, 1994.

43. Verdugo RJ, Campero M, Ochoa JL: Phentolamine sympathetic block in painful polyneuropathies: questioning the concept of sympathetically maintained pain, *Neurology* 44(6):1010-1014, 1994.

44. Elander G: Ethical conflicts in placebo treatment, *J Adv Nurs* 16(8):947-951, 1991.

45. Agency for Health Care Policy and Research: *Management of cancer pain,* Clinical Practice Guideline no. 9, pub no. 94-0592, Rockville, Md, 1994, AHCPR, pp 69, 223.

46. American Pain Society: *Principles of analgesic use in the treatment of acute and cancer pain,* ed 3, Skokie, Ill, 1992, APS, p 25.

47. Fox AE: Confronting the use of placebos for pain, *Am J Nurs* 94(9):42-45, 1994.

48. Brider P: Jury says neglect of pain is worth $15 million award, *Am J Nurs* 91:110, 1991.

49. Jaffe DT, Bresler DE: Guided imagery: healing through the mind's eye. In Shorr J, Sobel G, Pennee R, et al (eds): *Imagery: its many dimensions and applications,* New York, 1980, Plenum Press, pp 253-266.

50. Vines SW: The therapeutics of guided imagery, *Holist Nurs Pract* 2(3):34-44, 1988.

51. Stephens RL: Imagery: a strategic intervention to empower clients, part 1, *Clin Nurse Spec* 7(4):170-174, 1993.

52. Simonton OC, Matthews-Simonton S, Sparks TF: Psychological intervention in the treatment of cancer, *Psychosomatics* 21(3):226-233, 1980.

53. Benson H: *Timeless healing: the power and biology of belief,* New York, 1996, Scribner.

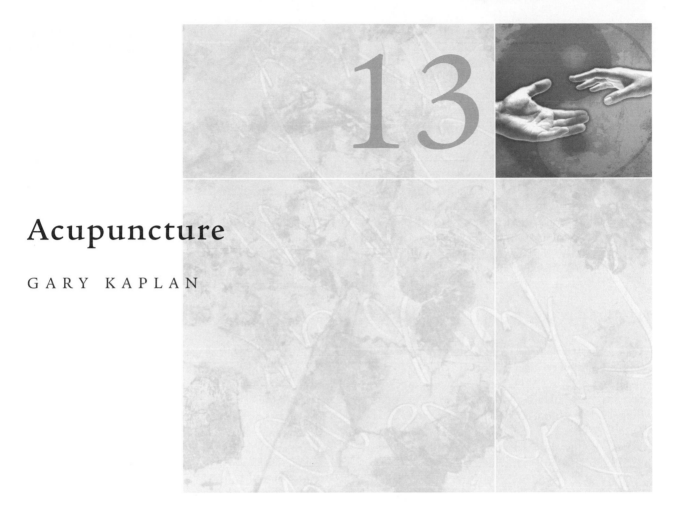

# Acupuncture

GARY KAPLAN

Acupuncture is one discipline or style of practice of a comprehensive system of health care known as Chinese medicine. Elements of traditional Chinese medical practice also include meditation and breathing exercises, musculoskeletal manipulation, herbal formulas, and magical correspondence.

Aspects of Chinese medicine, including acupuncture in particular, have been practiced throughout Asia for at least 1500 years; acupuncture entered European medical practices in the late seventeenth and early eighteenth centuries. As the treatment spread across the European continent, acupuncture theory and practice influenced and were influenced by the cultures and medical traditions of the countries in which it was adopted. The type of acupuncture first brought to the attention of American physicians in the nineteenth century was a European interpretation of traditional Chinese text.

With the opening of China in the late 1970s, however, Americans were able to gain more direct exposure to acupuncture as practiced in China. Today, in addition to the pure and hybrid forms of acupuncture adapted from Asian and European practices, U.S. medicine has also begun to see a further evolution of acupuncture as it becomes integrated into the mainstream healthcare system.

Common to all practices of acupuncture is the therapeutic insertion of solid (filiform) needles. The needles are placed in various combinations and patterns, with the intent of creating a positive effect on the health of the individual. The choice of placement of the needles may be based on traditional Chinese diagnosis, with the intent to modify the flow and balance of Qi (vital life force), or on the Western concept of modification of neurophysiology, or on a combination of these theories.

This chapter begins with a brief overview of acupuncture's history and its journey to Europe and the United States, followed by a discussion of the classical principles that inform the practice of acupuncture. We then look at current acupuncture practice in the United States, including an overview of the major schools of thought. Next, we explore the still evolving Western understanding of the mechanisms by which acupuncture may affect the body. Finally, we discuss the clinical uses of acupuncture, its potential complications, the qualifications and licensure of acupuncture practitioners, and its ongoing integration into the U.S. healthcare system.

## HISTORICAL PERSPECTIVE

The origins of Chinese medicine are ascribed to Huang Ti, the legendary Yellow Emperor. Huang Ti, the third of China's five legendary emperors, is reported to have ruled between 2696 and 2598 BC. The Huang Ti Nei Ching, or the *Yellow Emperor's Canon (or Classic) of Internal Medicine,* the oldest known purely medical text, established a foundation for theory and practice for all Chinese medicine.

The Nei Ching is divided into two sections. The first, Su Wen ("Simple questions"), focuses on the etiology, pathophysiology, diagnosis, and prevention of disease. The second, entitled Ling Shu ("The Mysterious or Spiritual Pivot"), addresses the clinical application of acupuncture and moxibustion (the burning of herbs, usually mugwort, to stimulate acupuncture points). The text is probably a compilation of written and oral traditions handed down throughout the centuries and first published as a unified tract during the Han Dynasty (206 through 220 AD).[1]

Over the centuries the Nei Ching has undergone numerous revisions, interpretations, and clarifications. One of the most significant occurred during the Western Jin Dynasty (265 through 361 AD), with the publication of the first comprehensive text devoted exclusively to acupuncture and moxibustion for the treatment of diseases and the maintenance of health. This new text underwent in turn further clarification and revision during the Ming Dynasty, between 1368 and 1644 AD. This book, *The Great Compendium of Acupuncture and Moxibustion,* is the basis for all mod-

ern Chinese texts on acupuncture.[2,3] Interpretation and translation of this text, in the latter half of the seventeenth century, provided Western physicians with their first substantial insight into the practice of acupuncture.

Chinese immigrants probably introduced acupuncture to the United States, but these early practitioners did not influence mainstream American medicine. In the early 1820s American medical journals began to report on European experiences with acupuncture. The first American physician credited with publishing and practicing acupuncture was Dr. Franklin Bache. Dr. Bache was the great-grandson of Benjamin Franklin and a prominent physician practicing in Philadelphia. In 1826 he published the first translation and studies by an American physician on acupuncture, in which he concluded that acupuncture could "be a proper remedy in almost all diseases whose prominent symptom is pain."[4] Despite Dr. Bache's work, and the later enthusiastic endorsement of Dr. William Osler for the use of acupuncture in the treatment of lumbago, acupuncture generally did not excite the interest of the medical community.[5] In 1971 *New York Times* writer James Reston, in China reporting on the opening of diplomatic relations between China and the United States, developed acute appendicitis and was rushed to the Anti-Imperialist Hospital in Beijing. There he underwent an appendectomy with conventional anesthesia. The next day he developed postoperative pain, and the house acupuncturist, Lee Chang Yuan, was able to provide near-immediate relief.[6] Reports soon followed of seemingly miraculous surgeries performed with acupuncture in place of general anesthetics.

Although the American public quickly became enamored of acupuncture's potential for the treatment of pain and other ailments, American physicians, however, were reluctant to endorse acupuncture. Their reasons were twofold. First, American physicians' attempt to replicate the Chinese reports on acupuncture proved, for the most part, unsuccessful. Second, the Chinese medical concepts of health and illness involving the flow and balance of Qi did not fit the American biomedical model and made little sense to many Western physicians.

Nevertheless, the initial skepticism of the medical establishment with acupuncture began to moderate in the late 1970s with the demonstration that acupuncture's analgesic affects may be linked to stimulation of various neuropathways and neurochemicals associated with control of pain. By 1991 it was estimated that approximately 9000 physician and nonphysician licensed acupuncturists were practicing in the United States.[7] At that time 23 states and the District of Columbia had established licensing requirements for acupuncturists.[7] In 1997 a Consensus Development Conference convened by the National Institutes of Health reviewed the research studies and concluded that acupuncture was useful for a number of specific medical conditions and suggested that further research would probably prove acupuncture to be useful as either a primary or adjunctive therapy for a wide range of medical problems.[7a]

## CLASSICAL CONCEPTS

According to the Nei Ching,[1] "A person is not sick because of disease, they are diseased because they are sick." The Chinese model of health and illness has its foundations in Taoism and in the agrarian society of ancient China. This model holds that harmony of an individual between his or her external physical environment and internal emotional environment is necessary for the maintenance of health. In this context, illness is caused by the individual's response to the assaults of external extremes, such as wind, cold, damp, and dryness, and to internal extremes, such as fear, anger, joy, worry, or sadness. Illness from a Chinese perspective, then, is a manifestation of the relations between a patient's constitutional makeup and the way that he or she is present in the world. Furthermore, illness is not of a part but always of the whole. In Chinese medicine, there is no separation of mind, body, and spirit. All symptoms, all illness, result from imbalances in quantity, distribution, and flow of the vital force referred to as *Qi*.

To define the movement, relative distribution, excesses, and deficiencies of Qi in the body, the Chinese apply the concept of yin and yang. Yin and yang represent the expression of a dynamic equilibrium between polarities, a concept applied in Chinese thought not only to health, to define Qi, but to all natural phenomena. Yin, literally "the shady side of the hill," is an expression of passivity and introspection. It is the feminine quality. In space, it defines inferior and the interior. With a yin illness, the patient appears withdrawn, frail, and pale. A yin pain complaint will be chronic, cool, and poorly defined. Yang evokes the image of the bright and sunny side of the hill. It is the male quality.

It is active, hot, and acute. In space, yang is the exterior and the superior. A yang illness may present with high fever, acute swelling, or severe muscle spasms made worse with heat and touch.

In the Chinese paradigm of health, the balance of yin and yang within the individual and in the individual's activities must be in balance. Qi must flow in the proper direction, and the yin and yang qualities must be in equilibrium. Identification of the imbalances of yin and yang refine the diagnosis of the patterns of disharmony in the individual and provide the Chinese practitioner with further guidance as to appropriate treatment.

Qi flows throughout the body in energy channels referred to in the West as *meridians*. There are six principal meridians, further subdivided into yin and yang divisions, each of which is named after an organ (Table 13-1).

Their areas of influences include the surface anatomical presentation of the meridian and the conventional Western anatomy and physiology of the organ for which the meridian is named, as well as functional and physiological qualities. Bladder, for example, influences the musculature of the back (over which its meridian travels) and the bladder itself; it is used in the treatment of people who may appear somewhat fearful, hyperanalytical, and reluctant in completing decisions. Kidney affects surface anatomical presentation of its meridian, the kidney organ itself, and bones, marrow, brain, hearing, head, hair, will, and motivation. In addition to the six principal meridians with their subdivisions, there are also two major meridians that bisect the body, the governor vessel and the conception vessel, as well as a network

TABLE 13-1

*Relationship of Principal Meridians and Yin/Yang Divisions*

| Principal meridians | Yang division | Yin division |
|---|---|---|
| Tai Yang | Small intestine | Bladder |
| Shao Yang | Triple heater | Gallbladder |
| Yang Ming | Large intestine | Stomach |
| Tai Min | Lung | Spleen |
| Shao Yin | Heart | Kidney |
| Jue Yin | Master of the heart | Liver |

of interconnecting vessels and reservoirs that allow Qi to flow throughout all the meridian systems.

Along the meridians are discrete areas referred to as *acupuncture points* (Figure 13-1). The Chinese literature describes 361 classical acupuncture points, and 1500 or more additional points have been reported. Each acupuncture point has unique characteristics and exerts both local and global influence over the flow of Qi in the body.

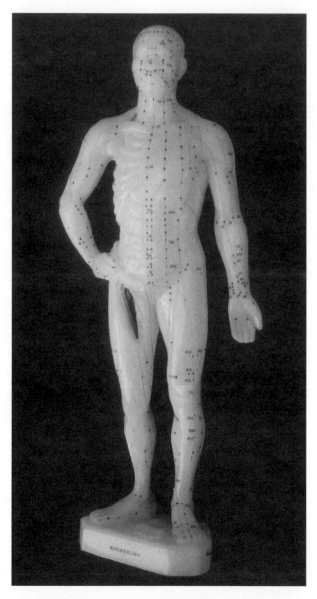

*Figure 13-1* Acupuncture points along the meridians of the human body.

Classical acupuncture physiology describes the role and function of each of the organ systems in the conversion of air, food, and water into the vital substances of blood and Qi. The health of each organ system depends not only on its interaction with other organ systems but also with the external environment. This principle is drawn from Chinese concepts of physiology. Health results from each organ maintaining its proper role and function in the environment. It is the concept of the microcosm and the macrocosm. Internal harmony of the emotional and physical being is balanced with the individual's external harmony, relations with others, and the elements. Because these relationships are so elaborately defined, reconciliation of a breakdown in any function is predictable and results in what the Chinese call a *pattern of disharmony*. A pattern of disharmony may be traceable to a constitutional weakness in the individual, present since birth, or to an unresolved emotional or environmental assault that left a weakness in the body and set up a compensatory homeostatic pattern, rendering the individual susceptible to future illness.

Historically, then, the Chinese practitioner views illness in the context of the entire life and lifestyle of the individual. Clues to diagnosis are found not only in the history of one's physical illness but in what one may be seeking from the environment to help reconcile the internal imbalances. Thus questions about a patient's preferences for and aversions to certain foods; cravings for specific tastes, such as salty or sweet; and environmental preferences, such as the dry desert or the verdant forest, provide important insights for formulating an acupuncture diagnosis. With knowledge of these homeostatic mechanisms, as defined by Chinese medicine, the acupuncturist determines the diagnosis and treatment plan.

Illness may be limited to a subdivision of a single meridian, may involve the entire meridian, or may have worked its way through the system of homeostasis, causing disturbances on multiple levels. Additionally, as previously discussed, problems may manifest at the anatomical zone of the meridian, in the functional governance of the meridian, or at the organ level itself. For example, an otherwise healthy individual with an acute ankle sprain may require only treatment of the involved gallbladder meridian (Yin portion of the Shao Yang meridian). An individual with an acute ankle sprain, a history of chronic anxiety, recurrent tendonitis, a craving for sour flavors, and a preference for green forest environments demonstrates a more involved disturbance on the Shao Yang energetic level and will require a more complex treatment approach. In such an individual the sprained ankle is seen as only the most recent manifestation of an underlying pattern of disharmony. Treatment with acupuncture will involve the placement of needles in select points in the appropriate meridians to reestablish the balance and flow of Qi addressing the problem at the root cause, as well in its current manifestations.

## ACUPUNCTURE PRACTICE IN THE UNITED STATES
### Common U.S. Models

In the United States the majority of physician acupuncturists are trained in a model called *medical acupuncture*.[8,9] Medical acupuncture is derived from European interpretation of the classic Chinese medical text blended with Western understanding of neuroanatomy, neurophysiology, and trigger points.[10] Chinese medical theory and treatments are combined with Western understanding of pathophysiology, enhancing diagnostic sensitivity and treatment options. Diagnostically, medical acupuncture seeks to understand how the flow of Qi has become disrupted in its movement through the meridian system. The manifestation of this pattern of disharmony is addressed by placement of needles designed to reestablish proper flow and balance of Qi. These needles are typically placed in acupuncture points on the extremities and along the two bisecting meridians (governor vessel and conception vessel). An enhancement is frequently made to these treatments by the placement of local needles, whose specific intent is to modify the response of the nervous system according the Western understanding of acupuncture's effects on our neurophysiology. Medical acupuncture can be used to address a wide range of medical problems. It is especially successful in the treatment of pain-related disorders.

The largest group of acupuncture practitioners in the country are licensed acupuncturists. The majority of licensed acupuncturists are trained in United States acupuncture schools, whose teachings are based on the Traditional Chinese Medical school (TCM) in China. TCM diagnosis is based on a theory of Chinese physiology. Treatment is rooted in the prescription of herbal formulas to address patterns of disharmony described in terms of pernicious assaults and subsequent imbalances created in the organ systems. Acupuncture points in the TCM system are selected on the basis of traditional functions. Although applicable to a wide range of medical conditions, TCM (especially with the use of herbal formulas) appears to be particularly useful for internal medicine conditions.

Five element acupuncture uses a theory of acupuncture that is a distillation of traditional concepts from Chinese medicine as interpreted by European practitioners.[10] This model has been championed by J.R. Worsley, Dr Ac (China) and imported from England. Diagnosis is based on understanding a specific construct of Chinese physiology called the *five elements*. The five elements (earth, metal, water, wind, and fire) represent different organ systems and systems of correspondence (i.e., environmental and emotional factors that interact with the elements). The elements have defined relationships to each other, and the theory defines how the balance of Qi is maintained and disturbances in the balance of Qi are reconciled. Acupuncture points are selected on the basis of their function to support or restore balance within the five element system. As a therapy, its strength appears to be greatest in its ability to affect change through its influence on the psychoemotional level of the individual.[11]

Acupuncture theory teaches that there are a number of microsystems, or subsystems, in the body; using one or more of these subsystems, a practitioner can look at a part of the body to diagnose and treat the whole. For example, examination of the tongue and radial pulse may provide insight into the flow of Qi in the whole body. Three types of acupuncture that have become popular in the United States are auricular acupuncture, Korean hand acupuncture, and Yamamoto new scalp acupuncture, which are based on the use of specific microsystems.

Auricular acupuncture was developed in France by Dr. Paul Nogier in the 1950s. Dr. Nogier created a representational map of the entire body on the ear, which can be used for both diagnostic and treatment purposes. When disturbances occur in the body, the corresponding ear point may exhibit an increased sensitivity to touch or an increased electrical conductance as identified by the use of an electronic point finder. Treatment of disturbed ear point is affected by placement of a small metal pellet or magnet taped over the area of disturbance, the use of fine acupuncture needles, or by application of a gentle electrical stimulation. It has been hypothesized that auricular acupuncture works via the nervous innervation of the ear through its effect on the autonomic nervous system, the brain, and subsequently the body.[12] Auricular acupuncture can be used alone but it is more commonly used in conjunction with whole-body acupuncture (Figure 13-2).

Korean hand acupuncture was developed by Dr. T.W. Yoo in the 1970s. He identified a reflex somatotopic system on the hand that corresponds to that of the entire body, as well as to the traditional Chinese points and meridians. In Korean hand acupuncture, hand acupuncture points are stimulated in a manner similar to that of body acupuncture points, and the treatment can be used for the same conditions as those treated with more traditional types of acupuncture.[13,14]

Scalp acupuncture was originally developed by Chinese researchers in the late 1960s. The technique now practiced most widely was developed by Dr. Toshikatsu Yamamoto in the 1970s. Yamamoto new scalp acupuncture (YNSA) appears to be particularly effective for treatment of painful disorders and neurological conditions such as stroke and Parkinson's disease.[15]

## The Acupuncture Treatment

In Western medicine, the method of arriving at a diagnosis is divided into two complementary parts: the patient history, which involves listening to the patient's story of his or her past and present medical problems, and the physical examination, or the actual inspection of the individual. The acupuncture interview likewise has a clinical history and a physical ex-

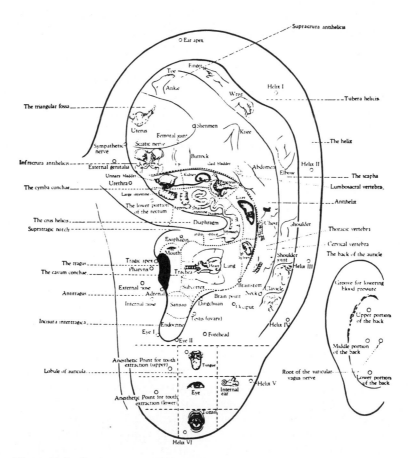

*Figure 13-2*  The corresponding regional anatomy of the auricular points.

amination component, yet these differ somewhat from those of the traditional Western medical examination. As previously discussed, historically, acupuncture practice allows for the incorporation of information not typically considered useful within a strict Western biomedical model of illness. Preferences for and aversions to various foods, tastes, seasons, colors, and climates add detail to the diagnostic tapestry. The acupuncturist's physical examination will involve palpation of specific acupuncture points, seeking areas of discomfort that indicate blockage of the flow of Qi. The color of the skin and odor of the body, as well as an examination of the microdiagnostic systems of the tongue and radial pulse, provide insight into the gross and subtle disruptions of the flow of Qi in the body. Combined with a comprehensive Western medical history and physical examination, the acupuncture history and examination provide for the creation of a richer, more dynamic tapestry of vivid colors and subtle depths describing the evolution of an individual's physical and psychological issues and the pattern of disharmony that caused him or her to seek medical attention.

Once the history and physical are complete, the practitioner will formulate a specific acupuncture diagnosis and treatment plan, influenced by his or her own background and training. As discussed, two principles are common to all acupuncture systems: affecting the subtle energies by harmonizing the flow of the life energy Qi; and inserting fine solid needles in various combinations and patterns to effect a therapeutic improvement in a patient's condition. Beyond a common reliance on these central principles, modern acupuncture practice is influenced by a variety of modes and techniques. Once a diagnosis is formulated, a treatment plan is outlined and initiated. U.S. acupuncture needles are typically very fine, 30 to 32 gauge, solid, and made of stainless steel. Most practitioners use presterilized, single-use needles, eliminating the concern for transmission of infectious diseases. The handles of the needles are usually made of a different material than the shaft itself, frequently copper, and twisted. Using two metals and twisting the handle is thought to facilitate stimulation of the acupuncture point because the needle both acts as a miniature battery (two metals in an electrolyte solution) and has a thermocouple effect.

The needles are inserted to a depth between 0.5 centimeters and 8 centimeters, depending on the location (Figure 13-3). When the needle contacts the acupuncture point, patients experience a brief sensation of dull ache referred to as the "Deqi," the "needle grab" phenomenon, or "obtaining Qi." Thereafter, no further discomfort should be experienced. Once inserted, the needles can be left in a neutral position, manually adjusted, heated (with moxibustion), or electrically stimulated. Moxibustion is accomplished by using a slow burning herb called *mugwort* (Figure 13-4). The herb can be applied directly to the acupuncture point itself or to the needle inserted in the acupuncture point. Electrical stimulation is accomplished with electrodes applied directly to the acupuncture needles and connected to a battery-powered generator. Different

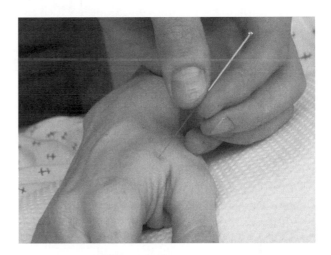

*Figure 13-3* Hand acupuncture.

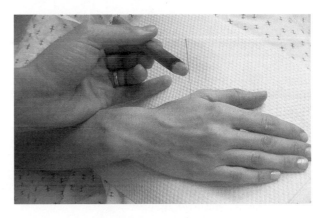

*Figure 13-4* Moxibustion.

electrical frequencies are selected according to the desired effect.

Treatment lasts from 5 to 30 minutes, depending on the desired effect and the condition of the patient. Elderly or physically exhausted patients will usually be treated for shorter periods to prevent further depletion of their energies. Patient visits are usually scheduled once weekly, although two to three visits a week initially is not uncommon. For an acute condition, such as bronchitis or a sprained ankle, as little as two or three treatments may suffice. For chronic conditions, 12 to 16 treatments are usually required. A patient will generally be treated weekly until improvement in his or her condition lasts between visits. Once this occurs, the treatments will be spread out to every other week, and so on, until the condition resolves or the maintenance level of treatment is reached. For chronic conditions in which significant improvement is obtained but a permanent resolution is not possible, maintenance treatments occurring at 1- to 3-month intervals may be appropriate. As with any therapy, patients and practitioners should have a clear set of goals at the outset of treatment and an agreed-upon timeframe in which improvement is expected. Acupuncture, like any therapy, is excellent for some conditions, is best used as an adjunct in other conditions, and is not effective at all in some cases.

As a treatment plan progresses, the placement of the needles changes. Acupuncture treatments are individualized and dynamic. Patients are reassessed at each visit, and treatment is modified according to the patient's response. Initially a mild, transient exacerbation of symptoms may occur and is considered a favorable response to acupuncture. In addition to improvement in presenting concerns, patients throughout the course of acupuncture treatment commonly report a feeling of increased vitality and overall improvement in their sense of well being. For example, in an individual who has been seeking treatment for chronic sinusitis, follow-up treatments may be recommended after resolution of the sinus problem to enhance continued well being. These treatments typically are given four times a year, at the change of seasons, and seek to prevent recurrence of the sinus problem. Thus acupuncture can be employed not only to treat chronic and acute medical illnesses but also as a form of health maintenance.

## A Case Study

### Painful Radiculopathy

John is a 71-year-old retired physician who presented to the office complaining of progressive pain and disability associated with a radiculopathy involving his left leg and foot. The leg pain began about 3 months ago, but he has become increasingly disabled over the last 2 years. Usually energetic with a sharp disciplined mind, he has become increasingly reclusive and preoccupied with his health. A slender gentleman to begin with, he has lost 15% of his normal body weight over the last 2 years. While discussing his medical history, John reported that he has a history of benign prostatic hypertrophy (BPH) and is taking Hytrin to address the symptoms associated with this condition. He noted that he is a good 1 to 2 inches shorter than he used to be, and he complained of difficulty sleeping. He also reported a significant decrease in his sexual libido. Extensive prior medical work-up showed the presence of osteoarthritis and degenerative disk disease with spinal stenosis of the lumbar spine and significant osteoporosis. He also suffered from a mild neurosensory hearing loss, which was particularly disturbing to him, given his passion for opera and the symphony. John was neatly dressed in dark colors, looked somewhat cachectic, with a sallow complexion, and was clearly apprehensive about his health. His hair was gray, and his voice had a low, groaning quality. On examination, his tongue was thin, pale, had a slight tremor, and appeared somewhat inflamed at the base. His radial pulses were weak, difficult to palpate, and absent in the kidney position.

This was a Shao Yin kidney presentation. This patient was manifesting problems at the organ, anatomical, functional, and psychological spheres of influence of the kidney meridian. At the organ level, John suffered from spinal stenosis, nerve damage, osteoporosis, and BPH, as well as hearing loss. Anatomically the kidney is a complement of the Tai Yang bladder meridian. Both bladder and kidney meridians influence the lower back and legs. Furthermore, the kidney influences the overall energy of the individual, which accounted for his pale, frail presentation, loss of sexual libido, and significant fatigue. Psychologically, kidney influences the will, and the emotion associated with kidney is fear. John sought to support his kidney energy from external sources with dark colors and music, both of which, according to traditional Chinese medical theory, nourish the kidney. Acupuncture treatments consisted of combining a French energetics and neuroanatomical approach focused on improving kidney energy in general and his radiculopathy specifically. Given his fragility and sensitivity to the needle, needling was done with great care. Moxibustion with and without needles was used early on in the treatment to support his kidney energy. As his overall energetic strength improved, a neuroanatomical approach was added to the treatment to specifically address the issue of radiculopathy.

After 12 weekly sessions, John reported a 95% improvement of his pain. Over that time he had gained 10 pounds. His energy, sleep, and sexual libido had all significantly improved. He also required less medication to manage the symptoms of his BPH. After 12 weekly treatments, the frequency of acupuncture treatments was tapered. Two years later, John now only receives maintenance treatments at 4- to 8-week intervals, depending on his symptoms. The pain remains well controlled. His activity level has returned to what it was before the onset of his illness. ∾

## ACUPUNCTURE AND WESTERN BIOSCIENTIFIC STUDIES

### General Trends

Western scientific studies are beginning to help us understand how the insertion of fine, solid needles can affect our physiology. A growing body of evidence supports the existence of acupuncture points as discrete anatomical areas with unique functional properties. Mechanisms by which acupuncture treatment can modify the body's perception of pain have been well documented. Imaging studies have shown that acupuncture can modify brain activity, giving us insight as to how acupuncture may be effective in the treatment of conditions such as depression and addiction. Studies that indicate acupuncture's possible effects on the immune system and hormonal system are helping us understand the clinically observed effects of acupuncture in conditions such as infectious diseases and menstrual disorders.

At the same time, our study of acupuncture is helping improve the West's understanding of physiology. Histological, histochemical, electrophysiological, and clinical studies, combined with data from sophisticated imaging studies, support the existence of acupuncture points.[16,17] Acupuncture points demonstrate increased neuronal innervations, with higher concentrations of substance P (a neurochemical necessary for pain perception) than the surrounding tissue.[18,19] Acupuncture points also have a significantly higher electroconductivity than surrounding skin areas.[20,21] Clinically, accurate placement of an acupuncture needle produces a significantly better effect than if needles are simply placed near the acupuncture point.[22] One functional magnetic resonance imaging (MRI) study showed a direct correlation between acupuncture points associated with the treatment of eye disorders and activity of the visual areas of the brain when these points were stimulated.[23] Though not conclusive, these data provide strong evidence that acupuncture points, as located by the Chinese, do exist.

Evidence demonstrating the existence of the meridians, although proving more elusive, has led to some intriguing hypotheses as to how the body is organized and the possible existence of a bioelectric communication system mediated through the connective tissues of the body. Electrophysiological studies have demonstrated a proximal-distal negative gradient along the channels not seen along nonmeridian lines. In studies of electrical impedance between acupuncture points, the resistance between the points was found to be lower and capacitance higher than between non acupuncture points and nonchannel areas.[24-26] From this data it has been hypothesized that channels might serve as direct-current analog communication channels and that the acupuncture system as a whole is "a primitive data transmission and cybernetic control system."[27] It has been further suggested that the channel system is a network of organizing centers. Ontogenically, it has been hypothesized that "the channel system evolved as an intracellular signal transduction system of growth control that preceded the development of the nervous, circulatory, and immune system," and that "its genetic blueprint might have served as a template from which the nervous system evolved."[28]

### Acupuncture Analgesia

The insertion of a needle into an acupuncture point produces a complex of local and distal neurochemically mediated events that may result in the relief of pain. Acupuncture analgesia induced by electrical acupuncture is the best clinically documented and physiologically understood effect of acupuncture. Acupuncture analgesia is mediated by the activation of the endogenous opioid peptide system, which influences the response of the spinal cord, the brain, and the sympathetic nervous system to pain. There are two distinct types of electrical acupuncture analgesia (EA): one induced by low-frequency stimulation (2 to

4 Hz), and the other induced by high-frequency stimulation (80 to 100 Hz). The low-frequency EA is mediated by enkephalins and β-endorphins in the brain and spinal cord and requires activation of specific opioid receptors to be effective. This analgesia can be reversed with naloxone. The analgesic response develops gradually, reaches a plateau, is generalized, and is maintained for a period after stimulation is terminated.[30-32] High-frequency electroacupuncture analgesia is mediated through the release of dynorphin and affects the release of monoamines. It depends more on the activation of different receptors than in low-frequency stimulation and is not reversible with naloxone. The analgesia develops rapidly but ends with the termination of the stimulus.[29-31]

The neural pathways that mediate low-frequency acupuncture analgesia are afferent (ascending) pathways, which, in addition to other nervous structures, stimulate the limbic system and the pituitary gland.[30,32] The limbic system is rich in neurotransmitters that are closely linked with the cravings that occur with substance abuse. Some imaging studies performed on addicts have demonstrated that cocaine infusion elicits a signal increase in many of the limbic structures that demonstrate a signal decrease with acupuncture treatments.[33] Studies have shown that acupuncture is effective in helping patients with cocaine and opiate addictions.[34-36] This observation begins to provide some understanding of the mechanisms by which acupuncture may act on the brain to reduce an individual's intense cravings after drug withdrawal (see Chapter 26). Further confirmation of acupuncture's action in these areas also provides support for acupuncture's reported usefulness in the treatment of neuropsychiatric disorders.[37] Acupuncture also has demonstrated the ability to affect the hormonal system. For example, acupuncture can induce the release of adrenocorticotropic hormone (ACTH).[29,31,32] ACTH stimulates the adrenal gland to increase production of cortisol, an important antiinflammatory hormone.

Acupuncture's ability to stimulate this hormone provides us with some insight into how acupuncture may be helpful in inflammatory diseases such as arthritis and asthma.[38,39]

High-frequency electroacupuncture analgesia stimulates efferent (descending) neural pathways and stimulates release of the neurotransmitters serotonin and norepinephrine.[29-31] Aside from their use in controlling pain problems, these neurotransmitters also have been implicated in conditions such as migraines and depression. Understanding the neural pathways and neurochemicals that are affected by acupuncture provides insight into how its effects can be extended beyond the treatment of pain and applied in a diverse array of medical conditions. This understanding of neurophysiology of acupuncture is complex and evolving. Acupuncture not only stimulates the release of neurotransmitters but actually causes an increase in their production.[40,41] This effect appears to be progressive with repetitive treatment. This observation provides some insight into how a short series of acupuncture treatments may provide long-term pain relief.

The use of sophisticated neuroimaging studies is beginning to confirm that the nervous system changes previously seen in animal studies also occur in humans. A team of researchers at the University of Pennsylvania demonstrated that an asymmetry in blood flow to the thalamic area of the brain in patients with shoulder pain could be resolved with acupuncture treatment.[42] Coincident with the changes in brain blood flow were the patients' reports of significant decrease in their pain. Another study, conducted at Massachusetts General Hospital, demonstrated acupuncture's ability to modify blood flow in the limbic and subcortical gray structures of the human brain.[43] The results of this study provide further support for the mechanism by which acupuncture can be useful in treating addiction and psychiatric disorders. This study also demonstrated the importance of stimulating the acupuncture point itself and not only the skin area over the acupuncture point to achieve the desired effect on brain metabolism.

## Other Applications

Although the mechanisms of acupuncture analgesia are the best researched of acupuncture's effects, an increasing body of literature documents acupuncture's ability to treat a wide range of physiological processes. In the immune system, acupuncture has been demonstrated to have wide-ranging beneficial effects on antibacterial and antiviral immune systems.[44-46] Studies have shown that acupuncture can modify the hypothalamic-pituitary-ovarian axis.[47,48] Studies of the gastrointestinal system have demonstrated electrical acupuncture's ability to suppress stomach acid secretions and affect gastrointestinal mobility.[49-51] In the cardiovascular system, acupuncture has been shown to decrease blood pressure in hypertensive patients, an effect partly mediated by decreased renin secretion.[52] Significantly increased blood-flow velocities in the right middle cerebral artery, with a slight increase in oxygen saturation, also have been documented.[53] This latter study may begin to give us insight into the mechanism through which acupuncture can be useful in treating of some types of stroke. Scientific evidence of acupuncture's physiological effects is wide-ranging and increasingly well documented. As we gain further insight into acupuncture's mechanism of action, this data will directly impact our clinical practices. Understanding the neurophysiological mechanisms of acupuncture has already allowed us to become increasingly sophisticated in our treatment of pain as we integrate traditional theories within Western research. As we study the body from an acupuncture perspective, we are also gaining new insights into how the body organizes itself and functions. The significance of the bioelectric properties of the human body as evidenced by the acupuncture points and channels is among the challenges for further physiological investigations.

## Global and U.S. Clinical Applications

A review of the world literature reveals that acupuncture has been used either as a primary or adjunctive therapy for almost every medical condition. Most of the literature, though, addresses reports of acupuncture's benefits for internal medical diseases. These diseases include conditions affecting the respiratory, cardiovascular, gastrointestinal, and gynecological systems. Examples of such conditions discussed in the literature are as diverse as asthma, pneumonia, cardiomyopathy, myocardial ischemia, ulcerative colitis, peptic ulcer disease, fibroids, dysmenorrhea, and dysfunctional uterine bleeding. A still substantial yet smaller percentage of world literature is devoted to acupuncture's efficacy for pain problems, surgical analgesia, neurological conditions, substance abuse, and psychiatric problems.[7] Although the literature is vast, its quality is highly variable and its conclusions can be unreliable. Many of the studies are single case reports, and most are not well designed. Therefore one cannot draw conclusions as to the efficacy of acupuncture in many of these conditions. At best, the breadth

of the world literature suggests that acupuncture may be useful for a wide range of medical conditions, but more study is required before conclusions can be drawn.

In 1997 the National Institutes of Health, seeking to address the issue of acupuncture's efficacy, held a Consensus Development Conference, which led to some general recommendations. The purpose of the conference was to "evaluate available scientific information and resolve safety and efficacy issues related to biomedical technology."[7a] The consensus process is one method by which the standard of medical care is influenced in the United States. The report concluded that "there is clear evidence that needle acupuncture is effective for adult postoperative and chemotherapy nausea and vomiting and probably for the nausea and vomiting of pregnancy."[7a] For a wide range of other conditions, the report concluded that acupuncture "may be useful as an adjunct treatment or an acceptable alternative or be included in a comprehensive management program."[7a] These conditions include pain problems such as headache, menstrual cramps, myofascial pain disorders, tennis elbow, and stroke rehabilitation, as well as addiction disorders and asthma. Additionally, the report concluded that further research is likely to uncover additional areas in which acupuncture intervention will be useful.

Clinically, in the United States acupuncture has found its greatest acceptance for the treatment of pain, especially that of musculoskeletal origin. Acupuncture is widely used for both acute and chronic musculoskeletal pain problems. In acute conditions, such as musculotendinous sprains, strains, and contusions, acupuncture, as the primary therapy, is frequently successful in facilitating resolution of the problems. Acute musculoskeletal problems in an otherwise healthy individual can be addressed with a short course of therapy (two to six treatments), with significantly faster resolution of the problem than that offered by other treatments.

## Acute and Chronic Pain

For chronic pain conditions, although acupuncture may be the primary therapy, it is most frequently used as part of a comprehensive medical program. The list of conditions in this category is extensive. Repetitive strain injuries (e.g., temporomandibular joint, neck, upper back, lower back, and regional shoulder problems), degenerative disc disease with or without radicular pain, postherpetic neuralgia, peripheral neuropathies, fibromyalgia, arthralgias (especially from osteoarthritis), postoperative pain, and headaches (both musculoskeletal and migraine) are some of the painful conditions in which acupuncture may be successfully employed. The advantages of integrating acupuncture into a comprehensive pain management program are numerous. In some cases, acupuncture treatment will resolve the pain problem. In other cases, although the pain problem may not be resolved, acupuncture treatment allows the patient to eliminate or significantly reduce the amount of medication required. Additionally, patients frequently report improvements in the quality and patterns of their sleep, as well as improvements of their overall energy, mood, and vitality.

## Other Conditions

Beyond pain, acupuncture in the United States is increasingly used for the full spectrum of medical conditions. Psychiatric problems (e.g., depression, anxiety disorders), digestive diseases (e.g., irritable bowel syndrome, nonulcerative dyspepsia), respiratory diseases (e.g., asthma, allergies, emphysema), gynecological problems (e.g., symptoms of menopause, infertility, dysmenorrhea) and well care, in which individuals seek to prevent the occurrence of illness, are among the frequent reasons individuals seek acupuncture treatment. For many of these conditions, acupuncture is best used as part of a comprehensive treatment program.

One of the areas in which acupuncture may be extremely useful is in the treatment of individuals suffering with what are referred to as *functional complaints* or *premorbid conditions*. In these cases, patients may complain of numerous ill-defined problems. Concerns such as fatigue, sleep disorder, mild depression, localized or generalized aches or pains, mild digestive disturbances, and ease of susceptibility to infections fall into this category. Typically, a medical work-up fails to produce a definitive diagnosis, and all laboratory testing is "normal" in these individuals. These types of presentations are common in a primary care physician's office. Although relatively mild, such symptoms in total frequently have a significant impact on the quality of an individual's life. Acupuncture provides a diagnostic system that can make sense of people who have these complaints and allows for the formulation of a rational treatment program. With its different diagnostic organizations and sensitivities, acupuncture can extend not only the treatment options of the Western practitioner but also his or her diagnostic sensitivity.

## A Case Study

### Acupuncture and Kidney Stones

Donald is a 45-year-old gentleman who presented on a cold January day complaining of a kidney stone lodged in his right ureter. He was seen in the emergency room over the weekend when the stone first developed and was discharged with the hope that it would pass without requiring surgery. The next day he was in pain, and the stone had not yet passed. He presented in the office dressed in dark colors, was thin and pale, and appeared to be apprehensive and fearful. In addition to his kidney stone, he reported that he had a history of chronic prostatitis, lower back pain, and a significant problem with fatigue. In the review of systems, he stated that his hearing is not as good as it used to be, which is particularly disturbing, given his passion for opera and the symphony. He also stated that he has been craving salty food. On examination, his tongue was thin and pale and appeared somewhat inflamed at the base. His radial pulses are weak, difficult to palpate, and absent in the kidney position.

This is a Shao Yin kidney presentation, in which the patient manifests problems in the organ, anatomical, functional, and psychological spheres of influence of the kidney meridian. At the organ level, he complained of a kidney stone and the recurrent prostatitis. Anatomically, kidney is the yin complement to the Tai Yang bladder meridian, which influences the lower back and hence the complaint of lower back pain. Functionally, kidney influences the overall energy of the individual, which accounted for the patient's pale, somewhat frail presentation and his complaint of significant fatigue. Psychologically, kidney influences the will, and the emotion associated with the kidney is fear. The energy of the kidney peaks during the winter, which is when the patient with deficient kidney energy finds himself most vulnerable to illnesses. He sought to support his kidney energy from external sources with dark colors, salty foods, and music, all of which, according to Chinese medicine, give nourishment to the kidney. Treatment consisted of a set of specific points, some of which were aimed to increase kidney energy at the organ level and some of which chose to elicit a reflex relaxation of the ureters so that the stone could pass more easily. Needling was done carefully because he was very sensitive to the needles. Some points were stimulated with moxibustion. At the end of the first treatment, the pain from the stone was dramatically improved, and within 6 hours the stone passed uneventfully. Additional treatments were undertaken in the following 6 weeks to address his other complaints. As these improved, the back pain resolved, and he reported that the quality of his sleep had improved. When seen for follow-up 3 months later, his demeanor had become more relaxed and outgoing, and he reported that his overall energy had increased as well.

## LIMITATIONS AND POTENTIAL COMPLICATIONS

Although acupuncture is ideal as the primary therapy in certain conditions and is best used as part of a comprehensive medical treatment program, its limitations in others must be recognized at all times. Chronic degenerative neurological conditions, spinal cord injuries, and cerebral vascular accidents require prolonged treatment and frequently respond only partially to acupuncture, if at all. Acupuncture as the primary intervention in conditions such as human immunodeficiency virus and cancer is inappropriate. Additionally, a small percentage of people may respond only minimally to acupuncture or not at all. This lack of response is also seen in animals and may be related to a decreased production of certain neurochemicals in the brain or an excessive production of substances that break down these neurochemicals.[54] Acupuncture's effects may also be limited by some medications. Steroids and certain antiseizure medications seem to interfere and may block the effects of acupuncture. In all cases, the practitioner and the patient must have a clear understanding of the medical condition and all available treatment options. Conventional medicine treatments may be better and more appropriate for any number of conditions.

As a modality, acupuncture is generally a very safe procedure, but side effects and complications are possible. Most of the potential complications are those that can be encountered any time a needle penetrates the body. Possible bruising, local contact dermatitis to the metal, or pain at the site of needle insertion are all mild and transitory problems. Acupuncture frequently induces a sense of relaxation; however, some patients become anxious, agitated, or tearful during treatment. Occasionally, patients may report a sense of depression or fatigue for several days after a treatment. Syncope, perforation of an organ, or infection, although rare, are among the more serious complications that have been reported.[55,56] In the hands of a well-trained practitioner using sterilized needles, the complication rate is extremely low, and acupuncture is widely acknowledged as a safe procedure.

## TRAINING AND LICENSURE

The regulation of acupuncture practice in the United States continues to evolve. Laws vary from state to state and according to the type of practitioner. In 36 states acupuncture is included in the scope and practice of a physician's medical or osteopathic license. Eleven states require physicians to obtain additional training to practice acupuncture, typically 200 to 300 hours of approved coursework.[57] The 200-hour training requirement is consistent with the guidelines adopted by the World Health Organization on basic training in acupuncture for physicians.

The American Academy of Medical Acupuncture (AAMA) represents the educational, legislative, and professional interests of physician acupuncturists. Full membership in the AAMA requires 220 hours of approved formal training in acupuncture and 2 years of experience. The AAMA has established a national examination and eligibility requirements for national board certification for physicians who wish to practice acupuncture.[58] The training and practice requirements established by the AAMA have become the basis for physician credentialing by the states, granting of hospital privileges, and insurance reimbursement.

The practice of acupuncture by nonphysicians is currently regulated in 33 states and the District of Columbia, with legislation pending in several other states.[57] The educational prerequisites for licensure required of nonphysician acupuncturists vary from state to state. All but two states (California and Nevada) require successful completion of the National Certification Examination developed by the National Commission for the Certification of Acupuncture and Oriental Medicine (NCCAOM) for licensure. Approximately 30 acupuncture and Oriental medical training programs have been certified by the Accreditation Commission of Acupuncture and Oriental Medicine (ACAOM), and a number of other programs are currently in candidacy status. The required core curriculum for accreditation is 3 academic years, including 1725 hours of training.[57] Two major organizations represent the professional interest of the licensed acupuncturists, the American Association of Oriental Medicine (AAOM) and the National Acupuncture and Oriental Medicine Alliance (NAOMA).[59,60]

Twenty-one states allow chiropractors to practice acupuncture. Most states that allow for the practice of acupuncture by chiropractors require additional training, typically 100 hours. Acupuncture training is offered by about half of the chiropractic colleges in the United States. Several states also allow for the practice of acupuncture by dentists, podiatrists, and naturopaths, but most have not established specific training or licensing requirements.[57]

The training and licensing requirements of all practitioners of acupuncture is in evolution. Given the variable requirements from state to state among the types of practitioners, it is important for the consumer to inquire into the qualifications and background of any practitioner. Where licensure requirements are established, the task is made easier. One consequence of the variability of licensure requirements across the United States is the difficulty in obtaining access to qualified acupuncture practitioners in many areas. With the establishment of more training programs, the increased standardization of training prerequisites, and the availability of national certification examinations, the overall quality and availability of acupuncture in the United States is improving.

## SUMMARY

In less than 30 years, acupuncture in the United States has evolved from a medical curiosity practiced predominantly in Chinese enclaves into a mainstream medical profession. As clinical research clarifies the best uses of acupuncture, basic research is revealing its mechanism of action and advancing our understanding of physiology. Although a number of schools of acupuncture have been imported to the United States, its evolution as a medical therapy in this country continues. The training, quality, and availability of acupuncture practitioners is constantly improving. Acupuncture holds the promise of offering treatment options that in some cases will decrease or eliminate the need for medications and in others will ameliorate conditions for which the approaches of Western medicine are unsuccessful or incomplete.

## References

1. Veith I: *The yellow emperor's classic of internal medicine,* Berkeley, 1973, University of California Press.
2. Unschuld PU: *Medicine in China: a history of ideas,* Berkeley, 1995, University of California Press.
3. Lu GD, Needham J: *A history and rationale of acupuncture and moxa,* Cambridge, UK, 1980, Cambridge University Press.
4. Bache F: Cases illustrative of the remedical effects of acupuncture, *North Am Med Surg J* 1:311-321, 1826.
5. Osler W: *The principles and practice of medicine,* ed 1, New York, 1892, Appleton.
6. Reston J: Now about my operation in Peking, *The New York Times,* July 26, 1971, p 1, 6.
7. Kaplan G: The status of acupuncture legislation in the United States: a comprehensive review, *Am Acad Med Acupunct Rev* 3(1):7-14, 1991.
7a. Acupuncture, *NIH Consens Statement* 15(5):1-34, 1997.
8. Helms JM: *Acupuncture energetics: a clinical approach for physicians,* Berkeley, 1995, Medical Acupuncture Publishers.
9. Helms JM: An overview of medical acupuncture, *Altern Ther Health Med* 4(3):40, 1998.
10. Moss CA: Five element acupuncture treating body, mind, and spirit, *Altern Ther Health Med* 5(5):52, 1999.
11. Kaptchuck TJ: *The web that has no weaver,* New York, 1983, Congdon and Weed.
12. Soliman N, Frank BL: Auricular acupuncture and auricular medicine, *Phys Med Rehabil Clin N Am* 10(3):553, 1999.
13. Joderkovsky R: Hand acupuncture, *Phys Med Rehabil Clin N Am* 10(3):563-571, 1999.
14. Yoo TW: *Koryo hand acupuncture,* vol 1, Seoul, 1988, Elm Yang Jin Publishing.
15. Yamamoto T: *New scalp acupuncture (YNSA),* Japan, 1998, Alex Springer Publishing.
16. Gunn CC: Acupuncture loci: a proposal for their classification according to their relationship to known neural structures, *Am J Chin Med* 4(2):183-195, 1976.
17. Lui YK, Varela M, Oswald R: The correspondence between some motor points and acupuncture loci, *Am J Chin Med* 3:347-358, 1977.
18. Heine H: Structure of acupuncture points, *J Trad Chin Med* 8(3):207-212, 1988.
19. Chan WW, Weissensteiner H, Bausch WD, et al: Comparison of substance P concentration in acupuncture points in different tissues in dogs, *Am J Chin Med* 26(1):13-18, 1998.
20. Comunetii A, Laage S, Schiessl N, et al: Characterization of human skin conductance at acupuncture points, *Exterprentia* 51:328-331, 1995.
21. Reichmanis M, Marino AA, Becker RO: D.C. electrical correlates of acupuncture points, *IEEE Trans Biomed Eng* 22(6):533-535, 1975.

22. Lewith GT, Vincent CA: *The clinical evaluation of acupuncture in medical acupuncture: a Western scientific approach,* Edinburgh, 1998, Churchill Livingstone.

23. Cho ZH, Chung SC, Jones JP, et al: New findings of the correlation between acupoints and corresponding brain cortices using functional MRI, *Proc Natl Acad Sci USA* 95:2670-2673, 1998.

24. Becker RO, Reichmanis M, Marino AA, et al: Electrophysiological correlates of acupuncture points and meridians, *Psychoenergetic Syst* 1:10-12, 1976.

25. Reichmanis M, Marino AA, Becker RO: D.C. skin conductance variation at acupuncture loci, *Am J Chin Med* 4(1):69-72, 1976.

26. Reichmanis M, Marino AA, Becker RO: Laplace plane analysis of transient impedance between acupuncture points LI-4 and LI-12, *IEEE Trans Biomed Eng* 24:402-427, 1977.

27. Reichmanis M, Becker RO: Relief of experimentally-induced pain by stimulation at acupuncture loci: a review, *Comp Med East West* 5(3-4):281-288, 1977.

28. Shang C: Electrophysiology of growth control and acupuncture, *Life Sci* 68(12):1333-1342, 2001.

29. Han JU: Central neurotransmitters and acupuncture analgesia. In Pomeranz B, Stax G (eds): *Scientific basis of acupuncture,* Berlin, 1989, Springer Verlag.

30. Pomeranz B: Scientific research into acupuncture for the relief of pain, *J Altern Complement Med* 2(1):53-60, 1996.

31. Hans JS: Review of thirty years of research, *J Altern Complement Med* 3:5101-5108, 1997.

32. Takeshige C, Oka K, Mizuno T, et al: The acupuncture point and its connecting central pathway for producing acupuncture analgesia, *Brain Res Bull* 30(1-2):53-67, 1993.

33. Breiter HC, Gollub RL, Weisskoff RM, et al: Acute effects of cocaine on human brain activity and emotion, *Neuron* 19(3):591-611, 1997.

34. Lipton DS, Brewington V, Smith M: Acupuncture for crack-cocaine detoxification: experimental evaluation of efficacy, *J Subst Abuse Treat* 11(3):205-215, 1994.

35. Avants SK, Margolin A, Chang P, et al: Acupuncture for the treatment of cocaine addiction: investigation of a needle puncture control, *J Subst Abuse Treat* 12(3):195-205, 1995.

36. Avants SK, Margoiln A, Kosten TR: Cocaine abuse in methadone maintenance programs: integrating pharmacotherapy with psychosocial interventions, *J Psychoactive Drugs* 26(2):137-146, 1994.

37. Cassidy C: Chinese medicine users in the United States part I: utilization, satisfaction, medial plurality, *J Altern Complement Med* 4(1):17-27, 1998.

38. Diehl DL, Kaplan G, Coulter I, et al: Use of acupuncture by American physicians, *J Altern Complement Med* 3(2):119-126, 1997.

39. Jobst KA: Acupuncture in asthma and pulmonary disease: an analysis of efficiency and safety, *J Altern Complement Med* 2(1):179-206, 1996.

40. Ma QP, Zhou Y, Yu YX, et al: Electroacupuncture accelerated the expression of c-fos protooncogene in serotonergic neurons of nucleus raphe dorsalis, *Int J Neurosci* 67:111-117, 1992.

41. Guo HF, Tian J, Wang X, et al: Brain substrates activated by electroacupuncture (EA) of different frequencies (II): role of Fos/Jun proteins in EA-induced transcription of preproenkephalin and preprodynorphin genes, *Mol Brain Res* 43(1-2):167-173, 1996.

42. Alavi A, LaRiccia PJ, Sadek AH, et al: Neuroimaging of acupuncture in patients with chronic pain, *J Altern Complement Med* 3(1):547-553, 1997.

43. Hui KK, Liu J, Makris N, et al: Acupuncture modulates the limbic system and subcortical gray structures of the human brain: evidence from fMRI studies in normal subjects, *Hum Brain Mapp* 9(1):13-22, 2000.

44. Zhou RX, Huang FL, Jiang SR, et al: The effect of acupuncture on the phagocytic activity of human leukocytes, *J Trad Chinese Med* 8(2):83-84, 1988.

45. Yu Y, Kasahara T, Sato T, et al: Role of endogenous interferon-gamma on the enhancement of splenic NK cell activity by electroacupuncture stimulation in mice, *J Neuroimmunol* 90:176-186, 1998.

46. Kasahara T, Amemiya M, Wu Y, et al: Involvement of central opioidenergic and nonopioidergic neuroendocrine systems in the suppressive effect of acupuncture on delayed type hypersensitivity in mice, *Int J Immunopharmacol* 15(4):501-508, 1993.

47. Chen BY: Acupuncture normalizes dysfunction of hypothalamic-pituitary-ovarian axis, *Acupunct Electrother Res Int J* 22(2):97-108, 1997.

48. Bo-yin C, Lianfang H: Electroacupuncture enhances activity of adrenal nucleolar organizer regions in ovarientomized rats, *Acupunct Electrother Res Int J* 17:15-20, 1992.

49. Jin HO, Zhou L, Lee KY, et al: Inhibition of acid secretion by electrical acupuncture is mediated via beta-endorphin and somatostatin, *Am J Physiol* 271:G524-530, 1996.

50. Sato A, Sato Y, Suzuki A, et al: Neural mechanisms of the reflex inhibition and excitation of gastric motility elicited by acupuncture-like stimulation in anesthetized rats, *Neurosci Res* 18(1):53-62, 1993.

51. Tougas G, Yuan LY, Radamaker JW, et al: Effect of acupuncture on gastric acid secretion in healthy male volunteers, *Dig Dis Sci* 37(10):1576-1582, 1992.

52. Chiu YJ, Chi A, Reid IA: Cardiovascular and endocrine effects of acupuncture in hypertensive patients, *Clin Exp Hypertens* 19(7):1047-1063, 1997.

53. Litscher G, Schwarz G, Eger E, et al: Effects of acupuncture on the oxygenation of cerebral tissues, *Neurolog Res* 20(1):528-532, 1998.

54. Tang NM, Dong HW, Wang XM, et al: Cholecystokinin antisense RNA increases the analgesic effect induced by electroacupuncture of low dose morphine: conversion of low responder rats into high responders, *Pain* 71: 71-80, 1997.

55. Norheim AJ: Adverse effects of acupuncture: a study of the literature for the years 1981-1994, *J Altern Complement Med* 2(2):291-297, 1996.

56. Bensoussan A, Myers SP, Carlton AL: Risks associated with the practice of traditional Chinese medicine: an Australian study, *Arch Fam Medicine* 9(10):1071-1078, 2000.

57. Leake R, Broderick JE: Current licensure for acupuncture in the United States, *Altern Ther Health Med* 5(4):94-96, 1999.

58. American Academy of Medical Acupuncture: 4929 Wilshire Blvd, Suite 428, Los Angeles, CA 90010; (323) 937-5514; Fax (213) 937-0959; www.medicalacupuncture.org.

59. American Association of Oriental Medicine: 433 Front Street, Catasauqua, PA 18032; (610) 433-2448; Fax (610) 264-2768; aaoml@aol.com.

60. National Acupuncture and Oriental Medicine Alliance: 14367 Star Road SE, Olalla, WA 98359; (206) 851-6896; Fax (206) 851-6883; www.acupuncturealliance.org.

## Suggested Readings

Helms JM: *Acupuncture energetics: a clinical approach for physicians,* Berkeley, Calif, 1995, Medical Acupuncture Publishers.

Liao SJ, Lee MHM, Ng LKY: *Principles and practice of contemporary acupuncture,* New York, 1994, Marcel Dekker.

Filshie J, White A, editors: *Medical acupuncture: a Western scientific approach,* Edinburgh, 1998, Churchill Livingstone.

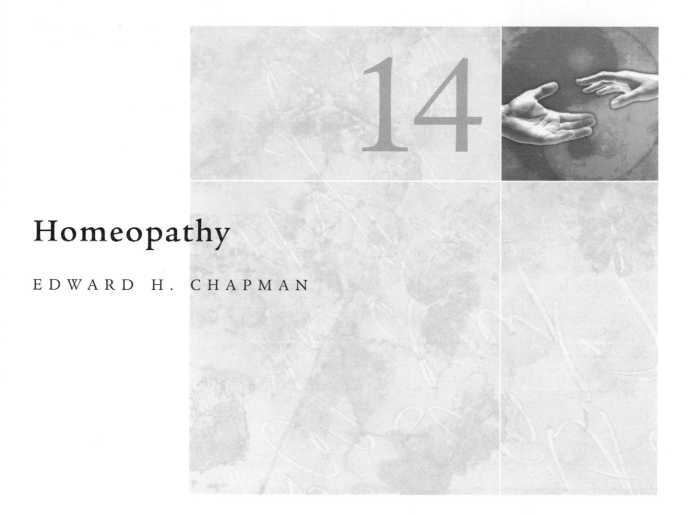

# 14

# Homeopathy

EDWARD H. CHAPMAN

When rehabilitation specialists are presented with a person who is afflicted following an injury or illness, they must assess not only the diagnostic entity but also the person who is sick—the physical, mental, emotional, spiritual, social, and occupational realities of the individual. Understanding the illness is less about the pathophysiological mechanism and more about function and how events have affected the patient's daily life. The rehabilitationist also understands the extent to which recovery and return to function are influenced by a variety of factors: the extent of organic change, the innate adaptive ability of the person, and the quality of the support the environment can offer. Fundamentally, outcomes are dependent on the patient's innate healing capacity, which the rehabilitationist tries to mobilize.

This understanding leads to a prescription that is holistic, addressing the person on many levels, incorporating pharmacological, physical, psychological, and even spiritual interventions. This appreciation of the multidimensionality of health and the need for a holistic perspective is increasing within modern rehabilitation medicine. Physiatrists are leading the way in the appreciation of the interdependence of therapists who collaborate in assisting a patient's healing process.

Understanding the holism involved in healing and confronting the limitations of conventional therapies have created an openness for the rehabilitation community to consider the usefulness of unconventional therapies, including the disciplines of homeopathy, osteopathy/chiropractic, acupuncture, mind-body therapies, and nutrition. Homeopathy is a therapeutic

177

system that has the potential to treat many people who find themselves at the door of the rehabilitationist. An attitude toward healing and the doctor-patient relationship that homeopaths share with their rehabilitation colleagues facilitates the incorporation of homeopathy in the practice of physical medicine and rehabilitation (PM&R).

Homeopathy, like PM&R, requires an assessment of the whole person and seeks to mobilize the individual's healing capacity. Preliminary data supporting the efficacy of a homeopathic approach for conditions that affect people seeking the services of the rehabilitationist are promising. Controlled clinical trials in mild traumatic brain injury (MTBI),[1] stroke,[2] vertigo,[3] fibrositis,[4] migraine headache,[5-7] sprains,[8] Parkinson's disease,[9] and arthritis[10] are discussed in detail, following a discussion of the fundamental principles of homeopathy. The emphasis on the individualized nature of the homeopathic prescription is the central theme of this discussion.

## WHAT IS HOMEOPATHY AND WHAT IS A HOMEOPATHIC MEDICINE?

Homeopathy is a system of therapy based on the observation that a medicine can cure the same symptoms in ill persons that it produces when administered to healthy subjects. Samuel Hahnemann articulated this correlation, known as the "principle or law of similars," 200 years ago in Germany.[11] A homeopathic medicine is one that acts according to this principle of similars. Homeopaths understand a person's symptoms to be clues to the workings of the homeostatic mechanisms of the body. These symptoms arise within a person spontaneously in illness or can be induced by giving medicines in experiments called *homeopathic drug provings (HDPs)*.[12-14] Homeopathic therapy depends on finding a homeopathic preparation whose proving symptoms are similar to the symptoms of the ill person. The capacity of homeopathic medicine to stimulate the innate healing capacity of an organism is person specific rather than diagnosis specific. This individualized nature of homeopathic prescription has important implications for therapy and the design of clinical research in homeopathy.

The homeopathic approach is unique. It differs from other systems of treatment, which act by suppressing bodily responses or inhibiting external disease agents (allopathy), replacing substances that the body is failing to produce (replacement therapy, e.g., hormones, insulin), or using attenuated doses of disease-producing agents to up- or down-regulate the immune system (isopathy, e.g., immunization or allergy desensitization). Homeopathy relies on the inherent capacity of an organism to heal itself. A homeopathic prescription provides the information an organism needs to bring about a healthier state of function using the minimum dose necessary.

## HOMEOPATHIC PHARMACY

In conventional medical circles, a dose of medication that is too small to have a clinical effect is jokingly referred to as a "homeopathic dose." Based on the concept of Avogadro's number ($6.03 \times 10^{23}$ molecules/gm molecular weight), any dilution below $10^{-23}$ molar (M) has an increasing probability of containing no molecules of the original substance. Homeopathic dilutions are prepared by a process of serially agitated dilution (SAD).[15] The processes of serial dilution and agitation confer both the therapeutic benefits and safety of homeopathic medicines. Therapeutically inert substances develop biological activity and toxic substances become safe. Very little data are available on the mechanism of action of homeopathic preparations. The most favored explanations stem from the recent data regarding the behavior of water and solute molecules in dilute aqueous solution.[16-20]

The preparation of homeopathic medicines follows a rigorous pharmaceutical process that in the United States is regulated by the Food and Drug Administration (FDA) (see "Homeopathic Regulation"). For soluble substances one part of the original plant, mineral, or animal substance is diluted in water or lactose on a decimal (X) (1:9) or centesimal (C) (1:99) scale, or the 50 millesimal (LM) (1:50,000) scale. Between each dilution the solution is vigorously agitated. For insoluble substances the material is serially diluted using lactose as the diluent, which is ground between each dilution using a mortar and pestle, a process referred to as trituration. Eventually the lactose triturate is dissolved in water, and the process of potentiation is continued using the liquid medium. Homeopaths refer to these dilutions as "potencies" or "remedies." Potency actually refers to the extent of dilution—low-potency remedies range from 2X (.01M) to 30C, and high-potency remedies range from 200X

($10^{-200}$M) to 100,000C ($10^{-200,000}$M). Therefore a 30C potency is diluted 1:99 30 times, equivalent to a $10^{-60}$M dilution of the original substance. A 12X is diluted 1:9 12 times and has a dilution of $10^{-12}$M.

Homeopathic medicines act like catalysts. A specific mechanism of action has yet to be determined, and the biological effects of a homeopathic medicine are inferred from the subjective and objective changes that occur following the administration of a dose. The evidence for a mechanism of action is further discussed in the sections on philosophy and research.

A well-studied example of the catalytic action of low dilutions in biological systems is the effect of pheromones. Pheromones are molecules secreted by animals; single molecules of a pheromone can stimulate specific receptors in animals of the same species, resulting in predictable and dramatic changes in the physiology and behavior of the animal. Similarly, homeopathic doses initiate effects on the homeostatic forces inherent to the organism. Once a desired response is initiated, the body completes the healing process. The dose needs to be repeated only when there is evidence that further stimulation is required. Consequently, following a curative response to a single dose, the medicine may not need repetition for months. The dose of homeopathic medicines is so minute that the risk of serious side effects or allergic reactions is minimal. Relative to conventional drugs, the cost of homeopathic medicines is also minimal.

# REGULATION OF HOMEOPATHY

The Homeopathic Pharmacopoeia of the United States[21] was one of two pharmacopoeias grandfathered into the 1938 Food and Drug Act that created the FDA. With few exceptions homeopathic medicines are classified and sold as over-the-counter (OTC) medicines[22] regulated by the FDA in consultation with the Homeopathic Pharmacopoeia Convention of the United States (HPCUS), the body responsible for setting standards for the manufacture of homeopathic medicines. Because of their safety, most homeopathic medicines are available to the general public for self-prescribing. Medicines in low potency (1X to 3X) that contain molecules that could have toxic effects, medicines formulated for injectable use, and medicines made from pathogenic organisms or those labeled for indications not considered OTC require prescription.

Two general categories of homeopathic medicines exist: single remedies and combination or complex remedies. The labeling requirements of the FDA poorly reflect the therapeutic reality of homeopathic medicines. Currently, single remedies, which are composed of only one medicine, are inaccurately labeled with common indications (e.g., headache, runny nose). The labeling of a single homeopathic medicine with a single indication is misleading. Accurate prescribing of single remedies depends on assessing the totality of the mental, emotional, and physical symptoms of the patient and prescribing the one medicine, or simillimum, that best matches that totality. Prescribing single homeopathic medicines is a skill that requires specific training and a basic understanding of homeopathic principles.

*Classical homeopathy* is a system of therapy based on the specific homeopathic principle, "the law of similars." Based on this principle, data that are patient specific rather than disease specific are used to prescribe single homeopathic medicines. The "minimum dose" principle of homeopathy refers to use of medicines produced by SAD.

The process of prescribing single or complex (combination) medicines using diagnosis-specific, allopathic indications is referred to as *homeopathic pathological prescribing*. Complex remedies combine several low-potency (usually 1X to 12C, but occasionally 200C) remedies commonly prescribed as single remedies in certain pathological conditions. One assumption behind homeopathic pathological prescribing is that the action of these complex homeopathic formulations comes from one of the ingredients acting as a simillimum (the most similar remedy) for the patient. Such medicines act like a shotgun shell as opposed to a carefully aimed single bullet. It is also possible that the ingredients act synergistically as in many conventional OTC pharmacological products. The design of these medicines allows prescription on allopathic, diagnosis-based indications such as premenstrual syndrome (PMS), sinusitis, allergy, cramps, and vertigo. While their labeling suggests efficacy for conditions, unfortunately, few manufacturers have performed efficacy testing of products for the specific indications for which they are sold.

Recent evidence demonstrated the effectiveness of a prescription homeopathic combination product for vertigo to be equivalent to that of an allopathic drug sold for the same indication.[3] Another clinical trial demonstrated the effectiveness of a homeopathic combination ointment for treatment of acute trauma.[23] Prescribing homeopathic preparations based on diagnosis or syndrome-based indications facilitates their use for the public and allopathic-trained healthcare providers who approach health and healing from this perspective. Consequently, complex homeopathic products represent 80% to 90% of the total sales of homeopathic medicines in the United States.[24]

Drug products supplied by homeopathic manufacturers are referred to as *homeopathic* because they are manufactured using the SAD process. However, because homeopathy has a unique status in the OTC market, the word *homeopathic* is sometimes loosely applied to other OTC products, herbal or nutritional. Although the majority of homeopathic medicines are derived from plants, they are not equivalent to herbal medicines. The two are often confused by the public because the common names on the label may be the same (e.g., chamomile or *Hypericum*). Herbal preparations are loose, compressed, or encapsulated plant materials or alcohol tinctures of the fresh plant and cannot have the HPUS designation on their label.

# SOCIAL/HISTORICAL CONTEXT

The current resurgence of interest in homeopathy by the general public and medical professions has arisen in the context of the public's frustration with conventional medical care.[25] Homeopathy is appropriate to consider as a therapy in a number of situations: when conventional therapy has had no or limited benefit, when the risk of conventional therapies is high (e.g., pregnancy), when side effects limit the usefulness of conventional medications, or when reduction of the dose of allopathic medications in the management of chronic conditions is desirable. Homeopathy also has an important role in managing many conditions commonly seen by specialists in physical medicine and rehabilitation.

Samuel Hahnemann first articulated the law of similars, *similia similibus curantur*, or *like cure like*, in Germany in 1796. His observations and discussion of this system of healing were described in the *Organon of the Medical Art*, first published in 1810,[11] with six editions published over the balance of his career (the last publishing in 1842, the year before his death). He also discovered that by serially diluting and succussing (vig-

orously shaking) medicines, the therapeutic efficacy could be increased while limiting the adverse effects of larger doses. Additionally, Hahnemann developed protocols for testing new medicines on healthy volunteers, which he called homeopathic drug provings. Minute repeated doses of medicines were given to healthy subjects. The symptoms that provers developed were recorded and published between 1825 and 1833 in the six volumes of *Materia Medica Pura*.[26] Through these experiments he expanded the number of medicinal agents used in the treatment of chronic and acute illness by the homeopathic process.

Hahnemann gathered around him a committed group of disciples who assisted and continued his work. Some of these students immigrated to the Americas, where homeopathy flourished throughout the rest of the nineteenth century.[27] The America Institute of Homeopathy (AIH) is the oldest national medical organization, founded two years before the American Medical Association.

During this past century many of the original provings of Hahnemann and his disciples were repeated and new substances were tested. These provings, together with toxicological and clinical observations of the effects of the medicines, were compiled in "materia medica." The most famous of these are *The Encyclopedia of Pure Materia Medica*[28] and *Guiding Symptoms*,[29] both of which are used daily by modern homeopaths. James Tyler Kent authored *Lectures on Homeopathic Philosophy*,[30] *Lectures on Homeopathic Materia Medica*,[31] and *Kent's General Repertory*.[32] *Kent's General Repertory*, an index of the symptoms contained in various materia medica, changed the way homeopathy was practiced and forms the basis for computerized repertorization systems developed in the last 20 years (an example is given later in this chapter).

A contentious relationship existed between homeopathic and the allopathic physicians during the nineteenth century. The code of ethics of the American Medical Association was designed to prevent medical practitioners from associating with homeopaths[33]:

No one can be a regular practitioner, or fit associate in consultation, whose practice is based on an exclusive dogma, to the rejection of the accumulated experience of the profession, and of the aids actually furnished by anatomy, physiology, pathology, and organic chemistry.

By 1900, 8% of American physicians incorporated homeopathy into their practice and there were 20 homeopathic medical schools,[34] including Boston

University, Hahnemann Medical School, New York Medical, and the University of Michigan. However, with the changes in medical education catalyzed by the Flexner Report in 1910 and the discovery of antimicrobials, the popularity of homeopathy steeply declined in the United States. The homeopathic schools either closed or, to maintain government funding and attract students, converted to the modern scientific paradigm espoused by the authors of the Flexner Report. The Hahnemann Medical School issued its last homeopathic diploma in 1950.

Currently an estimated 500 homeopathic physicians practice in the United States, and many more use homeopathy on a limited basis.[35] Extrapolation of data reported in December 1998 in the *JAMA*[36] suggested that 8.5 million Americans used homeopathic medicines, and of these about 16.5% actually visited homeopaths in 1997.

While the demise of homeopathic medical schools left a vacuum in homeopathic education and research in the United States, in Europe, India, Mexico, Argentina, and Brazil homeopathy continued to flourish. In the United States only a handful of medical doctors were practicing homeopathy by the 1960s.

## HOMEOPATHIC EDUCATION AND CERTIFICATION

Interest among healthcare professionals has spurred an increase in homeopathic educational opportunities. To date the only federally accredited undergraduate professional education program that teaches homeopathy is the naturopathic college at Bastyr University in Seattle. Outside of four naturopathic colleges, homeopathic education occurs through postgraduate programs, educating existing medical professionals to use homeopathic medicines. Basic courses require 30 to 100 classroom hours. To achieve specialty status requires a minimum of 500 hours, supplemented with preceptorship to develop homeopathic competence. The Council for Homeopathic Education accredits educational programs in homeopathy.

Board certification is available for medical (MD) and osteopathic (DO) physicians by the American Board of Homeotherapeutics (ABHT), founded in 1959; for naturopaths by the Homeopathic Association of Naturopathic Physicians; and for other homeopathic professionals, licensed and unlicensed, by the

Council for Homeopathic Certification. An entry-level Primary Homeopathic Certification for physicians, nurse practitioners, and physician assistants was inaugurated in 1997 by the ABHT. Three states—Nevada, Arizona, and Connecticut—have separate homeopathic licensure for physicians; otherwise healthcare professionals practice within their conventional licenses (MD, DO, RN-C [nurse practitioners], PA-C [physician assistants], LicAc [acupuncturists], DC [chiropractors], etc.).

There is a growing movement founded in the British tradition of professional homeopathy in which homeopathy is practiced as a separate profession with certification but without licensure. Arguing that homeopathy is safe in the hands of nonmedically trained professionals, this group, represented by the North American Society of Homeopaths (NASH), is petitioning for legislative change that would allow homeopathic practice outside of medical licensing statutes.

## HOMEOPATHIC PHILOSOPHY

Three principles encapsulate the heart of homeopathic philosophy: the law of similars, the minimum dose, and the totality of symptoms. In addition, the entire phenomenon of homeopathy is rooted in vitalism. Vitalism assumes an inherent, active, responsive intelligence that guides the workings of the living organism. Unlike the molecules and organs of the body, this "vital force"[37] cannot be directly measured. It is known only through its influence on the functions and expressions of the organism through the language of physical signs and symptoms, emotion, and thought. When homeopaths refer to treating the *totality* of a person, they are referring indirectly to a unique constellation that is greater than the sum of the individual symptoms and signs of illness. These expressions are specific to the individual; no two individuals with the same illness present with the same manifestations. These vitalistic roots give homeopathy its capacity to transcend the mind-body dualism of the biomolecular model and make homeopathy at home in the ambiguous and complex world of systemic thinking and chaos theory.[38]

Homeopaths learn the capacity of each substance to heal through toxicological data, information gained in HDPs, clinical research, and clinical experience. Pharmacological and toxicological data, as well as information gathered from the use of substances in indigenous healing systems, often provide an initial idea of the scope of a drug. To further elucidate the scope of a drug, provings are done that test a single substance by administering it in a homeopathic potency, usually 30C, in a controlled clinical trial to a group of healthy volunteers, or *provers*. The drug expresses itself in the symptoms that the provers develop. The recorded symptoms of provers form the basic symptom picture of the drug. Adding to it the symptoms that are repeatedly cured by the homeopathic medicine in clinical cases completes the full expression of each remedy. These data sets are combined into "remedy pictures," which are living, breathing portraits. The picture of each medicine is unique in the same way that each person is unique. The symptoms traditionally have been recorded in homeopathic materia medica and organized using an anatomical structure (e.g., mind, vertigo, head, eye). They are also available in other formats in computer databases.

Knowledge of the totality of symptoms for both a medicinal substance and a patient can be approached, but never known completely. The homeopath seeks to understand what is to be healed in a patient—the dysfunction that is represented by the noxious sensations and disturbances of feeling and thinking that cause suffering to the patient. Recognizing that patients' symptom clusters correspond to known pathogenetic patterns of medicines allows for the application of the law of similars. For example, the medicine *Belladonna,* the active ingredient of which is atropine, produces signs of cholinergic stimulation: lack of perspiration, flushing and heat of the skin, dilatation of the pupils, and visual hallucinations. Provers also develop throbbing pains, usually right sided, which come on suddenly and are associated with agitation. These symptoms and signs are very similar to those that a healthy young child might experience with an acute febrile illness, or an adult with a cluster headache. As a result, *Belladonna* is commonly prescribed in these cases. A detailed clinical example of the prescribing process is presented in a subsequent section of this chapter.

How homeopathic medicines act in the body is unknown. Hahnemann believed that the medicine creates an "artificial disease"[11] in the patient, which is similar in character to the natural disease. As the body mobilizes its defenses to eliminate the artificial disease, the natural disease, because of its resemblance to the medicinal disease, is also extinguished. This metaphor can be partially understood by the biological response to immunization or allergy desensitiza-tion. In homeopathy a medicinal substance and a disease are related by the similarity of symptoms they produce. Examples of the therapeutic action of similar medicines are observable in conventional medicine, for example, the paradoxical action of Ritalin. In most persons, Ritalin produces a hyperkinetic state, yet in those with attention deficit hyperactivity disorder (ADHD) it helps modify the same symptoms. Colchicine treats gout in material doses and SADs, but it produces symptoms of gout in homeopathic drug provings. Digitalis can produce any arrhythmia it can cure; the differing effects depend on the dose.

## A Possible Mechanism of Action

The lack of a defined mechanism of action for homeopathic medicines is at the center of the debate concerning the efficacy of homeopathy. "When a homeopathic medicine contains no molecules, what plausible mechanism of action can there be?" ask the critics. There is no answer at this time, only hypotheses. As stated earlier, the most popular theory is the "memory of water," which proposes that through the process of serial dilution and succussion, information in the original solute is transferred to the solvent and is maintained beyond dilutions in which molecules of the original substance can be measured. This information is transferred to the organism by the homeopathic medicine.

Homeopathic dilutions are prepared by a process of serially agitated dilution (SAD).[15] The process of agitation, or succussion, between consecutive dilutions appears essential to creating the crystalline-like structures necessary for the biological activity of SADs (see "Research"). SADs carry information transferred from the solute to the aqueous solvent. Agitation of the solution adds potential energy stored in altered bonding of the diluent molecules determined in part by characteristics of the solute. Information necessary for the catalytic property of homeopathic medicines is encoded in the altered molecular bonding of the homeopathic medicine.

This process of encoding information in water, a seemingly inert substance, is analogous to the record and playback functions of audiotape or videotape. When the tape is passed under the magnetic recording head, digital or analog information is encoded in the altered bonding angles of the ferrous emulsion on the tape. While chemically unaltered, enormous quantities of information are carried on the tape, which when passed through a tape deck are transformed into visual and/or auditory images. Likewise, the information encoded in the water used to prepare homeopathic medicines can be "read" by biological systems, which results in the transformation of the physiological processes of an organism. The specific mechanisms involved in this transfer of information have yet to be defined. The current data suggesting how this could happen are explained in the following section.

## RESEARCH

Research in homeopathy is in its infancy in many respects. A community of sophisticated homeopathic researchers, who are giving homeopathy a new respect within the scientific community, has evolved in the last decade. A recent publication edited by Ernst and Hahn[39] provides an up-to-date description of the status of homeopathic research and the issues facing researchers. The question most important to the scientific community is whether homeopathic medicines, which are so highly diluted, can have biological activity or efficacy in the treatment of disease. In other words, are they anything more than elaborate placebos? The general thrust of homeopathic research is currently focused on answering this question. The majority of high-quality homeopathic research has been done in Europe, although active research efforts are ongoing in India and the Americas. Evidence for the possible effectiveness of homeopathic medicines comes from a number of sources: epidemiological, clinical, and basic science studies.

In the realm of epidemiology, in 1997 Eisenberg estimated that 3.4% of Americans used homeopathy, an increase of more than 300% since 1991; only 16.5% of these saw homeopathic providers, suggesting that 85% of users self-prescribed OTC remedies. This number corresponds closely with the homeopathic manufacturers' figures for the percentage of their sales in the OTC category.[31] According to homeopathic pharmaceutical industry reports, sales of homeopathic medicines are increasing by 20% per year.[24] Berman[40] surveyed American primary care physicians and found that 13.8% refer, 15.9% use, and 49% want training in homeopathy. A survey[25] of homeopathic use in the Los Angeles area from 1994 to 1995 described the population seeking homeopathic services as predominately white, well educated, female, and in fair to good health. Subjects identified that they were seek-

ing care for more than one medical problem, mostly chronic problems for which they had already attempted conventional treatment. Of the survey subjects, 70% reported improvement, 18% reported complete resolution of their complaints, and 60% had improvement in general health status markers after 4 months of homeopathic treatment. These are indicators that the public and medical professions have a growing perception that homeopathy is effective and should be tried for "what ails you."

Laboratory research has demonstrated the activity of SADs beyond Avogadro's number ($10^{-23}$) in a variety of biological systems. Many of the significant experiments are reviewed in two recent publications.[41,42] A meta-analysis[43] of 135 experiments in toxicology found that 80% of the experiments showed positive outcomes, with an average 20% greater protective effect in SAD-treated animals than placebo. For example, mice were pretreated with a SAD derived from the hearts and livers of mice that had died from tularemia.[44] The mice were then exposed to tularemia organisms, a universally fatal disease in mice; 20% of the mice survived. In 1988 *Nature* published a report by Benveniste[45] in which human basophils were shown to degranulate when exposed to antiserum against IgE at dilution of $10^{-120}$. The accompanying editorial[46] summarized the incredulity of the scientific community to these findings that suggest that solutions containing no molecules can effect biological systems: "The principle of restraint which applies is simple: that when an unexpected observation requires that a substantial portion of our intellectual heritage should be thrown out it is prudent to ask whether the observation is correct." After a decade of controversy, Benveniste's findings were confirmed in a multicenter trial.[47,48]

The lack of a plausible mechanism of action for homeopathic medicines underlies the skepticism of modern scientists toward homeopathy. A number of hypotheses have been proposed, the most probable being that original substance leaves a "memory" in the water in which it is serially agitated and diluted. Experimental data supporting the theory of clathrates[49] have been recently confirmed by discoveries arising from research in catalyst chemistry[16,17] that serially agitated and diluted solutions contain 3 nm $I_E$ crystals composed of aggregated water molecules formed in response to the electrostatic forces around individual ions in solution. $I_E$ crystals are a proprietary product. The physicists who developed them have not as yet tested any manufactured homeopathic products but infer by analogy that homeopathic products may contain $I_E$ crystals because of the similarity of the process by which they are produced. At dilutions of $10^{-7}$ these $I_E$ crystals become self-replicating and increasingly stable; at dilutions of $10^{-16}$ they may compose almost 4% of the solution. Stable over a wide range of pH and temperature, $I_E$ crystals can be measured using UV spectroscopy, electron microscopy, and atomic phase microscopy. The physical characteristics of the aggregates appear to be dependent on the characteristics of the initial solute. It could be surmised that the serially agitated and diluted antiserum in Benveniste's experiments contained $I_E$ crystals capable of triggering the cell surface receptors on the basophils, resulting in degranulation. $I_E$ crystals have been shown to act as catalysts in a variety of systems, enhancing the combustion of gasoline and the production of cytokines by white blood cells.[18,19]

Randomized controlled clinical trials (RCCTs) in homeopathy number approximately 200. The bulk of this research has been conducted in Europe, where homeopathic researchers have the support of the government, including the European Economic Community, a well-established pharmaceutical industry, and private foundations. In the United States the federal government has funded only three clinical trials, and two have been published in peer reviewed medical journals.[1,50] Recognizing the deficiency of research in homeopathy and other alternative therapies, the Office of Alternative Medicine (OAM) at the National Institutes of Health (NIH) was created by Congress in 1992. This was the first time U.S. federal funding became available for research into any alternative therapies. In 1998 the OAM was upgraded by Congress to the status of a National Center of Complementary and Alternative Medicine (NCCAM), with independent granting authority. NCCAM's 1999 budget of $12 million was increased to $50 million in 2000 and to over $200 million in 2001. OAM and NCCAM have performed an invaluable service by legitimizing the links between academic institutions and alternative medicine providers. As a result, a number of promising research efforts are underway in the United States.

Clinical research on the efficacy of homeopathic treatments has increased over the last decade. High-quality[51] peer-reviewed RCCTs have suggested efficacy in a wide variety of conditions ranging from diarrhea,[50] asthma,[52] seasonal rhinitis,[53,54] mild head trauma,[1] otitis media,[55-57] fibrositis,[4] migraine,[5-7] and others. Two meta-analyses[51,58] of homeopathic RCCTs have similarly concluded that although the activity of homeopathic potencies cannot be explained by placebo, the lack of large-scale, independently replicated trials limits the conclusions that can be inferred from single studies.

The core clinical research in homeopathy is the HDP. Provings are analogous to Phase 2 clinical trials, which illicit the side effects of a drug at therapeutic doses. The symptoms (side effects) a homeopathic medicine produces when administered to healthy subjects provide a preliminary determination of the therapeutic potential of the drug. In Hahnemann's time, provings were informal experiments that tested medicines with potential therapeutic value based on information from toxicological reports or folk use. Contemporary HDPs employ modern methodology and statistical evaluation to define a set of symptoms that characterize each medicine and can be used to make homeopathic prescriptions.

## CLASSICAL HOMEOPATHIC RESEARCH SPECIFIC TO PHYSICAL MEDICINE AND REHABILITATION

Six areas of research are relevant to clinicians in rehabilitation: headache, acute trauma, vertigo, mild traumatic brain injury, fibrositis/arthritis, and stroke. Issues such as the size, quality, and reproducibility of the following RCCTs make definitive interpretation of this research premature.

### Migraine Headache

Brigo and Serpelloni[5] demonstrated that patients (n = 30) treated with classical homeopathy compared to placebo (n = 30) showed significant reductions in the intensity (p < .000001), duration (p < .001), and frequency (p < .000001) of migraine headaches. This study used an individualized classical approach with remedies in a 30C potency, which were administered four times at 2-week intervals over 6 weeks. Patients were followed for a total period of 4 months. Two attempts[6,7] to replicate this trial in chronic headaches, not specifically migraine, failed to find benefit for homeopathic treatment. Differences in methodology such as the use of prescription by a consensus of experts and inclusion of chronic headache patients rather than migraine subjects may account for the differences in outcome.

# Aphasia

There is evidence of the efficacy of homeopathic medicines for Broca's aphasia,[2] characterized by deficits in motor, verbal, and executive language functions in association with a dominant hemisphere stroke. A controlled clinical trial was performed in Bombay, India, and the outcomes presented at an international symposium in 1980. A randomized group of patients with a diagnosis of aphasia were treated with the appropriate homeopathic medication and followed for 120 days. Based on a bedside neurological examination and speech evaluation, 22 of 24 patients in the verum group improved, compared with 3 of 12 in the placebo group. Though the data is suggestive of benefit from homeopathic treatment, no formal statistical analysis was performed on this data.

*Bothrops lanceolatus,* a remedy derived from the venom of a snake, was used in more than 50% of cases. The symptoms produced by this venom are described as follows in the *Homeopathic Recorder*[59]: "Inability to articulate without any affection of the tongue. Hemorrhages, the blood being fluid and black . . . paralysis of one arm or one leg only." The similarity of these symptoms to those of a patient with Broca's aphasia is the key to the successful homeopathic prescription. The dilution of the venom by the homeopathic pharmaceutical process to potencies in the range of $10^{-60}$ to $10^{-400}$ make it safe while maintaining the desired effect. Unfortunately, this trial has never been replicated. The promising pilot data, lack of other treatment for this condition, and safety of homeopathy would make it an excellent candidate for RCCT.

# Fibromyalgia

A study of fibromyalgia[4] showed statistically significant outcomes in patients with chronic musculoskeletal pain treated with a single medicine, *Rhus toxicodendron* (poison ivy). This study was an attempt to emulate a single agent pharmaceutical trial. To do so patients were selected for inclusion only if their pains were similar to the symptoms of *Rhus toxicodendron:* worse from cold, wet weather and better from heat and continued motion. In a double-blind, placebo-controlled crossover design, 42% of potential subjects met these criteria and were treated with *Rhus toxicodendron* 6C tid. Subjective scoring of pain, sleep, and clinician-rated mean number of tender points was sig-

nificantly reduced, $(p < .005)$. Multicenter replication of this study is planned.

# Head Injury

Apparent efficacy of homeopathic treatment of MTBI[1] was observed in a pilot study of 50 patients conducted between 1994 and 1996 at Spaulding Rehabilitation Hospital in Boston. Statistically significant reductions in patients' symptom intensity ($p = .01$) and difficulty functioning ($p = .0008$) were found. MTBI is a devastating functional disturbance that persists in 5% to 15% of patients with mild closed head injury, resulting in considerable social and economic disruption. Because there is no conventional pharmacological therapy that stimulates the global recovery observed in patients in this study, the possibility that homeopathy could be helpful in MTBI patients needs further confirmation. The significance of the findings of this pilot study was limited because of the small sample size, the short-term duration of treatment, and questions about the validity and reliability of the measures used. A multicenter collaborative study is planned to validate the findings of the pilot study.

# Vertigo

Weiser and Strosser[3] demonstrated that patients (n = 59) treated with Vertigoheel, an oral combination formula for vertigo of various origins, fared equally well when compared with active treatment (n = 60) with the antihistamine drug betahistine hydrochloride. The Vertigoheel combination is as efficacious for the treatment of vertigo of various origins as this standard drug used widely in Europe. This RCCT was done in 15 general practice centers in Germany and measured the frequency, duration, and intensity of vertigo attacks over the 6-week treatment period. The tolerability of both treatments was very good.

# Sprains and Soft Tissue Injury

Zell and Connert[8] conducted an RCCT in the Department of Physical Therapy of the University Hospital of Homburg (Saar), West Germany. In this RCCT, 69 patients with acute ankle sprains were treated with 10 to 12 gm of the topical combination homeopathic product Traumeel. The ointment was applied under a compression bandage around the ankle. Changes were assessed on days 1, 3, 5, 8, 10, 12, and 15 after injury. The 33 patients in the active treatment group improved more than the 36 patients using a placebo ointment on several measures: range of motion, pain, and inversion angle (supination). While joint mobility and reduced supination angles improved in both groups, the improvement in the treatment group was significantly greater than in the placebo group: 17 of 33 in the treatment group compared with 9 of 36 in the placebo group by day 10. Pain was eliminated by day 10 in 28 of 33 in the treatment group and 13 of 36 in the placebo group ($p = .0001$) with Bonferroni adjustment and Fischer's Exact Test [$p = .0003$]). Difference in the inversion angle in the two groups showed a nonsignificant trend in favor of the Traumeel group.

The single most commonly used remedy in clinical practice to treat acute trauma is *Arnica montana*. A recent meta-analysis[60] of clinical trials using *Arnica* showed that half of the trials presented had a positive outcome, while half were negative. The authors of this meta-analysis point out that most of the trials had severe methodological flaws and therefore conclude that "the claim that *Arnica* is efficacious is not supported by rigorous clinical trials." Given the widespread use of *Arnica* clinically and the perception of benefit by the patients and clinicians using it, the issues defined by this meta-analysis point to the need for rigorous trials to settle the issue of the efficacy of *Arnica*.

## Summary

The need for rigorous trials has been the recommendation of all authors of the meta-analyses of homeopathic clinical trials done to date. Homeopathic researchers have begun to explore several areas of interest to rehabilitationists; these pilot studies are intriguing but await confirmation through larger high-quality independently replicated clinical trials. These findings represent only the beginning of the many areas in which integration of homeopathy into the field of rehabilitation could take place. To further illustrate the reality of homeopathic care, the case of a subject in the active treatment group of the study of the homeopathic treatment of MTBI is presented to exemplify the homeopathic prescribing process.

 *A Case Study*

### Mild Traumatic Brain Injury (MTBI)

A 32-year-old woman entered the study 2½ years after having a head-on automobile accident in which she lost consciousness for several minutes. She sustained fractures to her knees, cervical spine, clavicle, shoulder, and ribs, resulting in a 4-week hospitalization. Her intelligence was affected and she lost many skills, which prevented her from continuing gainful employment on discharge from the hospital.

Before the accident the patient had been employed in desktop publishing. After her MTBI she could not remember how to turn on a computer. Her math skills were severely affected: she was unable to conceptualize "3 inches" and no longer knew multiplication tables. When writing, her hand would tremble. Her concentration "stank." She could not think while speaking, and her short-term memory was poor.

She slept 19 hours a day for a year after the accident. The sleepiness, imbalance, and tremor were at least partly the effects of medications. Amitriptyline, Xanax, Klonopin, Prozac, and Stadol nasal spray had been prescribed to manage problems with mood and pain. She was weaned from these medications at an inpatient pain treatment unit. At enrollment she was taking no medications for MTBI; oral contraceptives, urinary tract infection prophylaxis with Bactrim and Nitrofurantoin, and vitamins were the only medications she used at that time.

At the time of enrollment in the study, the patient complained of left-sided headaches secondary to neck injury. Movement of her eyes caused pain, and her head felt as if it would explode. This was made worse by excitement; stress; stooping (she was "blacking out" and could "hear rushing in the neck"); noise; light; and the odor of perfumes, smoke, and paint fumes. It was made better by relaxation and quiet.

She experienced back pain and paresthesias in the legs when sitting. Her life was limited. The sounds of a voice irritated her. She experienced a driven feeling: "Things must be done now." She felt impatient when things got out of order. Everything had to be on time. Before the accident the patient had been happy-go-lucky and friendly. Because she did not like to spoil others' fun she did not say a lot about her symptoms. Only close friends knew.

Nine months after her accident, the patient had a psychiatric admission. While attending an auction she suddenly had become catatonic. She wasn't scared, just blank, like a zombie. For 3 months afterward she could not be left alone. Following a second accident she experienced a flashback of the original accident, with subsequent panic attacks, and was again hospitalized. This prompted her husband to call a meeting of her nine doctors and arrange for her transfer to a regional, inpatient pain treatment center. She had feared driving in a car, and her worst fears had come true. She had scary dreams. She feared taking drugs. She started from sudden noise. Since the injury she felt chillier and had night sweats. Her sex drive had disappeared.

*Assessment.* A 32-year-old woman who sustained MTBI. She was in an oversensitive state that appeared following treatment with polypharmacy allopathic medications. Her headaches and mental state were made worse by stimulation of all kinds. She was impatient, intolerant, and felt chillier than usual.

The process of a homeopathic prescription involves translating the patient's expressions of disease into language that can be used in the process of repertorization and materia medica study. The repertory[61] contains symptoms, or rubrics, organized anatomically. Each rubric is associated with a list of homeopathic medicines that have been associated with this symptom, based on data from provings or cured clinical cases. The following rubrics were chosen to represent her symptoms (numbers in parentheses indicate the number of remedies in the rubric).

MIND; IMPATIENCE (138)
MIND; HURRY, haste; tendency (138)
MIND; STARING, thoughtless (17)
MIND; MEMORY; weakness, loss of; mental exertion, from (14)
MIND; MEMORY; weakness, loss of; words, for (64)
MIND; MISTAKES, makes; calculating, in (21)
MEMORY; weakness, loss of; say, for what he is about to (41)
HEAD PAIN; GENERAL; injuries, after mechanical (24)
HEAD PAIN; GENERAL; noise, from (98)
HEAD PAIN; GENERAL; excitement of the emotions, after (58)
HEAD PAIN; GENERAL; odors; strong, from (22)
HEAD PAIN; GENERAL; stooping, from (140)
HEAD PAIN; LOCALIZATION; sides; left (197)
BLADDER; INFLAMMATION; chronic (53)
NUMBNESS, insensibility; lower limbs; sitting; while (22)
INJURIES, blows, falls, and bruises; concussion; actual or tendency (61)
MEDICAMENTS, allopathic medicine; oversensitive to (18)

When these symptoms are charted against the remedies included under each rubric, Figure 14-1 is generated.

| | Sulphur | Nux vomica | Puls | Nat-m | Sil | Calc | Belladonna | Lyc | Lach | Ph-ac | Arnica |
|---|---|---|---|---|---|---|---|---|---|---|---|
| MIND; IMPATIENCE (138) | 3 | 3 | 2 | 2 | 3 | 2 | 1 | 2 | 2 | 1 | 0 |
| MIND; HURRY, haste; tendency (138) | 3 | 2 | 2 | 3 | 3 | 1 | 2 | 1 | 2 | 2 | 0 |
| MIND; STARING, thoughtless (17) | 0 | 0 | 2 | 0 | 0 | 0 | 0 | 0 | 0 | 0 | 0 |
| MIND; MEMORY; weakness, loss of; mental exertion; from (14) | 3 | 3 | 1 | 2 | 2 | 2 | 0 | 0 | 2 | 1 | 0 |
| MIND; MEMORY; weakness, loss of; words, for (64) | 2 | 2 | 1 | 2 | 1 | 1 | 0 | 2 | 2 | 2 | 2 |
| MIND; MISTAKES, makes; calculating, in (21) | 0 | 2 | 0 | 0 | 0 | 0 | 0 | 2 | 1 | 0 | 0 |
| MEMORY; weakness, loss of; say, for what he is about to (41) | 2 | 0 | 0 | 2 | 0 | 0 | 0 | 1 | 0 | 1 | 2 |
| HEAD PAIN; GENERAL; injuries, after mechanical (24) | 1 | 0 | 1 | 2 | 0 | 1 | 2 | 0 | 1 | 0 | 2 |
| HEAD PAIN; GENERAL; noise, from (98) | 0 | 2 | 0 | 1 | 2 | 3 | 4 | 1 | 2 | 2 | 1 |
| HEAD PAIN; GENERAL; excitement of the emotions, after (58) | 1 | 3 | 3 | 3 | 1 | 2 | 2 | 2 | 2 | 3 | 2 |
| HEAD PAIN; GENERAL; odors; strong, from (22) | 2 | 1 | 0 | 0 | 2 | 0 | 2 | 2 | 0 | 0 | 0 |
| HEAD PAIN; GENERAL; stooping; from (140) | 3 | 2 | 3 | 2 | 2 | 2 | 3 | 1 | 1 | 0 | 1 |
| HEAD PAIN; LOCALIZATION; sides; left (197) | 2 | 2 | 1 | 1 | 1 | 2 | 2 | 1 | 2 | 1 | 2 |
| BLADDER; INFLAMMATION; chronic (53) | 2 | 0 | 2 | 0 | 0 | 0 | 0 | 1 | 0 | 0 | 0 |
| NUMBNESS, insensibility; lower limbs; sitting; while (22) | 1 | 1 | 0 | 0 | 1 | 1 | 0 | 1 | 0 | 1 | 0 |
| INJURIES, blows, falls and bruises; concussion; actual or ...(61) | 1 | 2 | 2 | 2 | 2 | 2 | 2 | 1 | 2 | 1 | 3 |
| MEDICAMENTS, allopathic medicine; oversensitive to (18) | 3 | 3 | 3 | 0 | 1 | 0 | 0 | 1 | 0 | 2 | 1 |
| Total | 29 | 28 | 23 | 22 | 21 | 20 | 20 | 19 | 19 | 17 | 16 |
| Rubrics | 14 | 13 | 12 | 11 | 12 | 12 | 9 | 14 | 11 | 11 | 9 |

*Figure 14-1* Graph shows intensity of correlation between symptoms and remedies.

*Repertorization of the head injury case.* In Figure 14-1, the patient's symptoms are listed to the left on the graph; abbreviations of remedies run across the top. The intensity of the correlation between the remedy and symptom is graded from one to four: 0 is lowest, 1 is second, 2 is third, and 3 is highest. The *Rubrics* row indicates the number of rubrics matched for each remedy. The *Total* row indicates the total score for each remedy. The remedy prescribed was Nux vomica, despite its not having numerically the highest score. Repertorization gives the homeopathic prescriber a sense of the remedies that might fit the case, but the actual selection is based on study of materia medica.

The study of materia medica leads to the prescription of the most similar remedy for the case. Prescribing is not simply matching specific symptoms but matching the characteristic "state" that is represented by the totality of these symptoms, sometime referred to as a "remedy picture." The following materia medica description of remedy Nux vomica[62] has a marked similarity to the essence of the case presented:

*It is often the first remedy, indicated after much dosing, establishing a sort of equilibrium of forces and counteracting chronic effects. Nux vomica is preeminently the remedy for many of the conditions incident to modern life. The typical Nux patient is rather thin, spare, quick, active, nervous, and irritable. He does a good deal of mental work; has mental strains and . . . leads to use of stimulants, coffee, wine, possibly in excess; . . . rich and stimulating food; . . . a thick head, dyspepsia, and irritable temper are the next day's inheritance. These conditions produce an irritable nervous system, hypersensitive and overimpressionable, which Nux vomica will do much to soothe and calm. Convulsions, consciousness; aggravated touch, moving; . . . patients are easily chilled, avoid open air. Nux vomica always seems to be out of tune. Inharmonious spasmodic action. . . . Tense contracted feeling. . . . Bruised soreness; of abdomen, brain. . . . Contractive pains throughout the body. General bruised feeling in the morning in bed. . . . Great debility, and oversensitiveness of all the senses. Everything makes too strong an impression. Stitches in jerks throughout the whole body. . . . Trembling all over; mostly of hands, especially in morning; in drunkards.*

*Therapeutic plan.* The similarity of this portrait to the patient's case, together with the matching of most of the specific symptoms displayed in the repertorization graph, led to the prescription of Nux vomica 200C once daily for 7 days.

*One-month follow-up.* The improvement was fairly sudden. She felt better, her mind was working again, and she stated that she could remember things more. She felt ready to try the computer and bought one 2 weeks before follow-up. She could read manuals and follow directions. Her husband commented, "She is sharper across the board." She had not tried math, and she still had difficulty conceptualizing "3 inches".

Her general energy level was changed; she was able to work from 8:00 AM to 3:30 PM on a computer. She was tired by evening and went to bed early. Her headaches were improved, coming on after maintaining steady concentration for 2 days, or significant excitement. Back pain had initially worsened after the remedy, peaking that same week, and had gradually improved since.

When asked about her irritability, she replied that she was in a better mood and felt more useful, although the driven feeling was still there. Insomnia and diminished sexual desire persisted. Performing multiple simultaneous tasks was still difficult. She continued to complain of chilliness.

*Assessment.* She rated her improvements in three areas on a scale of 10 (worst) to 0 (none) as follows:
- Cognitive dysfunction: From 10 to 4 and continuing to improve
- Physical dysfunction: From 10 to 8; continuing to have back pain
- Emotional dysfunction: From 10 to 0

She stated that her sense of usefulness had returned. There was a clear and dramatic improvement in her overall state.

*Plan.* Do nothing. Homeopathic medicines act as catalysts and do not need repetition unless the remedy reaction ceases. She was asked to call if she relapsed or stopped improving.

*Two-month follow-up.* She had a mild relapse of her symptoms 2 weeks after the visit and repeated the Nux vomica 200C in water daily for 3 days, after which she continued to improve.

*Three-month follow-up.* She had to repeat the remedy several times in water with minimal improvement. Her energy level was lower and she had fewer useful hours in the day. She was working 5 to 6 hours, 3 days a week. Memory remained an issue; she was unable to remember to take her oral contraceptive (OCP) or antibiotic. She had an unpleasant dream in which a friend was having a heart attack, and she didn't know what to do. Someone else was drowning. "I'm there and can't help." She had drenching night sweats at 1 or 3 am. She felt hot all over, especially her chest and thighs, and radiated heat when asleep; she left the window open while sleeping. Her moods were more stable: less cranky, agitated, and frustrated. She was craving fat, pizza, hot spices, and creamy foods.

*Assessment.* She was better but had reached the maximal benefit from the 200C potency of Nux vomica. The driven feeling and dreams of fatal accidents are characteristic of Nux vomica. Under routine circumstances the potency would be increased to Nux vomica 1000C (1M); but in the study protocol only the 200C potency was available. Some fundamental shifts in her state had begun to appear: body warmth, desire for spices, and an increase of her night sweats. The warmer body temperature was a return of a state normal for her before the accident.

*Plan.* In the absence of a higher potency of Nux vomica (because the study design only allowed a limited number of available remedies) she was given the complementary remedy Sulphur 200C daily for 7 days.

*Four-month follow-up.* "I'm excellent and have returned to work, on my own schedule, building up slowly, now averaging 20 hours per week." After taking the second remedy (Sulphur 200C), she developed intensive headaches; she then repeated Nux vomica 200C in water and gradually improved. In general she felt great. She went to bed by 9:30 PM, awoke at 6:30 AM with an alarm and on weekends at 8:00 AM. She was still waking between 1 and 2 AM with night sweats, and she still had nightmares. Her bladder was stable; she planned to speak to her primary care physician the next week about going off antibiotics. The "discs in her back felt swollen" in wet weather. A bad cold and possible pneumonia resolved; she used echinacea. Her short-term memory was still limited.

*Assessment.* Overall improved. The patient had an initial aggravation by the Sulphur, during which she took Nux vomica. It was unclear whether the subsequent improvement was due to the Sulphur or repeating the Nux vomica.

*Plan.* This patient was terminated from the study after the prescribed 4-month treatment period and referred to a local homeopathic physician for follow-up. Ideally a higher potency of Nux vomica will be given, and then possibly Sulphur, if indicated, but starting with a lower potency than previously given. Herbal support for her urinary tract infections might allow her to discontinue the antibiotics, which could be interfering with the homeopathic medicine. ∾

## PRESCRIBING COMBINATION HOMEOPATHIC MEDICINES

The use of combination homeopathic medicines requires knowledge of the patient's diagnosis, symptoms, and the etiology of the condition when known. Patient age, use of conventional medicines, and chronic disease, including cardiac and/or renal insufficiency, do not affect the choice of homeopathic product or dosage. The exceptions are those low-dose homeopathic drugs (1C, 2C, 1X to 4X) that are known to be organ toxic and only available by prescription.

Combination homeopathic medicines may be prescribed in injectable, topical, or sublingual forms. Several homeopathic pharmaceutical manufacturers have combined a number of homeopathic drugs known to be clinically helpful in trauma and label these combinations for treatment of symptoms of acute trauma.

Trauma combinations usually include official homeopathic drugs in OTC potencies such as *Aconitum napellus, Calendula officinalis, Hypericum perforatum, Arnica montana, Echinacea angustifolia, Hamamelis virginiana, Belladonna, Symphytum officinale,* and *Ruta graveolens.* The product is clearly labeled with the indications and how to take the homeopathic medicine. Usual dosage would be 2 tablets sublingually every 2 to 4 hours prn for pain, or a generous application of an ointment. While repetition of homeopathic combinations is determined by the patient's response, there is no danger with frequent use of the medicine. It may be used every 15 minutes initially, increasing the intervals between the doses as the symptoms improve.

Combination homeopathic remedies may be used for the following conditions: shin splints, strained calf muscle (gastrocnemius or soleus), iliotibial band strain, patellar tendinitis, quadriceps strain, strained adductor muscles, hematomas and contusions, sciatica, hamstring strain, and cramps. Homeopathic combination products are carried by many local and national pharmacies and health food stores and are available by mail order from homeopathic manufacturers. Some homeopathic combination medicines may be listed in the Physicians Desk Reference (PDR) in the alternative medicine product category index. Drugs listed in the PDR may require a prescription because they are used in injectable form or have an indication, such as vertigo, that is not an OTC indication.

Using combination homeopathic medicines is safe, easy, and affordable. Patient compliance is high. While side effects are minimal, efficacy is variable. It is wise to ask the patient if he or she has used homeopathic medicines in the past and what has worked in similar medical situations. Many patients have successfully self-prescribed homeopathic combination medicines and, given similar symptoms, would again like to try them.

## SUMMARY

From the research and clinical examples presented in this chapter, it is apparent that homeopathy has an important therapeutic role in rehabilitation medicine.

Two approaches exist for the use of homeopathy: classical and complex (combination), each with its merits and limitations. The combination approach allows the physician to practice in an allopathic mindset. While the results are likely to be palliative, the few published

 *Resources*

*Organizations*

The National Center for Homeopathy
801 Fairfax Street, Suite 306
Alexandria, VA 22314
(703) 548-7790
www.homeopathic.org
*Provides information on homeopathy and homeopathic practitioners for the general public.*

American Institute of Homeopathy
801 Fairfax Street, Suite 306
Alexandria, VA 22314
(703) 246-9501
www.healthy.net/associations/pa/aih
*The oldest national medical professional organization in the United States, dedicated to advancing healthcare through homeotherapeutics.*

American Board of Homeotherapeutics
801 N Fairfax Street, Suite 306
Alexandria, VA 22314
(703) 548-7790
*Provides specialty or primary care certification for MDs, DOs, RN-Cs, PA-Cs.*

Council for Homeopathic Education
801 N Fairfax Street, Suite 306
Alexandria, VA 22314
(212) 560-7136
www.chedu.org
*Accredits and maintains listing of homeopathic education programs.*

American Homeopathic Pharmaceutical Association
PO Box 2241
Southeastern, PA 19399
(610) 783-5124
*Provides information on manufacturing and distribution of homeopathic medicines.*

Homeopathic Pharmacopoeia Convention of the United States
PO Box 2221
Southeastern, PA 19399-2221
(610) 783-5124
www.hpus.com
*Provides the complete HPUS or abstracts.*

*Books/Tapes/Software*

Homeopathic Educational Services
2124 Kittredge Street
Berkeley, CA 94794
(800) 359-9051

Kent Homeopathic Associates, Inc.
710 Mission Avenue
San Rafael, CA 94901
(415) 457-0678
*Provides homeopathic software for the professional. The ReferenceWorks Library includes every notable homeopathic book published in the last 175 years.*

Minimum Price Homeopathic Books
PO Box 2187
Blaine, WA 98231
(800) 663-8272

*CAM Websites*

The website at www.nccam.nih.gov/ searches the National Institutes of Health, Center for Complementary and Alternative Medicine.

*Acknowledgment*

I would like to acknowledge Jackie Wilson, MD, for her input into the prescribing of complex homeopathic medicines.

Jacquelyn J. Wilson, MD, DHt, DABFP
Consultant in Homeopathy and Integrative Medicine
536 Brotherton Road
Escondido, CA 92025
www.homeopathicdoctor.com

trials of these products compare favorably with allopathic alternatives.

The application of the classical approach requires in-depth training in homeopathic prescribing and may lead to long-term, curative effects. Achieving competence in the classical methods has traditionally taken years of study. Recent initiatives in training in homeopathy have emphasized the recognition of the key patterns for remedies prescribed in conditions commonly seen in primary care. Physicians trained in this way have achieved clinically significant outcomes in 60% to 70% of their cases.

An evidence-based approach, using findings from clinical research in areas of interest to rehabilitationists, such as head trauma, stroke, fibromyalgia, and arthritis, will be necessary. Identification of commonly prescribed homeopathic medicines and the clinical indications for each specific medicine could lead to a simplification of homeopathic prescribing using algorithms. Alternatively, this data could be used to rationally design combination products that could then be tested for effectiveness.

Simplifying the classical homeopathic prescribing process would facilitate the use of homeopathic medicines in appropriate cases seen by rehabilitationists. The efficacy of combination products could be tested against both conventional alternatives and the classical homeopathic method. The curative potential of homeopathic medicines, together with their low cost and the minimal incidence of adverse reactions attending their use, makes collaboration between the rehabilitation and homeopathic communities an intriguing possibility.

## References

1. Chapman EH et al: The homeopathic treatment of mild traumatic brain injury: a randomized double-blind placebo controlled trial, *J Head Trauma Rehabil* 14(6):521-542, 1999.
2. Master FJ: Scope of drugs in the treatment of Broca's aphasia. In *42nd Congress of the International Homeopathic Medical League*, Washington, 1987, LIGA.
3. Weiser M, Strosser W, Klein P: Homeopathic vs. conventional treatment of vertigo, *Arch Otolaryngol Head Neck Surg* 124:879-883, 1998.
4. Fisher P et al: Effect of homeopathic treatment on fibrositis, *BMJ* 299:365-366, 1989.
5. Brigo B, Serpelloni G: Homeopathic treatment of migraines: a randomized double-blind controlled study of sixty cases, *Berl J Resin Homeopath* 1:8-105, 1991.
6. Whitmarsh THE: Double-blind randomized placebo-controlled study of the homeopathic prophylaxis of migraine, *Cephalalgia* 17:600-604, 1997.
7. Walach H et al: Classical homeopathic treatment of chronic headaches, *Cephalalgia* 17:119-126, 1997.
8. Zell J, Connert W, Feuerstake G: Treatment of acute sprains of the ankle: a controlled, double-blind study to test the effectiveness of a homeopathic treatment, *Biol Ther* 7(1):1-6, 1989.
9. Ericsson AD: *Homeopathic neurotropin: treatment of Parkinson's disease,* Houston, 1994, Institute of Biological Research, pp 1-12.
10. Gibson RG et al: Homeopathic therapy in rheumatoid arthritis: evaluation by double-blind clinical therapeutic trial, *Br J Clin Pharmacol* 9:453-459, 1980.
11. Hahnemann S: *Organon of the medical art,* Redmond, Wash, 1996, Birdcage Books, p 158. (Edited by WB O'Reilly.)
12. Riley D: Contemporary homeopathic drug provings, *J Am Inst Homeopath* 84(2):144-148, 1994.
13. Weiland F: The role of drug provings in the homeopathic concept. In Ernst E, Hahn EG (eds): *Homeopathy: a critical appraisal,* Oxford, 1998, Butterworth-Heinemann, pp 63-68.
14. Dantas F, Fisher P: A systematic review of homeopathic pathogenetic trials: methodological aspects and preliminary results from UK and US publications. In *51st Congress of the LHMI,* Seattle, Wash, American Institute of Homeopathy, 1996.
15. Kayne SB: *Homeopathic pharmacy: an introduction and handbook,* ed 1, Edinburgh, 1997, Churchill Livingstone, p 236.
16. Lo SY: Physical properties of water with IE structures, *Mod Physics Lett B* 10(19):921-930, 1996.
17. Lo SY: Anomalous state of ice, *Mod Physics Lett B* 10(19):909-919, 1996.
18. Bonavida B: Induction and regulation of human peripheral blood TH1-TH2 derived cytokines by IE water preparations and synergy with mitogens. In *Proceedings of the first international symposium of the physical, chemical and biological properties of IE clusters,* www.atcg.com/randd/workshop.html, 1997.
19. Sinitsyn A: Effect of IE solutions on enzymes and microbial cells. In *Proceedings of the first international symposium of the physical, chemical and biological properties of IE clusters,* www.atcg.com/randd/workshop.html, 1997.
20. Samal S, Geckeler KE: Unexpected solute aggregation in water on dilution, *Chem Commun,* 2224-2225, 2001.
21. Homeopathic Pharmacopoeia Convention of the United States: *Homeopathic pharmacopoeia convention of the United States—abstracts,* Washington, 1995, HPCUS.
22. United States Food and Drug Administration: *Compliance policy guide 7132.15: conditions under which homeopathic medicines may be marketed,* Washington, 1988, USFDA.
23. Bohmer D, Abrus P: Behandlung von sproverlletzungen mit Traumeel-Salbe kontrollierte doppelblndstudie, *Biologische Medzin* 21:260-268, 1992.

24. Borneman JP: Homeopathy in the United States and Canada: an analysis of the self-medication market for homeopathic drugs. In *Improving the success of homeopathy,* 1997.

25. Goldstein MS, Glick D: Use of and satisfaction with homeopathy in a patient population, *Altern Ther* 4(2): 60-65, 1998.

26. Hahnemann S: *Materia medica pura, vol 1,* New Delhi, India, 1980, B Jain, p 627.

27. Coulter HL: *Divided legacy, vol 3,* Washington, 1973, McGrath.

28. Allen TF: *The encyclopedia of pure materia medica,* Indian ed, New Delhi, India, 1982, B Jain.

29. Hering C: *The guiding symptoms of our materia medica,* Indian ed, New Delhi, India, 1972, B Jain.

30. Kent JT: *Lectures on homeopathic philosophy,* ed 2, Chicago, 1929, Ehrhart & Karl, p 288.

31. Kent JT: *Lectures on homeopathic materia medica,* ed 4, Philadelphia, 1932, Boericke & Tafel, p 991.

32. Kent JT: *Kent's general repertory,* Ottilien, Germany, 1994, Barthel & Barthel, p 1172. (Edited by J Klonzi.)

33. Rothstein WG: *American physicians in the 19th century,* Baltimore, 1984, Johns Hopkins University Press.

34. Ernst E, Kaptchuk T: Revisiting homeopathy, *Arch Int Med* 156:2162-2164, 1996.

35. Ullman D: *Discovering homeopathy,* Berkeley, Calif, 1991, North Atlantic Books.

36. Eisenberg DM et al: Trends in alternative medicine use in the United States, 1990-1997, *JAMA* 280(18):1569-1575, 1998.

37. Vithoulkas G: *The science of homeopathy,* New York, 1980, Grove Press.

38. Bellavite P, Signorini A: *Homeopathy: a frontier in medical science,* Berkeley, Calif, 1995, North Atlantic Books.

39. Ernst E, Hahn EG: *Homeopathy: a critical appraisal,* Woburn, Mass, 1998, Butterworth-Heinemann, p 240.

40. Berman BM et al: Primary care physicians and complementary-alternative medicine: training, attitudes, and practice patterns, *J Am Board Fam Pract* 11(4):272-282, 1998.

41. Endler PC, Schulte J (eds): *Ultra high dilutions: physiology and physics,* Dordrecht, The Netherlands, 1994, Kluwer Academic Publishers, p 268.

42. Bastide M (ed): *Signals and images, vol 1,* Dordrecht, The Netherlands, 1997, Kluwer Academic Press, p 299.

43. Linde K et al: Critical review and meta-analysis of serially agitated dilutions in experimental toxicology, *Hum Exp Toxicol* 13(7):481-492, 1994.

44. Jonas WB: Do homeopathic nosodes protect against infection? an experimental test, *Alternat Ther* 5(5):36-40, 1999.

45. Davenas E, Beauvais F, Amara J: Human basophile degranulation triggered by very dilute antiserum against IgE, *Nature* 333:816-818, 1988.

46. When to believe the unbelievable, *Nature* 333:857, 1988 (editorial).

47. Belon P et al: Inhibition of human basophile degranulation by successive histamine dilutions: results of a European multi-centre trial, *Inflamm Res* 48(13):17-18, 1999.

48. Belon P et al: *Inhibition of human basophile degranulation by successive histamine dilutions, Inflammation Res* 48(Suppl 1): S17-S18, 1999.

49. Anagnostatos GS et al: *Theory and experiments on high dilutions, in homeopathy: a critical appraisal,* Oxford, 1998, Butterworth-Heinemann, p 240. (Edited by E Ernst and EG Hahn.)

50. Jacobs J et al: Treatment of acute diarrhea with homeopathic medicine: a randomized clinical trial in Nicaragua, *Pediatrics* 93(5):719-725, 1994.

51. Kleijnen J, Knipschild P, ter Riet G: Clinical trials of homeopathy, *BMJ* 302:316-323, 1991.

52. Reilly D et al: Is evidence for homeopathy reproducible? a controlled trial of allergic asthma, *Lancet* 344:1601-1606, 1994.

53. Reilly DT et al: Is homeopathy a placebo response? Controlled trial of homeopathic potency, with pollen in hay fever as model, *Lancet* 2:881-885, 1986.

54. Taylor MA et al: Randomized controlled trial of homeopathy versus placebo in perennial allergic rhinitis with overview of four trial series, *BMJ* 321:19-26, 2000.

55. Jacobs J, Springer DA, Crothers D: Homeopathic treatment of otitis media in children: a randomized, placebo-controlled trial, *Pediatr Infect Dis J* 20(2):177-183, 2001.

56. Barnett ED et al: Challenges of evaluating treatment of acute otitis media, *Pediatr Infect Dis J* 19(4):273-275, 2000.

57. Friese KH et al: The homeopathic treatment of otitis media in children: comparison with conventional therapy, *Int J Clin Pharmacol Ther* 35(7):296-301, 1997.

58. Linde K et al: Are the clinical effects of homeopathy placebo effects? a meta-analysis of placebo controlled trials, *Lancet* 350:834-843, 1997.

59. Veneno de serpiente, *Homeopathic Record* 2:126, 1935.

60. Ernst E, Pittler MH: Efficacy of arnica: a systematic review of placebo-controlled clinical trials, *Arch Surg* 133:1187-1190, 1998.

61. Warkentin DK, van Zandvoort R: *MacRepertory: the complete repertory,* San Anselmo, Calif, Kent Homeopathic Associates, 1992.

62. Morrison R: *Desktop guide to keynotes and confirmatory symptoms,* Albany, Calif, 1993, Hahnemann Clinic Press.

## Suggested Readings

Bellavite P, Signorini A: *Homeopathy: a frontier in medical science,* Berkeley, Calif, 1995, North Atlantic Books. (Translated by A Steele.)

Castro M: *The complete book of homeopathy,* New York, 1990, St. Martins Press.

Hahnemann S: *Organon of the medical art,* Redmond, Wash, 1996, Birdcage Books, p 158. (Edited by WB O'Reilly.)

Jonas W, Jacobs J: *Healing with homeopathy: the complete guide,* New York, 1996, Warner Books.

Kayne SB: *Homeopathic pharmacy: an introduction and handbook,* Edinburgh, 1997, Churchill Livingstone.

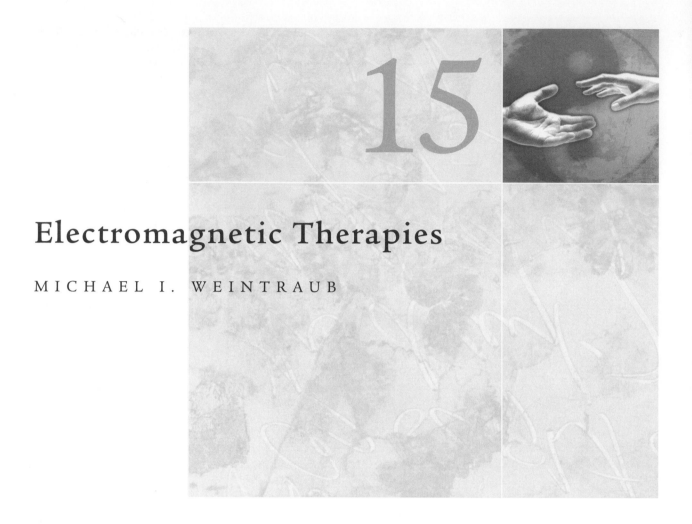

# Electromagnetic Therapies

MICHAEL I. WEINTRAUB

Light, magnets, and electricity—all forms of electromagnetic energy—have been used for thousands of years to improve health. This chapter discusses the history of the various types of electromagnetic therapy and the application of these therapies in rehabilitation today. In particular this chapter focuses on the therapeutic use of lasers, magnetic field therapy (both pulsed and static) and electrical stimulation via transcutaneous electrical nerve stimulation (TENS).

## PHOTOTHERAPY

Phototherapy (light applied for healing) has been used for thousands of years. The ancient Greeks believed that the sun was the center of the universe and

that exposure to sunlight induced strength and health. Over the ensuing centuries, the antiseptic and disinfectant properties of sunlight were used to combat the plague, tuberculosis, and other illnesses. In the twentieth century, light was used to treat psoriasis, hyperbilirubinemia, and seasonal affective disorder. It is now recognized that light energy produces biochemical and energetic reactions that are clinically useful.

## Definitions

Light consists of photonic energy bundles from one part of the electromagnetic spectrum. This spectrum is divided by specific wavelengths. The visible spectrum wavelengths range from 400 to 700 nm.

The smaller the wavelength, the greater the ability of this energy form to penetrate biological tissues. Thus x-rays, gamma rays, and ultraviolet rays have small wavelengths and are medically useful because of their ability to penetrate the body and interact with internal organs. Longer wavelengths such as infrared, short-wave diathermy, and microwaves have different characteristics but also are medically useful, largely because they affect the surface of the body.

The term *laser* is an acronym for *light amplification by stimulated emission of radiation*. It is an artificial light that has the specific characteristics of monochromaticity (one wavelength), collimation (a single beam), and coherence (all waves in the same phase). Thus the beams created consist of light with a specific frequency that is nondivergent, and all waves are parallel and in phase. Albert Einstein developed the basic theories in 1917, but the first instrument was not developed until the 1960s.

The power delivered by any of these radiation sources is measured in units of joules (J) or watts (W). The amount of radiation actually absorbed is measured in $W/cm^2$ or J.

## Historical Development of Phototherapy

Initial work with cold (nonthermal) laser therapy began in Hungary and Eastern Europe in the 1960s.[1] These studies were poorly controlled, using varying time, strengths, and types of lasers. However, the early reports demonstrated that low-power (<1 mW) nonthermal laser irradiation could alter cellular function (e.g., hair growth, bacterial growth, accelerated wound healing).[2,3] This was independent of heating. This positive laboratory evidence of efficacy was quickly extrapolated to human testing so that in Europe and Asia, laser therapy is currently used in 30% to 40% of sports clinics and physical therapy and dental facilities to promote wound healing and the reduction of pain and inflammation and to enhance recovery from soft tissue injuries.[4,5] While it has received widespread acceptance in Europe, the use of laser therapy has only recently been approved (2002). The U.S. Food and Drug Administration (FDA) accepts the gallium aluminum arsenide laser (830 nm) as a treatment for carpal tunnel syndrome and pain.

## Thermal Surgical Lasers

When light is directed onto an object, it can be reflected, scattered, transmitted, or absorbed. Every object has optic properties that determine the effectiveness of light and the subsequent reaction. For example, mid-infrared and far infrared lasers such as $CO_2$ and holmium or yttrium-aluminum garnet (YAG) are primarily absorbed by water in tissues. Thus absorption of the infrared light energy converts to heat, which leads to local vaporization of tissue. This as use in surgical oncology and in other surgical disciplines. Near infrared and visible light lasers, such as neodymium (Nd):YAG and argon, are poorly absorbed by water but are rapidly absorbed by pigments such as hemoglobin and melanin. These high-energy thermal lasers were found to be useful in surgery, and after appropriate human testing they were approved by the FDA.

## COLD LASER THERAPY

Cold laser therapy, or low-level light therapy (LLLT), is a safe, nonthermal therapy that uses a variety of lasers. The most popular include helium-neon (694 nm), which has a direct penetration of 0.8 mm and an indirect penetration and absorption up to 10 to 15 mm, and gallium aluminum arsenide (GaAlAs) (830 nm), which has a longer wavelength and a deeper penetration of up to 5 cm. In practice, these visible and infrared lasers have powers of 30 to 90 mW and deliver from 1 to $9 J/cm^2$ to treatment sites. Commercial laser pointers primarily use He-Ne wavelengths of 632 nm, which is in the visible spectrum. However, the longer wavelengths of GaAlAs are invisible and require a filter to warn individuals that they are in use.

Karu[6,7] demonstrated experimentally that $0.01 J/cm^2$ can alter cellular processes, but what is the optimal dosage for achieving a biological effect in humans? Basford et al[8] were able to reduce sensory and motor distal latency of median nerves in normal volunteers by a statistically significant amount in a double-blinded protocol using 1 J of energy. This suggests that human nerves can absorb photic light bundles and influence nerve conduction. Weintraub[9] used a similar laser but at higher energy levels of 9 J with significant reduction of sensory nerve action potential (SNAP) and compound muscle action potential (CMAP) distal latencies in carpal tunnel syndrome.

Naeser[10] and Branco,[11] using a He-Ne laser and TENS to stimulate acupuncture points, were able to achieve a statistically significant reduction of sensory latencies and reduction of pain by 92%. Recently Basford et al[12,13] have used a different laser of 1.06 nm Nd:YAG in musculoskeletal tissue for deeper penetration with 12 J, producing success in low back pain and failure in epicondylitis.

## Applications in Rehabilitation

Compelling evidence exists that cold lasers of various types are useful for the treatment of several conditions.

### Neurogenic Pain

The efficacy of laser therapy in various pain syndromes has been investigated by several groups. Walker,[14] in preliminary double-blind studies, demonstrated improvement in seven out of nine patients with trigeminal neuralgia, and two out of five patients with postherpetic neuralgia (shingles) improved. Baxter[5] also believed that laser therapy was helpful for postherpetic neuralgia. Moore et al,[15] in a double-blind crossover trial with 20 patients, using a GaAlAs laser, produced significant pain reduction. Hong et al[16] also validated this study with 60% of patients experiencing relief within 10 minutes. Friedman et al[17] used an intraoral He-Ne laser directed at a specific maxillary alveolar tender point to significantly abort atypical trigeminal pain.

### Carpal Tunnel Syndrome

Basford noted that one J of energy could significantly influence normal median sensory and motor distal latencies.[8] This led Weintraub to treat abnormal median nerves in carpal tunnel syndrome using 9 J of energy along five specific sites with up to 15 treatments (Figure 15-1).[9] Electrophysiological monitoring was done before and after each treatment. There was a 78% success rate resolving previously refractory symptoms for 48 hours. After each treatment, 40% of subjects displayed prolongation of distal latency (i.e., they showed worsening electrophysiologically but they remained clinically asymptomatic). By next visit they were back to baseline and/or improved from the electrophysiological standpoint. About 40% of subjects displayed reduction in the distal latency immediately, and 20% were unresponsive to treatment. Padua[18] has validated

these results and recently a 70% success rate was achieved in double-blind studies supported by Henley Healthcare.[19] This data was submitted to the FDA and felt to be both safe and effective (70%), leading to commercial approval for use in carpal tunnel syndrome and pain.

Naeser[10] and Branco[11] used a combination of red-beam He-Ne Laser and TENS to stimulate nerve and acupuncture points producing 92% benefit.

### Tarsal Tunnel Syndrome/Cubital Tunnel Syndrome/Meralgia Paresthetica

Lasers directed to posterior tibial nerve, ulnar nerve, and lateral anterior femoral cutaneous nerves in a repetitive manner have produced significant pain reduction in at least 50% to 85% of cases. Postoperative scar tissue, pain, and paresthesias also improve about 50%.[20]

### Migraine Headache

Using an intraoral He-Ne laser directed at a specific maxillary alveolar tender point, Weintraub[21] was able to abort acute migraine headaches in 78% of cases compared with sham controls. These findings support the trigeminal vascular theory of migraine with a maxillary V2 provocative site. It is presumed that the laser induces an inhibitory sensory potential in the trigem-

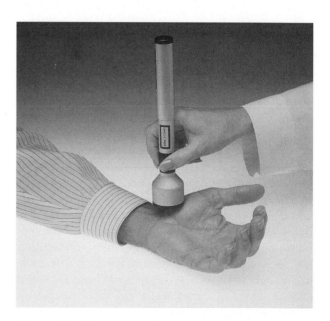

*Figure 15-1* Treatment of abnormal median nerves in carpal tunnel syndrome using 9 J of energy.

inal nerve, which influences thalamic firing. Use of laser acupuncture to the Hegu point, the Governor point, and the lower earlobe (auriculotherapy) has produced variable results.

## Cerebral Palsy/Spasticity

Asagai et al[22] used LLLT on acupressure points in 1,000 babies and children with cerebral palsy. The specific mechanisms of action were not identified, but tonic muscle spasms were significantly reduced.

## Stroke

Using CAT scan analysis, Naeser et al[23] reported improved blood flow in the brain using laser acupuncture.

## Vertigo and Dizziness

Weintraub has achieved benefits by stimulating the Naguien acupressure point with an 830 nm laser. Naeser, in a review of the *Highlights of the Second Congress World Association for Laser Therapy,* reported that Wilden treated inner ear disorders, including vertigo, tinnitus, and hearing loss, with a combination of 630 to 700 nm and 830 nm lasers. The total dose was at least 4,000 J. Daily 1-hour laser treatments to both ears were performed for at least 3 weeks. The lasers were applied to the auditory canal and the mastoid and petrous bone. Wilden stated that he used this approach for more than 9 years with 800 patients and accepted very severe cases; most patients reported improvement only in hearing.

## Arthritis

Rheumatologists in the United States have identified encouraging results in rheumatoid arthritis treatment,[24] and similar results have been reported in the Soviet Union, Eastern Europe, and Japan.[25] Walker[26] reported reduced pain in rheumatoid arthritis after a 10-week course of treatment. Asada et al[25] found 90% improvement in an uncontrolled trial of 170 patients. Despite these generally positive results, Bliddal et al[27] did not see any significant change in symptoms of morning stiffness or joint function. However, there was a slight improvement in pain scale scores. Similar positive results have been reported for osteoarthritis and other pseudoarthritic conditions. Critics have argued, however, that because rheumatoid arthritis is a disease of exacerbation and remission, it is difficult to assess efficacy. Nevertheless, pain relief, whether real or placebo, becomes a blessing to the sufferer. There are no biological markers to judge efficacy in pain re-

lief, only self-reported visual analog scale (VAS) pain scores.

## Soft Tissue Injuries

Soft tissue injuries are extremely common in sports and vehicular accidents. A number of reports document the apparent efficacy of laser therapy in reducing pain associated with sports injuries. These reports initially came from Russia and Eastern Europe and were subsequently confirmed by Morselli[28] and Emmanoulidis.[29] It is notable that in the latter study, improvement was accompanied by a decrease in thermographic readings.

## Tendinopathies

Lateral humeral epicondylitis (tennis elbow) has been studied by numerous groups, including the author's. There has usually been a relatively rapid response to therapy; however, Haker and Lundeberg[30] failed to show any effect with laser acupuncture treatment for tennis elbow. Similarly, a recent study by Basford et al[12] showed YAG laser therapy to be ineffective.

## Spasm and Myofascial Trigger Points

It has been reported that laser application to specific sites over the body can induce pain relief. The existence of these so-called trigger points is difficult to prove because of the absence of biological markers and poor definition of anatomy. A panel at the Institute of Medicine could not confirm the existence of these trigger points.[31] Trigger point identification is controversial and could not be reproduced initially in a 1990 publication by Wolfe on their fibromyalgia study.[31a]

## Radiculitis

Several groups have investigated the efficacy of laser therapy in the treatment of radicular and pseudoradicular pain syndromes. Bieglio[32] and Mizokami[33] have reported positive effects.

## Spinal Cord Injury

Dramatic results in the treatment of spinal cord injury have been reported in uncontrolled clinical trials in France. To view videotapes and MRIs of these patients, see Dr. Albert Bohbot's website at www.perso.infonie.fr/a.bohbot.infoni/english/home.htm.

## Safety

No detrimental effects are produced by low-output, nonthermal lasers, although it is obvious that direct retinal exposure is to be avoided. Pregnancy does not appear to be a contraindication with LLLT, but investigators have been advised to avoid treating pregnant women and individuals with local tumors in the area of treatment. Individuals taking photosensitizing drugs such as tetracycline or who have photosensitive skin should probably avoid this treatment.

## A Case Study

### Carpal Tunnel Syndrome

NH is a 51-year-old right-handed nurse with complaints of numbness and tingling with varying aches and pains for several years in the right first three fingers. The neurological examination revealed a positive Tinel's sign on the right hand without sensory changes. A nerve conduction study confirmed carpal tunnel syndrome with distal motor latency (CMAP) of 8.0 milliseconds (msec), prolongation of F-wave, and marked prolongation of SNAP of 5.8 msec. There was no evidence of denervation. The patient was started with laser therapy over the median nerve, and after one treatment she was able to open a new jar for the first time in over 2 years. Her fingers, however, still tingled and the Tinel's sign persisted. The right CMAP was significantly improved at 5.4 msec; the right SNAP was unable to be evoked. The patient continued to receive laser treatment and by the seventh specific treatment she was almost totally asymptomatic except for a rare episode of numbness and tingling during the day, which would last only a few minutes. There was no nocturnal pain and the right CMAP was noted at 4.7 msec. At her tenth and last treatment she was asymptomatic for over 48 hours. The right CMAP was 5.0 msec. The SNAP was still absent. ❧

The previous case study illustrates how carpal tunnel syndrome can be positively influenced by laser exposure with improvement of nocturnal symptoms, numbness and tingling, and motor strength, as well as improvement in the electrophysiological parameters.

## Summary

In conclusion, although there is a strong suggestion that laser therapy is beneficial for human pain, especially in carpal tunnel syndrome, it is clear that the quality of the studies has been highly variable and that there have been few properly controlled clinical trials. Over the years, research designs show that a variety of wavelengths, power and energy densities, frequencies, and duration of treatments have been employed. Objectives such as determining the optimum dosage for treatment have not yet been achieved. In addition, several publications have reported a lack of benefit from the use of laser therapy. Laboratory investigations of laser-mediated analgesia are sometimes contradictory, and critics have found it difficult to correlate animal pain with the more complex aspects of human pain. Finally, the lack of an obvious pathophysiological mechanism leads to confusion about such factors as the mechanism of action.

I believe that the distal latency of the median nerve, as demonstrated by nerve conduction studies, can serve as the biological marker in future studies. In our study of 800 physiological readings, it became apparent that the nerve itself absorbs light, which then produces a repolarization or hyperpolarization and, ultimately, faster neuronal conduction. The light can evoke a "foreign body response," producing localized edema and slowing of neuronal conduction temporarily, which then appears to marshal the reparative forces of the body and promote healing. It is hoped that future studies will be randomized and placebo controlled with a tight methodological design with regard to wavelength, frequency, and duration of treatment to determine the efficacy of laser therapy for specific conditions in physical medicine.

## MAGNETIC FIELD THERAPY

### Origins and History

Claims of magnetic healing have been traced back more than 2,000 years. The term *magnet* derives from the region of Turkey, known as Magnesia, where a mineral containing a magnetic oxide of iron ($Fe_3O_4$)—magnetite—was common.

Ancient peoples called these Herculean stones, lodestones, or live stones because they were active and meant to lead the way. People began to shape these stones and place them on various parts of the body with an acupuncture orientation to achieve healing. Over the ensuing centuries various theories abounded, but people were fascinated with magnetism and so blended science, quackery, sensationalism, and faddism. The lengthy history of magnetism in medicine is most interesting and controversial and has been described elsewhere.[34-36]

## Definitions

The term *biomagnetics* refers to the field of science that deals with the application of magnetic fields to living tissue. The human body is magnetosensitive and appears to have a threshold for the detection of these forces. Magnetic field strength is measured in gauss or teslas (10,000 gauss = 1 tesla). The earth's magnetic field is rated at 0.5 gauss, whereas a refrigerator magnet's field is 50-100 gauss in strength. Diagnostic MRI systems are usually in the 1-tesla range. These systems generate a time-varying field that easily penetrates the body and, based on appropriate sequencing patterns, can influence hydrogen, phosphate, and sodium ions. With the use of computers, MRI systems are able to generate pictures of tissue signatures with density readings of normal and abnormal tissue coefficients.

## Transcranial Magnetic Stimulation

Transcranial magnetic stimulation (TMS) uses a powerful time-varying magnet that can also be used diagnostically, as well as therapeutically. TMS is a suprathreshold high-intensity stimulation that has been in use since 1985 and has been applied transcranially to the motor cortex and peripheral nerves to stimulate sensory and motor axons. Based on the frequency of stimulation (e.g., 1 Hz vs. 5 Hz), neurons may demonstrate excitatory or inhibitory effects that may be either local or distal. Some therapeutic applications of TMS that are currently under exploration involve patients with multiple sclerosis, epilepsy, amyotrophic lateral sclerosis, ataxia, Parkinson's disease, dystonia, stroke, obsessive-compulsive disorder, and speech disorders. From these data, an improved understanding of brain and peripheral nerve functions is being generated. However, this is a relatively new field and is beyond the scope of this chapter.[37,38]

## Pulsed Electromagnetic Therapy

Pulsed electromagnetic fields (PEMF) is another form of electromagnetic therapy that influences biological systems. The application of electrical impulses has been investigated at the cellular membrane level, and studies have demonstrated ionic flux changes and stimulation of osteoblasts in nonunion fractures.[39,40] The original basis for the trial of this form of therapy was the observation that physical stress on bone causes the appearance of tiny electric currents (piezoelectric potentials) that are thought to be the mechanism by which the physical stresses of bodily movements are transduced into a signal that promotes bone formation. Thus direct electric field stimulation was felt to generate small induced currents (faraday currents) in the highly conductive extracellular fluid, mimicking the piezoelectric potentials. The FDA has approved PEMF for the treatment of bone healing and also incontinence. Interestingly, investigators who were treating a patient's symptomatic knee were impressed with the patient's statements that the weekly classic migraines with aura, which were previously poorly controlled, stopped shortly after initiating PEMF. Sherman et al[41] subsequently directed PEMF to the thigh, producing increased blood flow and significant reduction of headache.

### Pulsed Signal Therapy

As a logical extension of PEMF, which use a direct electrical current, pulsed signal therapy (PST) produces an alternating or changing rectangular magnetic pulse at a lower frequency. This is transmitted as a constantly changing pattern and seems to mimic the body's natural streaming potentials, working in the range of 1 to 20 gauss, with frequency ranges from 10 to 20 Hz. This type of therapy, given as nine 1-hour sessions, has been applied to over 100,000 patients, primarily outside the United States (mostly in Germany). It is safe and has successfully treated the following conditions[39-42]:

1. Osteoporosis
2. Arthritis
3. Carpal tunnel syndrome
4. Tendinitis
5. Fresh bone fractures and stress fractures
6. ACL postoperative repair and rehabilitation
7. Aseptic necrosis
8. Fibromyalgia
9. Sciatica
10. Postpolio syndrome
11. Metatarsalgia
12. Morton's neuroma
13. Atrophy of plantar metatarsal fat pad
14. Plantar fasciitis
15. Acute burns
16. Diabetic neuropathy
17. Migraine
18. Ankylosing spondylitis

19.  Meniscus tears
20.  Dupuytren's contractures
21.  Spinal cord injury

As clinical trials evolve and are developed in the United States, it is anticipated that the FDA will approve this type of treatment for more medical conditions. Suprathreshold, time-varying magnetic devices are accepted by the scientific community and by many physicians as biologically effective. They are also accepted by the FDA for investigational use in conditions such as epilepsy, pain, and Parkinson's disease. Use for the treatment of the previously listed conditions has received government approval in various European countries. Recent work with spinal cord injury patients has shown improvements in expiratory muscle strength and colonic peristalsis with functional magnetic stimulation.[43,44]

## Static Magnetic Fields

This category includes the common magnetic pads that are sold commercially. As a generalization, the scientific community and most physicians are skeptical about the ability of these ubiquitous, weak magnets to provide results similar to those described for pulsed fields. Despite the fact that there is a theoretical rationale, critics have attacked the anecdotal claims and the poorly performed studies without randomized placebo controls. However, one cannot ignore the significant literature and observations with regard to animals and infants with reduced pain, swelling, and ecchymosis that cannot be attributed to placebo.

The time is ripe to aggressively design studies in neurology and rehabilitative medicine that have valid and treatable parameters for diseases that have a known natural history. While the scientific method cannot be abandoned, researchers cannot be held hostage to a rigid demand for evidence of objective cellular changes or the presence of a biological marker when they may not be obtainable.

## Types of Permanent Magnet Designs

Permanent magnets are composed of different materials than those in the originally described lodestones. In addition to iron, they usually contain the rare earth metal neodymium and the mineral boron, which can be impregnated or combined as a ceramic or neoprene substance. Various commercial shapes and sizes are available, and manufacturers have claimed that combining several metals, such as gold, silver, copper or copper-zinc, nickel, and aluminum, can create an augmented resonance characteristic known as the *polarity agent effect*. Claims of increased clinical benefit, however, have not been proven.

It is important to recognize that all magnets are *not* equal with regard to strength, penetration, gradient, or design. The latter has been felt by many experts to be the most significant factor-producing efficacy.

In the unipolar design, only one magnetic pole surface, north or south, is applied to the body. It has been suggested that this design is more likely than other designs to activate the parasympathetic system.[45]

Philpott[46] believes that the negative magnetic field is equivalent to the earth's North Pole and the positive magnetic field is equivalent to the earth's South Pole. He claims that a negative energy field fights infection, improves mood, and increases cellular oxygenation whereas a positive magnetic field overstimulates biological systems to create an opposing effect. He categorically states that most human illness, including seizures, infections, and toxic states including psychopathology, are driven by positive magnetic energy, or overstimulation. Critics have argued about the lack of deep magnetic field penetration in his product design and the commercialization of his products, which makes his conclusions somewhat suspect.

Bipolar magnets have the north and south poles adjacent to each other on the same magnetic surface, and critics have stated that this leads to a cancellation effect and a lack of significant penetration. Nevertheless, Vallbona and Hazelwood[47] performed a placebo-controlled trial in postpolio syndrome with significant pain relief. Responses occurred within 1 hour with significant distal effects and placebo effects. Recently, however, Collacott et al[48] reported their negative experience with low back pain symptoms using bipolar devices.

The triangular or multipolar design consists of patterned arrays of magnetic fields shaped like isosceles triangles. Each pole is positioned contiguously to another identically shaped pole of opposite polarity. Strength is usually 300 to 600 gauss. It has been stated that this pattern optimally affects sensory nerves (pain afferents) because the sensory neurons are randomly oriented. The angular arrangement of alternating poles thus becomes an important factor because parallel flux lines predominate and induce a steeper field gradient of penetration. MacLean et al[49] describe an enhanced blockade of sensory neuron action potentials using this design compared with a unipolar design. Weintraub[50-52] performed two provocative pilot studies using this magnetic design for the treatment of neuropathic pain from diabetic peripheral neuropathy and peripheral neuropathy from other causes. Striking results occurred, with reduction of burning, numbness, and tingling. Subsequently, a nationwide, randomized placebo-controlled study of patients with Stage II/III diabetic peripheral neuropathy who continuously applied 450-gauss magnetic footpads for 4 months has been completed with statistical reduction of numbness, tingling, and burning (neuropathic pain) and improved quality of life scores.[58] These findings are provocative because benefits were not due to placebo effects, and this condition is usually refractive to treatment.

The first case study that follows demonstrates significant improvement in neuropathic pain in a Charcot foot with the constant wearing of magnetic foot devices. The next case study demonstrates improvement in long-standing symptoms of diabetic peripheral neuropathy with loss of autonomic functions.

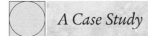 *A Case Study*

*Diabetic Peripheral Neuropathy*

WP is a 63-year-old male with diabetes mellitus for 24 years. Six months before evaluation, he developed a right Charcot foot with severe right foot pain, grade 5 to 6 (VAS = 0 to 10). He also was impotent with a history of hypertension. His examination revealed an awkward gait with pain in the right foot and a dorsiflexed posture to the right extensor hallucis longus (EHL). There was foot sensitivity on the right with hypalgesia over the right foot to pinprick, but vibration, position, and temperature were intact. The ankle jerks were absent. It was felt that he displayed aspects of a motor neuropathy and sensorimotor polyradiculopathy secondary to diabetes. On February 23, 2000, an electromyogram (EMG) confirmed axonal damage in the right foot and demyelinating damage in the left foot. The current perception threshold (CPT) (Neurometer) reading was right = 9.9, indicating severe hypoesthetic condition, and left = 7.0, a mild hypoesthetic condition. At that time, he was provided with magnetic foot devices that he wore for 24-hour periods. On March 20 he returned with a dramatic change in his level of pain. There was no burning, numbness, or tingling, and the examination revealed only hypalgesia over the

right foot. On April 24 he returned and indicated that there was improved feeling in the foot. On May 30 the improvement continued, but the examination again demonstrated hypalgesia to pin and now vibration was reduced bilaterally. A repeat CPT study revealed no significant change. On September 30 he had a myocardial infarction and stopped wearing the devices for 3 days. The right foot symptoms returned. His activity level had been markedly increased until that period. At his February 2001 follow-up examination, he had a low-grade discomfort with a definite improvement of the symptoms that he had 1 year earlier. There was also a return of symptoms when the device was stopped for 72 hours. The electrophysiological test did not improve during this course of treatment. ∽

 *A Case Study*

*Diabetic Peripheral Neuropathy*

RS is a 71-year-old man with a 20-year history of insulin-dependent diabetes mellitus (IDDM) with numbness and tingling of the feet and ankles and loss of erectile function. The examination revealed absent deep tendon reflexes and hypalgesia to pin and vibration in the feet. On January 28, 2000, an EMG confirmed axonal and demyelinating changes in the feet. Magnets were provided and, within 6 weeks, he experienced less foot pain and was not limping. By April 11 there was no pain in the arch of the left foot and he was not limping as before. He also described that the foot was now sweating intermittently, which had been absent for several years. There was no numbness, tingling, or burning and the feet began to feel normal, but there was a subjective "heaviness." The examination revealed better pinprick appreciation, but vibration and the reflexes were absent. A CPT (Neurometer) reading on April 11 was normal. Within 6 weeks he developed improvement in neuropathic pain and within 3 months experienced the return of some sweating. ∽

Weintraub and Cole[59] have used multipolar magnets for the treatment of carpal tunnel syndrome, producing a 57% reduction in pain and improved condition, although the underlying pathophysiology persisted. The proposed mechanism of benefit, similar to that in the Diabetic Peripheral Neuropathy Study, is that the C-fiber firing pattern is modulated. Weintraub and Steinberg[60] recently completed a randomized placebo-controlled study of failed back syndrome to determine if simultaneous wearing of back and foot devices reduces pain compared with placebo. This was not demonstrated.

Up to this point there have been no safety issues. However, it is recommended that patients who are pregnant or who wear pacemakers, cochlear implants, or insulin pumps avoid these devices. It should be noted that these are weak magnets and their successful application requires constant and close proximity to symptomatic sites because the magnetic field gradient falls off with distance.

## Potential Applications

The placement of magnets along acupuncture lines and inflamed areas has the potential to activate the musculoskeletal system. These tissues are well known to transmit electrical stimuli. Adey[53] believes that free radical production, especially nitric oxide (NO), can be significantly affected by weak magnetic fields (10 to 100 gauss). Other potential applications include the following.

1. Intraoral application for dental pain
2. Cervical and lumbar strains
3. Tendon strains
4. Epicondylitis
5. Swelling
6. Plantar fasciitis
7. Heel spurs
8. Diabetic peripheral neuropathy
9. Foot ulcers
10. Headaches

## Summary

Although magnetic therapy is currently creating great enthusiasm in the arena of alternative medicine, it is important to recognize that the current scientific literature must be considered anecdotal at best. Until large cohort studies with randomized, placebo-controlled designs are performed in patient groups suffering from homogenous disorders, there will continue to be speculation as to the efficacy of magnetic therapy. Weintraub's nationwide study[58] needs to be reproduced to gain more acceptance. Currently, the major skeptic of magnetic therapy is the FDA. No indications have been accepted by the FDA for the use of permanent magnets, and those who sell these devices are allowed only to indicate that they "may relieve pain" or "may feel good." Consumers must be cautious about these alleged claims. Progress will come only with appropriate funding for well-designed studies. Thus magnetic therapy with static magnets is still in the formative stages, and any serious student of neurology and rehabilitation medicine must remain skeptical until the definitive studies are published.

## ELECTRICAL THERAPIES

### Transcutaneous Electrical Nerve Stimulation

In 1965, Melzack and Wall[54] proposed a new theory to explain pain. In this famous "gate control theory," they postulated that selective stimulation of large diameter afferent nerve fibers could close a "pain gate" at the level of the substantia gelatinosa in the spinal cord and thereby inhibit the effect of the firing small-diameter fibers. This explanation served as the catalyst for the development of peripheral TENS units as a means of counterstimulation to alter pain perceptions. Initially, TENS was designed to serve as a screen for patients scheduled for spinal cord stimulation, although this predictive benefit has never been proven or documented. Commercial TENS units offer three different pulse frequencies, i.e., low (1 to 4 Hz), high (50 to 120 Hz), and burst (2 Hz), with the ability to adjust amplitude with timing. The use of different low- and high-pulsed frequencies and varying electrode placements by physicians and therapists has led to many claims in acute and chronic pain conditions.[55-57]

Despite its widespread use in rehabilitative and pain medicine clinics and its theoretical rationale, a great deal of controversy surrounds the merits of TENS. For example, critics indicate that the early studies lacked controls and randomization and used various frequencies, amplitudes, and electrode placements in cohorts that were not homogeneous. Thus the results were to be considered anecdotal at best. In addition, there were also complaints of possible fraudulent marketing techniques. When Deyo et al[55-56] performed a rigorous randomized placebo-control trial in chronic low back pain, they noted that there was no firm scientific evidence that TENS was more effective than placebo. Electrode positioning thus appears to be more art than science. Some advocates feel that the high frequency stimulus (up to 100 pulses per second) with electrodes placed in the center of the painful area should be preceded by induction of paresthesia in this area. If this is unsuccessful, treatment can then switch to low- or burst-pulsed frequencies, which are claimed to release endorphins, producing pain relief. Thus the optimal frequency, duration, and electrode placement has not yet been rigorously validated in randomized placebo-control trials.

While it is theoretically appealing that peripheral stimulation of afferent large A-fibers by TENS can reduce nociceptive pain by closing the gate, the literature demonstrates methodological flaws and shortcomings and also considers the role of placebo paramount. The use of TENS is at an all-time high and is considered safe.

## Summary

Electromagnetic therapies promise to play a larger role in the rehabilitation of the future, but adequate studies are only now coming to fruition.

## References

1. Mester E: The use of the laser beam in therapy, *Orv Hetil* 107:1012-1016, 1966 (Hungarian).
2. Mester E, Spiry T, Szende B, et al: Effect of laser rays on wound healing, *Am J Surg* 122:532-535, 1971.
3. Mester E, Toth N, Mester A: The biostimulative effect of laser beam, *Laser Basic Biomed Res* 22:4-7, 1982.
4. Gerschman JA, Ruben J, Gebart-Eaglemont J: Low level laser therapy for dentinal tooth hypersensitivity, *Aust Dent J* 39:353-357, 1994.
5. Baxter GD: *Therapeutic Lasers: theory & practice,* Edinburgh, 1994, Churchill Livingstone.
6. Karu TI: Photobiological fundamentals of low power laser therapy, *IEEE J Quantum Electron QE* 23:1703-1717, 1987.
7. Karu TI: Effects of visible radiation on cultured cells (review), *Photochem Photobiol* 52:1089-1098, 1990.
8. Basford JR, Hallman HO, Matsumoto JY, et al: Effects of 830 nm continuous wave laser diode irradiation on median nerve function in normal subjects, *Lasers Surg Med* 13:597-604, 1993.
9. Weintraub MI: Non-invasive laser neurolysis in carpal tunnel syndrome, *Muscle Nerve* 20:1029-1031, 1997.
10. Naeser MA, Hahn KK, Lieberman B: Real vs sham laser acupuncture and microamps TENS to treat carpal tunnel syndrome and worksite wrist pain: pilot study, *Lasers Surg Med* (suppl 8):7, 1996.
11. Branco K, Naeser MA: Carpal tunnel syndrome: clinical outcome after low-level laser acupuncture, microamps transcutaneous electrical nerve stimulation and other alternative therapies—an open protocol study, *J Alt Comp Med* 5:5-26, 1999.
12. Basford JR, Sheffield CS, Harmsen WS: Laser therapy: a randomized, controlled trial of the effects of low-intensity Nd—YAG laser irradiation on musculoskeletal back pain, *Arch Phys Med Rehabil* 80:647-652, 1999.
13. Basford JR, Sheffield CS, Cieslak KR: Laser therapy: a randomized, controlled trial of the effects of low intensity Nd:YAG laser irradiation on lateral epicondylitis, *Arch Med Rehab* 81:1504-1510, 2000.
14. Walker JB: Relief from chronic pain by low-power laser irradiation, *Neurosci Lett* 43:339-344, 1983.
15. Moore KC, Hira N, Kumar PS, et al: A double-blind crossover trial of low level laser therapy in the treatment of post-herpetic neuralgia, *Lasers Med Sci* 6:301, 1988 (abstract).
16. Hong JN, Kim TH, Lim SD: Clinical trial of low reactive level laser therapy in 20 patients with post-herpetic neuralgia, *Laser Ther* 2:167-170, 1990.
17. Friedman MH, Weintraub MI, Forman S: Atypical facial pain: a localized maxillary nerve disorder? *Amer J Pain Mgt* 4:149-152, 1994.
18. Padua L: Laser biostimulation: a reply, *Muscle Nerve* 21:1232-1233, 1998.
19. Henley Healthcare: Personal communication.
20. Weintraub MI: Laser stimulation in neurologic disease. In Weintraub MI: *Alternative and complementary treatment in neurologic illness,* New York, 2001, Churchill Livingstone, pp 268-277.
21. Weintraub MI: Migraine: a maxillary nerve disorder? A novel therapy—preliminary results, *Am J Pain Manage* 6:77-82, 1996.
22. Asagi Y, Kanai H, Miura Y, et al: Application of low reactive-level laser therapy (LLLT) in the functional training of cerebral palsy patients, *Laser Ther* 6:195-202, 1994.
23. Naeser MA, Alexander MP, Stiassny-Eder D, et al: Laser acupuncture in the treatment of paralysis in stroke patients: a CT scan lesion site study, *Am J Acupunct* 23:13-28, 1995.
24. Goldman JA, Chiapella J, Caser H, et al: Laser therapy of rheumatoid arthritis, *Lasers Surg Med* 1:93-101, 1980.
25. Asada K, Yutani Y, Shimazu A: Diode laser therapy for rheumatoid arthritis: a clinical evaluation of 102 joints treated with low reactive laser therapy (LLLT), *Laser Ther* 1:147-151, 1989.
26. Walker JB, Akhanjee LK, Cooney MM: Laser therapy for pain of rheumatoid arthritis, *Lasers Surg Med* 6:171, 1986.
27. Bliddal H, Hellesen C, Ditleusen P, et al: Soft laser therapy in rheumatoid arthritis, *Scand J Rheumatol* 16:225-228, 1987.

28. Morselli M, Soragni O, Lupia BP: Effects of very low energy-density treatment of joint pain by $CO_2$ lasers, *Lasers Surg Med* 5:149, 1985.

29. Emmanoulidis O, Diamantopoulos C: CW IR low power laser applications significantly accelerate chronic pain relief rehabilitation of professional athletes: a double blind study, *Lasers Surg Med* 6:173, 1986.

30. Haker E, Lundeberg T: Laser treatment applied to acupuncture points in lateral humeral epicondylalgia: a double-blind study, *Pain* 43(2):243-248, 1990.

31. Osterweiss M, Kleinman A, Mechanic D (eds): *Pain and disability: clinical, behavioral and public policy perspectives,* Washington, DC, National Academy Press, 1987.

31a. Wolfe F: Fibromyalgia, *Rheum Dis Clin North Am* 16(3): 681-698, 1990.

32. Bieglio C, Bisschop C: Physical treatment for radicular pain with low-power laser stimulation, *Lasers Surg Med* 6:173, 1986.

33. Mizokami T, Yoshii N, Ushikubo Y, et al: Effect of diode laser for pain: a clinical study on different pain types, *Laser Ther* 2:171-174, 1990.

34. Mourino MR: From Thales to Lauterbur, or from the lodestone to MR imaging: magnetism & medicine, *Radiology* 180:593-612, 1991.

35. Macklis RM: Magnetic healing, quackery and the debate about the health effects of electromagnetic fields, *Ann Int Med* 118:376-383, 1993.

36. Armstrong D, Armstrong EM: *The great American medicine show,* New York, 1991, Prentiss Hall.

37. George MS, Wasserman EM, Williams WA, et al: Daily repetitive transcranial magnetic stimulation (rTMS) improves mood in depression, *Neuro Rep* 6:1853-1856, 1995.

38. Pascual-Leone A et al: Study and modulation of human cortical excitability with transcranial magnetic stimulation, *J Clin Neurophysiol* 15:333-343, 1998.

39. Connolly J, Ortiz J, Price R, et al: The effect of electrical stimulation on the biophysical properties of fracture healing, *Ann NY Acad Sci* 238:519-528, 1974.

40. Farndale R, Murray J: Pulsed electromagnetic fields promote collagen production in bone marrow fibroblasts via athermal mechanisms, *Calcif Tissue Int* 37:178-182, 1985.

41. Sherman RA, Robson L, Marden LA: Initial exploration of pulsing electromagnetic fields for treatment of migraine, *Headache* 38:208-213, 1998.

42. Trock DH, Bollet AJ, Markoll R: The effect of pulsed electromagnetic fields in the treatment of osteoarthritis of the knee and cervical spine: report of randomized, double blind, placebo controlled trials, *J Rhematol* 21: 1903-1911, 1994.

43. Liu V et al: Functional magnetic stimulation for conditioning of expiratory muscles in patients with SCI, *Arch Phys Med Rehabil* 82:162-166, 2001.

44. Liu V et al: Functional magnetic stimulation of the colon in persons with SCI, *Arch PM&R* 82:167-173, 2001.

45. Hannemann H: *Magnetic therapy: balancing your body's energy flow for self-healing,* New York, Sterling, 1990.

46. Philpott WA, Taplin SL: *Biomagnetic handbook,* Oklahoma City, Okla, 1992, Envirotech Production.

47. Vallbona C, Hazelwood CFD, Jurida G: Response of pain to static magnetic fields in post-polio patients: a double-blind pilot study, *Arch Phys Med Rehabil* 78:1200-1203, 1997.

48. Collacott EA, Zimmerman T, White DW, et al: Bipolar permanent magnets for the treatment of chronic low back pain: a pilot study, *JAMA* 283:1322-1325, 2000.

49. McLean MJ, Holcomb RR, et al: Blockade of sensory neuron action potentials by a static magnetic field in the 10 mT range, *Bioelectromagnetics* 18:20-32, 1995.

50. Weintraub MI: Chronic submaximal magnetic stimulation in peripheral neuropathy: is there a beneficial therapeutic relationship? Pilot study, *Am J Pain Manage* 8: 9-13, 1998.

51. Weintraub MI: Magnetic biostimulation in painful diabetic peripheral neuropathy: a novel intervention—a randomized double-placebo crossover study, *Am J Pain Manage* 9:8-17, 1999.

52. Weintraub MI: Magnetic biostimulation in neurologic illness. In Weintraub MI (ed): *Alternative and complementary treatment in neurologic illness,* New York, 2001, Churchill Livingstone.

53. Adey WR: *Resonance and other interactions of electromagnetic fields with living systems,* Oxford, Oxford University Press, 1992.

54. Melzack R, Wall PD: Pain mechanisms: a new theory, *Science* 150:971-979, 1965.

55. Deyo RA, Walsh E, Martin DC, et al: A controlled trial of transcutaneous electrical nerve stimulation (TENS) in low back pain, *N Engl J Med* 322:1627-1634, 1990.

56. Letters to the editor: TENS for chronic low back pain, *N Engl J Med* 323:1423-1425, 1990.

57. Walsh DM, Lowe AS, McCormack K, et al: Transcutaneous electrical stimulation: effect on peripheral nerve conduction, mechanical pain threshold and tactile threshold in humans, *Arch Phys Med Rehabil* 79:1051-1058, 1998.

58. Weintraub MI, Wolfe GI, Barohn RA, et al: Magnetic field therapy for symptomatic diabetic neuropathy: a randomized, double-blind, placebo-controlled trial. (Submitted for publication.)

59. Weintraub MI, Cole SP: Neuromagnetic treatment of pain in refractory carpal tunnel syndrome: an electrophysiological and placebo analysis, *J Back Musculoskel Rehab* April 2002.

60. Weintraub MI, Steinberg R, Cole SP: Role of constant static magnetic stimulation in failed back syndrome: a randomized placebo-controlled trial. (In preparation.)

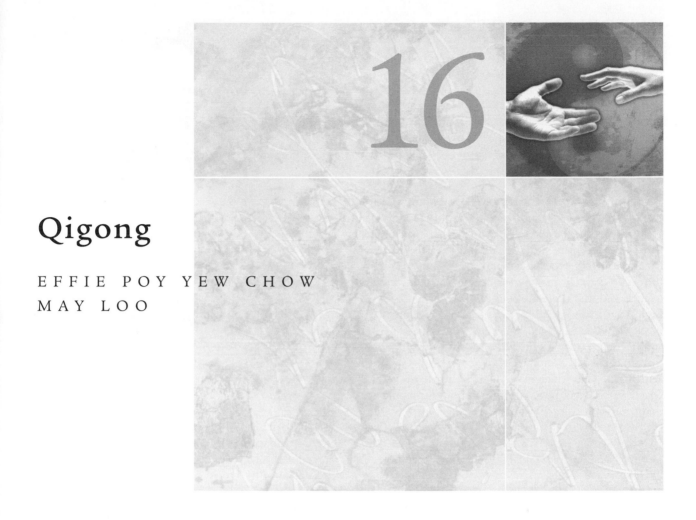

# Qigong

EFFIE POY YEW CHOW
MAY LOO

*Look, it cannot be seen*
*It is beyond form*
*Listen, it cannot be heard*
*It is beyond sound*
*Grasp, it cannot be held*
*It is intangible*
*It is called indefinable and beyond imagination*
*Stand before it and there is no beginning*
*Follow it and there is no end*
*Stay with the ancient Tao, move with the present.*

TAO TE CHING

## HISTORICAL ROOTS

We invite the reader to keep an open mind and enjoy the challenge of seeing the human being from a very different theoretical perspective, that which seems to be unbelievable and difficult to understand. That which seems to be unscientific, yet has much history and science, one where the word "danger" also means "opportunity." Hopefully this chapter will begin your exciting journey of exploration into the lesser-known and the exotic.

With the above ancient words of wisdom of Tao Te Ching, Dr. Chow and the East West Academy of Healing Arts (EWAHA) applied the principles and practice of Qigong (a part of Traditional Chinese Medicine [TCM]) to elicit remarkable results for rehabilitative conditions where all else has failed. It has been stated that there are over 5,000 styles of Qigong, each having been developed in its own village or town or city in ancient China. Of course, electronic media did not exist then to easily transmit knowledge instantly to all parts of the country or world. The presenting theories (the Laws of the Five Elements, a different way of looking at the human body—integrating body, mind, and spirit with nature, microcosm within a macrocosm, Yin and Yang, the Qi, all to be presented later), are those used in a System known as the *Chow Integrated Healing System and Qigong,* which is responsible for the outcomes of the cases presented in the beginning of this chapter. These cases are only a few of the many thousands of EWAHA clients and students. They all have tried unsuccessfully all means of Western medical treatment and other alternative therapies. Fortunately, everyone who wishes to can learn the methods of Chow Integrated Healing System and Qigong to help oneself and others.

Qigong is an ancient system of harmonious integration of the human body with the Universe. It is an exercise that maintains and strengthens health, prevents and treats diseases, impedes aging, and prolongs life.

Qigong is derived from two Chinese words, Qi and Gong. *Qi* has no English equivalent, but it can be roughly translated as "vital energy." The Chinese character consists of two radicals or components: the top radical signifies air or vapor, and the lower radical is the word for rice (Figure 16-1). These represent the two sources of Qi: the air we breathe and the food we eat. *Gong* means discipline, work, or skill. *Qigong* can roughly be defined as "energy work" and "breath skills."

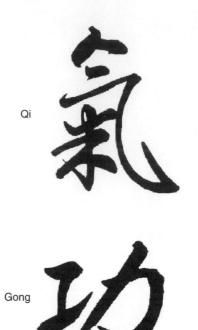

Qi

Gong

*Figure 16-1* Chinese characters for Qi and gong.

Historically, Qigong has a long tradition that predates acupuncture and the martial arts. It can be traced verbally as far back as 10,000 years. Written records about Qigong date back 4,000 years. In the sixth century BC, a contemporary of the Taoist philosopher Laozi wrote, "Inhaling and exhaling helps to rid one of the stale and take in the fresh. Moving as a bear and stretching as a bird can result in longevity." In the second century AD, the famous physician Hua Tuo invented a series of Qigong routines called the "Frolics of Five Animals" (Wuqinxi), which imitate the movements of tiger, deer, bear, monkey, and bird. These animal-like Qigong exercises and their variations are practiced widely today. Fortunately, over 100 ancient books have survived to modern times, providing a long history of Qigong.

Many Qigong exercises have been developed over the past 3,000 to 4,000 years, and new ones continue to be unearthed. Fortunately, for general health purposes, only a few exercises need to be learned. There are both moving and stationary exercises that can be done in various positions: lying, sitting, or standing. There are Qigong exercises that can develop "internal Qi" and "external Qi."[2]

# THE FLOW OF QI

The philosophy of Qigong shares these key concepts with Traditional Chinese Medicine:

1. The system of Qi channels, or meridians, that course throughout the body.
2. The principle of Yin-Yang or "dynamic opposites" in the way the body functions.
3. The Five-Element relationship of organ systems.

Qi circulates in the human body within channels called *meridians*. It is also part of blood and moves within blood vessels. It permeates organs and tissues. Qi is therefore the foundation of our being and is behind all of our physiologic functions. Within the meridians, Qi flows in one direction. Health is the harmonious, uninterrupted flow of Qi, and disease ensues when there is disruption of Qi flow. The power of Qigong lies in its ability to restore normal Qi flow. For example, several major Qi channels flow through the neck. Any interruption of the Qi flow can result in a variety of symptoms, ranging from headaches to inability to think clearly. Simple Qigong exercises can resolve headaches and restore mental function.

The homeostasis of Qi flow also balances the dynamic opposites of the human body: the Yin and the Yang. Both Qigong and Chinese medicine view humankind as a small replica of Nature, a microcosm to Nature as the macrocosm. Everything in Nature and within humans can be classified as opposites; for example, night and day, cold and hot, female and male, deficiency and excess. The Yin-Yang opposites are not exclusive of each other, but each is moving along a continuum to be in balance with the opposite so that there is no absolute Yin or Yang, but within Yin there is Yang, and within Yang, there is Yin. The dynamic balance between the opposites keeps all of Nature in equilibrium instead of chaos. The most common manifestation of Yin and Yang in diseases are excess and deficiency states. Qigong can redirect Qi from excess accumulation to areas of Qi deficiency, thereby restoring the body to a healthy balance.

The organs in the human body are grouped as six Yin-Yang couplets, consisting of Yin organs that carry out the physiologic process of production and transformation of Qi and hollow Yang organs that carry out the lesser functions of storage and of transport of Qi. These organs are further classified according to the Five Elements: Fire, Earth, Metal, Water, and Wood. The Elements interact according to the natural laws governing nurturance and destruction, which explains

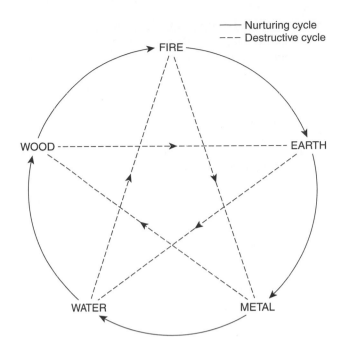

*Figure 16-2* The cycle of the Five Elements.

the progression of healing and disease process in the human body.

The Yin-Yang couples are as follows: Heart-Small Intestine; Kidney-Bladder; Lung-Large Intestine; Spleen/Pancreas-Stomach; Pericardium (Master of the Heart)-Triple Heater (a division of the body into three parts). The meridians of the Yin-Yang organs connect with each other, so that the first point on the Large Intestine channel follows the last point on the Lung channel, and the last point on the Stomach channel connects to the first point on the Spleen channel. Both the Yin and Yang organs in a couplet belong to the same Element, each having numerous physical and metaphoric correspondences, such as emotions, voice, taste, and color preferences. Universally, the Five Elements have symbolic correspondences that connect man with the natural world (Figure 16-2). Each element is the primary nurturer of another element and at the same time is the primary controller or destroyer of another element in a cycle such as the following:

The nurturing cycle operates as each element nurtures the succeeding element. The nurturer is the Mother element to the nurtured, Son element:

- Fire creates the ashes that become Earth.
- Earth stores Metal.

- Metal can be transformed into Water. (This is true for metals being melted down to liquid and for biochemical processes such as the metabolism of glucose [sugar], which gives off water as an end product.)
- Water feeds Wood, as all trees need water to grow.
- Wood provides the substance for Fire.

Within the human body, the Mother organs nurture the Son organs to make sure that they do not become too weak or too deficient:

- Heart (Fire) nurtures Spleen/Pancreas (Earth).
- Spleen/Pancreas (Earth) nurtures Lung (Metal).
- Lung (Metal) nurtures Kidney (Water).
- Kidney (Water) nurtures Liver (Wood).
- Liver (Wood) nurtures Heart (Fire).

The cycle also has a destructive, controlling component, a sort of checks-and-balances system to make sure that no one element becomes too excessive or too strong:

- Fire melts Metal.
- Metal destroys Wood, as when an ax cuts down a tree.
- Wood breaks up Earth, as when a root tears into earth.
- Earth controls Water, as the earth defines the shapes of oceans, lakes, and the direction of flow of rivers.
- Water puts out Fire.

Within the human body, the controlling organ prevents the controlled organ from becoming excessive, which can throw the body into a state of imbalance:

- Heart (Fire) controls Lung (Metal).
- Lung (Metal) controls Liver (Wood).
- Liver (Wood) controls Spleen/Pancreas (Earth).
- Spleen/Pancreas (Earth) controls Kidney (Water).
- Kidney (Water) controls Heart (Fire).

## Organ Function in Qigong

The power of Qigong lies in its ability to direct Qi to a specific organ and meridian, to rectify the deficient and reduce the excess according to the nurturing and destructive sequences of the Five Elements. Of all the organs, the Heart is especially central to Qigong. Chinese medicine regards the Heart as the "Emperor," the irreplaceable organ that rules the body in all aspects of our being: energetic, physical, emotional, and spiritual. Heart governs the movement of blood—it is the vitality of Heart Qi within the blood vessels that moves blood. Heart influences sweat and other body fluids. Our facial complexion reflects the condition of our Heart: rosy cheeks indicate good blood flow and a healthy Heart, whereas a pale complexion indicates anemia, poor blood flow, and an unhealthy Heart.

The Heart opens onto the tongue and therefore influences speech. We are articulate when our Heart is calm, and we have a hard time finding the right words when our Heart is restless. The Heart is at the center of our emotional being, since all emotions eventually affect the heart. The primary emotions that correspond to the Heart are joy and passion.

The most important function of the Heart, however, is being the House for Shen. There is not a precise translation for Shen. It is both the Mind and the Spirit—our eternal, Ethereal Soul. Through the Soul, the Mind extends to thoughts and ideas from the Soul World and connects all beings from eternity. When the Heart is balanced and the Shen or Emperor is properly housed, we can think and articulate clearly. We can appropriately experience joy and passion. When we are at peace within ourselves, we can then connect with one another. The Heart is very vulnerable and can easily become imbalanced by all stresses and emotions. Simple Qigong exercises can specifically and directly bring Heart Qi into balance, which can in turn influence the harmony of Qi flow in all the other organs and meridians. Regular practice of Qigong can maintain health and vitality by preventing further Heart Qi disruption.

Qigong also exerts important influence on all the other Yin organs: Kidney, Liver, Spleen, and Lung. In Chinese, the Kidney is the foundation of life, the root of all organs. The Kidney stores Essence, or Jing, which exerts powerful, global effects that include growth, development, maturation, sexual function, conception, pregnancy, childbirth, and aging. Jing is quickly expended with stress, with aging, and with ejaculation in the male and menstruation in the female. Jing is therefore precious and not easily replaced. The Kidney influences bone growth and is associated with the emotion of fear. Liver Qi can easily become stagnated, especially with stress. The Liver is the "General" who directs smooth and proper Qi movement in all directions. The emotional correspondences with Liver are frustration, irritability, anxiety, and smoldering anger. When the Liver Qi is out of balance, the emotions become exaggerated, and the person feels confused and lost, not knowing which direction to take. Liver also controls tendons and sinews, which are important for movement. The Spleen represents the Earth element and should be designated as Spleen/Pancreas, since it is the major Yin organ for digestion. It transforms food into Qi and transports Qi throughout the body. It influences muscles, so that when there is Spleen Qi deficiency, the person feels weak and tired. The emotions that correspond to the Spleen/Pancreas are empathy and worry. The Lung takes in pure Qi from the air, from Heaven, and gets rid of impure Qi from the body. The pure Qi from the air combines with the Qi from food to form the nourishing Qi that circulates in our bodies. After forming Qi, the Lung then has the important function of governing or overseeing the movement of Qi. The emotion that corresponds to Lung is sadness. Qigong can augment Kidney Qi and Jing, diminish Liver Qi stagnation, and tonify Spleen/Pancreas and Lung.[1,3-4,7,12-13,15-16,19]

## SCIENTIFIC RESEARCH

Qigong first gained scientific validity in 1953, with the establishment of the Shanghai Qigong Research Institute. Since 1982, Qigong research has spread throughout the world.[2] Many Traditional Chinese Medicine hospitals incorporate Qigong in their core curriculum. The National Center of Complementary and Alternative Medicine at the National Institutes of Health has conducted and encourages research in Qigong. However, there is still a paucity of randomized controlled scientific data available.

Current data indicates that Qigong has healing properties and can be integrated and incorporated into the maintenance of health and the management of various medical conditions. Qigong is considered as part of mind-body techniques, which have been found to be efficacious as complementary treatments for musculoskeletal disease and related disorders.[10] Many consider Qigong to be valuable in the care of both ambulatory and nonambulatory patients in physical medicine.[6]

An extensive review of research on mind-body techniques conducted at Stanford University revealed that Qigong and other mind-body techniques were found to be efficacious as complementary and sometimes as stand-alone alternative treatments for cardiovascular disease-related conditions. Studies provided evidence for treatment efficacy, but the need for further controlled research was evident.[11]

One clinical study investigated the changes in blood pressure, heart rate, and respiratory rate before, during, and after a form of Korean Qigong. All the parameters were found to be significantly decreased during Qigong training. The results suggest that Qigong has the potential to physiologically stabilize the cardiovascular system.[9]

The Qigong Institute, a nonprofit organization, developed the Qigong Bibliographic Database in 1994. An extensive review from the Database of approximately 1,300 references dating back to 1986 revealed clinical reports and scientific studies from China, Asia, the United States, and Europe that demonstrate and support the efficacy of Qigong, although many studies do not conform to the strict scientific protocol of randomized, controlled clinical trials. Controlled studies revealed that Qigong has a definite therapeutic role for hypertension, respiratory diseases, and cancer. In studies where patients on medication were divided into two groups; one group that practiced Qigong and another group that did not, the results strongly suggested that practicing Qigong exercises favorably affects the physiologic functions of the body, consequently permitting the reduction of the dosage of drugs. In hypertensive patients, combining Qigong practice with drug therapy not only resulted in reducing the required drug dosage, but also reduced the incidence of stroke and mortality. In asthmatics, the combination of Qigong with medication resulted in reduction in the dosage of medication, the need for sick leave, the duration of hospitalization, and costs of therapy. In cancer patients, those who practiced Qigong manifested fewer side effects of potent cancer therapy. One study revealed that Qigong helps to rehabilitate drug addicts.[17]

Another review of 30 studies on Qigong and hypertension also criticized the numerous problems and weaknesses in the design and methodology of research protocols but concluded that the evidence does suggest that practicing Qigong may have a positive effect on hypertension and that Qigong should be considered as part of an integrated, multifaceted management program for hypertension.[14] One review of physiotherapeutic breathing techniques—a scientific term for Qigong—suggested that Qigong may be beneficial for asthmatics and again comments on the necessity for rigorous clinical trials.[5]

Other studies examine the role of Qigong in diabetes, paralysis, and psychological disturbances. One study compared the effects of conventional walking with Qigong walking on blood glucose levels in diabetes. Although both forms of walking decreased serum glucose levels after lunch, the pulse rate markedly increased after conventional walking, but

Qigong walking was more beneficial in that it reduced plasma glucose without significant increase in the pulse rate.[8] One study indicates that Qigong may be beneficial as an adjunct to psychotherapy.[18]

Chow Qigong is not only used with the very seriously ill, but also has helped those in superb health, such as business executives and world class athletes. For example, the British representative to the women's World Triathlon nearly stopped training because of physical, mental, and spiritual fatigue. In a 1-week period of training with Chow Qigong, she redeveloped her stamina and drive, continued her training, and subsequently won the Gold Medal.

*Giving individuals the power to determine and manage their own health and destinies is the secret of true healing.*

EFFIE POY YEW CHOW

## PRINCIPLES OF QIGONG PRACTICE

Following are some examples of the use of Traditional Chinese Medicine and Qigong with rehabilitation cases.[2]

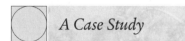

### A Case Study

*Parkinson's Disease*
Ten years with Parkinson's disease made me totally dependent upon my wife for all activities of daily living (ADL). I am 60 years young, over 6 feet tall, and a retired Royal Canadian Mounted Police (RCMP). My symptoms included very severe tremors with rigidity, "freezing," stooped posture 80% hunched over, poor balance, and no longer driving. Prior to treatment with Chow Integrated Healing System and Chow Qigong, I had tried all medicine means and had just spent $40,000 for a one-month experimental program and had further deteriorated.

Approximately once a month I had 2 or 3 days of therapy when Dr. Chow came to Ottawa. Then in between times I practiced what I was taught and had Chow Qigong therapy with Dr. Chow's assistants. Many things improved simultaneously, but I will highlight only some major first time improvements. In June 1998 after the first 1½ hours of therapy with Dr. Chow and her team, tremors were reduced. In July, movement improved, with less "freezing." In August, for the first time in 6 months,

I drove my car accompanied by my wife; for the first time in more than 2 years, I read some books, shaved with safety razors, and carried out some self-care. In October, I was rolling and crawling, playing, and closed up the pool with grandchildren. In November, I got up from and down to the floor readily. In December, for the first time in a year, I drove my car alone. From December 1998 to now, July 2001, I have continued to improve; in fact, some things I am doing even better than before I became ill. (Such as lying on the floor with my feet simulating riding a bicycle up in the air!) I now lead a normal life handling all my own ADLs. I golf, climb ladders to prune trees, sleep well, have spent 4 hours shoveling snow off my roof this winter, and opened a new business with my wife—the only gift shop at the new casino. I also can think of others better and be more thoughtful, whereas I was quite centered onto myself in the height of my condition. ❧

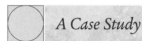

### A Case Study

*Head Injury*
I was a second-year engineering student and an aspiring champion in the International Indy Auto Races. In January 1999, my world collapsed when I suffered a brain injury in a motor vehicle accident along with a fractured pelvis, broken collar bone, and a torn urethra. I remained unconscious for almost 3 months.

For 1 year my recovery progressed well under the care of a good rehab team. With my strong will and desire to get back on my feet, I regained my ability to speak, and although in a wheelchair most times, I was able to use a walker unsteadily for short stints with close surveillance. By the second year my progress had leveled off. In spite of the expert team and for undetermined reasons, severe intentional tremors impeded and even made me regress.

My family and I were very frustrated and angry. I now used a wheelchair more often and needed total assistance to dress and eat. My whole body had moderate shaking when I tried to take steps to walk. My right hand was gripped and rigid with a fixed elbow and wrist, making it almost useless. My left arm had severe tremors so that I could not hold it up and had to hold my upper arm pressed to my body in order to have any control. I had some drooling, and my speech was unclear.

In March 2001, we were introduced to the Chow Qigong Healing System. Immediately I felt my body responding. Dr. Chow showed me how to breathe using my diaphragm to control my spasms. My drooling stopped, and my speech was clearer. She used Qigong massage with my right wrist, which was very tight, making it nearly useless. Within about 10 minutes, Dr. Chow had my wrist bending easily. My mother cried seeing this and we were both convinced of the magic of the Chow Qigong Healing System.

Under Dr. Chow's training I started noticing that I could do things I hadn't been able to do since my accident. In 3 short months of seeing Dr. Chow each month for 3 to 4 days, 3 to 4 hours per day, I have been able to achieve many "firsts" and complete many activities of daily living. Whereas before I had to be fed most of my meals, now I can eat independently with a regular fork and spoon. A caregiver or my mom would dress me and now I get dressed independently. I can put on my belt, shoes and socks and even tie my waist ties. I spent most of my time in a wheelchair before and needed close supervision when I walked with a walker. Now I walk using only a walking stick with supervision for occasional loss of balance. I would never answer the phone but let the caller leave a message; now I can write phone messages and even make journal entries that are legible with smaller printing. Because of the urethra tear, I was impotent. After 2 and a half years, now with Qigong, I have regained some sexual sensations.

This list of "firsts" is lengthy, and I will achieve more each day. I continue to look forward to my sessions with Dr. Chow, convinced that I will soon return to a life which is full, rich, and independent. ◈

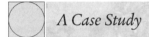

## A Case Study

### Spinal Cord Injury (Cervical)

The physician explained that Mr. P. sustained a head injury, C5 fracture, and spinal cord injury, and he received surgical intervention to fuse and stabilize his cervical spine. With respect to his spinal cord injury, Mr. P. had no power in his legs and only large muscle movement in his arms. He had no independent trunk movement. In addition to his permanent quadriplegia, Mr. P. also suffered from poor sleep, neurogenic pain in his shoulders and arms, and bladder incontinence. Overall, Mr. P. demonstrated mild to moderate loss in memory, more in nonverbal memory.

The physician also indicated that Mr. P. would experience further recovery around the level of his spinal cord but not below. Therefore it was expected that Mr. P. would recover further function/movement of his shoulders and increased strength bilaterally to his arms. Less recovery was expected, however, of his wrists and hands, and it was not likely that Mr. P. would recover further trunk or leg function.

Mr. P. first saw Dr. Chow on July 13, 1999. At that time, Mr. P. could lift his right arm to shoulder height and his left to half that height with a lot of pain in the neck and shoulders. He had very little wrist movement and feeling only on the inner side from his elbows down. When he was touched, he went into spasms and had to be held down. Exercising was impossible because of this. He also had an ulcer on his left foot, which would not heal. He was depressed and cranky, would speak very little and made no eye contact. He was very apathetic.

After his first session with Dr. Chow, Mr. P. could control his spasms with his new breathing technique, he could sit by himself on the side of the bed for a few minutes, and he could pull himself up from lying to sitting with help.

Six months later, after seeing Dr. Chow every month and having two practitioners work with him twice a week at home, Mr. P. has made significant physical and mental improvements:

- The ulcer on his left sole has healed.
- He controls spasms with Qigong breathing techniques.
- He is free from shoulder and neck pain at rest or during exercise.
- He sleeps a lot better.
- He can turn on his side in bed by hooking his arm over the side rail.

Because of the above improvements, the need for an overnight attendant was eliminated. Assisted exercise involving Mr. P. pulling himself up from a lying to a sitting position has strengthened his back muscles. He can now bend down to touch his toes while sitting in his wheelchair and get back to the chair by himself. Rolling with only a little assistance on the floor mat continues to strengthen his upper torso and helped him regain some sense of his body movement and alignment. His endurance has increased to the point where he can roll 200 times in 52 minutes without resting.

For the first time in his life, he can hold his 20-month-old son, Chris, in his arms. Chris has also changed from a shy boy to a very warm and joyous fellow. He eagerly watches Dr. Chow working with his father, and he uses some of the English words he has learned to encourage him.

Massage and Cupping has resulted in feeling on the outer part of his upper arms and he has more feeling in his upper chest and back. His urine stream is now strong.

Mr. P. has a more positive outlook on life now. He eagerly participates in his exercise program. He is also thinking about learning computer skills or other possibilities to improve his chances of working again.

It is strongly believed that with the continuation of the intensive therapy with the Chow Qigong Integrated Healing System, Mr. P. could regain much more mobility and independence and lead a happy and fulfilling life. With all the improvements achieved in the last few months, recovery potential can be unlimited as long as he is willing to work hard. ◈

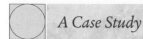

## A Case Study

### Stroke

*Before treatment.* The 62-year-old patient from North Carolina suffered a stroke 2 years before coming to see Dr. Chow, and she manifested right hemiplegia requiring a shoulder sling and right hand and leg braces. The prognosis was that of continued deterioration and that she would never be able to drive a car again. She could walk only about 10 feet with a quad cane with her right leg dragging. Her right hand and arm hung useless by her side, and she could not move her right arm or leg at all. She was told that unless she used the sling and braces, arms, hands, knees, and ankles would come out of their sockets. Her energy level was extremely low, she tired easily and was very depressed. Medical treatment had not helped her, and the acupuncture she received elsewhere gave no results.

*After treatment.* In 9 days of treatment, Dr. Chow used a strong Qigong component in her therapy, and she immediately accomplished the following: The patient could walk seven blocks in San Francisco, including hills, she did not need braces or slings; lying down she could totally move and exercise her right arm and leg; she could use her right hand to hold a cup to drink; she could balance well with both feet together, and she could walk around home without support. She felt optimistic, happy, and energetic.  ∾

## Components of the Integrated Approach

The Chow Integrated Healing System and Qigong (The Chow System) is a pragmatic system that combines modern Western health practices, ancient Traditional Chinese Medicine, and Qigong, and Dr. Chow's original concepts of a total integrated approach to health of the body, mind, and spirit. Qigong is the basic underlying component of The Chow System.

In this integrated approach, a person's body, mind, and spirit are one, interacting with people, the immediate environment, and the Universe. Clients play a central role in their therapy. Fitness and preventive health are emphasized, and stress and tension often are seen as common precursors to disease. Another concept is that all true healing originates from a higher power, and that effective healing occurs only when a healer or practitioner has facilitated the flow of Qi from this higher source.

The Chow Integrated Healing System and Qigong is comprised of many important components, theories, and principles. As a summary, 10 of the most important basic concepts for initial practice are as follows:

1. Get at least eight hugs a day, and be "in touch."
2. Get at least three Belly-Aching-Laughs-A-Day.
3. Maintain proper posture and breathe with the diaphragm (not the chest).
4. Maintain a positive mental attitude.
5. Meditate daily.
6. Use good nutrition, supplements, and perhaps herbs.
7. Practice the right type of exercise, especially Qigong exercises.
8. Be at peace with yourself and others.
9. Live the Qi energy concept.
10. Give and receive lots of love.

A good Qigong master or "healer" must be free from the self-ego.[20] People who come to see the Qigong master are referred to as *clients* instead of *patients.* The healing process is a mutual educational experience rather than the usual patient-practitioner relationship. When clients schedule appointments, they are asked to prepare a self-written chronology of their condition(s) and bring records of a recent evaluation by a physician.

Writing the chronology forces clients to sit down and think through their condition and its evolution and about life events. Frequently, they gain new insight into a problem. Clients are requested to keep a written daily journal during therapy and note all of the positive things that take place.

The usual Traditional Chinese Medicine diagnostic steps (observation, energy scanning, auscultation, and pulsation) are taken, including a medical-social history, blood pressure, and vital signs. Body, mind, spirit, and environmental concepts are discussed. Emotional or spiritual problems may be an underlying cause of a physical problem, and the converse is also true. Major and often even minor events in people's lives have great significance: events 5 years before the beginning of the current situation, or even from childhood, may be related causally. Individuals have a chance to explore past events or relationships.

In carrying out the previous steps, therapy has already begun. Next, clients begin to learn proper breathing, posture, and meditation. Usually they will begin to feel a little better after the first session; pain may diminish, and their energy level may rise enough for them to notice a difference. Even in clients with serious problems, such as paralysis, dramatic progress has occurred in the first session, such as being able to stand up and walk by themselves.

Next, they learn one or two Qigong exercises, such as the "Heavenly Stretch," and "Hip Rotation" exercises (described in Chapter 7). Different exercises may be selected according to what is indicated by the client's condition. Clients might learn how to apply Qipressure (acupressure) on themselves. Usually acupuncture needles are not used in the first session. Clients need to sense that they are helping themselves and becoming responsible for their own therapy.

Everyone needs to realize that he or she is the greatest instrument ever created, and the greatest miracle on earth! The job of the healer is to help the clients maximize their own instrument, not to depend on the instruments of others.

People need a support system, whether it consists of families, selected friends, or associates. Clients who are seriously ill need to establish whether they want to live or die. Whatever they choose is not to be judged; it is all right, it is their choice. We then help them to live or die well.

Part of the healing process involves being at peace with yourself and others. It is important to settle conflicts with parents, brothers, sisters, friends, other family members or associates, and so on. Harboring deep, dark, fearful secrets constricts Qi, which in turn affects the body, mind, and spirit and can make a person ill or impede the healing process. Having dreams and fantasies is important because they open Qi to feelings of freedom of expression.

EWAHA has a learning package for people who want to learn Qigong, consisting of the book *Miracle Healing from China Qigong* by Dr. Charles McGee and Grandmaster Effie Poy Yew Chow, two Chow Qigong Videotapes, and one audiotape to learn the Chow Qigong meditation. There are progressive training workshops for people who wish to excel in Qigong or Medical Qigong and learn to heal oneself or others with Qigong.

EWAHA and Dr. Chow have sponsored, along with many co-sponsors, the four World Congresses on Qigong and The Qigong Summit, formed the American Qigong Association (AQA) and the World Qigong Federation (WQF) to bring about a solid Qigong community for both the professionals and the public—a clearing house—and to promote scientific research into Qigong so that it may be better understood by the Western medical and scientific population and to better serve the people.

The overall consensus of the investigators and reviewers of current data is the dire need for more sound research in all areas related to Qigong: to decipher the mechanism of Qigong for the scientific community, to demonstrate the efficacy of Qigong, to determine the appropriate type and amount of Qigong needed for health and for various medical conditions, and to assess cost effectiveness of Qigong. Supported by the rich background of thousands of years of history and a myriad of anecdotal evidence, it will only be a matter of time before Qigong is fully integrated into the conventional regimen of health maintenance and healing.

## References

1. *China Zhenjiuology:* series of video teaching tapes produced by "hundreds of renowned professors and specialists" from numerous Chinese Medical Colleges, Chinese Medical Audio-Video Organization and Meditalent Enterprises, Ltd, 1990-1999, China.
2. Chow EPY, McGee CT: *Miracle healing from China: Qigong,* Coeur d'Alene, Idaho, 1996, Medipress.
3. Ellis E, Wiseman N, Boss K: *Fundamentals of Chinese acupuncture,* revised ed, Brookline, Mass, 1991, Paradigm Publications.
4. *English-Chinese encyclopedia of practical traditional Chinese medicine,* vol 1-14, Beijing, 1990, Higher Education Press.
5. Ernst E: Breathing techniques: adjunctive treatment modalities for asthma? a systematic review, *Eur Respir J* 15(5):969-72, 2000.
6. Farrell SJ, Ross AD, Sehgal KV: Easter movement therapies, *Phys Med Rehabil Clin N Am* 10(3):617-29, 1999.
7. Helms J: *Acupuncture energetics: a clinical approach for physicians,* Berkeley, Calif, 1995, Medical Acupuncture Publishers.
8. Iwao M, Kajiyama S, Mori H, et al: Effects of qigong walking on diabetic patients: a pilot study, *J Altern Complement Med* 5(4):353-8, 1999.
9. Lee MS, Kim BG, Huh HG, et al: Effect of Qi-training on blood pressure, heart rate, and respiration rate, *Clin Physiol* 20(3):173-6, 2000.
10. Luskin FM et al: A review of mind/body therapies in the treatment of musculoskeletal disorders with implications for the elderly, *Altern Ther Health Med* 6(2):46-56, 2000.
11. Luskin FM et al: A review of mind/body therapies in the treatment of cardiovascular disease. Part 1: implications for the elderly, *Altern Ther Health Med* 4(3):46-61, 1998.
12. Maciocia G: *The foundations of Chinese medicine: a comprehensive text for acupuncturists and herbalists,* London, 1989, Churchill Livingstone.
13. Maciocia G: *The practice of Chinese medicine: the treatment of diseases with acupuncture and Chinese herbs,* London, 1994, Churchill Livingstone.

14. Mayer M: Qigong and hypertension: a critique of research, *J Altern Complement Med* 5(4):371-82, 1999.
15. Nei Ching: *The Yellow Emperor's classic of internal medicine,* Berkeley, 1949, University of California Press (translated by Ilza Veith).
16. O'Connor J, Bensky D (eds): *Acupuncture: a comprehensive text,* Seattle, 1981, Eastland Press.
17. Sancier KM: Therapeutic benefits of qigong exercises in combination with drugs, *J Altern Complement Med* 5(4):383-9, 1999.
18. Shang C: Emerging paradigms in mind-body medicine, *J Altern Complement Med* 7(1):83-91, 2001.
19. *The English-Chinese encyclopedia of practical traditional Chinese medicine,* Beijing, 1999, Higher Education Press.
20. Zhu Master: *Qi Gong for long life,* HangZhou, 1999, China (in Chinese).

## Suggested Readings

Chow E: Chow qigong and rehabilitation: chronic degenerative diseases, paralysis, and disabilities, *2nd World Congress Qigong,* 38, 1998.

Dixhoorn JJ, Duivenvoorden HJ: Effect of relaxation therapy on cardiac events after myocardial infarction: a 5-year follow-up study, *J Cardiopulm Rehabil* 19:178-85, 1999.

He Q, Zhang J, Li J: Effect of different qigong exercises on EEG manifested by computer analysis, *1st World Conf Acad Exch Med Qigong,* 37, 1988.

Huang M: Effect of the emitted qi combined with self-practice of qigong in treating paralysis, *1st World Conf Acad Exch Med Qigong,* 95, 1988.

Li M et al: 100 cases of neurogenic myophagism cured by Taihu qigong through correspondence, *2nd Int Conf on Qigong,* 157, 1989.

Li X: Clinical analysis of cervical spondylopathy and its rehabilitation by Tuina qigong in 267 cases, *2nd World Conf Acad Exch Med Qigong,* 136, 1993.

Lin H: Preliminary experimental results of the investigation on the basis of qigong therapy, *2nd Int Conf on Qigong,* 61, 1989.

Liu G: Effect of qigong state and emitted qi on the human nervous system, *1st Int Cong of Qigong,* 107, 1990.

Ma X: Infantile paralysis treated by qigong, *3rd World Conf Acad Exch Med Qigong,* 174, 1996.

Omura Y: Simple method for evaluating qigong state: reversible changes in qigong master and subject; effect of qigong on bacteria, viruses, and acupressure points, *1st Int Conf of Qigong,* 129, 1990.

Sancier K, Chow E: Healing with qigong and quantitative effects of qigong measured by a muscle test, *J Am Coll Trad Chin Med* 7(3):89, 1989.

Sun J, Yuan R, Yang C: Analysis of 51 cases with coronary heart disease treated by qigong, *1st World Conf Acad Exch Med Qigong,* 135, 1988.

Wan S et al: The study of traumatic paraplegia in canine model treated by Bagua Xun Dao Gong, *Chin J Somat Sci* 1:115, 1991.

Wan S, He Y, Hao S, et al: Repeated experiments by using emitted qi in treatment of spinal cord injury, *2nd World Conf Acad Exch Med Qigong,* 97, 1993.

Wang C, Xu D, Qian Y, et al: Research on antiaging effect of qigong, *1st World Conf Acad Exch Med Qigong,* 85, 1988.

Wang C: Effect of qigong on cardiovascular disease, *6th Int Sym on Qigong,* 14-16, 1996.

Wang C, Xu D, Qian Y, et al: Effects of qigong on preventing stroke and alleviating the multiple cerebro-cardiovascular risk factors: a followup report on 242 hypertensive cases over 30 years, *2nd World Conf Acad Exch Med Qigong,* 123, 1993.

Wei S, Liu T, Yang J, et al: A clinical observation on the recovery of extremity motion function in hemiplegic patients promoted by hypnosis and acupoint pressing, *4th World Conf Acad Exch Med Qigong,* 166, 1998.

Xia H, Xu F, Cui C, et al: Effect of qigong exercise on electromyogram of poliomyelitis paralysis, *3rd Nat Academy on Qigong Science,* 90, 1990.

Xu L, Yu H, Yan X: Investigation of physiological characteristics on qigong eigen state, *1st World Conf Acad Exch Med Qigong,* 10, 1988.

Xu X: Marked effect on facial paralysis treated by Yoga, *4th World Conf Acad Exch Med Qigong,* 154-155, 1998.

Yu H, Yan X, Xu L: Systematic investigation of the qigong state, *1st World Conf Acad Exch Med Qigong,* 8, 1988.

Zhao B: Effects of qigong on cerebral blood flow and extremitic blood flow, *1st World Conf Acad Exch Med Qigong,* 83, 1988.

Zhou Y, Yan X, Zhang L: Effect of emitted qi on the change of antibody dependence cell-mediated cytotoxicity (ADCC) of K cell of mice caused by injury of left and right brain cortex, *2nd World Conf Acad Exch Med Qigong,* 109, 1993.

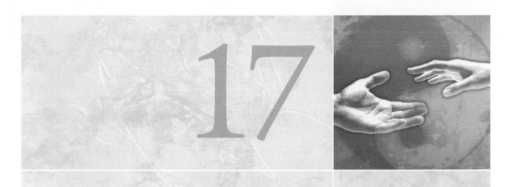

# Meridian-Based Psychotherapy

FRED P. GALLO

Psychological treatment traditionally has focused on unconscious psychodynamics; behavioral techniques such as respondent and operant conditioning, flooding, systematic desensitization, reinforcement, and modeling; and humanistic approaches that attend to values and choice, such as gestalt therapy, phenomenology, and cognitive therapy. Recently the new paradigm of energy psychology has emerged, which can be called psychology's *fourth force*. This theoretical and practical approach offers the field some interesting and stunning findings because it views psychological problems from the perspective of bioenergy fields and provides treatment alternatives that directly and efficiently address these substrates.

This chapter covers some of the historical development and theoretical implications of energy psychology, with specific attention to meridian-based psychotherapy (within the wider context of energy and energy psychotherapy). Case illustrations and treatment protocols are provided to detail how this approach can be applied to the treatment of psychological trauma, physical pain, and other conditions of relevance to the rehabilitation professional. Research on meridian-based therapy is also highlighted. Additionally, the distinction between global treatments and causal energy diagnostic approaches to treatment is addressed.

## THE PHYSICS OF ENERGY

In 1905, a 26-year-old patent clerk, Albert Einstein, published four epoch-making, original papers that have transformed the way scientists perceive reality.

215

His paper on the photoelectric effect, which won him the Nobel Prize, introduced the quantum of light. He also wrote about Brownian motion, helping further to establish the reality of atoms, and then there were the paradigm-shaking special and general theories of relativity. In these papers, Einstein established that while the speed of light is a constant, there are no absolute reference frames or absolute velocities—that the position of the observer determines what can be observed. He also concluded that matter and energy are interconvertible aspects of the same basic reality. Fundamentally, everything in the known universe, including, obviously, matter, is reducible to energy organized into fields. (Although I consider subtle energies as field phenomena, currently physics recognizes only four fields: gravity, electromagnetism, the strong or nuclear force, and the weak force.) While subatomic phenomena, such as electrons and photons, can manifest as particles or waves, physicists researching atoms with particle accelerators or "atom smashers" have been unable to discern the most essential particle, again pointing to energy and fields as fundamental to the structure of our material reality and more.

Quantum theory is the best attempt yet to explain energy and the mysteriousness of our universe. For example, it has been discovered that, rather than existing as a continuous phenomenon, energy exists discontinuously or in packets referred to as quanta. Additionally, quantum physicists have had to contend with other odd findings about reality, especially the phenomena of complementarity, uncertainty, nonlocality, and information fields.

*Complementarity* is illustrated by the fact that an electron paradoxically will reveal itself as either a particle or a wave, depending on the experiment conducted to observe it. Electrons and other subatomic elements appear to be simultaneously particles and waves. Perhaps this also points to an integral interaction between subject and object, to the extent that a distinction between subjective and objective reality is profoundly blurred. It seems that the very act of observing affects, and possibly even creates, what is being observed. These conclusions would be impossible in a Newtonian universe.

*Uncertainty* is evident by the fact that if we know the location of a subatomic "particle," then we can only make probability statements about its speed. Conversely, if we know the speed of a subatomic particle, we can only make probability statements about its location. Our ability to know is profoundly limited.

Also, rather than being simply deterministic, the quantum universe is open to probability and a whole lot of possibility. In the spirit of Alfred Adler, soft determinism becomes the rule.

Regarding *nonlocality,* there appears to be a holographic interconnection throughout the universe that transcends time, space, and velocity. A number of physics experiments have demonstrated that the communication exchange between "intimately" related photons occurs astronomically faster than light speed, although speed really has nothing to do with it.[1-3] The interconnection is practically instantaneous.

Another interesting finding, explicit in the work of Davies[4] and Prigogine,[5] is that systems become information rich as they are forced farther from equilibrium or symmetry. Conversely, symmetrical systems are information poor. Information appears to be a function of structure and shape and, similar to atoms and molecules, information, I believe, is fundamentally a manifestation of energy and fields.

The phenomena of complementarity, uncertainty, nonlocality, and information fields reveal that the universe does not conform to our logic and that perhaps it is saturated with consciousness and choice. Complementarity alone brings to mind the humorous Far Side cartoon in which cows only behave as cows when humans drive by and otherwise engage in human-like conversation. Cow one does not equal Cow two. Only instead of cows, we are observing electrons. We might have to ask Newton what those electrons are doing when we are not watching them.

## BIOENERGY FIELDS

Approximately 7,000 years ago, an anonymous person or persons in India entertained the idea that the human body has an energy system extending beyond its visible boundaries—namely, biofields (radiating auras) and chakras (vortices extending out from or into the material body at key locations). Another indication of biofields showed up in portraits of saintly people with halos about their bodies. Perhaps the artists simply imagined such radiation, or possibly they were psychically attuned to see the biofields.

From a more scientific approach, Burr[6] employed electronic devices to investigate Life fields or L-fields, which he demonstrated as surrounding humans, animals, trees, and inanimate objects. Hunt[7] also used sophisticated electronic equipment to study various biofield manifestations that occur during healing. In seminars I have led participants through procedures that seem to provide sensual validation of biofields. For example, producing a circular motion of one hand in opposition to the other will generally result in the sensation of a tingling electromagnetic field, which appears to sensitize one's hands to detect the chakras and biofield emanating from various physical bodies. While biofields may be seen as epiphenomena of the body, from another perspective they precede and are more fundamental than the physical body. That is, biofields may be similar to molds, which account for the form that the physical body assumes. This position is partly supported by the fact that over the course of every 4 years the human body sheds every atom and molecule and yet maintains its essential physical structure.

## ACUPUNCTURE MERIDIANS

About 4,500 to 5,000 years ago, the Chinese discovered that there exist pathways of energy, also called *meridians,* within the physical body. The Chinese designated twelve primary meridians involving organ systems, two collector meridians or vessels, and eight extraordinary vessels. Each is a distinct pathway, along which are tiny portals where electrical resistance is lower than in the surrounding skin. The meridians and vessels were described in the *Nei Jing,* or *The Yellow Emperor's Classic of Internal Medicine.* This 24-volume work details two ways of working with the meridians: needles and moxa (an herb that is caused to smolder at the location of acupoints). The basic notion is that *chi* energy flows through the meridians and vessels and that they can develop imbalances that result in illness.

We can only guess about how the Chinese discovered the energy meridians and vessels. To the best of our knowledge, they did not have sophisticated electronic equipment in those days (unless advanced cultures existed for which we have no historical documentation). One guess is that the pathways were mapped out as a result of soldiers being injured in battle. For example, given an injury in a location related to a specific meridian, another physical malady might improve or clear up. Another theory is that tailors accidentally stuck their patrons with needles and then came to speculate whether being stuck in those locations accounted for the resolution of a physical malady. Still another theory is that the discoverers of

meridians possessed extrasensory perceptual abilities that made it possible for them to actually see the energy pathways.

The goal of meridian therapies is to reinstate balance (and thus health) by addressing key acupoints along the disrupted meridian(s). It should be noted that each meridian has a tonification point, which is used to stimulate the meridian; a sedation point, which is used to sedate the meridian; a source point, which is used to activate the whole of the meridian; and a number of additional types of acupoints. Although the meridians are integrally interconnected (in effect functioning as one continuous meridian or meridian system), there appears to be some specialization among specific meridians and acupoints. For example, Diamond[8] has suggested that the lung meridian is associated with humility vs. intolerance, the gall bladder meridian with love vs. rage, and the spleen meridian with confidence vs. anxiety about the future. Concerning specific acupoints, research has shown that the sixth acupoint on the pericardium meridian (PC-6), which is located 2 inches above the transverse wrist crease at the middle of the palmar side of the forearm, is effective in treating motion sickness, morning sickness, and nausea.[9]

In the early 1970s, Becker[10,11] researched electrical skin resistance related to acupoints. He found that many of the acupoints along the pericardium meridian and large intestine meridian lines on the forearms of his subjects evidenced lower electrical resistance as compared with surrounding skin. Additionally, researchers in France[12] have provided radiological evidence for the existence of meridians.

## APPLIED KINESIOLOGY

Beginning in 1964, George A. Goodheart, Jr., a chiropractor from Detroit, Michigan, began to carve out a field that is referred to as applied kinesiology. He used manual muscle testing from physical therapy[13] to assess the integrity of various systems throughout the body, not merely the physiological strength of the isolated muscle. The commonsense assumption here is that the body is an integrated whole and that interconnections exist among the various organ systems, which are fundamentally useful but artificial distinctions. If a muscle tests "strong," obviously this has different implications than if it tests "weak." In addition to discovering that weakness in a muscle can be caused by hypertonicity in an opposing muscle, he also found that the hypertonic or hypotonic muscle can be respectively relaxed or strengthened by addressing neurolymphatic reflexes, neurovascular reflexes, cranial faults, exogenous substances, emotional reactions, and the acupuncture meridian system.[14,15]

Not surprisingly, Goodheart also found that emotions could be causal in the development, exacerbation, and sustaining of a physical condition. He discovered that he could employ emotional neurovascular reflexes, located at the frontal eminence on the forehead, to treat emotional factors. This is referred to as the emotional stress release (ESR) procedure. If there is an emotional component to a physical condition, testing an associated indicator muscle while challenging the emotional neurovascular reflexes (a procedure called *therapy localization*) will result in a change in the indicator muscle response. Either the patient or the therapist can hold the ESR points for a period to treat the emotional component. It may be helpful for the patient to think about the emotional issue while the ESR procedure is being employed, but it is not essential. This procedure appears to be effective with patients who do not have conscious access to the emotional issue.

In a psychotherapeutic context, ESR can be used to reduce the stress associated with issues in the patient's life without having therapy to localize and perform manual muscle testing. The patient simply attunes or thinks about the issue (e.g., traumatic memory, phobia, feelings of depression) and lightly holds the emotional neurovascular reflexes with his or her fingertips while monitoring the decrease in emotional distress. While ESR will usually result in a significant temporary decrease in the level of emotional distress associated with the treated issue, also at times it results in ongoing emotional relief. I have found that it is often useful and effective to combine ESR with relevant affirmations. For example, while using ESR to treat anger, concomitantly the patient may find it beneficial to affirm, "At the deepest level I release myself of this anger," or "There is forgiveness in my heart."

## LIFE ENERGY ANALYSIS

In the 1970s, John Diamond, a psychiatrist involved in preventive medicine, studied applied kinesiology and integrated these findings with psychoanalytical understandings, using the acupuncture meridian system to diagnose and treat psychological problems.[8,16] This was the beginning of modern meridian-based psychotherapy. Diamond's method, referred to as behavioral kinesiology (BK) to distinguish it from applied kinesiology, involves assessing the integrity of the patient's acupuncture meridian system and drawing conclusions about prominent emotional issues involved in the individual's functioning. He employs a wide array of techniques and modalities to treat emotional issues, including the thymus thump, positive affirmations, music, sounds, gestures, postural adjustments (Alexander technique), nutritional supplements, Bach flower essences, and others. He also introduced the concept of "reversal of the body morality," which represents a significant block to treatment effectiveness. The "reversed" person responds as though what is good is bad and what is bad is good. Diamond has explored various ways of correcting for this problem, including the use of nutritional supplements, altering negative life decisions, and resolving relevant negative feelings in relationship to one's mother (à la Melanie Klein).

## THOUGHT FIELD THERAPY

In 1979, psychologist Roger A. Callahan began to elaborate on certain aspects of Diamond's work. He also studied applied kinesiology and used Diamond's straight arm technique for manual muscle testing.[17] His approach was initially referred to as the Callahan techniques, later as thought field therapy (TFT), and presently as Callahan techniques—thought field therapy (CT-TFT) to distinguish it from other approaches to TFT. Using double-negative testing,[8] the therapy localizes meridian alarm points while the patient attunes to the thought field associated with a phobia or trauma. In Callahan's view, this procedure makes it possible to define the energetic elements or sequences of meridian points involved in a psychological problem. He found that percussing or tapping on beginning and ending points of meridians would reinstate harmony in the meridian by neutralizing the negative emotion(s) associated with the psychological problem. He also developed diagnostic and treatment procedures to correct psychological reversal, which is essentially a block to treatment effectiveness (similar to Diamond's reversal of the body morality).

TFT (and energy psychotherapy as a whole) has gone in a myriad of directions, with various theorist-researcher clinicians offering their refinements and advancements.[18-23] Many of these approaches have roots in TFT and BK, combined with other methods.

## ENERGY DIAGNOSTIC AND TREATMENT METHODS

Influenced by the work of Goodheart, Diamond, Callahan, and others, I began to develop energy diagnostic and treatment methods (EDxTM) around 1993. EDxTM is similar to BK and TFT in the use of alarm points to diagnose meridians in need of treatment. However, it also offers a wider range of corrections for psychological reversal and criteria-related reversals, as well as an expansion of relevant treatment points. EDxTM entails a number of protocols for assessing the energetic structure of the problem, the status of the individual's energetic state at the time, and various means of treating psychoenergetic problems. Additionally, unlike CT-TFT, EDxTM does not assume that a sequence of meridian points is needed to correct a problem. (I have not found any one sequence of meridian points to be essential, although, as in acupuncture, clusters of meridian points are often needed.)

While EDxTM is a meridian-based psychotherapy, it also addresses other aspects of the energy system (e.g., chakras) and incorporates a wide variety of energy-based procedures to treat psychological problems. Other modalities include visualization, creative activities such as music and song, affirmations, redecision, addressing core beliefs, and thought recognition.[19,20,23] For example, the healing energy light process (HELP) combines corrections for neurological disorganization and psychological reversal with a yoga-style visualization, the negative affect erasing method, HeartMath, and affirmations to treat psychological issues.[20]

## EYE MOVEMENT THERAPIES

Eye movement integration,[24] rapid eye technology,[25] eye movement desensitization and reprocessing,[26] and one-eye techniques[27] are eye movement therapies that have been found to be effective in the treatment of trauma and a number of other conditions. Essentially these methods have the patient access a trauma or other emotionally charged issue while moving his or her eyes bilaterally in various patterns. Eden[28] reports that "versions of this technique have been passed down in various cultures for thousands of years." While Shapiro[26] posits an information processing model to account for the effectiveness of eye movement desensitization and reprocessing (EMDR), other researchers and theoreticians have offered energetic hypotheses to account for their mechanism of action.[19,23] Although eye movement methods possibly promote cerebral hemisphere balance to treat the presenting problem, an interrelationship of cerebral hemispheres, meridians, and psychological problems has been observed by Diamond.[8]

It should be noted that many of the results obtained with bilateral eye movements are also achievable with bilateral tapping on shoulders or hands and alternating finger snapping adjacent to both ears.[26] Additionally, Johnson[25] has explored the therapeutic effects of light, sound, color, and eye blinking. It should be further noted that quality training in these therapies is imperative because severe abreaction commonly occurs even in the hands of the most skilled practitioner. Considerable research has supported the effectiveness of eye movement therapies, specifically EMDR.[26]

## NEGATIVE AFFECT ERASING METHOD, CAUSAL DIAGNOSIS, AND TRAUMA

Many meridian-based psychotherapy approaches and techniques are highly effective and efficient in treating psychological trauma and a wide range of psychological conditions and issues. The negative affect erasing method (NAEM), which I developed, has been found to be especially safe and effective. When providing NAEM, the therapist asks the patient to briefly think about the trauma (or other emotionally charged issue) and then tap on or otherwise stimulate the following treatment points: governing vessel-24.5 (the third eye point on the forehead between the eyebrows), governing vessel-26 (under the nose), conception vessel-24 (under the bottom lip), and governing vessel-20 (on the upper sternum). (In some cases having the patient position his or her free hand on or above the occipital ridge in the vicinity of governing vessel-17 can enhance treatment effects.) After each round of tapping, the patient reevaluates the subjective units of distress (SUD). In most cases I have found that several rounds of NAEM will resolve most single-incident traumas. For highly complex and multiple traumas, NAEM is used to treat the various components involved. NAEM is often usefully combined with simple cognitive procedures such as the instillation of positive outcomes and beliefs.[20]

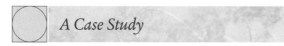

## A Case Study

### Posttraumatic Stress Disorder

A 19-year-old female college student was referred to me for treatment of posttraumatic stress disorder (PTSD) as a result of an automobile accident. The driver in the opposing car went over the medial strip and struck her vehicle head-on, killing him and both of his passengers. My patient was pinned under the dashboard for several hours while a rescue team cut her out of her car. She incurred broken ankles, a broken arm and shoulder, and back injuries. Since the accident she had been suffering frequent nightmares, flashbacks, panic, generalized anxiety, and feelings of guilt and anger. She was also regularly abusing alcohol.

Initially we focused on her experience of being pinned under the dashboard. After she thought about it and rated the SUD level as a 9, I then had her dismiss the memory from consciousness while following the NAEM protocol, intermittently reassessing the SUD level. (Rather than assuming the necessity of exposure to promote desensitization, NAEM and other meridian-based therapies do not require this. It is not the abreaction that promotes therapeutic results.) After about five rounds of NAEM, she was able to think about the event without experiencing distress. Follow-up sessions at 1 week, 2 weeks, and 2 months revealed that after the initial session, nightmares and flashbacks no longer occurred. Additionally, if she were asked to think about the event, she would no longer experience distress.

During the course of treatment, other aspects of the trauma were treated, including the feelings of anger and guilt she experienced concerning the people who died. That distress was also successfully resolved in one session.

During intake she also revealed that her grandfather molested her from ages 5 to 12 years. After successfully treating the vehicular trauma, we treated several of her distressing molestation memories. These were easily resolved by employing NAEM and a more specifically focused EDxTM diagnostic-treatment protocol involving manual muscle testing.[20] Even after treating the memories that she

was conscious of, she reported a lingering "dirty and disgusting" feeling, which she reported as being localized in the vicinity of the lower abdomen. Employing an EDxTM diagnostic-treatment protocol, we were able to alleviate this sensation in a single session as well. Follow-up several months later revealed ongoing relief of this and other issues treated with these modalities. ∿

It is commonly accepted among psychotherapists that psychological trauma results in a variety of psychiatric problems and can lead to physical disease and interfere with physical and psychological healing. Such was the case with the patient discussed in the case study, as well as with other patients I have treated. With this patient, resolution of the psychological trauma yielded many benefits, including alleviation of intrusive thoughts, flashbacks, and nightmares of the trauma, as well as resolution of clinical depression and a tendency to abuse alcohol. In addition (and of particular interest to rehabilitation professionals), through the use of these efficient techniques the patient's physical rehabilitation was enhanced. Because she was no longer plagued with the trauma symptoms that tended to be activated during the course of physical therapy, the rehabilitative process was facilitated.

## CHRONIC PAIN TREATMENT

Although meridian-based psychotherapies are most often used in the treatment of psychological problems, these methods are also useful in the treatment of physical pain. In addition to relieving negative emotions and physical tension associated with the patient's pain condition, meridian-based psychotherapy can be used to alleviate, reduce, and control the pain symptoms themselves. I have found this to be particularly useful in treating headaches and migraines, in addition to pain of the lower back, neck, shoulders, knees, and heels. However, in my experience these methods are not as consistently effective in treating physical pain as they are in treating emotional issues.

When treating pain, I have the patient rate the pain level on a 0 to 10 scale and observe various features of the physical symptoms while tapping on specific acupoints. For example, a headache sufferer would be asked to describe changes in the intensity, location, shape, color, and other dimensions of the pain while stimulating acupoints such as triple energizer-3 (TE-3), large intestine-4 (LI-4), kidney-27 (K-27), pericardium-6 (PC-6), or whatever other treatment points are discerned via energy diagnostics. In many cases NAEM alone, or in combination with other treatment points, has been found useful for effectively treating many pain conditions. However, it should be noted that TE-3 (on the dorsal side of the hand, between and approximately 1 inch above the knuckles of the little finger and ring finger in the direction of the wrist) and LI-4 (on the dorsal side of either hand between the thumb and index fingers at the midpoint of the radial margin of the second metacarpal bone) are particularly potent treatment points for various pain conditions.

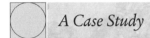

### A Case Study

*Failed Back Syndrome*
A middle-aged female patient entered treatment because of incessant nail biting, which also occurred nocturnally. History revealed that she had a chronic back pain condition and had undergone four back surgeries, including laminectomies and a fusion. The fusion also resulted in pain at the location of her right donor hip.

She reported the pain level at the time of the initial session as being an 8 on a 10-point scale. She indicated that she had not experienced appreciable relief from oral pain medications, injections, or physical therapy. Although the patient initially requested hypnosis to help her stop biting her nails, I questioned whether possibly her incessant pain contributed to the nail biting. I suggested that we attempt to reduce her pain, which might eliminate the nail biting as well. She agreed.

Employing standard EDxTM diagnostic procedures, I found that she was psychologically ready to alleviate the pain (i.e., there was no psychological reversal). Diagnostics also suggested that treatment of the triple energizer and kidney meridians would help to treat the problem. Initially I had her visually observe the pain symptoms three dimensionally and report ongoing changes in the location, dimensions, color, and weight of the pain while she tapped on specific acupoints. I directed her to tap on the TE-3 acupoint, alternating this with stimulating the kidney meridian K-27 (under either collarbone next to the sternum). Over the course of 10 minutes, the patient's physical symptoms dissipated and she reported a "warm tingling" at the base of her spine. She was able to move about and bend without experiencing pain. This session resulted in pain relief for approximately 5 hours. At follow-up, the pain was successfully alleviated and she was educated in detail about how to repeat the treatment procedure herself. Over time she experienced increasing periods of relief from the pain, with little need for medication. She was able to discontinue the use of a cane and found that she could walk distances comfortably. Also shortly after beginning treatment, she quit biting her nails. In all, treatment involved five sessions. About a month and a half after treatment concluded, she came to my office sporting her beautifully manicured fingernails. ∿

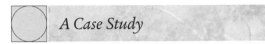

### A Case Study

*Chronic Angina*
A chronic back pain patient had a history of coronary artery disease and suffered from chronic angina. Energy diagnosing of a meridian-based treatment regimen alleviated the back pain for 4 to 5 hours after each application; pain relief lasted the entire day within a few months of regular treatment. Interestingly, the patient's episodes of angina significantly decreased and eventually remitted, making it possible for him to discontinue the use of nitroglycerin patches. ∿

## MERIDIAN-BASED THERAPY AND REHABILITATION

Meridian-based therapy has many uses of interest to rehabilitation personnel. When a patient is experiencing psychological distress related to a trauma, it can interfere with other aspects of treatment. The associated tension and other emotional features can aggravate muscle functioning and block optimal benefits from physical therapy. Similarly, when a patient has been given an unfavorable diagnosis and told of the need for surgery or other medical procedures, it can be traumatic for the patient and can interfere with his or her cooperation with and motivation for treatment. Diagnostic procedures such as MRIs pose a problem for claustrophobic patients, and meridian-based techniques can be employed to rapidly alleviate such phobic responses. A common problem is general compliance with treatment. Meridian-based therapies can be employed to efficiently alleviate obstacles to compliance. They can also be used to alleviate needle and blood phobia and anxiety related to surgical procedures.

Finally, let us not forget the rehabilitation professionals themselves. The stress of one's work can interfere with professional effectiveness and personal enjoyment. Self-treatment with various meridian-based protocols can be of tremendous benefit in alleviating stress and preventing compassion fatigue.

## RESEARCH

Several studies have documented the effectiveness of meridian-based techniques, specifically TFT, in the treatment of phobias and anxiety,[29,30] phobias and self-concept,[31] PTSD symptoms,[32] and acrophobia.[33]

Uncontrolled pilot studies by Callahan[29] and Leonoff[30] revealed significant decreases in SUD ratings of subjects treated on radio call-in shows. Of course the subjects could not be randomized, nor did the studies include control groups, placebos, follow-up, or other evaluative measures. Some might want to dismiss these results because of the methodology; nevertheless 132 of the total 136 subjects were successfully treated in this way—a 97% success rate. The mean decrease in SUD was 6.43 across both studies, and the total treatment times ranged from 4.34 to 6.04 minutes.

At Florida State University, Figley and Carbonell[32] conducted a systematic clinical demonstration study on four innovative approaches to treating PTSD symptoms: TFT, visual/kinesthetic dissociation (VK/D), EMDR, and traumatic incident reduction (TIR). This study included various evaluative measures, not merely SUD ratings, and follow-along and follow-up measures were also taken. Significant positive results were obtained for all four approaches.

The study by Wade[30] included 28 experimental subjects and 25 controls. Two self-concept questionnaires were employed: the Tennessee Self-Concept Scale (TSCS) and the Self-Concept Evaluation of Location Form (SELF). Approximately 1 month after these instruments were administered, the experimental subjects were treated with a TFT algorithm within a group setting. Sixteen of the subjects evidenced a drop in SUD ratings of four or more points, while only four of the no-treatment controls showed a decrease of two or more points. Two months after treatment, the TSCS and SELF were again administered. Statistical analysis revealed modest but significant improvements in three of the scales: the self-acceptance scale of the TSCS, the self-esteem scale, and the self-incongruency scale of the SELF. Results support the effectiveness of the treatment and its possible impact on one's self-concept.

Carbonell[33] investigated TFT in the treatment of acrophobia. All 49 subjects completed a behavioral measure that involved approaching and possibly climbing a 4-foot ladder. A 4-foot path leading to the ladder was also calibrated in 1-foot segments. As the subject approached and climbed the ladder, SUD ratings were taken at each floor segment and rung. Subjects were permitted to discontinue the task if necessary. After obtaining these measures, each subject met with another experimenter in a separate room and a SUD rating was obtained while the subject thought about a situation related to height. Subjects were then randomly assigned to treatment and placebo groups. After these procedures were conducted, SUD measures again were obtained. If the subject did not obtain a rating of zero, the respective procedure was repeated. Posttesting was conducted after the second administration of the procedure. Afterward the subject returned to the initial experimenter, who was "blind" to the treatment received by the subject, for posttesting. Posttesting was the same as pretesting, which involved in vivo assessment of SUD ratings as the subject approached and possibly climbed the ladder. Before data analysis, comparison of the groups on pretreatment measures revealed that the groups were essentially equivalent. While both groups improved, the treatment group demonstrated significantly more improvement, which was even more pronounced while climbing the ladder.

## MECHANISMS OF ACTION

How can we account for the therapeutic results achieved by stimulating acupoints while attuning a psychological problem (or even physical pain)? Are the specific acupoints relevant or does it not matter where we tap? What does the tapping (or other forms of stimulation) really do?

A myriad of explanations can be offered to account for the results that we observe with meridian-based psychotherapies and several other energetic approaches. *Placebo effect* is one suggested mechanism of action. While this has some merit, if acupoint stimulation produces the rapid, consistent, and profound results that many clinicians report, it would seem that placebo has little to do with it. Rather, something is being efficiently harnessed by these modes of treatment that occurs only occasionally when a "genuine placebo" is administered. After all, that "something" that occurs with the placebo effect is not simply an illusion. Perhaps it can be said that these therapies consistently activate the placebo effect, but then that would negate the essential definition of such a term.

Another explanation is that these methods and techniques simply *distract* the patient from psychological or physical distress. While some degree of distraction undoubtedly occurs because it is often difficult to maintain focus on the emotional or physical sensations while tapping on various locations on one's body, this explanation appears to be insufficient when ongoing relief is experienced after the treatment has been completed. Could the tapping result in ongoing resonating distraction long after the tapping has ceased? Perhaps, but then we should wonder about the basis of such resonating.

*Cognitive restructuring* can also be posited as a viable explanation because changes in thought and perception regularly occur as a result of these treatment modalities. However, it would seem that the cognitive shifts represent a secondary or tertiary effect after the negative emotion has been relieved. While a positive shift in cognition can serve to support and further actualize healthy psychological functioning, energetic treatments per se do not directly address cognition as the lever for change. Also, while awareness of the associated thoughts and cognitive restructuring are useful in the treatment of pain patients, they are insufficient to account for the alleviation of nociceptive sensations that often occurs with this form of treatment. (It should be noted that EDxTM protocols regularly incorporate the outcome projection procedure [OPP], a cognitive-energetic technique, to increase the probability that treatment effects will last.[20])

Because acupoints are used with meridian-based psychotherapies, neurotransmitters, such as *endogenous opioids,* may play a role in the treatment effects, similar to what has been proposed with acupuncture.[34] While it is likely that peripheral nerve stimulation activates the central nervous system to release endorphins, this hardly discounts the involvement of energetic effects. The question remains about the relationship among specific problems, specific acupoints, and the release of specific neurochemicals. There appears to be a signaling mechanism associated with the acupuncture meridians that figure into such action.

My preferred theoretical explanation is that invariably a whole range of aspects is involved in psychological functioning, healthy or otherwise. While the brain, neurochemistry, and cognition are implicated in psychological problems, these conditions are also perpetuated energetically. I believe that the distinctions among energy, brain, chemistry, emotions, consciousness, cognition, and behavior are arbitrary (but useful) distinctions at best.

## THEORETICAL MUSINGS

Psychological problems can be viewed as energetic informational structures similar to the electromagnetic configurations that adhere to audiotapes and computer hard drives. The nervous system electrochemically captures, stores, and replicates sensory information at various levels of abstraction—subtle energy, electromagnetic, chemical, brain physiology, emotion, cognition, linguistic, and external behavior. Because nature constructs complex structures from fractals, at a fundamental level psychological problems are energetic configurations or field structures. By destabilizing the energetic informational field, the system is prepared to transform into another, preferably healthier, structure. Tapping on or otherwise stimulating specific acupoints while the field structure is attuned serves to destabilize it and removes or collapses those features within the thought field that trigger the chain of events that result in the psychological or other health problem. Before it can transform into another stabilized informational field, the field must be destabilized. Often simple pattern interruption and disruption via energy therapies is sufficient for the system to leap to a higher order of organization. At other times it is useful to instill or reinforce a healthier structure.[20,22]

This informational field has also been referred to as a thought field.[35] In this respect, a thought is literally a specific kind of field, having a physical reality. It is composed of electromagnetic features, as well as subtle energetic markers that can activate emotions. When the field is attuned, these energetic markers are available for treatment. Concurrently, all of the other features of the problem are activated. This includes brain structures, neurochemistry, internal dialogue and other cognitive features, and various behaviors consistent with the state. The application of causal diagnostic procedures, which are germane to more sophisticated meridian-based psychotherapies, makes it possible to elicit the structure of the thought field.

For the most part, emotions are congenitally hardwired,[35] with brain structures such as the thalamus and amygdala designed to produce the myriad of emotions. When a trauma or other distressing event occurs, the input is represented in multimodal sensory form. Simultaneously these emotion-producing brain structures become bonded to the visual, auditory, tactile, gustatory, olfactory, and motor information (respondent conditioning). A trauma gestalt is formed, fundamentally held together energetically. When the memory of the trauma is attuned (even at a low signal strength), the entire informational network comprising the trauma is activated. While this structure is activated, tapping on key acupoints sends electromagnetic impulses into the energetic informational field, destabilizing it, collapsing the energetic markers, and severing the stimulus-response bond to the limbic system. Informational structures, similar to other systems, are maintained within a range of energy balance—too much or too little energy causes the structure to collapse. The tapping destabilizes the structure by diverting or overloading the adhesive energetic field. It now becomes possible to view the traumatic event calmly and to incorporate the calmness into a new, transformed gestalt. The memory is basically the same; the experience is transformed. The patient comes to view the event from a higher perspective, with neutrality or deeper positive feelings predominating. Mindfulness prevails.

I think that theoretical explanations along these lines are relevant with regard to any psychological problem. I also think that psychological problems account for the genesis of many, if not all, physical diseases. Fundamentally there is an energetic field structure at the basis of any physical form, whether that form consists of psychological or more obvious physical phenomena. A vision of energy medicine may be the diagnosis, treatment, and prevention of disease at the energetic level. Energy psychology and meridian-based psychotherapies energetically address what have been historically referred to as psychological problems. I think that the distinction between mind and body will blur and rightly so. Or should I say that their fundamental oneness will come into focus?

## References

1. Aspect A, Grangier P: Experiments on Einstein-Podolsky-Rosen-type correlations with pairs of visible photons. In Penrose R, Isham CJ (eds): *Quantum concepts in space and time,* New York, 1986, Oxford University Press,
2. Clauser JF, Horne MA, Shimony A: Bell's theorem: experimental tests and implications, *Rep Prog Physics* 41:1881-1927, 1978.
3. Tittel W, Brendel J, Zbinden H, et al: Violations of bell inequalities more than 10 km apart, *Phys Rev Lett* 81:3563-3566, 1998.
4. Davies P: *The fifth miracle: the search for the origins and meaning of life,* New York, 1999, Simon & Schuster.
5. Prigogine I: *The end of certainty: time, chaos, and the new laws of nature,* New York, 1996, The Free Press.
6. Burr HS: *Blueprint for immortality: the electric patterns of life,* Essex, England, 1976, Saffron Walden.
7. Hunt VV: *Infinite mind: science of the human vibrations of consciousness,* Malibu, Calif, 1989, Malibu Publishing.
8. Diamond J: *Life energy,* New York, 1985, Dodd, Mead.
9. McMillan CM: Acupuncture for nausea and vomiting. In Filshie J, White A (eds): *Medical acupuncture: a western scientific approach,* New York, 1998, Churchill Livingstone.
10. Becker RO: *Cross currents,* New York, 1990, GP Putnam's Sons.
11. Becker RO, Selden G: *The body electric,* New York, 1985, Morrow.
12. de Vernejoul P, Albarede P, Darras JC: Study of the acupuncture meridians with radioactive tracers, *Bull Acad Natl Med* 169:1071-1075, 1985.
13. Kendell HO, Kendell FMP: *Muscles: testing and function,* Baltimore, 1949, Williams & Wilkins.
14. Goodheart GJ: *You'll be better,* Geneva, Ohio, 1987, Author.
15. Walther DS: *Applied kinesiology: synopsis,* Pueblo, Colo, 1988, Systems DC.
16. Diamond J: *Behavioral kinesiology and the autonomic nervous system,* New York, 1978, Institute of Behavioral Kinesiology.
17. Callahan RJ: *Five minute phobia cure,* Wilmington, Del, 1985, Enterprise.
18. Durlacher JV: *Freedom from fear forever,* Tempe, Ariz, 1994, Van Ness.
19. Gallo FP: *Energy psychology: explorations at the interface of energy, cognition, behavior, and health,* Boca Raton, Fla, 1998, CRC Press.
20. Gallo FP: *Energy diagnostic and treatment methods,* Oakland, Calif, 2000, New Harbinger.
21. Furman ME, Gallo FP: *The neurophysics of human behavior: explorations at the interface of brain, mind, behavior, and information,* Boca Raton, Fla, 2000, CRC Press.
22. Gallo FP (ed): *Energy psychology in psychotherapy: a comprehensive source book,* New York, 2001, Norton.
23. Andreas C, Andreas S: *Eye movement integration (applied with a Vietnam veteran who has been experiencing intrusive memories),* Boulder, Colo, 1995, NLP Comprehensive (videotape).
24. Johnson R: *Rapid eye technology,* Salem, Ore, 1994, Rain Tree Press.
25. Shapiro F: *Eye movement desensitization and reprocessing: basic principles, protocols, and procedures,* New York, 1995, Guilford.
26. Cook A, Bradshaw R: *Toward integration: one eye at a time,* Vancouver, 1999, One-Eye Press.
27. Eden D, Feinstein D: *Energy medicine,* New York, 1998, Putnam/Tarcher, p 330.

28. Callahan RJ: Successful psychotherapy by radio and telephone, *Int Coll Appl Kines* Winter 1987.

29. Leonoff G: The successful treatment of phobias and anxiety by telephone and radio: a replication of Callahan's 1987 study, *The Thought Field* 1(2), 1995.

30. Wade JF: *The effects of the Callahan phobia treatment on self concept*, San Diego, Calif, 1990, The Professional School of Psychological Studies.

31. Carbonell JL, Figley C: A systematic clinical demonstration of promising PTSD treatment approaches, *Traumatology* 5(1), 1999.

32. Carbonell JL: An experimental study of TFT and acrophobia, Indian Wells, Calif, *The Thought Field* 2(3):1-6, 1997.

33. Pomeranz B: Acupuncture and the raison d'etre for alternative medicine, *Altern Ther Health Med* 2(6):84-91, 1996.

34. Callahan RJ, Callahan J: *Thought field therapy and trauma: treatment and theory,* Indian Wells, Calif, 1996, Author.

35. Nathanson DL: *Shame and pride: affect, sex, and the birth of the self,* New York, 1992, Norton.

# Compassion-Based Rehabilitation*

LAURO S. HALSTEAD

In April 1983, Jerome Gans, a physician at Braintree Hospital in Massachusetts, published an article, "Hate in the Rehabilitation Setting."[1] His thesis was that hate is an intrinsic part of the rehabilitation process and had been overlooked as a clinical issue in most rehabilitation hospitals. Common manifestations, he believed, include patient self-hatred, patient hatred of staff, and staff hatred of patients and their families.

I realize these sound like harsh words; however, I believe Dr. Gans was right. In my own experience, hate was not something I had ever heard discussed in the hospitals where I had worked. Anger, maybe. Dislike, definitely. But hate? No! Yet I knew it was there, and his article struck a responsive chord.

Six years later, a second discussion on this topic appeared by Larry Mullins, a psychologist at the University of Oklahoma. This article was titled, "Hate Revisited: Power, Envy, and Greed in the Rehabilitation Setting."[2] Now there were two articles on hate in the rehabilitation literature and no similar articles I knew of on more positive emotions to provide some balance. With this in mind, I pulled out a folder and labeled it "Compassion and Caring in the Rehabilitation Setting." Over the past decade I have added articles and clippings to the folder with the idea of someday writing an article or giving a talk on this topic—and I believe Dr. Coulter would be pleased to know his lecture made that "someday" finally arrive.

---

*This chapter is adapted from the *Archives of Physical Medicine and Rehabilitation* article, "The power of compassion and caring in rehabilitation healing," by Lauro S. Halstead, MD, and appeared in the February 2001 issue on pp 149-154 as the Harris Coulter Memorial Lecture.

It is not my intention, however, to minimize the importance of hate, anger, and envy in settings where we work with individuals who have sustained major trauma and life-changing losses. Rather, as the title of this chapter indicates, I would like to focus on some of the complementary qualities I believe play a much larger role in the rehabilitation experience—qualities such as caring, compassion, and empathy that are life-enhancing and create a healing environment.

First, however, let me explain what I mean by compassion and caring. Webster's Dictionary says compassion is "to feel sorrow for the sufferings of others accompanied by an urge to help." As for caring, it is "being responsible for, looking after, providing for." It is worth noting that both these words convey the twin concepts of feeling *and* action that I think are essential to promoting a healing environment. However, these definitions do not capture everything I believe is conveyed by the words "compassion" and "caring" in settings where I have worked. Rather, these words encompass all the countless, unnamed acts of providing comfort and therapy by nurses and occupational therapists, acts of teaching and nurturing by speech and recreational therapists and by the whole array of service personnel and professionals—individually or together as a team, scripted or spontaneous. These acts and words of kindness, empathy, and understanding are part of the person-intensive, complex interaction between patient and caregiver, between someone who feels his or her body is broken and in-valid and someone whose job it is to respond to those feelings and relieve the suffering, to mend and heal, to make whole. This is what all of us try to do, each in our own imperfect way—professional to patient, person to person, human to human. This, and much more, is what I mean by compassion and caring.

With this introduction, I now want to outline a conceptual model that will provide a framework to discuss rehabilitation healing. This framework is expressed in terms of scientific and humanistic health care (Table 18-1).

# SCIENTIFIC AND HUMANISTIC HEALTH CARE

Scientific health care refers to the rapidly expanding and often dazzling body of objective and reproducible knowledge developed using the scientific method. It is empirical, rational, and quantitative and comprises

TABLE 18-1

*Comparison of Scientific and Humanistic Medicine for Selected Health Care Elements*

| Health care elements | Scientific medicine | Humanistic medicine |
|---|---|---|
| *Structure* | | |
| Physical setting | Impersonal | Personal |
| | | |
| *Process* | | |
| Problem orientation | Disease | Illness |
| Physician's role | Doer, knower | Teacher, learner |
| Patient's role | Passive | Active |
| Care orientation | Physical (staff)-oriented | Patient-oriented |
| Physician's relation to patient | Reserved | Empathetic |
| Physician's relation to health team | Dominant | Facilitative |
| Physician's relation to colleagues | Competitive | Collaborative |
| Therapeutic approach | Treatment of disease | Management of illness |
| *Outcome* | | |
| Objectives | Enhancing physiological function | Enhancing functional performance |

Modified from Halstead LS, Halstead MG: *Arch Phys Med Rehabil* 59:53-57, 1978.

the enormous repository of information contained in the basic sciences along with the skills required to apply that information in a clinical setting to diagnose, cure, and prevent pathologic conditions. Historically, scientific health care has come into its own over the past century and is the dominant force in American medicine today.

Humanistic health care, by contrast, refers to the broad accumulation of human experience and knowledge that has evolved over the centuries in each culture and in the life events of each individual.[3] It is subjective, intuitive, and empathetic and encompasses all the skills of personal interaction and caring that have characterized the best tradition of healers in all societies and ages. For most of recorded history, humanistic health care was the dominant force in medicine until the latter part of the 19th century. Since then, it has slowly and steadily given way to scientific medicine until the present, when most health care is perceived as largely scientific. In a sense, then, the pendulum has swung from one extreme to the other.

These variables are divided into three groups using the conceptual framework originally proposed by Donabedian: structural, process, organizational, and outcome.[4] To illustrate what I mean by the terms *scientific* and *humanistic* health care, let us consider two examples. The first is the process variable "Problem Orientation." The general orientation of scientific health care is toward *disease,* whereas humanistic health care is toward *illness.* Disease is defined as the interaction of a pathologic process with individual molecules, cells, and organs. It is essentially a *biologic* event. Illness, on the other hand, is essentially a *human* event. It represents the resulting interaction of a person with a disease.

The second example is the outcome variable "Objectives." Scientific health care is generally concerned with *curing* disease and enhancing *physiological* function, whereas humanistic health care is focused on *healing* the person and enhancing *functional* performance. Curing is defined as removing or reversing a disease process, whereas healing is defined as decreasing discomfort and enhancing a sense of physical and psychological well-being. For both patient and staff, healing is more *active,* whereas curing is more *passive.* Healing does not exclude curing but extends beyond it to include *caring.*

It is important to stress that nothing I have said implies a value judgment. In fact, both the scientific and humanistic components in medicine are essential for good health care and both are necessary in a system that acknowledges the strengths and limitations of each. Although professionals in any specialty can practice a blend of humanistic and scientific medicine, rehabilitation as a field is uniquely suited to achieving this balance. From its inception, the philosophy of rehabilitation has been strongly oriented toward the humanistic approach while developing an ever-expanding scientific and research base.

## HUMANISM IN REHABILITATION MEDICINE

With this model in mind, I want to turn next to a discussion of the humanistic qualities I believe are an intrinsic part of rehabilitation healing—qualities that emerge from the kind of catastrophic patient problems we often deal with and the range of responses they evoke from caregivers, both emotional and behavioral.

Table 18-2 outlines three aspects of the healing process that can occur in an acute rehabilitation setting: "What Happens to the Patient," "What the Patient Experiences and Feels," and "What the Caregiver Feels and Does." Under "What Happens to the Patient," I have listed four potential responses to a devastating illness or injury. Starting with "Physical and Psychological Loss," there is sometimes a loss of one or more limbs, as with a man who is a quadruple amputee. Sometimes there are losses that are not physical but you know are there, as with a man with tetraplegia who is unable to stand and walk or stop the flow of his urine.

What do these patients experience and feel? To begin with, there is a significant alteration in body image, in one's sense of self. So much of who we are is determined by our physical body, the way it looks and feels and works without the slightest thought—especially when young. And then all that is transformed in an instant—an auto accident, a fall, a fire—and we are changed forever. Self-esteem plummets, and for a time we may feel worthless, broken, and beyond repair.

What do the caregivers feel and do? Fortunately, what we do (or I should say what the nurses, the nurse technicians, the aides, and the therapists do, for they provide the great majority of acute rehabilitation care) is fairly well prescribed. They turn the patients, give them food and slack their thirst, exercise their limbs, and wash their feet. This is at one level. At another level, however, they are tending to a wounded human, a person whose feelings of self-worth are shattered. By tending to these wounds, the caregiver comes to know at some level a sense of his or her own loss, grief, and sorrow.

It is this knowing and understanding that empowers and leads to the thousands of undocumented, selfless acts of caring and compassion. From experience, caregivers know where the hurt places are; they can ask questions without prying because they know what the patient's concerns are. From experience, they

TABLE 18-2

## Catastrophic Illness and the Dynamics of a Healing Environment

| What happens to the patient | What the patient experiences and feels | What the caregiver feels and does |
| --- | --- | --- |
| Physical and psychological loss (paralysis, amputation, loss of function) | Changes in body image | Empathy, sorrow, compassion |
| | Diminished self-esteem | Attends to bodily needs |
| | Worthlessness | Validates the whole person inside the "broken" body |
| Physical and psychological pain | Sense of suffering, isolation | Caregiver as witness |
| | Grief, despair | Decreases isolation |
| Loss of autonomy, self-actualization (increased dependence) | Helplessness, depression, anger | Teaches information, skills, training |
| | Changes in roles (family, career, community) | Specific tasks, progress, goals |
| | Past becomes more important | |
| | Future, dreams uncertain | |
| Moral and spiritual pain | Hopelessness, guilt, shame | Provides nonjudgmental adult |
| | Challenges transcendental self, life of the spirit | Helps connect with other patients: individuals, groups |
| | | Helps integrate mind, body, spirit |

know that in time healing will occur. By their confidence and acceptance they *validate* the person inside the broken body. This is the caregiver as *witness* and allows the patient to say, "If you can accept me, and in all the ways I am wounded, maybe, just maybe, I can accept myself."

What else happens to the patient? As outlined in Table 18-2, there is pain—both physical and psychological—that is almost palpable in a little girl who has lost both arms because she touched a high-tension wire. For most of us, comprehending her sense of physical loss and devastating change in body image is impossible; and if that is beyond our reach, who can understand her emotional pain and her isolation and despair, which one imagines is without measure? Although this girl's loss is hardly typical of what we deal with in most acute rehabilitation settings, it still would be difficult to say whose grief is more, whose suffering runs deeper. Consider a 26-year-old tetraplegic father of three, hit by a drunken driver. He has his arms but cannot tie the bow in his daughter's hair. He has his legs but cannot move his toes. There is no convenient scale of grief, no way, in Reynolds Price's phrase, to measure "the bottomless

mystery of suffering."[5] All of us feel we have suffered in one way or another, and haven't there been times when you felt your suffering was the worst of all?

How does the caregiver respond to this kind of pain? It is hard to answer such a question. I know of no studies that address this issue, only anecdotes and our own experience. Surely there are moments for all of us, however fleeting, when we are overwhelmed by powerful emotions such as hate, frustration, and bitterness, emotions that are often seen as negative but are part of a defense that allows us to cope with our own fears, our own black nights, our own mortality. For an instant, we are in that bed, reclined in that "Tilt-in-Space" wheelchair. I would contend that the best caregivers among us experience at some level, even if only subconsciously, the other person's grief. When this happens, there is the potential for our compassion to rise to the level of the other's suffering.

By the nature of what takes place in an acute rehabilitation environment, day in and day out, from morning to night, it is inevitable that the physical isolation is diminished. Patients have a schedule to follow. They have to get up and get dressed. They have to move from their hospital room to the therapy areas.

Rehabilitation is a *physical* process. There is a lot of touching and body contact. As a society, we do not indulge in hugs very often, but there is a lot of power in the hug from a parent, spouse, or friend. When a nurse helps someone sit up in a wheelchair or a therapist massages someone's back—all that touching is a kind of hug. There is a tactile warmth, a feeling of the caregiver's energy as his or her hands work the patient's body; there is a person-to-person contact that momentarily, at least, breaks through the isolation and transfers energy from one to the other.

I know I felt this when I was recovering from polio years ago and a nurse would wash my face or a therapist would massage and stretch my legs. This kind of touching does not happen just once but countless times throughout the day. When you think of the professionals on the rehabilitation team—many of them are young and healthy, vibrant with energy with a "can-do," optimistic attitude and no shortage of smiles—is it any wonder that patients often come back from therapy with a smile themselves and say they feel better?

In addition to the touching and body contact, caregivers do a lot of listening: listening to the grief, anguish, and confusion, listening to all the voices that cry out from the dark night of the soul. Sometimes caregivers listen without responding, knowing that just talking can be therapeutic, and just listening is a way of affirming that what a patient is feeling is understandable, normal, and natural. The patient can ask the same questions, have the same doubts, tell her story a hundred times and spread out her grief in a thousand ways. She will talk to everyone on her team and others as well, professionals with MSWs and PhDs, the people who bring the food and clean the toilets, or other patients and their families. They are all part of the healing community, and each contact has the potential for a therapeutic lift: older people, young people, people of the same or different ethnic group or socioeconomic class. It is an extraordinary mix and all part of the power and magic of rehabilitation healing. Is it any wonder that it is hard to study, hard to prove how it works or that it works at all?

What else does the patient experience? Many persons with severe neurotrauma experience a loss of autonomy and a dramatic, unimagined increase in physical dependence on others: suddenly one is unable to bring food to the mouth, clean the loins, and avoid soiling the sheets. The patient often feels infantilized. In addition, at least during the period of acute recovery, many social roles are lost or changed: in the family, at work, in the community. The past takes on a disproportionately large part of one's life, as if to say, "That's who I once was. That was what I could do. That was the *real* me." Then he shows you pictures of when he was in a football uniform or a wedding tuxedo or on graduation day: all smiles, and health was a never-ending sunny day. Now that future, those dreams are uncertain—possibly gone forever.

What is the caregiver's response? It is impossible not to feel some anger, some resentment, and some depression ourselves: "Why did he do that? Why wasn't she more careful? Look at the work it means for me! I have my own worries, my own problems, my own burdens to carry. Who cares about me?" We would not be human if we did not feel these and other strong emotions. I would argue that to be compassionate we must be able to recognize and respond to our own feelings of loss and suffering as well as the patient's. In this way, the caregiver moves from feeling to action: from caring *about* to caring *for*.

Because there is a formal program with a set of learning expectations, the patient becomes a student. Monday morning he or she learns how to recognize urinary tract infections; Wednesday afternoon he or she is taught wheelchair transfers; Thursday morning there is a class on sexuality; Friday afternoon a trip downtown to buy a shirt in a clothing store. The patient is learning new information, practicing new skills, and strengthening muscles to achieve specific tasks. Goals are set. Sometimes they are micro-goals like eating one bite of food at dinner or learning how to teach someone to turn herself in bed; but they are goals that convey a forceful message: you are making progress, you are moving forward, you are less dependent, more autonomous. It is an accumulation of power: knowledge as power, strength as power, independence as power. Of course it is never enough, everyone wants more; unfortunately, it is rare to restore someone to how he or she appeared in his or her wedding picture.

The fourth response in Table 18-2 under "What Happens to the Patient" concerns a patient's moral and spiritual pain. Many excellent resources exist that discuss this and related issues.[5-10] However, readers of this chapter know as well as I that there are no easy answers in this realm of patient care. Patient responses vary depending on numerous factors: age, life experience, family support, and ethnic and religious background, to name a few. Regardless of upbringing, most undoubtedly feel, at some stage in their recovery, a sense of hopelessness, that nothing can be done. Perhaps this is mixed with a feeling of guilt or shame for transgressions, real or imagined. I know when I contracted polio at the age of 18 and was lying in an iron lung, I kept asking myself, " Why me? Why did this happen to me?" All my Judeo-Christian conscience could fathom was that I had lusted in my heart. For most, such feelings are deep inside us and not easily verbalized to others much less ourselves. Yet these questions penetrate to the very core of who we are. In Eric Cassell's phrase, these issues challenge "the transcendent self," the life of the spirit.[10]

What does the caregiver feel and do? This aspect of the patient's suffering is undoubtedly the most challenging for the caregiver. She must be in touch with her own spirituality and her own transcendence. And with that understanding take an inward journey, as it were, that leads to compassion. As with the patient, the caregiver's response to this kind of challenge, this crisis of the spirit will vary depending on her age, her life experience, and her ethnic and religious background. In the best tradition of medical practice, the response is nonjudgmental. Even if we are dealing with a gunshot victim, wounded by a drug dealer in the midst of a robbery, our response is not to a criminal but to a human being whose life is now in our hands. Perhaps for the first time in his chaotic life on the streets, he is surrounded by adults who have no hidden agenda nor wish to harm. Rather, they are mature, knowledgeable professionals who have chosen this specialty and elected to be at his bedside, seeking to ease his pain and sorrow, to identify his strengths, to find ways to rebuild his life and restore his dignity.

Not everyone responds to these opportunities in the same way. We have all witnessed individuals for whom rehabilitation can be a life-enhancing, even life-transforming experience. For some this occurs early in the process; for others it comes later, maybe years later; for others, never. However, everyone is offered an extended hand that says in effect, "We want to work with you—not just to get the pain under control or teach you to transfer independently—but to help heal *all* the parts of you that have been injured and bleed." In this sense, of all the specialties, rehabilitation attempts, however imperfectly, to deal with the whole person: the physical, the emotional, the social, and the spiritual, although we do not do nearly as much as we might in ministering to the life of the spirit.[11]

## IS THERE A SCIENTIFIC BASIS FOR REHABILITATION HEALING?

I began this presentation with a discussion of the scientific-humanistic model of health care and how in the rehabilitation setting the humanistic interactions between patients and caregivers help create a healing environment. Now I would like to return to the scientific-humanistic paradigm and address a question I believe is especially relevant to this audience: "Is there a scientific basis for some of the humanistic elements of rehabilitation healing?"

A review of the literature over the past 25 years reveals many anecdotes and philosophical discussions. Only in recent years has there been a serious attempt to use scientific methods to explore humanistic elements or what is now called *complementary and alternative medicine*. Table 18-3 summarizes seven articles that illustrate examples of research-based interventions with potential for enhancing outcomes in traditional rehabilitation populations. These studies cover a broad spectrum of diagnoses and therapies but provide only a small glimpse into what might be applied to our clients. As you will see, they range from fairly traditional research interventions to the "outer edge of the envelope" of alternative medicine.

The first article describes a study I and others did back in the mid-1980s.[12] Our goal was to look at the behavioral impact on individuals with spinal cord injury (SCI) and team members using a team conference format that deliberately made the conference client-centered. Rather than the traditional medical model illustrated in Figure 18-1, with the subject lying passively in bed and team members standing around the bedside talking primarily to each other, we had the participant dressed, sitting at the table, and actively engaged as a member of the team (Figure 18-2).

One team experienced this intervention for 18 months with two control teams. Baseline recordings were made before the study and then during and after the intervention. Verbatim transcripts of all conferences were scored by blinded evaluators and a Group Environmental Scale (GES) was used to assess clients' and team members' subjective feelings about different aspects of the team conference experience. As shown under results, there was increased participation by individuals with SCI and decreased participation and domination of the agenda by the staff during team

TABLE 18-3

## Research-Based Interventions With Potential for Enhancing Rehabilitation Healing

| Intervention | Research design | Results |
| --- | --- | --- |
| Patient-centered team care × 18 mo (patients with SCI)[13] | Intervention team, 2 control teams, verbatim transcripts; GES baseline; 20-mo FU | Rx team: increase team conference participation by patients and 20-mo FU decrease by staff; improved staff GES rating and patient satisfaction with team care |
| Health promotion to modify risk factors in patients with stroke during comprehensive rehabilitation[14] | 105 consecutive patients in FU: asked to demonstrate knowledge/awareness of goals | 68%-91% knew blood pressure, cholesterol, blood glucose, medication goals |
| Acupuncture treatment in 41 patients with subacute stroke[15] | Randomized Rx vs control groups; Acupuncture 30 min × 3-4 wk × 6 wk | Rx group: increase in ADLs, motor scores, QOL scale at 1 yr |
| Massage therapy in 20 patients with juvenile rheumatoid arthritis[16] | Randomized groups: massage vs. relaxation 15 min/day × 30 days | Decrease in pain, anxiety, cortisol levels postmassage therapy |
| Supportive group therapy in 86 patients with metastatic breast cancer[17] | Random assignment to weekly support groups or control groups × 1 yr | Rx groups: mean survival time doubled at 10 yr |
| Transcendental meditation in 21 patients with coronary artery disease[18] | Single-blind, randomized transcendental meditation group 20 min/day × 7.6 mo | Rx group: increase in exercise tolerance, maximum workload and cardiac function on stress testing |
| Distant healing in 40 patients with AIDS[19] | Double-blind, randomized distant healing vs. control group × 6 mo | Rx group: fewer/less severe AIDS complications, fever, doctor visits, hospitalizations: CD4 counts unchanged |

*ADLs,* Activities of daily living; *CD4,* HIV helper cell; *FU,* follow-up; *QOL,* quality of life; *Rx,* treatment.

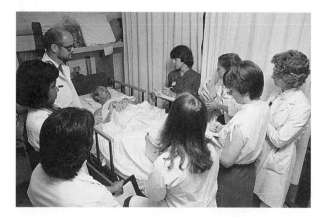

*Figure 18-1*  Traditional medical team visiting a hospitalized patient.

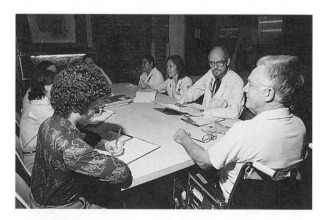

*Figure 18-2*  Meeting between medical team and patient around a table instead of in a hospital room.

conferences. There was significant improvement in GES ratings and increased satisfaction by the clients and staff with team conferences compared with the control groups.

In response to the question, "What does this have to do with compassion and caring?" I would answer that team conferences are at the heart of an inpatient rehabilitation program. It is the one time each week when the team gets together with the client to review progress, problems, and goals. By making the conference deliberately client-centered and client-focused, this group of six, eight, or 10 professionals communicates collectively and individually their concern for how that individual is doing. For the duration of that conference, their time, energy, and expertise are focused on nothing else but that person—his or her concerns, complaints, and progress. It is an example of "team caring" and can be a powerful experience that helps reinforce other caring activities throughout the week.

The second study was conducted by Ozer, Materson, and Caplan, who implemented a health promotion program for stroke victims during comprehensive rehabilitation.[14] The intervention consisted of education regarding risk factors and risk-factor modification among persons with strokes and their families to help prevent a second stroke. The results for a group of 105 individuals at the time of follow-up showed that between 78% to 90% knew what their blood pressure, cholesterol, and medication goals were. The unspoken message was of staff caring and personal empowerment: We care enough about you and your health that we want you to know how to change your behaviors so you can reduce the risk of more disability or even death.

The third article by Kjendahl et al reviews the effects of acupuncture in a group of individuals with subacute stroke in a traditional rehabilitation setting.[15] Patients were randomized into treatment and control groups, and acupuncture was performed according to the schedule described in Table 18-3. Follow-up of the treatment group at 1 year revealed a significant improvement in activities of daily living and motor and quality-of-life scores compared with the control group.

The next studies (the fourth through sixth articles in Table 18-3) describe three preliminary reports in outpatients using interventions that, depending on your perspective, nudge the "envelope" even further.

For example, massage therapy was provided in a research project to individuals with juvenile rheumatoid arthritis.[16] Twenty children were randomly assigned to receive either massage or relaxation therapies for 30 days. The results demonstrated a significant decrease in pain, anxiety, and cortisol levels in the massage group compared with the control subjects. The other two investigations assessed the effect of group therapy in 86 women with metastatic breast cancer and transcendental meditation in 21 individuals with coronary artery disease.[17,18] Despite limitations of sample size, duration of treatment, and other factors, the research designs in all three of these studies used traditional scientific methodologies to assess the effectiveness of each intervention. As summarized in Table 18-3, the results demonstrated positive outcomes for all treatment groups. Although each study is provocative in its own way, the serendipitous finding in the breast cancer report (discovered only in retrospect) is simultaneously breathtaking and humbling: women randomly assigned to weekly support groups for 1 year survived, on average, *twice* as long as members of the control group 10 years after the intervention. Although none of these three studies was in a rehabilitation setting, I do not believe it requires undue optimism to foresee researchers using any or all of these modalities in groups of traditional rehabilitation patients, or even, for that matter, among staff members to help them cope with stress and the daily challenges of providing compassionate rehabilitation care.

If you believe massage therapy, support groups, and transcendental meditation are esoteric, wait until you hear about the seventh article in Table 18-3. This article concerns what is known as *distant healing (DH)*, which in effect is prayer.[19] In this study, prayer was offered up by ministers and other religious persons without the individuals' knowledge in a double-blind, randomized group of 40 AIDS patients over 6 months. The results demonstrated that the treatment group had fewer AIDS complications, complications were less severe, and there was less fever and fewer doctor visits and hospitalizations.

In addition to this report, numerous other studies have looked at the effects of distant healing. A critical review of this literature published last year in the *Annals of Internal Medicine* evaluated 23 studies that met strict scientific criteria.[20] Of these, 57% demonstrated a positive treatment effect.

Whatever you think about these studies and distant healing, my own view is that we all have a spiritual self and a spiritual life, regardless of our affiliation with organized religion, and that we do not pay enough attention to this aspect of our patients when they are going through the worst crisis of their lives.

## RESEARCH CHALLENGES AND CONCLUSIONS

I have already discussed several research challenges for the future. I would like to end by mentioning a few more, along with some general observations and recommendations:

1.  Find ways to increase our involvement with each patient in terms of the life of the spirit. One concrete way would be to include the chaplain or spiritual adviser on a regular basis in team conferences. Although it does not always happen, this is now a requirement of the Joint Commission on Accreditation of Healthcare Organizations (JCAHO).
2.  A recent article described the impact on the staff who work in an Intensive Care Unit entitled, "The Phenomenon of Compassion Fatigue in Perioperative Nursing."[21] I have not talked about this problem, but my guess is that "compassion fatigue" is a common phenomenon in rehabilitation settings too—particularly among nurses and nurse's aides. We should pay more attention to this phenomenon and learn how to recognize it and how to develop strategies to prevent and treat it.

    Many hospitals have chapels for patients and staff. A recent informal survey at our hospital found that 8 out of 10 personnel either did not know there was a chapel or know where it was located. Few had used it. The majority also believed the chapel was reserved for the exclusive use of patients and their families. I doubt these are unique findings. With this in mind, I believe we should develop programs to encourage the staff to use this resource more frequently for meditation, prayer, or just quiet time. In addition to coffee breaks, hospital administrations could promote "meditation breaks." Another recommendation is to set aside space as a staff "recovery" room. This would be a place where personnel could lie down for a few minutes, listen to quiet music, and perhaps get a massage from other staff on a volunteer basis.

3.  Increase research efforts into the application of complementary and alternative health care in various rehabilitation settings. Specifically, we need to identify what types of alternative therapies are effective and for what kind of problems.[22-27] It is encouraging that there are currently a number of Institutes or Centers of Complimentary and Alternative Medicine connected with traditional departments of physical medicine and rehabilitation. This new area appears to be already evolving as a subspecialty within our field and perhaps could be the topic of workshops, instructional courses, or even the theme of an entire conference in future meetings of the Congress. In October 1999, Spaulding Rehabilitation Hospital in Boston and Harvard Medical School sponsored a 2-day conference on Complementary and Alternative Medicine in Rehabilitation.

    In our urgent desire to prove to ourselves and third-party payers that rehabilitation works and is a good investment, I have no concern that the scientific side of rehabilitation will continue to prosper and grow. However, I am worried about the humanistic side. No health maintenance organization (HMO) I know of has ever called to complain that their patients were not getting enough humanistic care. One way of ensuring that they do is to place a higher priority on research studies that use some of the treatments discussed today and are listed in Table 18-3. It is a curious but hopeful irony that in this age of scientific medicine there is now a movement, however small, to use scien-

### Resources

The George Washington Institute for Spirituality and Health
www.gwish.org

Duke University Center for the Study of Aging and Human Development
www.geri.duke.edu

International Center for the Integration of Health and Spirituality
www.nihr.org

Dharma Haven
www.dharma-haven.org

tific methods to demonstrate that humanistic treatments might improve outcomes. Perhaps this will be the next frontier for rehabilitation medicine in this new century. In closing, I would like to say in response to Dr. Gans and his 1983 article, "Yes, there is hate in rehabilitation settings but there is also an abundance of compassion, caring and, dare I say it, even love."

## References

1. Gans JS: Hate in the rehabilitation setting, *Arch Phys Med Rehabil* 64:176-179, 1983.
2. Mullins LL: Hate revisited: power, envy, and greed in the rehabilitation setting, *Arch Phys Med Rehabil* 70:740-744, 1989.
3. Halstead LS, Halstead MG: Chronic illness and humanism: rehabilitation as a model for teaching humanistic and scientific health care, *Arch Phys Med Rehabil* 59:53-57, 1978.
4. Donabedian A: Evaluating the quality of medical care, *Milbank Q* 44:166-203, 1966.
5. Price R: *Letter to a man in the fire: does God exist and does He care?* New York, 1999, Scribner.
6. Campo R: *The poetry of healing,* New York, 1997, WW Norton.
7. Spiro H: *The power of hope,* New Haven, Conn, 1998, Yale University Press.
8. Siegel BS: *Love, medicine, and miracles,* New York, 1990, HarperCollins.
9. Scofield GR: Ethical considerations in rehabilitation medicine, *Arch Phys Med Rehabil* 74:341-346, 1993.
10. Dossey L: *Healing words,* New York, 1993, HarperCollins.
11. Cassell EJ: *The nature of suffering and the goals of medicine,* New York, 1991, Oxford University Press.
12. Anderson JM, Anderson LJ, Felsenthal G: Pastoral needs and support within an inpatient rehabilitation unit, *Arch Phys Med Rehabil* 74:574-578, 1993.
13. Halstead LS, Rintala DH, Kanellos M, et al: The innovative rehabilitation team: an experiment in team building, *Arch Phys Med Rehabil* 67:357-361, 1986.
14. Ozer MN, Materson RS, Caplan RL: *Management of persons with stroke,* St Louis, 1994, Mosby-Year Book.
15. Kjendahl A, Sallstrom S, Osten PE, et al: A one-year follow-up study on the effects of acupuncture in the treatment of stroke patients in the subacute stage: a randomized, controlled study, *Clin Rehabil* 11:192-200, 1997.
16. Field T, Hernandez-Reif M, Seligman S, et al: Juvenile rheumatoid arthritis: benefits from massage therapy, *J Pediatr Psychol* 22:607-617, 1997.
17. Spiegel D, Bloom JR, Kraemer HC, et al: Effect of psychosocial treatment on survival of patients with metastatic breast cancer, *Lancet* 10:888-891, 1989.
18. Zamarra JW, Schneider RH, Basseghini I, et al: Usefulness of the transcendental meditation program in the treatment of patients with coronary artery disease, *Am J Cardiol* 77:867-870, 1996.
19. Sicher F, Targ E, Moore D, et al: A randomized, double-blind study of the effect of distant healing in a population with advanced AIDS, *West J Med* 169:356-363, 1998.
20. Astin JA, Harkness E, Ernst E: The efficacy of "distant healing": a systematic review of randomized trials, *Ann Intern Med* 132:903-910, 2000.
21. Schwam K: The phenomenon of compassion fatigue in perioperative nursing, *AORN J* 68:642-645, 1998.
22. Luskin FM, Newell KA, Griffith M, et al: A review of mind/body therapies in the treatment of musculoskeletal disorders with implications for the elderly, *Altern Ther* 6:46-56, 2000.
23. Fridlund B, Pihlgren C, Wannestig LB: A supportive-educative caring rehabilitation programme: improvements of physical health after myocardial infarction, *J Clin Nurs* 1:141-146, 1992.
24. Ornish D: *Love and survival,* New York, 1998, Harper-Collins.
25. Faughnan JG, Lagace EA: Science and the alternative, *J Fam Pract* 47:262-263, 1998 (editorial).
26. Benson H: *Timeless healing,* New York, 1996, Simon and Schuster.
27. Wood JD: Compassion 101, *Am J Hosp Pall Care* 1997:10-11, 1997.

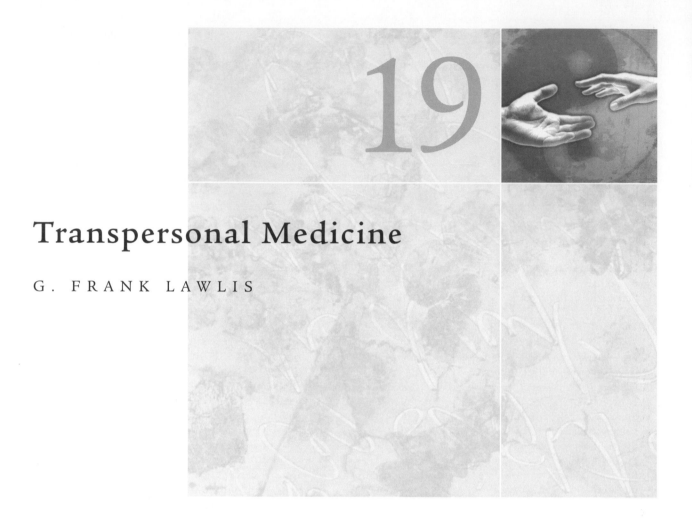

# Transpersonal Medicine

## G. FRANK LAWLIS

## HISTORICAL BACKGROUND

The history of Western psychology is often divided into four phases or forces: (1) Watson's behaviorism; (2) Freud's psychoanalysis; (3) Roger's self theory; and (4) the outgrowth of Maslow's work, now called transpersonal psychology. The current era of psychology is the result of the acknowledgement that there are more forces of influence on a person's consciousness than those considered totally bounded within any single brain. The evidence clearly supports the principle that we receive wisdom from sources other than purely environmental learning or insight into our own experience.

The term *Transpersonal Medicine* was coined to bridge two major concepts: *transpersonal*—beyond the self, and *medicine*—to make well. The underlying prin-

ciple of Transpersonal Medicine is that power from a source beyond the self or beyond what we consider consensual reality is available, and this power can be called upon to help heal ourselves and others. *Trans* denotes not only "beyond" (as in "transcendental") but also "across" (as in "transfer"). It implies change or action. The three aspects of transpersonal process: the *cross-personal*, the *extra-personal*, and the *beyond-personal*, as well as the *ever-changing-personal*, are all encompassed in the approach of Transpersonal Medicine.[1] In a larger sense, Transpersonal Medicine can be seen as an important outgrowth of the new consciousness evolving throughout the world, with its renewed respect for ancient methods that allow us to draw on broader realms of wisdom than the merely personal. Examples of these broader realms can be seen in all spiritual traditions of healing, which universally acknowledge that there are three general paths to wholeness: love, wisdom, and power. *Love* is how we transform each other and ourselves. It is what bonds our relationships. *Wisdom* is the path of learning that which is beyond knowledge and intelligence. It is the insight that sees the inner connection among all aspects of existence. *Power* is not power over others but rather the power to bring forth energy from oneself and others. Power has the potential for transforming every level of our being.

Spiritual traditions have been considered major contributors to the healing professions for generations. For example, the Christian teachings embrace healing as a missionary path, and there are several studies verifying the results of prayer and compassionate applications of spiritual counseling. Dr. Larry Dossey[2] has written extensively about the validity of prayer for health benefits, and he has intimated that the weight of the evidence is so strong that if a healthcare professional does not pray for his or her patients, it might be considered malpractice.

# DEVELOPMENT OF REHABILITATION

The work of Dr. Howard Rusk brought much visibility to the field of rehabilitation. His work with World War II veterans, as well as polio patients, led to the establishment of the medical specialty of physiatry. Visibility for the field of rehabilitation was also heightened by the passage by Congress of several bills to support rehabilitation efforts in the areas of mental retardation, cardiovascular disease, and limb reconstruction, among others.

Dr. Beatrix Cobb guided my entry into the field of vocational rehabilitation. Dr. Cobb led the nation to the recognition of rehabilitation from a psychological point of view, formulating the ingredients for the preparation of professional counselors in this regard. During the 1960s and 1970s there was a tremendous amount of passion and fervor around the development and training of this new professional. The *vocational rehabilitation counselor* was supposed to be a combination nurse, social worker, and psychologist who would have the medical background to understand the extent to which various types of physical and emotional limitations might impede an individual's lifestyle, particularly with regard to vocation. Moreover, this professional would have an in-depth understanding of various treatments and resources that

would enhance the rehabilitation of the individual. Although Dr. Cobb's vision for the field of vocational rehabilitation might not be fully manifested, it is still very clear in the minds of those of us who participated in the early stages with her. It was truly ingenious of Dr. Cobb and her colleagues to establish a fully developed discipline so quickly. To those of us fortunate enough to have been under her mentorship, it is obvious that this field includes the ingredients of mind, body, and spirit in its definition of rehabilitation.

The traditional definition of rehabilitation comes from the architectural concept of reconstructing homes. The intention of rehabilitation after a trauma is to rebuild or reconstruct the individual so that he or she is in as good or better shape as he or she was before the trauma. With this definition in mind, therapists attempt to rebuild limbs or create prosthetics that will enable the individual to function as before. The psychologist attempts to help the individual cope with the crisis. In essence, the individual gains the resources to compensate for the earlier compromise that the trauma created. Although this definition contains the ingredients for the creation of scientific and clinical applications, it falls short of the spirit of rehabilitation from a transpersonal perspective. It lacks the spiritual component that is apparent when one becomes involved with the true process of rehabilitation.

Rehabilitation is defined differently by the shamans of indigenous cultures.[3] I studied with these natural healers over a period of 20 years, and during that time I discovered that when they speak of what we call rehabilitation, they define the process not as the person reaching the same level of functioning as before the trauma but as the person becoming *better, wiser,* and *more spiritual*. I find this definition to be much more satisfying because in my clinical and research experience, individuals who are rehabilitated do in fact become more than they were before the trauma. They get "weller than well." For many cultures a shaman is a person who has survived a severe disease and recovered, thus learning the path of rehabilitation.

It is within this broad definition of rehabilitation that I approached this chapter, in which the dynamics of Transpersonal Medicine are readily applied. Transpersonal Medicine has been practiced for many generations, yet only within the last decade have we begun to acknowledge its practice. This may be largely because the mention of anything other than very concrete influences on healing would be embarrassing to the academic professional. Or perhaps

Transpersonal Medicine would be considered "flaky" and therefore the practitioner might be drummed out of business. It also might mean that we as professionals have been embarrassed. Nevertheless, clients and patients know that Transpersonal Medicine is the essence of rehabilitation.

## MEANINGFULNESS

In Transpersonal Medicine, as it relates to Jung's works, the essence of a person's soul is expressed in the meaningfulness of his or her experience. This is not just a personal perspective. It is an acknowledgement that the individual is not isolated but instead is a part of something larger, thereby giving hope to the individual by focussing on the greater good. The individual has a responsibility not only to himself or herself but also to the community and all of humankind to strive for optimization.

One of the primary lessons that Dr. Beatrix Cobb taught her clients is that it is not the specifics of the trauma that are important in the rehabilitation of an individual but instead it is the meaning the individual assigns to the trauma. In 1978 Dr. Jeanne Achterberg and I developed the Health Attribution Test (HAT).[4] This 22-item questionnaire attempts to measure how much a person believes that various sources are responsible for his or her disease or condition. We developed the HAT as a means to predict how effective rehabilitation efforts would be, especially in the rehabilitation of chronic pain patients.

The HAT measures what a person attributes his or her health to: internal resources, powerful others, or chance/fate. Applied to rehabilitation, the *internal resources scale* measures how much a person believes that his or her behaviors or thoughts affect the outcome of rehabilitation, the *powerful others scale* measures how much a person believes that external sources (powerful others) affect the outcome of rehabilitation (these external sources usually are the patient's doctor, enemies, and God), and the *chance/fate scale* measures how much a person believes that the outcome of his or her rehabilitation is left up to chance or fate ("health roulette"). The chance/fate scale is the most predictive of negative outcome: the greater the score, the more negative the outcome.

The HAT has been used in a variety of studies; however, we have used it primarily as a means of advising the various insurance carriers on the probability of successful rehabilitation for a variety of conditions that require a high level of motivation on the part of the client. We have found that we can predict positive outcome about 50% of the time and negative outcome about 80% of the time.

One thing we have found is that regardless of the type of trauma a person has experienced, if he or she has a very clear sense of having some measure of control, the outcome of rehabilitation is significantly improved. Another finding, which might be somewhat surprising, is that if a person has a tremendous amount of faith in an external source, such as a doctor or therapist, the outcome is also improved, regardless of whether it is a mental or physical condition. Whether the faith is primarily in oneself or in another, there is an underlying sense that the healing source is relevant to the disease and therefore there is hope.

As stated previously, the most significant prediction has to do with the chance factor. If the person has no hope or expectation of getting any help for his or her condition, then there is a very high probability of failure despite rehabilitation. This result relates not only to the psychological level of hope and expectation but also to the imagery of the dysfunction. In other words, if the person does not have images to help him understand the cause of his condition, he will not understand the intention of the therapeutic approach or his responsibility as patient. The clinical outcome is likely to be dismal at best, and the long-term effects will definitely become chronic.

The HAT profiles of two patients follow.

*A Case Study*

*Failed Back Syndrome*

"Bob" is a 52-year-old carpenter with a 7-year history of back pain. His medical evaluation revealed severe scarring of the tissues emerging from L4/L5 and L5/S1. The scar tissue apparently resulted from two earlier surgical interventions. Bob's HAT profile is shown in Figure 19-1. Bob's *internal* scale score of 8 is high, his *powerful others* score of 5 is average, and his *chance* score of 3 is below average (mean = 5.5; standard deviation = 2).

During our discussions, Bob described intense pain and depression. He also exhibited a high degree of insight and intelligence. He constantly requested articles and books that might explain his chronic pain syndrome and

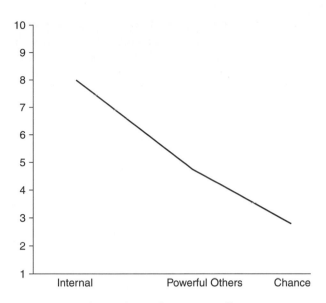

*Figure 19-1* Bob's HAT profile.

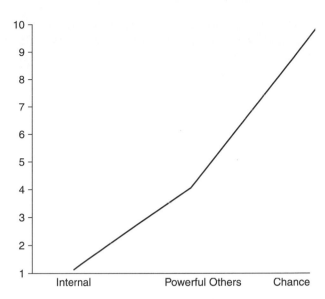

*Figure 19-2* Francis' HAT profile.

help him understand why he was experiencing it. After approximately 10 days of therapy, Bob concluded that this pain emanated from a chronic imbalance of his muscles. He also concluded that this imbalance of his muscles emanated from an imbalance of his emotions. His life story spoke of long-term stress as a result of feeling overworked and overburdened with responsibilities. He revealed that he has had many bouts with depression as a result of some early family history. In essence, he felt that the chronic pain began as a function of the imbalance of his life. More importantly, he concluded that he could reverse his condition by creating more balance in his life and consequently his muscle system. Bob was exemplary in terms of his efforts to improve his health and left the clinic with moderate pain syndrome that on follow-up of 1 year had become very mild and did not interfere with his ability to function. ❧

The following is an example of a person with a lower level of insight or meaningfulness attribution.

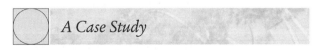

### A Case Study

#### Chronic Low Back Pain

"Francis" is a 53-year-old psychiatrist who came into the clinic with a condition resulting from an injury that occurred 5 years ago while she was lifting furniture. This injury involved the L4/L5 area. No medical interventions had been conducted because there were no significant

pathological findings to the internal bone structure; however, it was felt that she did have symptoms of nerve compromise. In her visit to the pain clinic, Francis did not have any intention of finding an explanation for her pain. All she could say was, "I hurt, and I want somebody to take care of this pain. The doctors are worthless and I feel like that I should be getting better treatment than I have." Her HAT profile is presented in Figure 19-2 and shows the scale scores of *internal* = 1, *powerful others* = 4, and *chance* = 10.

In her rehabilitation efforts, Francis made no effort to understand her condition and continued see it in terms of functionality. She felt that she could not perform any kind of work either in the home or in the competitive workplace. She felt that treatment made her pain worse. The benefit of the therapy was considered to be nonexistent, but the tragedy is that Francis felt that her entire rehabilitation experience was a waste of time. ❧

These two cases illustrate very clearly that unless patients can attribute some meaning to their experience, it is unlikely that they will benefit from rehabilitation. As a clinical practitioner in the field, I consider it mandatory that patients find some sort of positive meaningfulness, a personal reason for their disease or pain. Chronic pain is significant in the rehabilitation field in that the patients often have to endure more pain before they feel a lessening of the pain.

One of the major benefits of exercise is the alleviation of depression. However, to reap any benefits from exercise one has to extend oneself energetically, and this initially creates more pain and discomfort. For a person to be able to endure the road to rehabilitation, he or she must find some deeper meaning in the process.

Most of my clinical stories of success are really stories of transcendence and the breaking down of barriers between a person's premorbid self and postmorbid reality. There are many stories in which the patient has far exceeded his or her own expectations in terms of vocational success as well as relationship success. Many patients have found new and more satisfying careers. Many patients have found much more loving relationships. In fact, 90% of my patients who have achieved successful rehabilitation admit that their particular trauma might be the best thing that could have happened to them. The differences between the HAT profiles of successfully rehabilitated patients (60% of my patients) and those not successfully rehabilitated are striking. Successful patients show higher scores on internal resources and lower scores on fate/chance attributions.

## THE USE OF RITUAL IN TRANSPERSONAL MEDICINE

At its foundation, Transpersonal Medicine draws on another ancient healing source: ritual. According to Jeanne Achterberg, ritual is "the universal foundation for all Transpersonal Medicine."[5] The true essence of ritual is the empowerment of the individual through the personal and collective use of symbols. A young man undergoes the rite of passage into adulthood in the bar mitzvah; a wedding ceremony or a graduation exercise grants a person new privileges and status. There are familiar rituals that mark turning points in people's lives, the *trans-process*. In each ritual there is some homage paid to the power greater than the individual, be it humanity or a spiritual power. In these rituals the individual is given the hope and dream of success, or the grace of love and forgiveness. A ritual articulates the ongoing connection between an individual and the universal. During ritual the person knows that he or she is part of the fiber of life, a component and recipient of the love of God or supreme consciousness. The ritual serves as a reminder that everything and everyone has meaning.

Ritual is often seen as an unconscious act of consistent behaviors, such as shaving or brushing one's teeth. In reality, this is the opposite of the true definition. A ritual is a prescribed set of events and behaviors that have significant symbolism to the individual performing them, as well as to any other persons who are participating in that particular ritual. Rituals bring about extended meaningfulness to people's lives; they also empower people. There is definite evidence that through the practice of rituals there is an elevation in self-esteem and at the same time a relaxation of the sense of stress and disconnectedness.[1]

Whenever human beings gather together to ward off danger, to worship, or to acknowledge major changes, they develop rituals. These rituals honor life transitions and passages, providing form, substance, and guidance in their lives. They often prescribe behavioral methods of dealing with important physical, social, and mental changes. Without rituals we have no map for how to act, no occasion for people to share their common bonds and experiences.[1]

In 1984 I began to explore shamanic ritual as a process for promoting change and personal growth that embraced a belief in a higher truth, i.e., a truth beyond our individual egos and personalities. I did this exploration because our psychological treatment for chronic pain, primarily counseling and psychotherapy, simply was not working as well as I wanted it to. In the challenge that was offered to me by Dr. Vert Mooney of Southwestern Medical School, I had great license to perform whatever psychological techniques I could to increase the likelihood of rehabilitation for chronic pain patients. My purely psychological techniques simply were inappropriate. For example, my Rogerian approach to counseling left many of my patients puzzled. The attempt at in-depth understanding also met with a great deal of confusion, if not outright disregard and disrespect. I needed something more powerful. I began the pilgrimage of learning from Michael Harner and a variety of other shamans around the world. Shamanic ritual is unique in that it offers ways to integrate spiritual with psychological and physical healing. From my perspective as a psychologist, it seemed that rituals could give shape and meaning to the aspect of human behavior we know as volition or will, from which intention springs. Intention allows us to determine our own path and to change that path when necessary for healing and personal growth.

A recent article in *Science* by House, Landis, and Umberson[6] cited 62 studies that reveal strong supportive documentation that "lack of social support constitutes a risk factor for mortality," and that social relationship protects health and promotes healing.[7] Through the practice of ritual in a social context, intention becomes more tangible. Ritual allows us to step outside of our normal life, which is guided by complex, individualized habits of thinking, feeling, and acting. We can now gain new perspective on what we are doing and how we are living, which allows us to define ways to support changes that we might desire. Because ritual is clearly directed to the inner world, it offers a more holistic approach to human change then analytical methods that attempt to reduce the human experience to a medical or psychological model.

## Spiritual Aspects of Ritual

Another aspect of ritual that appeals to me is that it views change as normal and sees all conflict as lessons on a spiritual, rather than a material, life plane. Within this system, the body is seen not as the be all and end all of our lives; rather, it is a vehicle for the spirit, which is not limited by time and space. A subtle but extremely important aspect of this vision is that spirit is seen as ongoing, not limited to its present form, which is attached to the body or personality. Healing, or working with the change on the individual level, has a higher purpose—to benefit the ongoing spirit of life on earth. Thus all of our struggles and their healing have meaning beyond our individual self, and the purpose of healing has less to do with the adjustment (as we often say in psychological circles) to painful situations.

I have found that there is a higher energy produced when people gather together that can appear to generate a healing as well as a destructive power. If the ritual contains participants who have a genuine positive feeling toward an individual, there is a definite sense and perhaps even a demonstrable power that can influence our healing on the visible and certainly the mental level.

The idea that health can be enhanced by strengthening personal supportive relationships is now widely accepted. William Braud [8] has taken this concept further in studies that suggest that intention, a primary component in ritual, has a direct bearing on health and healing. While this influence may be accounted for in human consciousness models, it cannot be totally accounted for in current scientific models of energy exchange.

I conducted many experiments on the occurrence of physiological changes in individuals from the distant influences of groups. Between 10 and 15 patients admitted for the treatment of cancer care participated in each study group. In each experiment one member of the group was selected as the focus patient. The focus patient would then leave the group and go into a separate room, where he or she was hooked up to biofeedback monitors to measure psychophysiological responses. At random times and unbeknownst to the subject, the prayer group would focus on the patient, sending him or her love and support. At these times the biofeedback devices measured an elevated skin temperature, indicating a physical change in the subject. Subjects reported an increased sense of well being indicating a psychological change.

These experiments and others have objectified clinical perceptions; however, what was not documentable were the number of extraordinary changes that occurred. Extraordinary psychological changes took place and some very remarkable "spontaneous remissions" occurred. For example, one woman's neck bone fractures healed in 1 week in spite of clear documentation of years of nonhealing union. Another woman's leg fracture healed in 3 weeks, although this condition had been a focus of surgery and electrical attempts for 3 years. Tumors dissolved, and healings nothing short of miraculous occurred.

When patients were discharged from the hospital, the exit interview would always request information about what they remembered as being their most positive and most negative experience. Among the successful patients the consistent description of the most important and unforgettable experience was the love they felt from the staff and patient group. When asked to articulate the central elements of the rehabilitation program, 90% could not describe them in concrete terms. Most would discuss some magical moment when they felt a strong wave of love that helped them through the discomfort and discouragement. Some defined it as a spiritual experience while others would relate the feeling of being part of a family where people "really cared." However love is defined, it is at least expressed through some altruistic energy intending the well-being of another person. This evidence is extremely persuasive with regard to the healing power of love within the context of community ritual.

Rituals can create conditions necessary for transformation. Whether transformation is a part of any rehabilitation program, I believe that individuals who can transform themselves and transcend their problems do reach a higher level of rehabilitation. The integration process of transformation is extremely difficult without ritual. To change one's life requires tremendous courage, and to have this change honored and respected by those around one is critical. Much research comparing individual with group psychotherapy supports this conclusion.[9]

Rituals are used to honor a person's transition from one state to another. Without ritual there is no specific time or place that one can pinpoint as initiating the change, and there is no respect given to the person's new role. The lifestyle that enhanced disease state must die for the person to establish a state of harmony and health. For example, the person with the diagnosis of alcoholism must change; however, to change independently within the context of community is difficult because of role expectations. The strength of the habit that the body and mind have created is reinforced by external forces. It is the alcoholic whose life is difficult to change; however, the problem of alcoholism is a community and family problem. The principles underlying the rehabilitation experienced in Alcoholics Anonymous are ritualistic in nature. Rituals for healing have a purpose of giving freedoms and significance to transition; they provide maps of form for guidance during perilous times for minds and spirits that are broken. Rituals allow people to share common experiences and give visible support to one other. The symbols and events of healing rituals cement bonds and engender faith that the passage into the place of wholeness, harmony, or relief from suffering will be achieved.

## ALTERED STATES OF CONSCIOUSNESS

One of the principles of Transpersonal Medicine is the search for wholeness and harmony beyond the rational self. The process of moving into those realms is aided by altered states of consciousness, a major pathway to physical and psychological healing.[10] In general terms, an altered state of consciousness is a state of reality that is separate from our normal, day-to-day reality, defined as a sufficient deviation in subjective or psychological functioning from certain norms for that individual.[11,12] To have hope, there must be a breakage of obstacles to healing and some possibility of wellness. We must dismiss our self-imposed limitations of our daily reality, and when we are in trance, we have that opportunity. In our dreams we can leap tall buildings and heal ourselves by sheer imagination. There are many ways to achieve an altered state of consciousness. One of the most powerful is rhythmic stimulation, such as drumming to a specific rhythm, which stimulates theta brain waves. Powerful music has been shown to be very successful for moving consciousness into new and healing streams of thought. Also, studies have shown that certain meditation techniques can bring about significant results. We have used environmental stimulations, such as tuning beds and vibrational techniques. Our techniques have also included the use of chants and tones to stimulate a person's pain (self-disclosure) and the use of individual music selections.

When I was searching for ways of achieving this level of consciousness for my patients, I personally experienced sensory deprivation in a flotation tank, a large tub totally enclosed in darkness with approximately 18 inches of salt water heated to 95° F. The experience impressed me. The flotation tank helped me to become acutely aware of my body and my thoughts. I reached a deep state of relaxation and experienced a profound sense of peace. After intensely exploring the applications of flotation devices, I began the search for a suitable tank for the hospital.

Having flotation tanks in the hospital was problematic from the start. There were concerns about maintaining hygiene and constant temperature, as well as the wax-dissolving properties of the salt solution on the floors of the hospital. I was always worried about leakage and had to clean up spills from time to time. When I finally decided to abandon the flotation tank model, the hospital engineer became interested in our work and volunteered to help me design a workable apparatus. The result was something of a combination sensory deprivation chamber and waterbed. It finally met the specifications of the hospital, and we began to experiment with its benefits to the patients.

As I had suspected, patients who used this chamber became more relaxed. However, something even more important happened. Patients would be gently and safely introduced to what many of them referred to as a "different world where there was a sense of peace and a total loss of personal boundaries." One patient explained that she "felt God's love" while floating in the chamber. Another patient described the sense that she understood "everything" from her experience. We discovered that some of the patients would often slip into the chamber, sometimes all night, and spend long hours in the peacefulness and the safety of the enclosure without our knowledge. Later it occurred to us that we were providing an environment to induce altered states of consciousness.

The staff and I became very concerned that we might have instigated some form of psychotic behavior, and we were afraid that patients' physical condition would also deteriorate. We were seriously considering disposing of the chamber. However, as it turned out, just the opposite proved to be true, and certain conditions significantly improved. Reports of decreased pain, insomnia, and depression were highly correlated with the use of the chamber. Moreover, patients appeared to make psychological gains. Less depression, more energy, and more insight were evidenced. What symptoms remained, such as pain and tissue damage, became almost a secondary concern to the patients as feelings such as love and peace emerged.

Regardless of our intentions, patient feedback revealed the following results.

1. A feeling of spiritual love
2. A connection to universal community
3. A deeper sense of self
4. A sense of goals beyond personal needs
5. An understanding of problems
6. An understanding of many levels at once
7. A sense of being "real," yet with no boundaries
8. A general frustration with trying to express their experience in words

## OTHER FORCES: TRANSPERSONAL BEINGS

In the transpersonal psychology literature, it is a common occurrence that one is in another level of reality; one needs other beings for guidance and support.[13] These beings can be in the form of a spirit animal, God, Jesus Christ, ancestors, angels, and other entities that are not necessarily of our reality. This phenomenon appears to be mostly beneficial. However, there are some instances in which paranoid schizophrenics tend to view the experiences as extremely harmful and dangerous. Nevertheless, when our patients are in a relatively good psychological state, visits from these entities appear to bring wisdom and comfort.

The presence of these entities appears also to provide very positive motivations for patients. One of the common findings with the flotation chamber was that when a person would spend long periods in that deprivation environment, he or she would get a strong sense of support from the "other side." Some of these visitations were from persons significant to the person, and the relationships seemed to benefit from the experience.

 *A Case Study*

### Chronic Headache

One day I arrived at the clinic and met one of our most intractable patients walking at a very quick pace. She was a 51-year-old secretary who had severe headaches for 10 years. She could not work and her marriage suffered. She was delighted when she met me, and said to me that she had just had a long, wonderful visit with her mother.

When I asked the patient what it was about her mother's visit that seemed to be so helpful, she indicated to me that through her visit her mother had assuaged the patient's sense of guilt for not being with her mother as much as she should have. The mother also told the patient that she had married the right person after all. While she was telling me of this visit, tears came to her eyes and she seemed to be very excited in a positive way. I asked her where her mother was, and she indicated that she had died 5 years earlier.

Being somewhat surprised by this, I inquired how she came to be talking to her mother, expecting to hear a story about a dream visitation. The patient reported that she had spent the night in the isolation chamber and sometime during the night her mother had come to her. They had discussed their relationship all night long. She was eventually able to return to her job as a secretary and appeared to have a greater appreciation for whatever gifts she had at that time. Her pain eventually decreased to zero levels. From all indications, this result continued into the 1-year follow-up. ∾

The presence of other entities may or may not be scientifically proven. However, for many patients these entities do exist, and they exist for the beneficial concern of the patient. The sense of transpersonal community is a major factor in many patients' resolution to overcome their pain and disease. In some cases of terminal cancer patients, these entities appear to be extremely valuable in terms of transitioning into the death process.

Inasmuch as the presence of theses other entities has proven to be very helpful to patients overall, the question arises: "Should we encourage the seeking of support from such 'others'?" This practice has been encouraged by a variety of Native American and Celtic approaches. It has been my feeling that if these entities appear to show support, then certainly I would not discourage the patients from discussing them. However, I have observed that these entities may not have such beneficial effects. In this regard, I have found it necessary from time to time to enter the patient's reality by developing a mutual imagery trance, sometimes with the help of a drum rhythm or music. If I can be in communication with their experience, it is possible to challenge the intentionality of both the person and the entity.

## HUMOR AS TRANSPERSONAL MEDICINE

Some years ago I met with Pete Conchos, spiritual leader of the Taos Pueblo in New Mexico. When I asked him what ingredients go into the healing process, he replied, "Forgiveness and laughter." He then explained that if we do not forgive each other, we are caught in a time trap in the past. Laughter helps us break out of that particular prison and allows us to march forward.

Forgiveness is a primary therapeutic activity with all the patients with whom I have worked. The power of humor has greatly impressed me with its transformative potential. When patients are asked what components of the program were the most significant in their recovery, group support and humor are common responses. "Once I can begin to laugh, my pain starts to recede and I can see life from a different perspective."

From a Transpersonal Medicine perspective, humor is definitely a transpersonal dynamic. Humor shifts one's awareness and realities and meets the sudden change in this perspective with laughter. Although on the surface humor may be incongruous with any given situation, the shift often reduces tension in trying to solve whatever problem the situation presents.[14,15] The change in orientation or interruption of linear logic can reorder the energetic field or response to a broader perceptual field, offering new problem-solving strategies or at least a shift in attitude. Even the language and emotions we use in approaching the problem may change the logical patterns and physio-

logical transformation is changed by laughter; a healthier response to any situation can result.[16]

Humor can evoke a childlike authenticity and a simplification of values, which can be helpful in conflict resolution. For example, the need to "win" an argument or debate may be dissipated as both parties see the humor in their disagreement. That in itself creates a new plane of understanding, reducing fear of loss of self-esteem.

There have been many research efforts to demonstrate that although short lived, the physiological effects of humor can be demonstrated through changes in blood chemistries and breathing patterns.[16] There have also been extensive studies done on the psychological effects of humor, showing reduction of stress and improvement in self-esteem. The literature points to 10 basic contributions of humor, at least in functional methods for conducting a process of any kind of psychological approach.

1. Providing clarification of self-defeating behavior
2. Providing a means to explore new solutions to problems
3. Relieving monotony of ongoing problem solving
4. Shifting conscious of broader perspective from seriousness of fear to courage
5. Interrupting paradoxical or irrational thinking
6. Reducing grandiosity
7. Reducing helplessness
8. Inducing better interpersonal relationships
9. Reducing anxiety stress and its tension
10. Redirecting or reducing hostility and aggression

Using humor is an art. It requires judicious choice of subject, word choice, and method of delivery. It is an important way to teach rational emotions, reinforce self-esteem, share thoughts and creativity, and express joy. With humor we can transcend ordinary reality. The shifting of perception is a natural outcome of having fun.

As elsewhere, in a clinical study humor can be accidental or programmed. However, it is harder to plan humor. The very nature of humor is rooted in surprise. In the clinical setting, a sudden shift in reality may be confusing, and the patient may misunderstand the healthcare worker's efforts. Sensitivity and intelligence are crucial to using humor constructively.

Situations that present opportunities for "accidental" humor are blessings. One example that comes to mind concerns a time when we were experiencing some racial tension in one of our clinics. The patients included two Hispanics and six whites. One white man was very prejudiced and outspoken, which created a definite sense of unease in the group.

One day I was demonstrating the therapeutic use of massage for stress and pain management, with instructions for breathing and relaxation. While I was working on one of the Hispanic women, I put some mild pressure on her back. She passed gas loudly. Silence prevailed for what seemed a very long time, but then she began to laugh. I hugged her and we laughed together. The prejudiced man soon joined us, saying, "We are all human. I can respect that." Soon, the whole group was laughing and shouting, "We are all human, after all." That became the group slogan, and the group became a community.

## Transpersonal Techniques in the Hospital: Cautions

I must warn the enthusiastic practitioner about employing these techniques in the traditional medical setting: all that I do within the realm of transpersonal medicine is set in standardized medical language. It is not that the approaches lack scientific or clinical validation, but they are not usually stated in words and terminology that a traditional healthcare professional would want to hear. It is important to understand medical language and use these terms to ground the methods scientifically. I have found that it is imperative to know the language of neurology, orthopedics, and oncology. If you can express your methods in terms that harmonize with your associates' realities, there are enormous opportunities for the application of Transpersonal Medicine. For example, I remember the first day I carried my drum into the hospital. As I stepped onto the elevator, the hospital administrator and chief of staff entered. This was a rather large brass drum so it was not very easily hidden.

The hospital administrator looked at me and my drum and asked, "Frank, what do you have there under your arm?"

I was not invisible, as I had hoped I would be, so I replied, "This is a new neuroacoustical stimulator. It has a membrane that when applied in the right frequency stimulates the brain into trance rhythms, such as theta, and we suspect that endorphins are released

to relieve pain and depression. A steady administration of this acoustical effect can be very healthful for constructive imagery, perhaps hypnosis. This is a very old concept, but we have had very good results."

The hospital administrator and chief of staff looked at each other for a moment, then the chief of staff said, "I can understand your approach, but it looks like a drum to me."

Rather than become defensive, I replied, "Yes, this could be a special type of drum, but this is used just for entrainment of brainwaves."

The hospital administrator looked concerned, "Does this thing use electricity, and is it safe? Any side effects we need to clear with the committee?"

"No, it is very safe and besides a little noise, there is absolutely no problem. It has been tested thoroughly."

Both of them shrugged as they stepped off the elevator. I heard the administrator say as the doors closed, "If you need any help, let me know."

I want to explain that the administrator and chief of staff were no dummies, but they have their responsibilities to the patients, as well as to the staff. They want to know in their language what I am doing, and they have that right. It is my obligation to use standard terminology so that the methods would be honored.

## SUMMARY

Transpersonal Psychology has been a very critical dimension of therapy in my clinical and research experience. I feel that traditional psychological terminology and therapy process are only relevant to about 10% of the population. The Freudian approach certainly is limited in its prospects, and other approaches also have limited application. Although various new cognitive psychological approaches have been examined in Alcoholics Anonymous, none have been actually applied on a day-to-day basis. However, it is the transpersonal elements discussed in this chapter that are the most profound in this work.

I have learned a great deal about the deeper application of Transpersonal Medicine to my own situation, as well as the situations of my clients. I have rediscovered the power of love and healing, not only for myself, but also for the planet, and I am convinced that this is the major constructive force in our world. Because it is gentle by nature, this force is usually less obvious than aggressive methods, but by its focus on consensual goodness, it is our best hope in redemption of what true living is about. For lack of a better name, the principle underlying this effective love could be called Transpersonal Medicine.

Transpersonal Medicine goes beyond the view of disease as merely a mechanical breakdown of some tissue or biochemical response, containing a time and place. Instead, Transpersonal Medicine looks at disease and the healing process from an entirely different perspective, one that integrates larger emotional and spiritual factors. Disease is the tear in the fabric of an individual's connection with the universe and the community at large. Rather than seeing disease simply as a malfunction of a body part, those involved in the transpersonal process regard disease as an integral part of personal development, an opportunity for growth and transformation.

Disease and health are viewed as lifetime processes. Too often a disease is seen to be contained in a time capsule: "I had measles when I was 4." "I had arthritis when I was 50." Treatment has also been placed in the time capsule: "I will be well in 2 weeks." From a transpersonal perspective of health and disease, time and space are disregarded.

Today's concept of preventive medicine emphasizes denial and self-discipline. Passion and joy are the most preventive emotions in care. The present prevention philosophy operates on the assumption that when we are doing something that promotes disease, everyone has to stop doing it or get sick. But the basic law of behavior is that we behave for a reason. There is a deeper reason for destructive behavior, other than we want to die or become ill. For example, we all know that smoking is correlated with a number of diseases, but there is little recognition that smoking serves as an important coping mechanisms for some people. I am not suggesting that smoking be continued for the sake of coping measures, but I do suggest that if we are going to ask people to stop smoking, we should present them with a better way of coping based on higher needs. Prevention should consist of finding better ways of dealing with the problems of the world, rather than trying to eliminate behaviors that serve some purpose. Two of the best preventive behaviors (and the main therapeutic approach in some cultures) are dancing and singing, which are often related to religious ritual. Successful health spas around the world have built their programs around activities of passion such as music, art, exercise, and writing. Passion's forms can even be diagnostic to unlock healing symbols and energies from the unconscious.

Disease can be equated with the breakdown of the relationship between body, mind, and spirit. Unlike the present medical practice of defining disease in terms of measurable cellular function, the transpersonal approach identifies spiritual and emotional precursors to disease and implants deeper healing as a result. These precursors include internal factors such as loss of connectedness to others; loss of connectedness with a spiritual being; and loss of joy, passion, or hope. Healing comes when the relationship between the body, mind and spirit are repaired.

## References

1. Lawlis F: *Transpersonal medicine,* Boston, 1996, Shambhala.
2. Dossey L: *Healing words,* San Francisco, 1993, Harper.
3. Sankar A: Ritual and dying: a cultural analysis of social support for caregivers, *Gerontologist* 31(1):43-50, 1991.
4. Achterberg J, Lawlis GF: *The health attribution test,* Champaign, Ill, 1989, Institute of Personality and Ability Testing.
5. Achterberg J: Transpersonal medicine: a proposed system of healing, *ReVision* 14:127, 1992.
6. House JS, Landis KR, Umberson D: Social relationships and health, *Science* 29:540-550, 1988.
7. Bright MA: Therapeutic ritual: helping families grow, *J Psychosoc Nurs Ment Health Serv* 28(12):24-29, 1990.
8. Braud W: Distant mental influence on rate of hemolysis of human red blood cells, *J Am Soc Psychical Res* 84(7):1-24, 1990.
9. Achterberg J: Ritual: the foundation of transpersonal medicine, *ReVision* 14(3):158-164, 1992.
10. Ludwig A: Altered states of consciousness. In Tart C (ed): *Altered states of consciousness,* New York, 1969, Wiley.
11. Searle JR: Consciousness, *Ann Rev Neurosci* 23:557-578, 2000.
12. Tart C: Putting the pieces together: a conceptual framework for understanding discrete states of consciousness. In Zinberg NE (ed): *Alternate states of consciousness,* New York, 1977, Macmillian, pp 158-219.
13. Harner M: *The way of the shaman,* San Francisco, 1990, Harper.
14. Habrentz M: The effects of humor on the initial client-counselor relationship, PhD dissertation, University of Southern Mississippi, *Dissertation Abstracts Int* 34:3875, 1974.
15. Huber AT: The effects of humor on client discomfort in the counseling interview, PhD dissertation, Lehigh University, *Dissertation Abstracts Int* 35:1980, 1974.
16. Davidhizar R, Bowen M: The dynamics of laughter, *Arch Psychiatr Nurs* 6(2):132-137, 1992.

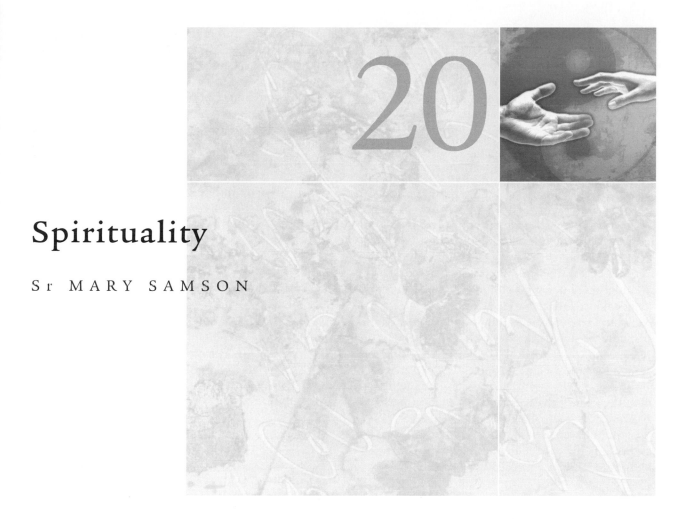

# Spirituality

Sr MARY SAMSON

$\mathcal{N}$ot too many years ago a medical literature search on the topic of spirituality yielded very few articles. Currently there is a noticeable increase both in interest in and in writing on the topic. A recent search of articles from 1998 to the present yielded 277 citations on Medline, compared with 300 during the previous 30 years. The "critical, comprehensive, and systematic" analysis in the *Handbook of Religion and Health,* published in 2001, includes "more than 1,200 studies and 400 research reviews conducted during the twentieth century."[1] The word *spirituality* as used in the studies cited, and as used in this chapter, is very broad in concept. It is the guiding principle in a person's life but is not necessarily doctrine oriented. It is unique to each person and is present in each in some form or another. *Religion* is the expression of one's spirituality in a formal, organized manner. *Theology* may be said to be the movement between the two. These three words are related but not synonymous.[1] In other words, we are speaking of the universal search for meaning and purpose in the life of every human being.

## SPIRITUALITY

Verna Benner Carson, in her book *Spiritual Dimensions of Nursing Practice,* states

Providing spiritual care is much more than recognizing a client's religious beliefs and incorporating those beliefs into our planned interventions. Spiritual care is anything that touches the spirit of another. . . . People may express their spirituality in unique ways, but everyone has a spiritual dimension that can be touched through the ministrations of another.[2]

247

Another definition states that "spirituality deals with the search for meaning and purpose in life and is that part of the psyche that strives for transcendental values, meaning, and experience."[3]

Perhaps a clearer definition is stated in the *Handbook of Religion and Health*[1]:

Spirituality is the personal quest for understanding answers to ultimate questions about life, about meaning, and about relationship to the sacred or transcendent, which may (or may not) lead to or arise from the development of religious rituals and the formation of community.

Spirituality is essentially the inner person. It is part of the uniqueness of each individual. Spirituality is expressed through one's body, thinking, feeling, judgments, and creativity. It motivates one to choose meaningful relationships and pursuits. The spiritual can be said to be that part of a person that allows one to give and receive love, to respond to the beauty of a symphony or sunrise, and to respond to and appreciate God and other living beings. It can drive a person forward in spite of pain and allows a person to reflect on the self and discover that one is indeed more than the sum of one's physical parts. Spirituality provides motivation and enables a person to value, worship, and communicate with the holy, the transcendent.[2] In essence it is the core of one's being—a sense of personhood, a sense of who one is and is becoming.

## RELIGION

Some people do choose to express their spirituality in a religious context. In so doing the person expresses individual spirituality within a social context as a member of a specific religious denomination and faith. This includes an organized belief system with religious ritual that influences the actual living of one's life. Many people speak of their religion and remain within the confines of formalized religion. Religion thus deals with the external and social aspects of belief in the supernatural, while spirituality refers to an internal state or interior life that is fueled by such beliefs.

A more formal definition would be

Religion is an organized system of beliefs, practices, rituals, and symbols designed (a) to facilitate closeness to the sacred or transcendent (God, higher power, or ultimate truth/reality) and (b) to foster an understanding of one's relationship and responsibility to others living together in community.[1]

Spirituality and religion are not necessarily synonymous, yet they are both almost always present in some form in the rehabilitation setting. It is not unusual for a person to say that he or she does not go to church or no longer belongs to the religion in which he or she was reared. Yet, when asked, or even when not asked, the person is quick to say that he or she prays in the morning and evening and believes in God, saying that God may well have had a role in his or her survival of a catastrophic event. Why? Why me? Why did this happen to me? Why did God do this to me? are questions that are commonly asked. The first three may or may not have a religious basis, but the last one usually does have religious overtones.

## THEOLOGY

When a person begins to find some connection between his or her religion and the answers to these questions, one may say that this becomes a form of theological reflection. It is an effort to find meaning in what would otherwise be meaningless.

Theology is not abstract musing about unintelligible mysteries, but it is a challenging and thoughtful reflection on the way God's hand is involved in the day-to-day experiences of men and women. In other words, theology is not a series of conjectures and propositions about a "God" who is existing in unseen celestial spaces. . . . The task of theological reflection is to peer into one's "house of experience" through that "window of theology" and begin to articulate what is being observed in this relationship of a God with us. One's notion of "mystery" prevents or allows this task of theological reflection to take place. If one understands mystery as unknowable ideas and complicated theories, the window of theology is indeed useless. If one perceives mystery as an event, which continues to unfold around and within us, however, the beginnings of theological reflection are taking root. The window of theology is becoming a clearer piece of glass through which one's experience is observed and interpreted.[4]

## THE INTERRELATEDNESS OF RELIGION, THEOLOGY, AND SPIRITUALITY

It would be a mistake to underestimate the role of religion, theology, or spirituality in the healing process. Religion can be either a positive or a negative force, and it can be a very strong one. Hence it is extremely important that it not be neglected nor demeaned by anyone, be it a member of the rehabilitation team or the chaplain.

*Religion* is perhaps the most observable of the three. A person will often verbalize, quite easily, religious needs. Hence it is the one of the three terms most thought of and sometimes the only one addressed. Someone coming into a medical setting may request a visit from a chaplain for prayer, sacraments such as reception of Communion, or counseling. Many times a person has said after receiving Communion in the morning, "You know, this is the reason I am getting better." Morning prayer upon awakening is not only a longtime habit for many, but it may also bring a sense of hope and peace to a day. It is a link to the familiar, to a life before and after illness, to a sense of well-being. Observing the room may give an indication of the importance of religion in the person's life. A bible or other religious books in a place of prominence, greeting cards with religious themes, and religious articles are all indications of a person's religious devotion. These should be affirmed and supported as a very powerful part of the healing process. Their presence could be considered an invitation to inquire about what religious/spiritual interventions might be helpful to the patient. Several studies are underway on the power of prayer in the process of healing. My comment would simply be to not underestimate the power of such religious faith in bringing the person through the rehabilitation process to true healing. The positive influence of religion is a thread that weaves in and out of most of the cases cited in this chapter.

On the other hand, there are times when religion can have a negative effect on the healing process. These incidents tend to be in the minority, but they are significant nonetheless.

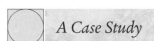

*A Case Study*

### Negative Influence of Religion: Amputation

Years ago a man in his early thirties from the Virgin Islands had a below the knee amputation. In addition, he was diagnosed with vascular disease. In his religious belief system, God, not the doctors, was in charge. This belief was so ingrained that he absolutely believed that God was going to cause his limb to grow back. Because of this belief, he refused therapy and the use of any assistive devices, and he would not even consider the possibility of a prosthetic leg. He never was transferred to a rehabilitation setting.

There was no way that he could be convinced, cajoled, or enticed to think otherwise. Needless to say, in this case religion played a very negative role in his healing process. The leg wound healed but he left the hospital a wounded man in so many other ways, at least to our way of thinking. There was not even the possibility of inviting him to see his God and religion in a different light. Fortunately this is not the usual scenario. ✑

Religion can also become a negative influence when a person believes that one's well being is dependent on one's own faith and/or prayer. It would follow that if the person does not get well or improve, it is his or her fault. If illness is thought to be a punishment from God, it is time for an invitation to rethink one's image of God. Psalm 118 is sometimes translated, "If God is for us, who can be against us?" or "With the Lord at my side I do not fear. What can mortals do to me?"[5] But the reverse can be a very negative influence and a very frightening thought. What if I believe that God is indeed punishing me?

*Theology* can be defined as belief about God and one's relationship to God. Rudolf Bultmann is the source of some of the most significant theology in recent years. According to Bultmann, "We have no way of speaking conceptually about the God who encounters us, but we can speak of the impact of the encounter upon our understanding of our self and our situation. The proper object of theology is, then, not God but man."[6]

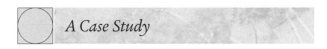

*A Case Study*

### Failure of God: Traumatic Injury

Jane, in her late sixties, made the statement, "My catechism doesn't work anymore." Her God was still the God of childhood innocence who protects the good and sees that no evil befalls them. Here she was, someone who had lived according to the rules but who was hit by a truck on the way home from church! She was religiously devastated, if you will. Her faith and her God had failed her. ✑

Sometimes when these questions arise, it is the person's faith, as well as his or her body, that needs rehabilitation. When the religious beliefs of the child do not mature with age, one often is left with a theology that is no longer life giving, which can indeed be a negative rather than a positive force in one's life. Why did God do this to me? Why is God punishing me? What did I do to deserve this? I spent all my life caring for my parents and as soon as they died I got sick. These are religious questions, which invite a person beyond the catechism or basic religious beliefs to a spiritual place, a place of a deeper understanding of and relationship with God. If God has indeed done this to me, then what did I do to deserve it? Of what am I guilty? For what do I need forgiveness? These are the questions that surface when one has hours, days, and months during which one lies in bed and thinks at a deeper level than ever before. Some people will say, "I have too much time to think." It is often a struggle, sometimes with the demons in one's life. At times it is a struggle with questions to which there appear to be no answers. If God has indeed arbitrarily done this to me, then do I even have a chance of recovery? There can be the fatalism of the ancients. In the course of rehabilitation there is often time and often an invitation to ponder/theologize, to gain insight as a result of "man's passionate concern to understand himself in his history where myth and reason are practical means for that reflective activity."[6] It is an invitation to theological reflection and to spiritual maturity.

# RELIGION AND PSYCHOLOGY

There are times when the religious and psychological aspects become so intertwined that one cannot be successful without the other. At times it is best for the patient when the psychiatrist or psychologist can work in concert with the chaplain.

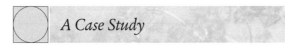

### A Case Study

*Religion and Psychology: Sexual Abuse*
One of my friends, a Jewish psychiatrist, approached me one day and explained that he was treating a 25-year-old Roman Catholic client who had been sexually abused at age 12 by her uncle, a priest. The psychiatrist felt that he had reached an impasse and was unsure exactly how to proceed.

While listening I began to sense that not only was the client feeling responsible, as most victims do, she was also seeing herself as estranged from God. This was com-

pounded by the fact that the abuser was a priest. My suggestion was to approach the situation using the conditions within the Catholic religion that would constitute serious or mortal sin. Naturally the psychiatrist and I agreed that the client was indeed in no way responsible for what had transpired. However, she believed herself to be responsible. I explained that one requirement of responsibility was obviously missing: full consent of the will. Although the psychiatrist was in unfamiliar territory, he followed through on the suggestion and found that it was indeed the key that allowed him and his client to continue the road to healing. ❧

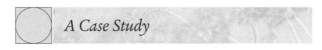

### A Case Study

*God's Intention*
A middle-aged woman was being referred for a psychiatric consultation but absolutely refused. In her strict religious upbringing, she had been taught that God never gives a person more than he or she can handle. Therefore God should be a sufficient guide or support through this hospitalization. It was only in her discussion with the chaplain about who the psychiatrist is, why God gave some people the ability and desire to become psychiatrists, and God's intention for us to use all reasonable means at our disposal to become well that she came to accept the idea that speaking to the psychiatrist was really not in conflict with her religious beliefs. ❧

Some patients absolutely refuse the intervention of a psychiatrist, for whatever reason. Often it is because they attach a stereotypical stigma to even the possibility of mental illness of any kind. However, it is not unusual for these patients to agree to speak to a chaplain. Going to a clergyperson for counseling is much more acceptable in their mind and, I dare say, in the mind of society. In all of these situations it is imperative that the chaplain know the limits of his or her expertise. It is equally important for the psychiatrist or psychologist to recognize when the intervention of a clergyperson would be beneficial to the patient. Respect for the role of other healthcare professionals is so important in achieving the common goal of healing. It is possible to work together, to the benefit of the patient, without compromising the boundaries of confidentiality. An excellent example of this is in the case of a person who chooses to stop medical treatment such as dialysis. It should be determined that the person understands the implications of his or her choice and that depression is not the reason governing the decision. This is the proper role of the psychiatrist. In addition, the question of suicide very often enters the picture. In choosing to refuse treatment, the person is choosing to die. Because suicide is not acceptable in many religions, a discussion with a member of the clergy is most appropriate and helpful to the patient and family.

One woman, a nurse, perceiving the need for psychological counseling in her own life, specifically requested the name of a therapist who would include her spirituality in the healing process. A woman in her late twenties, who suffered with chronic pain and whose father was a minister, became indignant and refused to see a clinical social worker who had told her that her religious faith had no place in her healing process.

The belief or nonbelief of the caregiver should not become part of the equation. The important factor that is present as a resource is what the patient believes. This must be respected and attention must be given to the impact a person's beliefs have on his or her healthcare decisions. Feeling that their spiritual needs are not being taken seriously can drive people away from standard medical treatment.

## SPIRITUALITY AS RELATIONSHIP

Experience has taught me that spirituality is caught up in relationship, be it relationship to oneself, God, others, or the environment. "The person's relationships are grounded in expressions of love, forgiveness, and trust and result in meaning and purpose in life."[2] These virtues exist even in a purely humanistic framework. In general, people seek meaning and purpose in life, regardless of whether it is directly linked to belief in God. Hence spirituality is a dimension of every person. Some people choose to seek and live out these virtues within a specific religious community or religion. In religious bodies, various tenets place particular emphasis on ritual, prayer, and specific ways of conducting one's life, elevating the human to a higher plane, at least for the individual. The virtue of forgiveness, which is so important in life, becomes the Virtue of Forgiveness when God or one's religious beliefs become a primary guiding force in life.

## RELATIONSHIP TO SELF AND OTHERS

In actuality, relationship to oneself and others cannot be separated because no one lives in isolation.

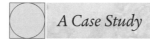 *A Case Study*

*Relationships/Forgiveness: Arthritis*
A few years ago Mary was readmitted due to an exacerbation of her arthritis. Over the course of several admissions I had gotten to know Mary as a lovely Irish Catholic woman who very much appreciated the rituals and prayers of the Catholic Church. One afternoon Mary and I had a conversation in which she told me of her recent need to seek a nursing home placement for her sister, who had lived with her for many years. As many do, she had promised her sister that she would never place her in a nursing home, but the time had come when Mary, in her eighties, could no longer care for her sister at home. She spoke of her sadness. Her guilt about not having been able to keep her promise was taking a toll on her. We spoke at length about how she felt, the many avenues she had considered, and that she had just run out of viable options. Her decision had been the only one possible and she had indeed done all she could over the years. When I was leaving, Mary's comment was very telling. When expressing her thanks she simply added, "Now I know why I had to come into the hospital." ❧

Religion was part of the equation, but an even more important part was Mary's feeling of having let her sister down. Are there things in life for which I need the forgiveness of others or, even more importantly, for which I need to forgive myself? Forgiving another is usually the easier of the two. It has been my experience that exploring such depths can be very frightening for a person.

For this reason it is important that the clinician listen very carefully to what the client is saying or is leaving unsaid. An immediate expectation in visiting Mary would have been to surmise that she might be expecting to participate in a specific ritual from her usual religious activities such as the reception of Holy Communion. However, by allowing Mary to continue her train of thought, I came to understand that she was struggling and had been struggling with her feeling that she had betrayed her sister's trust. Her need was not only to know her sister's forgiveness but also to be able to forgive herself. It is just about impossible to underestimate the role some spiritual factor may play in a person's ability to participate in the rehabilitation process. Once Mary realized that she had followed the only course open to her, she was able to better participate in therapy and prepare to return to a home without the companionship of her sister.

### A Case Study

*Forgiveness of Self*
One Catholic woman in her eighties confided to me that her children had never forgiven her for remaining with an abusive, alcoholic husband. One would never have surmised this because the children and their families were loving, attentive, and very caring. Was it really they who needed to forgive, or was it she who needed to forgive herself? According to her religion, divorce was not permissible. In the society in which she lived in the early twentieth century, a divorced woman would have been looked down upon and she would have had few avenues open to her to pursue any economic means of properly raising four growing children. It was so necessary for her to discover that she had done what was possible for her to do in that era, when a woman had limited opportunities for employment and could not even establish credit on her own. She had, for all intents and purposes, raised her children as a single parent, raised them to be the fine adults they showed themselves to be, and, in the process, she herself had a very difficult life. Recognizing this allowed her to forgive herself. ✍

It is so important that a person be enabled to gain some perspective on the reality of the times. Providing answers or simply offering words of forgiveness are usually not that helpful. A person needs to be able to forgive himself or herself before he or she can accept the forgiveness of God or others. The adult children had long ago come to understand the circumstances of their upbringing and had not only "forgiven" their mother but had the greatest respect for her. In the telling of her story she could finally acknowledge that God had indeed been there for her all along, as her faith had told her, and she had done what was possible for her in that time and place. She progressed in the rehabilitation process and became a resident of a nursing home chosen by her children and close enough that they and their families could visit daily.

There are times when it is difficult and time consuming to facilitate this process. It would be easier to simply give our objective view of the situation, but that ignores what the person needs. In this case it was self-forgiveness. Most of the time it is necessary to talk things out and arrive at a conclusion that can be owned by the person. Is that not the premise of talking therapy?

## FAMILY SYSTEMS

Relationships are at the center of family systems theory. What toll is the rehabilitation process taking on the respective members of the family? Is the spouse being overly demanding or has fear taken over? It may be as important to meet the spiritual needs of the family members as it is to meet the medical needs of the patient. As we know, people's feelings and emotions play off each other.

### A Case Study

*Family Relationships: Brain Tumor*
The mother of a 40-year-old man with a brain tumor sat beside her son and stroked him by the hour. She became angry with her daughter-in-law, who had difficulty staying in the room for any length of time. The wife would be in the room with her husband for a short time and would then become involved in helping other patients, watering their plants, or engaging in other helpful activities. What the mother did not understand was that her unresponsive son had, in a sense, died in the eyes of his wife about 6 months earlier. His situation placed him in the role of an infant but also had deprived his wife of her husband. ✍

Generations may need to be brought together in understanding of each other. In rehabilitation we speak of the quality of life. The patient does not live in a vacuum. Neither do the family members. The quality of life of one will influence the quality of life of the whole. The unit of care must be the patient and the family or significant others. In reality a person, especially an older person, who is bereft of family and friends will have a more difficult time and may lack the motivation for a successful recovery. Other times it is the caretaker who has need of understanding and support. One woman, a teacher, wrote during her husband's illness

I, too, feel that I am in overdrive all the time. I looked at the first grade bulletin board in school on Friday. It was a leafless tree with many branches going out in all directions and I thought to myself that that tree is just like I feel—spread out in all directions. Sometimes I feel so frazzled.

On the other hand, working may have been the only "normal" activity in her life and may have been her saving grace. All too often older spouses left to their own devices will spend hours in the hospital. When they do go home they are often tired. Phone calls need to be made or answered. Left to their own devices they may not eat or sleep well. They may need help from the staff in organizing their time to conserve energy. Because they are so close to the situation they may lose any objectivity.

## SELF-IMAGE AND SELF-ESTEEM

When speaking of a person's relationship to self, we are often speaking about a person's self-image and sense of self-worth. It is important to recognize that the only one who has complete access to the impact and meaning of an event is the one who has experienced it. Some aspects of the rehabilitation process may be taken in stride by the staff, and we may have no concept of the monumental impact of what appears to us to be inconsequential.

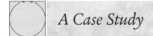 *A Case Study*

### Self-Image: Cervical Fracture
One woman in her nineties with a neck fracture was wearing a halo to stabilize her neck. During every visit she would make the comment, "But I don't really look like this." Her self-image had been fractured along with her neck. Finally I thought it might help her if a family member brought in a picture of her and put it on the board in her room so that we could indeed see what she really looked like. It was a very simple intervention but put her in a frame of mind that allowed her to, in a sense, relax into the healing process and be much more amenable to the interventions of the therapists. Her appearance was no longer an issue. ∾

It is so important to assess a patient's awareness of the emotional, psychological, and spiritual, as well as the physical, impact of the event. What of the man who consistently shows and caresses the stump that

remains after an above the knee amputation? Before any success can be achieved using a prosthesis, this person must grieve the loss of part of who he has been and discover who he now is. Who is this man? Did he require both limbs to accomplish his work in life? What is really important? When these issues are addressed, the person is then able to move on.

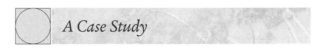 *A Case Study*

### Self-Esteem: Amputation
One beautiful 47-year-old woman demanded that her artificial limb have an interchangeable foot. Needless to say, many of us were a bit puzzled. Isn't the ability to walk primary? Not for her! She explained to us that she loved to go dancing and that she certainly was not going to be seen dancing with those flat shoes! Ingenuity prevailed and she was fitted with a leg that had a foot for a flat shoe and one that would allow her to wear "good shoes" and be graceful on the dance floor with her husband. She returned home to Virginia on "dancing feet." This is the spiritual, the uniquely individual person who finds meaning in what is important to him or her. ∾

Discovering just who this person is can become even more complicated in this twenty-first century world when, unfortunately, so many people define themselves by what they do rather than who they are. What happens to the "person" when he or she is no longer able to perform the same work or engage in the same endeavors that basically defined his or her sense of being, of self-identity?

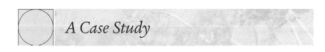 *A Case Study*

### Self-Identity: Lupus
A pediatric neuropsychologist and associate professor of neuropsychology in her mid-forties finds her body taken over by lupus and several other complicating diseases. Because of her compromised immune system, there is essentially no way in which she will be able to treat children again or even be involved in the normal social and academic circles that were her lifeline. Are there ways to enable a very intelligent woman to maintain some sense of her self-esteem and self-worth in the face of such devastating circumstances? Is it possible to tease out threads of

inner strength that can be positive resources? Intelligence, a drive to competitiveness, a desire to teach, a sense of humor, responsibility for an aging parent, and a sense of responsibility to maintain some stability within complicated family relationships are all parts of this woman. Though the physical part of her is in essence failing her, she must find a way to hold all of these other parts of her psychosocial being intact. Fortunately these strengths could be fostered and other avenues of engaging in life could be found. Needless to say, she was a challenge to members of the healthcare team and not solely because of her complicated medical condition. Perhaps her major strength, which has enabled her to manage in the face of such devastating medical illness, is a mature theology and spirituality. Even the development of these became an activity engaging those parts of her being that were in a sense most sacred to her, her mind and her ability to teach. ☙

Another woman said that she lives near a church and each morning she looks out at the steeple and finds the strength and hope to face another day. There is an innate need to find meaning in our lives. There are times when the only meaning one can find is that this, whatever it is, is God's will. The need to find meaning can have a very positive effect on some. If indeed this is God's will, then it is part of a divine plan and therefore there is a reason for whatever is happening in the present. Very profound theological reflection may follow. A more philosophical outlook on life may take shape. Victor Frankl, in *Man's Search for Meaning*, alludes to the fact that when one knows the "why," one can put up with any "how."[7] Finding meaning is inextricably bound to a person's sense of self-esteem, self-worth, reason for being, and even one's faith. Meaning is not simply the ability to cope with illness and suffering but the ability to put together broken, seemingly meaningless pieces and develop a meaningful whole. It is mending, healing, searching for a new meaning, new purpose, and making sense of circumstances, events of the day, relationships, and life itself.

## RELATIONSHIP TO GOD

One often needs to be able to experience the forgiveness of one's self before being able to develop a relationship with God, which is often intertwined with forgiveness. Many people who consider themselves religious and belong to a particular religion need to know God's forgiveness but have been reared with the image of a punishing God. The "why" questions often arise out of this concept. Why is God punishing me? is not an uncommon question. The person then proceeds to enumerate the many good things they have done and are at a loss to find an answer. Harold Kushner's book, *When Bad Things Happen to Good People*,[8] is one of the most popularly read books dealing with this very question.

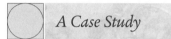

## A Case Study

*Forgiveness: Amputation*

A few years back a Vietnam veteran who was a double amputee was hospitalized. He had developed a habit of sitting alone in the corner of the sunroom between therapy sessions. I wondered if he was just someone who liked time alone or if something deeper was going on. We developed a rapport over time and he shared his story. He began by talking about his time in Vietnam. He told of his various experiences then, one day, he began sharing his feeling about having killed people, military and civilian. He had spoken to the military chaplain of his feelings. The "Padre" told him that they were engaged in a war and, under the circumstances, killing was acceptable. That has been said to many in the military over the centuries, but this man could not accept that and had carried the guilt for many years. Finally he was able to confess his feelings of guilt and accept the fact that God had probably forgiven him long ago. Now he could forgive himself. He also had to forgive himself for not living up to his image of what a father should be. As an amputee there were so many activities he would not be able to engage in with his son. He had missed his son's earlier years and felt that he was now not able to be what he felt the father of a teenager should be. ☙

So many people are plagued by memories of past events over which they had little or no control. There is a saying that hindsight is 20/20 vision, but it is not always so. First there may be a need for the healing of memories.

Given the cultural and religious diversity of our clients, it is impossible for us to know all the facts. Beliefs and practices can differ within the same religious tradition (e.g., Orthodox, Conservative, and Reformed Judaism). People do not expect us to be all knowing, but they do expect us to be respectful of their beliefs. At times the most respectful thing to do is admit our lack of knowledge and ask the person to explain what is important to him or her. In addition, there are a number of resources available in print to help us understand our clients.

## RELATIONSHIP TO THE ENVIRONMENT

For survival we need to be needed, to matter to someone or something, even to a beloved pet. At one time I met a hobo, the black sheep of his family, who had chosen to live that lifestyle. He was a very interesting character. Much to our surprise and dismay he had befriended a mouse who had discovered that his room was a welcome refuge from nearby construction! The man was terminally ill but became very angry when his sister sent him a beautiful plant. In voicing his anger he said, "Now I have to stay alive to take care of this plant." He regained his peace when not only was he assured that the plant would be taken care of but also he had the opportunity to demonstrate exactly how the plant should be cared for. He died within the next week.

Is it possible to make the hospital environment more pleasant? What will enhance the person's sense of being in the right place, especially when he or she would much rather be at home?

## PSYCHOLOGICAL/ EMOTIONAL/HUMAN NEEDS

### Hope

What is there to hope for when there is no apparent meaning in life? Can a person live without hope? Hope is considered essential for human life and is associated with meaning and value. It is part of one's life, religious or not. Hope is the expectation that there can be a better tomorrow. Hope does change. That is quite apparent when a person moves from acute care to a rehabilitation facility. In the immediate wake of a catastrophic experience, energy is focused on survival. For some people hope may even exist on an unconscious or subconscious level. Perhaps it is better termed the will to live. At that time conscious hope is the prerogative of the family or significant others because the patient is often in a coma. A person may say, "I don't even know what to hope for, what to pray for." Perhaps one can only hope "for the best" because nothing is clear. This is so often true in the case of trau-

matic injury, especially brain injury. Can one presume to know what should be hoped for? Yet hope is present in some form. In many cases the person involved does not even remember the event. This complicates matters because when a person does not understand what happened, there can be anger at one's own body for not acting as it should and/or toward those persons who are not acting as one believes they should. In not remembering the trauma the person has no real recollection of the extent of physical damage sustained. Hence discouragement and depression, rather than hope, can become the order of the day. It is so important that even small physical gains be affirmed. It is also sometimes necessary to remind the person that he or she is making a comparison with who he or she was before the injury because he or she does not have any sense of the actual physical impact of the injury. Once gains, though small, become apparent, sustained, and obvious to the person, hope may begin to return. Hope changes as levels of recovery are achieved. It is important to discover a person's hopes and help sustain them. Even when a hope appears to be unreasonable or impossible, it is important not to destroy it. It may be necessary to encourage that the hope be modified or channeled, at least for the time being. One needs to walk before one can run, and one may need to use a walker before graduating to a cane or to independent mobility. However, there are some people who cannot and will not compromise. For some a life without hope for complete independence is a life without meaning.

We also live in a world of ever-changing technology. Research depends on hope. There is hope for a better tomorrow, for new advances in technique and technology. Even when there is no hope for a cure, hope can exist in the expectation or hope that one's own illness can somehow be used to help others. Technology is constantly improving, and the impossible hope of 5 or even 2 years ago is now possible. Hope must be sustained.

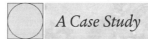

*A Case Study*

#### The Power of Hope: Amputation
One man whose life was intertwined with running both as an author and athlete had a below the knee amputation. Ray left the hospital walking with a prosthesis. However, his hope, his determination was to run again. The rehabilitation team did not take this hope quite as seriously as

he did. To them it seemed like an unreasonable expectation. Today he wears a prosthetic leg that looks and feels like a natural leg. Not only that, he engages in karate and is indeed a runner once again. There is a saying, "Never say never." For some people, like Ray, difficulties are simply challenges meant to be overcome. Today Ray also produces motivational videos. The road to recovery was long both in and out of the hospital, but his goal was achieved. There were days when his hope seemed impossible, yet our not accepting that hope would have put him into a depression that warranted clinical intervention. ✍

## Meaning

Hope and meaning can be intertwined and solidly grounded in one's religion. It is not unusual to hear a person say, "I know I shouldn't ask 'Why?' Whatever happens is God's will." They believe that somehow this is part of God's divine plan. Many have grown up with the saying that God never gives you more than you can handle. This can be a positive force, and it is very important that this resource be cultivated. Somehow, if what is happening is part of a divine plan then there is a purpose, a reason. Why? or Why me? are questions that most often defy an answer. They are questions to be pursued. Seeking an answer can somehow give meaning to apparent meaninglessness. Religion is often the context in which a person seeks answers to the ultimate questions about the meaning of life, illness, and death. Theological reflection can lead to seeing God as present in all the experiences of life. God is strength to sustain one through whatever the future may bring.

## Control

One of the driving forces in life is to be in control of our own body, if not our destiny. Life, especially illness, teaches us that we cannot control our destiny. Whether it is an addiction or an accident, we learn that there are powers greater than we. This is often an invitation to turn to God or to a "higher power." What is achieved may be a religious rebirth and/or a depth of spirituality previously unknown. There has to be a locus of control somewhere and the person arrives at the stark realization that it is not within himself or herself. We cannot control what happens to us, but we can control how we respond. A sense of some control opposes a fatalistic approach to life. There may be more precise definitions of resignation and acceptance. To my mind

resignation is more passive. It is possible to view oneself as a helpless victim of circumstances. In practice I try to facilitate a movement from resignation to acceptance. In resignation one simply gives over control to what is. One patient put it so well.[9]

Although I was in a state of physical and spiritual chaos, I tried to gain control of my environment. If only I could get firmly in control of what was going on, what was wrong, I thought I would be safe. If only I could get all those ducks in a row. But always one or two (or more) would stray, would stay out of control. This was happening not only physically but spiritually. As I tried to get answers from doctors I was met with, "We just don't know." . . . I could not connect with familiar spiritual supports.

I was tempted to give up totally, to hand it over. "It's the doctor's job to get me well. It's God's job. If it doesn't happen, then they are to blame, not me. They are in control." I knew I certainly wasn't. I didn't know; they must know. It was easy to think it was their fault if it didn't turn out all right. It would be their failure. It seemed almost logical that God couldn't be good, loving, kind, just or supportive if this was happening to me for no good reason. My catechism didn't work anymore.

It was so imperative when working with this woman to facilitate movement from this resignation to what I term *acceptance*. It is a taking of "what is," the reality, and seizing some control by making conscious decisions about how one chooses to respond to the reality. It is a sense of reality in admitting that this is indeed "what is." Now, what do I do about it?

A patient in the hospital is certainly not in control and usually feels very vulnerable. Often the patient, much to his or her embarrassment, may not even be in control of the most elementary of bodily functions. It may not be possible for the patient to be in control completely, certainly not of his or her body, but it is often possible to give the patient some control in other ways. One very important way is to involve the patient in setting goals, even in small ways, and discussing ways of achieving those goals. A patient can often choose the order of therapeutic exercises. The result will be the same, but the patient will have some sense of being in charge. Often with the most uncooperative patient this technique can achieve positive results.

## Respect

All interactions must convey a respect for the patient. One gentleman remembered many years later that what impressed him about the chaplain was that she immediately reached out to shake hands in the ordinary way, the normal way, of meeting a new person. This was at a time when everything around him felt anything but normal. He went in for cardiac surgery and suffered a stroke. The outcome was far from what he expected as a 50-year-old Navy veteran and teacher. In this case, and in every case, it was also important to respect the members of the family and their feelings. What came across as a demanding, angry wife was really a young woman who was angry at what had happened to her husband and who was feeling extremely vulnerable. When she was included in the treatment plans and kept informed by the doctor and staff, her anxiety level decreased. She then felt better able to control her own responses to the healthcare team.

No matter what the disability, it is important to remember that we are treating a person, not a disability. Because a person cannot speak does not necessarily mean that he or she cannot understand and communicate in some way. It is up to us to find the way.

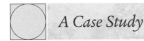

## A Case Study

### Regaining Control: Head Injury

A woman in her forties and in good physical condition had the misfortune to be hit by a bus, sustaining a serious head injury and many broken bones. She was a licensed social worker and in a position of leadership and management. When she finally reached the rehabilitation phase of her recovery, she found that group therapy was not only not helpful but also very frustrating. She found herself "frustrated and beginning to fight the word games and exercises for 'finding language'." Because of her brain injury, most of the therapy was focused on language recovery. She stated "as for my disposition, I believe I grew up as a 'can do' person. Early on, I began asking the rehabilitation director if I could use some of my time for tasks that I did want to do. The language groups were not helpful to me. I asked to begin organizing some of my paperwork and communications that I wanted to do. That director did give me a period each day to bring that work and do it at the center. She also asked me to put together a presentation to her staff on the social work I had done in the past years. Well, my memory was not able to pull that together very easily (memory had been hampered by the head injury). I asked if I could use a library or computer to work on some research. The computer was a terrific tool for me. It was via Internet research that I was able to research and relearn much of what I had wanted.

"Just prior to the accident I had made reservations to attend a continuing education workshop. I continued to lobby the director to take a few weeks off from the rehab program to attend the workshop. Eventually she relented. The benefit was to listen to lectures on theories of clinical social work that also gave me the opportunity to get my mind moving. It also gave others the confidence that I could travel on my own and not get lost. I believe that one of the biggest challenges I faced had to do with others' concern for me." ∾

This rehabilitation director is an example of someone who could listen to the patient and adjust her treatment plan to one that would fit. She respected the person and allowed her to take control as much as possible. Frustration was causing the patient to resist attending the rehabilitation as an outpatient. She could not see the value in the original mode of therapy. She indeed had no recollection of the accident or of the seriousness of her injuries. Combining the therapy with productive activity allowed the patient to become more involved. The difficulty encountered in preparing a presentation for the staff not only caused her to face her deficits, which had not been obvious to her, but also helped her relearn how to use the tools that would be helpful to her, i.e., the library and the computer. The workshop was in her hometown in California and her parents had been supportive from the time of the accident. Allowing her to travel from Boston was a calculated risk, but there are times when risk must be taken to allow for healing. Today, 3 years later, she can give a public presentation with relative ease and takes what residual effects remain in stride.

## Values

People will live or die in relation to their value system. At times healing is not just within the self but involves others.

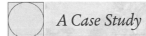

## A Case Study

### Value Systems: Musculoskeletal Injury

A woman facing at least a year of rehabilitation after a bicycle accident said that the gifts that helped her keep up her spirits and keep life in perspective were her faith, family, and friends. Life had not recently been kind to this 50-year-old. Loss of a seemingly secure position as a professional woman and the illness and death of her mother had spoken to her of the uncertainties of life and led her back to the religious practice of her mother and her younger days. Family and friends had been supportive through the year and she knew that they would be there through her recuperation. We need to know someone cares, that we are important to someone, that we are indispensable. For our own survival we need to be needed, to matter. Faith, family, and friends were indeed her support. ∾

Some people are not quite as articulate and therefore it takes listening, observation, and insight to discern what is going on behind the scenes. It may take time to develop a rapport, a sense of trust, before a person can say what is really bothering him or her. One woman finally said, "If one more person tells me how strong I am, I am going to scream."

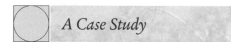

### A Case Study

#### All May Not be Well: Amputation

A young woman was admitted from an acute care facility. From the discharge summary the team received the impression that all was well. Yet the patient was noticed crying on several occasions. Speaking with her left one with the feeling that all was not well. However, she was reluctant to share how she was feeling because, medically, all was going well and she should have been pleased. The cancer was contained, the amputation went well, her stump was healing, and she was ready to be fitted for prosthesis. What was she not saying? The patient was from out of state, married, and the mother of a 5-year-old. The chaplain, a former teacher, inquired about how the child was coping with her mother's illness. What was not being said was that the child had not seen her mother since the amputation. Part of her unspoken anxiety was a concern about how her daughter would respond to her mother's amputation. Another fear was that other children would tease the little girl about having a mother with only one leg. As a weekend visit to her sister's home approached where her husband and daughter would be visiting, there were tears, sleeplessness, and signs of depression that, of course, interfered with her therapy sessions. The appropriate nonmedical intervention was actually a serious discussion about child psychology. Glimmers of hope began to appear. The weekend came and went. Her husband and sister were wonderfully supportive, but her daughter's curiosity carried the day. Even better, the child decided that she would be the one to take care of "Mommy's boo-boo leg" even though it was too heavy for her to carry! ∾

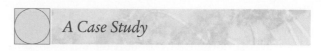

### A Case Study

#### Hidden Effects of Injury

A 68-year-old woman who had been injured in a car accident said, "No one dealt with the effects of the trauma. The physical therapist came closest when she said not to be surprised at the emotional impact of the experience. That was during my meeting with the therapist for the first time. Had I known her better, as I do now, I might have responded. I hesitated to share my spiritual experience with anyone—there just did not seem to be an opportunity. I dealt with all the effects by acknowledging them to myself, offering them and the physical discomfort for others worse off than me, and realizing that in time they would diminish." Simultaneously this woman, a former teacher and one who had counseled others so many times was struggling with the reality of the accident, flashbacks, and residual "terrors of the night." A religious woman, she adds that she could not pray to God, understood the feeling of abandonment by God, and struggled with her felt need to "forgive the driver who had caused the accident and had gone off unhurt and unapprehended." Waiting for an ankle, wrist, and ribs to heal again left her with hours in the day and night to struggle with these emotional and spiritual issues. ∾

## Summary

The values of the patient need to be considered but are often not readily observable. What are the motivating forces influencing this patient's decisions and responses? What is most important to this individual? In every case study in this chapter, there are implicit values that governed the person's response. What does this person value most in life? The answer to this question could be and probably should be an important factor in setting up goals with the patient and in developing the individual care plan.

Unfortunately, unless the need for psychological, psychiatric, or spiritual intervention is apparent, this part of the injury may be left untreated as well. There are people who never have the opportunity to recover from the "terrors of the night" and never achieve the quality of life that could so easily be theirs.

The fact is that in the busy, real world of healthcare, concentration is on the physical. The emotional and spiritual are considered secondary, if considered at all, as though a person is made up of various parts that function independently of each other. We know that is not true, but how does one fit everything into a limited time slot? It is a challenge, true. However, I have overheard therapists during their rest period have wonderfully therapeutic conversations with patients.

## CARING FOR THE TERMINALLY ILL

What has been said so far in this chapter is also true in the care of the terminally ill patient. The patient may be dying, but he or she is still a person with physical, spiritual, and emotional needs. The dying patient may have some unfinished business that must be attended to in order to arrive at a sense of peace. Family members may also have needs that must be considered because they are the ones who will have to live with the memories.

### A Case Study

*The Healing of Memories: Terminal Cancer*

A relatively young woman was dying from cancer. Each day her ex-husband drove their two children to the hospital but would not go in to see the patient. Some things cannot be forced. On the day the mother was very close to death, the nurses suggested that the children, in their early teens, be allowed to stay. It was agreed that if anything happened the father would be called immediately. When the chaplain spoke to the children it was apparent that there was a need for mutual forgiveness. It was important that they have the opportunity to create more positive memories if they chose to. Discussion centered on their obvious love for their mother, that some memories may have been in need of healing, and that they could decide how the relationship might end. In other words, we spoke of what, after she died, they might wish they had said or not said. The chaplain was called away to the phone and the children were left to themselves. Shortly thereafter they went to their mother's room and asked the nurse that they be left alone. They closed the door. When the son opened the door it was obvious all three had been crying. However, there was a newly found sense of peace in and about the three. ✺

Insight and sensitivity are indispensable at times like this. Grief counselors often speak of the healing of memories. This is even more important if the healing can take place before a person dies because it is possible in terminal illness to create good memories.

This also suggests that there are ways of taking some control over whatever time remains.

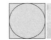

### A Case Study

*Creating Memories of Grace: Stroke*

Anne and Bob were completely devoted to each other. Bob suffered a debilitating stroke while undergoing heart surgery. After months in rehabilitation and against the advice of the team, Anne took Bob home. They knew Bob's time was limited. It was a monumental task, but Anne engaged caretakers to care for Bob so that she could continue working, which she needed to do because he was on her health insurance. Life did not end. Friends were devoted and helped in any way they could. They continued to go out to church together and sometimes to social events. Fortunately both had a sense of humor. (How does one decide whether to use the ladies or the men's room?) Anne is a realist and a very determined woman. She was determined that they would have a life together as long as Bob was alive. One time the physician told Anne that she was the reason Bob was still alive.

Religious faith was a very powerful force, and they could trust God in the midst of very difficult circumstances. They truly lived as a couple until the moment Bob died 5 years later. Anne shares these thoughts about her feelings. "I have to tell you that at Bob's funeral, when the casket was rolled down and we were all in the pews, I had a very profound feeling. I guess I would call it a grace-filled moment. I can't really explain it except that I was completely relaxed and at ease and I knew that I had done all that I possibly could for Bob in many ways—physically, emotionally, spiritually. I had told him the day before his death that he had been a wonderful husband and I could not have had a better life as a wife with anyone else. I told him not to hang on just for me and that I would be fine. I would miss him like crazy but I would survive. I told him that I was a survivor for sure. During this peace-filled moment in church, all this flashed through my mind and I knew that it was all true. I felt very much at peace. I felt grace and faith and courage to go on with my life, whatever might come. It was truly a profound feeling and moment for me." ✺

In many ways this was an ideal situation. Not every family has the financial means or the physical strength to accomplish what Anne and Bob did. They had supportive friends and caring religious guides in their lives. They also had personalities that allowed good things to happen despite what was, in reality, a bad situation. It is important that physicians, clergy, and caregivers be in tune with what is happening. It may be uncomfortable but, with care and concern, healing takes place even when curing is impossible.

Koening says, "Our calling as physicians is to cure sometimes, relieve often, comfort always."[10] We may not always be able to cure, but we can always care. There are some problems that just cannot be fixed. The amputated limb will not grow back, but we can see and treat this person as a complex human being, like us, with similar feelings, thoughts, emotions, loves. I do not have to have cancer to understand the person with cancer, but I do have to know love of life and family, meaning and purpose in life, and the fear that the loss of any of these would instill in my heart.

The word "healing" comes from the Greek word heilen, which means "to set right" or "to restore." . . . "Religion" comes from the Latin word, religare which is composed of two roots re and ligare. Re means "back" and ligare means "to bind, bind together." Thus, the word "religion" literally means "to bind back together." When our patients become physically ill or mentally out of balance, they need to be bound back together.[1]

It has always been believed that "not only does healing bring wholeness to the inner person but also that the power of healing comes from within the person seeking healing."[11] In *Timeless Healing,* Herbert Benson calls it "remembered wellness."

But as disconcerting as the news may be for some, my medical pursuits maintain that it really makes no difference where this capacity for wellness came from, from God or from some evolutionary mandate, only that it is very good for health and humanity. It is a win-win situation to believe in an Infinite Absolute.[12]

Benson's studies have taken him to many countries, countries of Eastern and of Western religious traditions, and he comes to the same conclusions stated in this chapter. Once we discover that spirituality is a very powerful force/resource in the healing process, we do not need to understand it but we do need to support it. We do not use computers because we understand them—we use them because they work. It does not matter if the person's belief is the same as mine. What matters is that I listen and respect the person's belief and affirm the presence of the divine in every human person.

Perhaps this 22-year-old woman sums it up best:

Family and friends are dear to me and really helped me get through. . . . My church was also supportive. I also believe in the power of prayer. Not only my prayer but also the prayer of others. A friend who lives in West Virginia got a group of people together and prayed for me. My minister knew people in other countries who were saying prayers for me. It was awesome to know that people I don't even know half way around the world cared about me.

Even though my father had already passed on, I thought about him. I knew that I did not want to leave my mom, if I could help it. Getting mad at God helped. I felt as though a big sigh of relief had come over me and I'd wondered why I hadn't done it earlier. Being able to go to the chapel also helped, as it was peaceful and reviving in my thoughts and strength to see another day.

I would have to say, though, the biggest way I got through was not thinking that I wasn't going to. I knew I was sick and really sick, but I never knew just how sick I was or how close to not making it I was.

Another part of it is like describing the spirit. I just can't. It just happened. I guess it wasn't my time yet. Things happen for a reason and we, as humans, can't always say why they happen or what they happened for. I believe though that I am a lot stronger person for it. I take great joy in the simplest of things.

Journeying through her illness with her, we traveled the way of the spirit, through religion, theology, and spirituality.

## ROLE OF THE HEALTHCARE PROFESSIONAL

There are discussions in the medical literature about whether a physician should inquire about a person's spirituality or offer to pray with the patient. Many feel it is intrusive, and many are uncomfortable in the realm of the spiritual. If we regard spirituality in the broad definition presented here, it may be easier to make inquiries of a patient.

In his essay, *Religion, Spirituality, and Medicine: Application to Clinical Practice,* Harold Koening delineates four questions suggested by a panel of the American College of Physicians. They are (1) Is faith (religion, spirituality) important to you in this illness? (2) Has faith been important to you at other times in your life? (3) Do you have someone with whom to talk to about religious matters? and (4) Would you like to explore these matters with someone?[10]

If religion or spirituality is important to a person, supporting his or her beliefs will aid the person in coping with present circumstances. It is also well documented that people who place a value on religious beliefs and practices, on the whole, live a happier, healthier lifestyle.

Especially in the rehabilitation setting, the simple question, Where are you finding the strength to help you through this time? will elicit responses similar to the responses to Koening's four questions without seeming to be intrusive. This question is more open-ended than those and may yield even more useful information. The 50-year-old mentioned earlier very quickly answered, "Faith, family, and friends." Sometimes the answer will have religious overtones, i.e., God, prayer, my minister, people from my church.

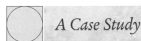

## A Case Study

### Caring From a Distance: Multiple Sclerosis

One 24-year-old woman showed me a prayer that a minister had composed for her and sent over the Internet at the request of her mother. This prayer led to a sharing that her mother was in Alabama, the minister was in another state, and the woman had recently moved to Massachusetts. She had recently been diagnosed with multiple sclerosis. Complications during a surgery had left her unable to walk, and there was a possible need for additional surgery. Fear of additional complications increased her incidence of headaches and sleepless nights.

Despite her numerous medical problems, this woman knew that, although geographically separated from her family, she was not alone. She found that it is easier to struggle on through uncertainty and fear when there is tangible support, whether it is emotional, spiritual, or psychological. ❧

Rehabilitation hospitals have discovered the myriad benefits of having technology, especially computers, available for the use of the patients. It allows the person to keep lines of communication open with family, friends and even the workplace. A sense of belonging, a feeling of hope and connectedness that can be facilitated by computer technology has become a valuable resource in the rehabilitation process.

## SUMMARY

One simple question may be the key to discovering who a person really is. If the clinician does not feel comfortable following up on religious matters, it may be possible to make a referral to the chaplain, who can provide religious support. Koening states:

> Patients want to be seen and treated as whole persons, not as diseases. A whole person is someone whose being has physical, emotional, and spiritual dimensions. Ignoring any of these aspects of humanity leaves the patient feeling incomplete and may even interfere with healing. . . . More than 850 studies have now examined the relationship between religious involvement and various aspects of mental health. . . . Between two thirds and three quarters of these have found that people experience better mental health and adapt more successfully to stress if they are religious.[10]

Studies also show that people who are religious are physically healthier, lead healthier lifestyles, and require fewer health services than others.[13]

It is of the utmost importance to treat the person who comes for medical care. This person is a physical, emotional, spiritual, psychological, and social being. No one of these facets of an individual can be isolated from the others. One facet affects the others, consciously or unconsciously. How often does someone, we included, develop a cold, flu-like symptoms, lethargy, or some other condition and upon reflection discover that there is an inordinate amount of stress, overwork, lack of sleep, or super-human demands in his or her life?

In other words, it is important to see this unique individual in relationship to these many facets. There are so many ways a person conveys a sense of personal self-esteem and self-image, both verbal and nonverbal. Who are the important people in this person's life? Does he or she feel needed or put upon? Does God, religion, or faith fit into the picture? Does he or she believe that there is meaning in life? What is the environment in which this person lives? Is this person alone, part of a large extended family, homeless? The answers to all of these questions will influence a person's response to treatment and ability to heal.

It is important that healthcare professionals, including those in rehabilitation medicine, not lose sight of these truths. The goal of rehabilitation is to help the patient achieve all that is possible, to allow the patient a life that is both full and fulfilling in as many ways as possible. Spirituality is a part of the healing process. When discounted, it is the patient who suffers.

## References

1. Koenig HG, McCullough MC, Larson DB: *Handbook of religion and health,* New York, 2001, Oxford University Press.

2. Carson VB: *Spiritual dimensions of nursing practice,* Philadelphia, 1989, WB Saunders, p vii.

3. Ellis MR, Vinson DC, Ewigman B: Addressing spiritual concerns: family physicians' attitudes and practices, *J Fam Pract* 48(2):105-109, 1999.

4. Wicks RJ (ed): *Handbook of spirituality for ministers,* Mahwah, NJ 1995, Paulist Press, p 309.

5. *Holy Bible: the new revised standard version,* Nashville, 1989, Thomas Nelson, p 565.

6. Brauer J, Homans P (eds): *Essays in divinity, vol III: The dialogue between theology and psychology,* Chicago, 1968, University of Chicago Press, p 12.

7. Frankl V: *Man's search for meaning: an introduction to logotherapy,* New York, 1952, Simon & Schuster.

8. Kushner H: *When bad things happen to good people,* New York, 1981, Schoken Books.

9. Samson M, McColgan S: Chaplaincy in action . . . and inaction, *J Religion Disabil Health* 3(3):43, 1999.

10. Koenig HG: Religion, spirituality, and medicine, *JAMA* 284(13):1708, 2000.

11. Nicosia JF: Healing the human spirit: the healing paradigm, *J Relig Disabil Rehabil* 1(3):65-74, 1994.

12. Benson H: *Timeless healing,* New York, 1996, Scribner, p 216.

13. Dossey L: *Healing Words: The power of prayer and the practice of medicine,* New York, 1993, Harper Collins.

## Suggested Readings

Wicks RJ, Parsons RD, Capps D (ed): *Clinical handbook of pastoral counseling, vol 1 and 2,* Mahwah, NJ, 1993, Paulist Press.

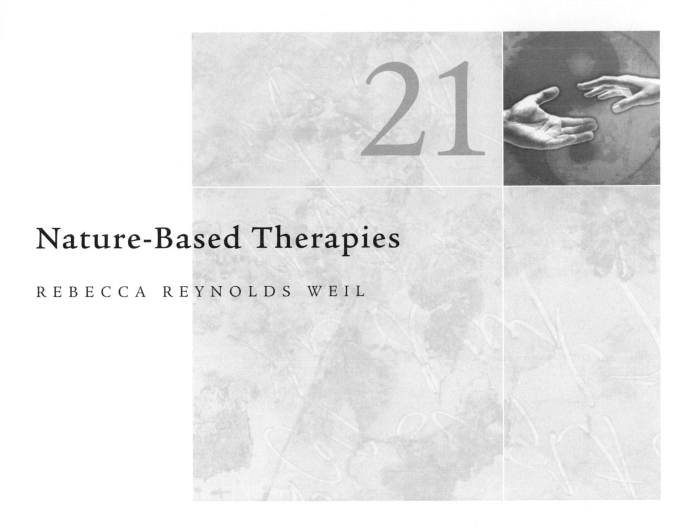

# Nature-Based Therapies

REBECCA REYNOLDS WEIL

*There is something infinitely healing in the repeated refrains of nature—the assurance that dawn comes after night, and spring after the winter.*

RACHEL CARSON, *THE SENSE OF WONDER*

The purpose of this chapter is to provide guidance to healthcare practitioners who wish to incorporate the natural world and animals in efforts to improve the lives of patients in short- and long-term rehabilitation settings. The field of Nature-Based Therapies (NBTs) encompasses many approaches and specialties. These approaches and specialties offer rich resources for clients, families, and practitioners.

One of the basic tenets and a great strength of NBTs is that nature itself is infinitely diverse. Such is the ubiquity and simple power of nature—it is at our fingertips and is awesome, wherever we reside on this earth.

This chapter offers an overview of NBTs, a contextual definition of NBT, the basis for adding NBT to therapeutic venues, and some examples of how NBT can be applied. Introductions to considerations of safety, including gaining reasonable credentials and experience before practice, are proposed. Resources are included to guide the interested practitioner to further information.

263

## GENERAL DEFINITIONS

NBT uses two primary approaches: (1) Nature-Assisted Therapy (NAT)—working with plants; natural environments; and natural materials, or biofacts, and (2) Animal-Assisted Therapy (AAT)—working with animals.

These two subcategories may be further divided into specialties. For example, NAT includes such specialties as Horticultural Therapy, while AAT includes such specialties as Therapeutic Riding. As an overarching term, NBTs include many specialties of practice.

While each specialty may be developed further, this chapter is designed to describe the intersection of NAT and AAT, or the combination of both nature and animals in rehabilitation settings.

## ORIGINS AND HISTORY

Integrating nature and animals in therapy is based on the historical premise that people have evolved as part of a community within nature and that ongoing contact with nature and animals may be essential in some intrinsic way to our understanding of community. Our earliest origins had us in constant, direct contact with the natural world and its living creatures. Nature and animals were synonymous with our survival. Long before we were considering what was good for our health, our lives were inextricably interwoven with the lives of animals and plants. Through cave paintings, oral history, and the written word, people have described and questioned the meaning of interaction with nature and animals. Despite such a long history, our connection with nature and animals remains a living mystery pursued by philosophy, science, and the arts.

In healthcare, the documented use of horticultural therapy for treatment may be traced as far back as ancient Egypt, when gardens were designed for members of royalty who were mentally disturbed.[1,2] The documented use of animals in healthcare settings has been traced as far back as the ninth century AD, in Gheel, Belgium, where animals were included as part of the therapeutic process.[3]

In recent years, the practice of including nature and animals in therapeutic approaches has been expanding. In the context of integrative medicine, it is a model that offers diverse resources to the practitioner.

## WHAT IS THE HYPOTHETICAL BENEFIT OF NATURE-BASED THERAPY?

In 1984, E.O. Wilson suggested that our basic connection with nature "is the innately emotional affiliation of human beings to other living organisms."[4] He said that our link with nature "began hundreds of thousands of years ago with the origin of the genus *Homo*. For more than 99% of human history, people have lived in hunter-gatherer bands totally and intimately involved with other organisms. During this period of deep history, and still farther back, into paleohominid times, they depended on an exact learned knowledge of crucial aspects of natural history."[4]

Along with the publication of Wilsons' *Biophilia*, substantial literature has emerged examining our affinity for nature and theorizing the cause and effect. The cornerstone of NBT emerges in the form of two questions: If people are inherently a part of nature, what happens for someone who is removed from nature and animals by hospitalization or treatment? What is to be gained when this interaction is restored?

Incorporating nature and animals into the context of a rehabilitation setting supports a full range of interaction for an individual undergoing challenge and recovery. An older person confined to a nursing home after a hip fracture has lost far more than mobility. A child in a locked psychiatric unit is removed from contexts that may support him emotionally. NBTs are based in the premise that restoration, if only in part, of other missing elements will improve quality of life, preserve meaning, and may enhance and hasten healing (Figure 21-1).

## WHAT IS THE EVIDENCE SUPPORTING NATURE-BASED THERAPIES?

Practitioners interested in working with nature and animals in healthcare settings find a unique approach, with unique complexities. Unlike some methods of treatment, work with nature and animals largely resists standardization as each animal is different in personality, nature is widely varying, and the practitioner themselves will share their methods with different style. The diversity of such

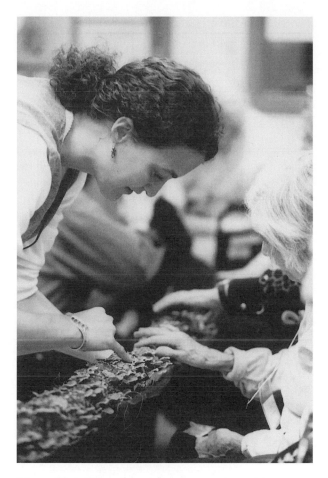

*Figure 21-1* Elder shares her connection with nature. (Courtesy Atsuko Otsuka.)

may actually be one of the strongest benefits: although some standardization of training and technique is possible, diversity is actually one of the merits of NBTs. After all, community, connection, and inspiration are dynamic forces that are supported by creative surroundings. However, the question of therapeutic effect from nature remains widely debated, and understudied. As a basis for implementing NBTs in healthcare, only one of three possible elements of success need be demonstrated: (1) that contact with nature improves objective endpoints of healing above and beyond conventional therapies; (2) that contact with nature provides motivation; or (3) that contact with nature simply improves the quality of life during the time of confinement, independent of objective measures of improvement.

## Objective Support for Nature-Based Therapy

Over the past 20 years numerous studies have been conducted on the effects of nature and animals on the health and well-being of humans. It has been proposed that even the simple viewing of nature scenes may have health benefits in a hospital setting. In 1984, Ulrich examined patients following gallbladder surgery. He contrasted the recovery of patients who had a view of trees to that of patients who had a view of a brick wall. The study showed that "patients with the natural window view had shorter postoperative hospital stays . . . and tended to have lower scores for minor postsurgical complications such as persistent headache or nausea requiring medication. Moreover, the wall-view patients required many more injections of potent painkillers, whereas the tree-view patients more frequently received weak oral analgesics such as acetaminophen[5,6] In a review of studies about affiliation with nature and its benefits, Kahn says, "Even minimal experiences with nature can reduce immediate and long-term stress, reduce sickness of prisoners, calm patients before and during surgery, and promote healing after surgery."[7]

Studies suggest that the health benefits of people interacting with animals are wide-ranging. Evidence suggests that stroking an animal can lower one's blood pressure.[8] Freidmann et al[9] studied survival rates following myocardial infarction for pet owners and non–pet owners and found greater survival rates in pet owners.

While other studies exist, reviews have criticized many as too limited in scope to provide evidence of clear therapeutic advantage.[10,11] Definitive prospective, randomized clinical trials defining the therapeutic benefits of NBTs remain to be performed. For collections and descriptions of key studies, this author suggests books by Fine,[12] Wilson,[13] Arkow,[3] and Simson.[1]

## Subjective Support for Nature-Based Therapy

Beyond published studies, a substantial body of anecdotal experience with NBTs exists in print. For many years these collected stories from therapists, family members, and clients have created a "commonsense" understanding of the benefits of nature and animals.

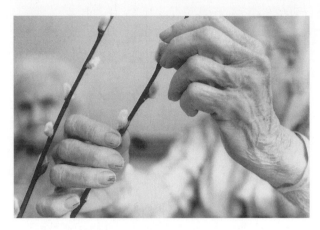

*Figure 21-2*  Spring comes indoors. (Courtesy Sue Huszar.)

An older woman says "Thank you for bringing the spring inside, it made me feel so much better". A young man unwilling to get out of bed because of pain and fear asks to see the dog and walks down the hall with the therapy dog for the first time in a week of hospitalization. A child who is distraught and anxious in a psychiatric hospital visibly calms down when stroking the rabbit and says, "I am calmer now." For family members and clinicians it is often enough to have a person say it matters to them, that it is of value to them (Figure 21-2).

A multitude of therapists have described anecdotal benefits in terms of attitude and motivation, making the rehabilitative process easier and less painful. In addition, the time spent in a rehabilitative setting—time that is a part of the cumulative life experience of those thrust into such settings—is often observed to be improved by contact with nature. In virtually any institutional setting, there are people who tell us so.

## Summary

A body of objective evidence supporting NBTs exists, but additional randomized controlled trials that isolate the effect of nature and animals from other potentially confounding factors and compare it to conventional therapies are needed. These studies will be critical if availability of NBTs is to broaden, because funding, for example, through Medicare, will depend on them. In the meantime, there is strong support from the therapeutic community and from many patients for the introduction of nature and animals into rehabilitative settings.

## THE THERAPEUTIC CHALLENGE AND THE ROLE OF NATURE-BASED THERAPY

*To insure health, a man's relation to Nature must come very near to a personal one; he must be conscious of a friendliness in her; when human friends fail or die, she must stand in the gap to him. I cannot conceive of any life which deserves the name, unless there is a certain tender relation to Nature. This it is which makes winter warm and supplies society in the desert and wilderness. Unless Nature sympathizes with and speaks to us, as it were, the most fertile and blooming regions are barren and dreary.*

HENRY DAVID THOREAU, *JOURNAL*, JANUARY 23, 1858

Rehabilitation may be painful, depressing, slow, worrisome, and isolating. Often, the greatest barrier to recovery is the seeming lack of motivation. The puzzle for the practitioner is to create a treatment plan that is based on safety, aptitude, and efficacy; is geared for success and graded for difficulty; and addresses the body, mind, and spirit of the individual in a way that holds meaning for him or her beyond the hospital or clinic.

In view of this, the person has first suffered a primary loss which puts them in rehab (e.g., stroke) but suffers secondary profound losses from being there. These secondary losses can include the loss of self-sufficiency, dignity, attractiveness (at least in the patient's own eyes), self-control, choice, purpose, income, vocation, community/family/friends/pets (companionship), and environment. Any one of these losses can add up to an individual's losing connection with meaningful parts of his or her life. It is perhaps self-evident that restoration of missing parts in a patient's life will make the rehabilitation process less difficult. Restoration of such elements may avert the malaise, or even depression, which so often accompanies challenging events.

When one considers the lives of most individuals before entering rehabilitation, most have had daily links to both nature and animals, if only on the unselfconscious level of moving through their local environment. Most people see the sky, hear birds, smell the rain, or walk under trees on a daily basis. Some have had a highly developed connection with nature

TABLE 21-1

*Examples of Integrated Approach*

| Treatment areas | Traditional approach | Additional NBT integrated approaches |
|---|---|---|
| Fine motor skills | Sorting items: paperclips, buttons, plastic bobbins | Planting seeds in garden bed; pinching off old flower heads; bridling a horse; painting a bird house |
| Gross motor skills | Weight machine; therapy ball; pushing weighted sledge | Turning soil with shovel; carrying water buckets to a garden; pushing a wheelbarrow; throwing a ball for dog; brushing a rabbit; riding a horse |
| Speech increased vocal clarity; language production | Repeating words from flash cards | Asking a dog to fetch ball; asking questions about horse's history; requesting time with the rabbit |
| Short- and long-term memory | Knowing the date and day; relearning relearning the names of presidents | Learning the names of animals or plants; learning how to care for an animal. |
| Ambulation | Walking up/down hospital corridor | Walking dog outside to play |

*NBT,* Nature-based therapy.

and animals, through vocation, such as farming, or through avocation, such as hiking or birding.

As the individual enters rehabilitation, often he or she enters a building, ascends to the fourth floor, and does not leave for 3 months. A holistic assessment of that person's losses would take account of this, and the practitioner would inquire if the absence of the natural world may undercut recovery.

NBTs may bring motivation, connection, and orientation to treatment approaches. Contextual experience and learning, drawing on themes based on the seasons and patterns of the natural world and animals may provide unique support for individuals who are in rehabilitation for either physical or emotional reasons. To paraphrase Thoreau, the nature in NBTs may "fill the gap."[14]

## NATURE-BASED THERAPIES IN PHYSICAL REHABILITATION
### Goals

In concert with traditional rehabilitation approaches, one may combine the benefits of NBT. The possibilities are vast, with only a few listed in Table 21-1.

When using a combined approach, the practitioner and client will still assess progress toward goals in a measurable, time-honored manner. Standardized tests may be administered to evaluate progress. Essen-

tially, by adding the additional integrative approaches, one is enriching the traditional approach with more motivation, meaning, and purpose. One is not changing the goal(s) of recovery; one is both reaching therapeutic goals and adding meaning to the process.

In developing the treatment plan, the therapist has the opportunity to keep the plan specific (e.g., lifting weights) or broad (e.g., lifting weights and interacting with animals and nature). Lifting a set of weights 10 times has no context other than the specific health benefit to the individual. The person has only lifted a weight on a machine 10 times. In contrast, if you add in things of interest to the person that are real, that occur outside of the hospital or treatment setting, the individual is more likely to invest in his or her treatment and to engage in the activity.

 *A Case Study*

*Nature-Based Therapy*

Jonathan, a 45-year-old male, has been undergoing therapy treatment in a rehabilitation hospital and states that he is "tired" with his therapy plan. He is status post-traumatic brain injury (TBI) and previously worked as a computer programmer. He says that he is depressed and that the therapy is meaningless. The therapy team stops, reevaluates the initial treatment plan, and with Jonathan develops new goals that include more of his interests and a number of possible ways to reach these goals. The occupational therapist finds that Jonathan loves to garden and that one of his goals is to resume building a vegetable garden when he returns home. The occupational therapist and physical therapist coordinate a series of treatment sessions using the hospital patio, where there is a rooftop garden. Jonathan begins caring for the garden, which involves multiple activities that address his own personal goals, his motivation, and his treatment plan. The social worker becomes involved with finding community resources in his hometown, while the vocational rehabilitation counselor considers potential jobs Jonathan might find in garden centers, and the psychologist finds that Jonathan is better able to frame his change of abilities using the example of the garden work.

The rehabilitation goals achieved are multilevel: Jonathan articulates what he needs each day for the garden (speech initiation, problem solving); plans the activity with the therapist (cognition/sequencing/memory); waits for the water bucket to fill (impulse control, perception); walks to and from the garden (ambulation); carries buckets and supplies to the garden (gross motor, proprioception, weight bearing, and coordination/balance); waters the plants, digs holes, dead-heads plants, plants seeds (using discrimination and coordination, fine-motor and gross motor, visual tracking, range of motion); plans for work after leaving the hospital (vocational); and ultimately achieves the satisfaction and distraction of doing something that adds beauty to the area and leads him to be further prepared for returning home. Overall, the garden offers effective therapeutic gains, may be tailored for specific meaning to the individual, and is multileveled and interdisciplinary.  ∿

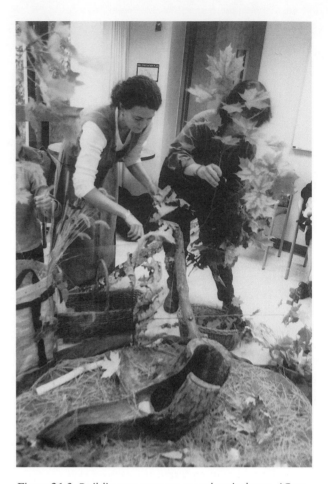

*Figure 21-3*  Building an autumn meadow indoors. (Courtesy Atsuko Otsuka.)

## INTEGRATION IN PSYCHOSOCIAL REHABILITATION

### Therapeutic Metaphor and Motivation Drawn from Nature-Based Therapy

The integration of NBTs in cases of recovery from psychological and emotional trauma is a rewarding area of NBT practice. Often individuals will respond when traditional methods have reached their limitations. Because of the therapeutic metaphors available with nature and animals, an individual can draw support from the dynamic and the soothing elements of the natural world (Figure 21-3).

Nature and animals are rich resources for drawing on an individual's intrinsic (1) curiosity, (2) inspiration, (3) meaning and sense of purpose, and (4) hope.[15]

1. **Curiosity:** In the natural world, the living dynamic qualities of nature and animals can encourage an individual's curiosity through the following:
   a. *Mystery:* In nature there is the constant tension between the known and the unknown, the mystery between predictable patterns and novel experience. Often clients are in a state of uncertainty and can gain insight from the intricacies of nature, and support from the steady, known patterns.
   b. *Beauty:* Nature and animals can evoke meaning and connection through the compelling quality of their beauty.

c. *Wonder:* Experiencing the complexity of nature can evoke wonder and awe, a sense of perspective on the relationship between self and nonself.

2. **Inspiration:** Once curiosity is evoked, an individual may find more inspiration through the following:

   a. *Creativity:* NBTs are inherently creative Nature does not hold one shape and can model creative approaches to life.

   b. *Awareness:* The vibrancy of nature can lead to awareness of our surroundings, including other people and their interactions, increasing sensory engagement.

   c. *Active participation:* An individual may be more likely to actively participate in groups or in individual treatments if he or she is interested and curious. Increased participation in ones surroundings can increase the likelihood of increased inspiration from contact with others and ones surroundings.

3. **Meaning and Purpose:** As the individual engages in his or her surroundings, he or she may find a reframing of experience, the ability to compare and contrast, greater perspective and reality orientation, and engagement.

   a. *Reframing experience:* Nature offers a broad range of what is normal in the world; there is every possible example of experience to see and learn from, normalizing experiences and framing them within a larger experience.

   b. *Comparing and contrasting—therapeutic metaphor:* Experience with NBTs can offer therapeutic Metaphors to our own experiences. For an individual, developing an understanding of how an animal stays safe, or the way a tree grows, can be a reflective area for therapeutic metaphor. An individual may draw comparisons, for example, when looking for the inner resiliency to adjust to challenge. Nature and animals show many examples of resiliency in the face of extreme circumstances, such as how the landscape recovers after a fire, or how animals survive through winter. For the individual needing rehabilitation, life has changed and adaptation to this change holds a particular challenge.

   c. *Perspective and reality orientation:* The physical, tangible presence of natural materials and animals provides an orienting and real experience for the child who is having difficulty with reality, or for an older person who may be struggling with orientation.

d. *Engagement:* As a group of individuals explore nature, animals, and the arts, they are sharing an experience together, building a template for community. An older person who previously was focused on the pain in his or her hip or the medication schedule now has something dynamic to talk about with family and with others in the hospital. The individual can check on the newly planted seeds in the window box, water them, and talk about flowers or spring or the animal he or she has met. The focus shifts to include the larger world in addition to the specifics of healing. Community can be drawn from the resources of nature.

 *A Case Study*

*Quahog*

Elaine, an 80-year-old woman in a chronic care nursing home, was escorted to the group by two staff members. They described her as unable to see and disoriented. On this visit we had created a small ocean environment in the nursing home, bringing in buckets of salt water, seaweed, baskets of sand and shells, and had built an environment for the elders to experience. We brought the ocean around to each person: the kelp with its slippery fronds, the salt water still cold from the sea, the sand and rocks and shells with their many textures and weights. As Elaine laid her hands on the large quahog shell, she ran her fingers over the ridges and the wing joints of the bivalve, recognizing the shape, remembering, and declared with clarity and knowledge, "This would make great clam chowder!"

When other parts of the human world had become confusing, the solid, real experience of handling a quahog shell gave Elaine a moment of orientation and lucidity, connecting her with something familiar and linking her to the present through her senses. The staff and Elaine spoke of the simple gains. The staff had more ideas how to help Elaine stay oriented with tangible items, and Elaine was pleased to experience something and know what it was. ❧

4. **Hope:** As meaning and purpose are supported with nature and animals, hope or faith may be renewed.

   a. *Orientation through patterns, cycles, and seasons:* As an individual enters rehabilitation, he or she often experiences disorientation as a result of changing roles and environment. NBTs can offer compass points for retaining the larger

### A Case Study

*Shared Nature-Based Therapy*

Maureen, a 65-year-old woman, was feeling isolated by her stroke. Maureen had been a science teacher and a poet before living in the nursing home. Her greatest delight had been teaching and learning about science, and communicating this with her art. After a stroke, she used a communication board and had no access to walking in the woods or simply getting outside. Betty, 68 years of age, had also been a science teacher. Betty felt isolated by her recent blindness and also missed being outside and seeing nature. During numerous visits with nature and animals, Maureen and Betty found that they could communicate about the nature and animals brought indoors to them. Maureen scratched letters into Betty's hand, and Betty would discuss the things Maureen was spelling. They began teaching other people in the nursing home about nature and animals. They each found ways to express their profound interests. They built friendships, and kept an engagement with life outside the nursing home. ∾

picture around an individual and stabilizing patterns from which he or she can draw support.

(1) *The four seasons*
   (a) The stabilizing knowledge of seasonal rhythms. Spring will come after winter.
   (b) The dynamic understanding of change through the seasons. Each season offers something vital to the next season.
(2) *Context*
   (a) Exploring how an individual's sense of place fits into the larger context of the world.
   (b) Interconnection of all living and nonliving things; a sense of belonging to a larger system. We learn from nature to generalize again, reminded of the whole, while at the same time being utterly specific. The natural world is very specific with regard to how things work together and where they thrive. Nature offers the perspective of interrelationships.
(3) *Circadian Reassurance:* Circadian means the behavioral or physiological rhythm associated with the 24-hour cycles of the earth's rotation. When an individual is trying to make sense of a world while experiencing change, physical/emotional challenge, betrayal, violence, or chaos, nature can offer

patterns and rhythms that are steady despite the arbitrary qualities of human experience. The sun will always come up in the morning. The tides are always on a regular sequence. These cycles will continue despite other changes in our human lives. *Circadian Reassurance*[16] then is the reassurance that may be derived from the knowledge that another day is coming, that the sun will rise as it always does.

### A Case Study

*Tangible, Real, and Alive*

A child feeling the heartbeat of a dog knows that it is real and alive. This child may follow the gaze of the dog as it hears a sound—alert and attentive, focusing his awareness to his surroundings. This same child may be inspired to learn through curiosity and upon being engaged in inquiry may follow this exploration to being more connected with self, others, and surroundings. For a child, connection can lead to a perception of orientation, a way of making sense of the world.

Eight-year-old Tyler was in a unit for children with severe emotional and behavioral issues. When we passed the small sweetgrass basket with moss bedded inside bright yellow maple leaves, Tyler wanted to know if it was alive. "What is it?" he inquired. He listened to the moss, putting it close to his ear. He smelled the rich earthy scent, looked underneath at the fine roots, then stroked the moss as if it were a small animal. His body became quiet—he was focused and calm.

We moved from the moss to an environment of a meadow in fall—the group of six boys eagerly anticipating the arrival of the rabbits. Responding to our question, "What do the rabbits need in order to live?" the boys created a meadow including grass to eat, water to drink, and a log for shelter and safety. They worked together, exchanging ideas, and their excitement began to build as the meadow took shape in front of them. We asked the boys another question: "What would you and the rabbits need to feel safe here in this room?" They offered ideas for the rabbits, saying that they would need to be gentle with them, to not crowd them, to use quiet voices and hands, and to not make big movements. On asking them how we would get to this quiet place, Tyler replied clearly to the group, "I need to touch the moss again, to feel still in my body. Maybe we all need to hold the moss again to get still." We brought out the moss once more, and as it was passed around the circle again we were all stilled.

Tyler was in an institutional setting because of his violence toward others. He had a difficult time controlling his impulses, being aware of social behavior, and respecting other people. The therapists were working to determine how he could reintegrate into society, where he would go next. As Tyler identified something that helped him to settle himself, something as simple and accessible as a piece of moss, he was learning how to find and replicate calmness, developing the tools to better interact with the world. ∾

Each simple experience like this can build toward another. For children in psychiatric facilities, the natural world offers an essential voice to the process of recovery. These children are familiar with chaos; what is less familiar to them is a way to find calmness. They often lack the pathways to settle themselves or to order their internal process. For children being prepared to reenter the world outside of treatment, it is imperative that they learn internal skills to self-calm, to focus, to read the world around them, to find the inner resources to interact with others. For many children, experiences with nature and animals, can trigger and identify unexpected abilities and provide a reason for them to access these abilities.

A piece of moss may become a link that leads to gentleness with self and others; a rabbit seen in the context of its meadow may build inquiry, stewardship, and community. Children may be able to see the direct cause and effect of their actions, to feel the success of making the rabbits, and later a dog, feel safe, and of identifying and solving the problem. The immediacy of this feedback is very helpful for children as they are trying to learn better social cues and interactions. As they read the animals, they respond and create a safe environment for them. The children, following their natural curiosity, may be inspired to work together to create a safe environment, connecting with each other and with the natural materials, orienting to how they could be active participants in building a trusting environment together. It is often less complicated than human interaction, and readily accessible for them, endorsing their ability to observe, read, and respond. Such success may be helpful both in the assessment of a child, but also in that child's ability to translate difficult human emotions into something that they can work with and learn from.

Connection with nature does not always happen on its own. Simply placing a rabbit in a room does not mean a child will learn stewardship or kindness. In fact, often the opposite will occur. It may take an intermediary; it may take modeling and intentional support for this engagement to work. Thematic work with nature-based programs may fill this gap, supporting learning and healing in a safe environment.

## SAFETY

NBTs are relatively safe and noninvasive addition to the traditional treatment model; however, the practitioner must have solid training and supervision from an organization or other individuals in the field. The practitioner must be aware of laws, contraindications, and procedures for safety. Guidelines for such safety have been developed by many organizations.[3,17,18]

There are issues that are common to both nature and animal approaches. A few examples of these are (1) What are the health laws for the state? (2) What are the regulations for the specific facility? and (3) What medical concerns are there regarding allergies, wounds, fears, dislike of nature/animals, infection (risk to individual or animal), misuse of animal, grief at separating from material or animal, previous history (e.g., dog bite, phobias), rare/endangered plants, poisonous plants and animals (e.g., ticks, poison-ivy, poison sumac), and laws regarding gathering of plants?

State and local laws must be followed carefully when involving animals in institutional settings. Animals must be free of communicable diseases and external parasites and must receive regular vaccinations. They must be checked for stress, behavior, and suitability for this work. Certain animals are better suited for this work than others.[24]

In NBTs, animals and natural materials should not be considered modalities. The animal or natural materials are not "tools" and should not be "used" as such. NBTs may be viewed more ethically as relationships and interactions that assist the goals of therapy. Ethical consideration must be high on the list of any practitioner. The welfare of the animal, natural material, and client is a complex and interrelated issue in healthcare settings.[19-21]

If the medical intervention and outcome-based models are applied to animals and natural materials, the pressure to increase revenue, publicity, or even benefits for people can outweigh the considerations needed for the animals and natural materials. Simply put, what is needed at the core of interactions in NBTs is safety and respect for the client, safety and respect for the animal, and care for the natural materials.

Objectivity is also important to the success of this work. A frequent, incorrect assumption is that everyone likes animals and nature, or that they should. It is vital to respect an individual's choice. Professional responsibility is needed for a good, safe program to develop. Preparation, training, and thoughtful development will lead to high quality programs.

Facilities often have an initial reluctance to initiate programs, liability and safety issues being the most commonly cited concerns. Once these concerns have been appropriately addressed and the site is deemed suitable, the administration must be highly involved and the staff willing to participate actively in order to develop and maintain a high-quality program.

 ## Resources

American Horticultural Therapy Association (AHTA)
909 York Street
Denver, CO 80206
(303) 370-8087
www.ahta.org

American Humane Association
63 Inverness Drive East
Englewood, CO 80112-5117
(800) 227-4645
www.americanhumane.org

Animals as Intermediaries (AAI)
Seabury School, Inc.
PO Box 155
Concord, MA 01742
(978) 369-2585
www.aai-nature.org

Center for Animal and Human Relationships
    (CENTAUR)
Virginia-Maryland Regional College of Veterinary
    Medicine
Virginia Polytechnic Institute and State University
Duck Pond Drive
Blacksburg, VA 24061-0442
www.vetmed.vt.edu

CENSHARE
University of Minnesota Gateway
200 Oak Street SE, Suite 350
Minneapolis, MN 55455-2040
(612) 626-1975
www.censhare.umn.edu

Delta Society
289 Perimeter Road East
Renton, WA 98055-1329
(425) 226-7357
www.deltasociety.org

International Association of Human-Animal
    Interaction Organizations (IAHAIO)
c/o Delta Society
289 Perimeter Road East
Renton, WA 98055-1329
www.iahaio.org

The Latham Foundation
1826 Clement Avenue
Alameda, CA 95401
(510) 521-0920
www.latham.org

North American Riding for the Handicapped
    Association (NAHRA)
PO Box 33150
Denver, CO 80233
(800) 369-RIDE
www.narha.org

People-Plant Council
Virginia Polytechnic Institute and State University
Blacksburg, VA 24061
www.hort.vt.edu/human/PPC.html

People, Animals, Nature (PAN)
1820 Princeton Circle
Naperville, IL 60565
(630) 369-8328
www.pan-inc.org

Tufts University
Center for Animals and Public Policy
200 Westboro Road
North Grafton, MA 01536
www.tufts.edu/vet/cfa/

As the field grows at a rapid rate, it is important that individuals have training and adhere to generally recommended standards for safety and procedure. Each time a person with good intentions but no training takes an animal into a hospital, clinic, or school, that person jeopardizes the client, the animal, himself or herself, and the field as a whole. It is up to each individual to develop his or her professional skills and add to the thoughtful, ethical, quality programs that are available.

## CREDENTIALING

NBTs are rapidly growing in numbers of organizations, service programs, and practitioners. Each discipline within the field of NBTs has approached training and credentialing differently. Generally, for it to be considered *therapy,* the practitioner should be a health/human service provider certified/licensed/recognized in his or her specific field (e.g., social work, psychiatry, occupational therapy). The practitioner would then apply the specialty training in NAT or AAT within the scope of his or her profession.[22,23]

## TRAINING

Certification and masters degree courses are expanding in numbers throughout the country and abroad. Coursework ranges from semester-long graduate level work, to 1-day certifications. There is currently no consensus on the amount of training needed to work with NBTs. Each discipline and association has developed its own criteria. Several specialties have created certifications (e.g., Therapeutic Riding and Horticultural Therapy). As a resource, various organizations are listed at the end of this chapter.

## SUMMARY

In a time when staff turnover rates are high and concern is expressed for retaining staff, the application of NBTs can be as helpful for renewing the engagement of staff members as it can be supportive for clients. Often staff members will have interests in animals and plants; connecting them with creative programs that encompass their own interests can lead staff members to renewed commitment to and interest in their work.

The very diversity, beauty, and intricacy of nature and animals offer unique possibilities for the practitioner. Creative and dynamic treatment plans can be developed, addressing meaning and healing in an integrated manner. As practitioners consider the environment their patient has come from, the losses they may be experiencing, and the ways to provide multileveled resources for their recovery: nature and animals bring with them the broad spectrum of connection and community. Ultimately, working with nature and animals can benefit not only the patient, caregiver and family, but may also have a positive impact on how individuals interact with nature and animals and the world around them.

## *References*

1. Simson S, Straus M (eds): *Horticulture as therapy: principles and practice,* Binghamton, NY, 1998, Food Products Press.
2. Davis S: Development of the profession of horticultural therapy. In Simson S, Straus M (eds): *Horticulture as therapy: principles and practice,* Binghamton, NY, 1998, Food Products Press.
3. Arkow P: *Pet therapy: a study & resource guide for the use of companion animals in selected therapies,* Stratford, NJ, 1998, Author.
4. Wilson EO: *Biophilia,* Cambridge, Mass, DC, 1984, Harvard University Press.
5. Ulrich RS: Biophilia, biophobia, and natural landscapes. In Kellert SR, Wilson EO (eds): *The biophilia hypothesis,* Washington, DC, 1993, Island Press, p 107.
6. Ulrich RS: View through a window may influence recovery from surgery, *Science* 224:420-421, 1984.
7. Kahn PH: *The human relationship with nature: development and culture,* Cambridge, Mass, 1999, Massachusetts Institute of Technology.
8. Beck A, Katcher A: *Between pets and people,* New York, 1983, Putnam Publishing Group.
9. Friedmann E, Katcher AH, Lynch JJ, et al: Animal companions and one-year survival of patients after discharge from a coronary care unit, *Public Health Rep* 95:307-312, 1980.
10. Beck A, Katcher A: A new look at pet-facilitated therapy, *JAMA* 184(4):414-421, 1984.
11. Rowan A, Thayer L: Foreward. In Fine A: *Handbook on animal-assisted therapy,* San Diego, 2000, Academic Press.
12. Fine A: *Handbook on animal-assisted therapy,* San Diego, 2000, Academic Press.
13. Wilson C, Turner D (eds): *Companion animals in human health,* Thousand Oaks, Calif, 1998, Sage Publications.
14. Thoreau HD: *Journal,* January 23, 1858.
15. Reynolds RA: Proceedings, Tufts Animal Expo, Boston, Mass, 2000.

16. Reynolds RA: *Bring me the ocean: nature as teacher, messenger, and intermediary,* Acton, Mass, 1995, VanderWyk & Burnham.

17. Delta Society: *Standards of practice for animal-assisted activities and animal-assisted therapy,* Renton, Wash, 1996, Delta Society.

18. Fredrickson M, Howie A: Guidelines and standards for animal selection in animal-assisted activity and therapy programs. In Fine A: *Handbook on animal-assisted therapy,* San Diego, 2000, Academic Press.

19. Beck A: The use of animals to benefit humans: animal-assisted therapy. In Fine A: *Handbook on animal-assisted therapy,* San Diego, 2000, Academic Press.

20. Hart L: Understanding animal behavior, species, and temperament as applied to interactions with specific populations. In Fine A: *Handbook on animal-assisted therapy,* San Diego, 2000, Academic Press.

21. Iannuzzi D, Rowan A.N: Ethical issues in animal-assisted therapy programs, *Anthrozoos* 4(3). 1991

22. Delta Society: *Animal-assisted therapy: therapeutic interventions,* Renton, Wash, 1997, Delta Society.

23. Nebbe L: *Nature as a guide: nature in counseling, therapy, and education,* Minneapolis, 1995, Educational Media.

24. Centers for Disease Control and Prevention: Draft guidelines, Atlanta, 2000, CDC.

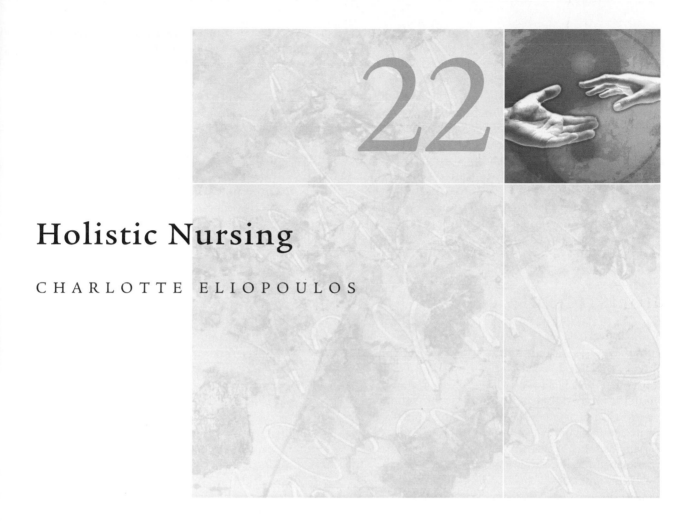

# Holistic Nursing

CHARLOTTE ELIOPOULOS

egardless of the nature of the condition, disability affects the whole person—body, mind, and spirit. There are changes in function, roles, and relationships. Old competencies need to be regained and new skills learned. Priorities are shifted and values clarified. Emotional and spiritual issues arise, often calling for as much attention as physical symptoms. Repair and restored function of a damaged body part are essential to the rehabilitative process, but these activities only begin to address the multifaceted needs that commonly arise. At the core of achieving a meaningful, satisfying life in which independence and quality of life are optimized is the process of assisting the client in the process of healing.

## HEALING VERSUS CURING

In the biomedical system, healing often has been viewed synonymously with cure; however, they are different processes. Curing implies the elimination of a disease and its signs and symptoms. Usually, curing focuses on finding and treating the physical cause of the disease. The probability of cure can be determined by comparing the person's progress to expected, predictable outcome measurements, such as reduction in size of an inflamed organ or return of electrolytes to a normal range. It is not always possible to cure, and death is seen as the consequence of a failure to cure.

On the other hand, healing implies living in harmony with a disease. Elimination or cure of the

275

disease may not be possible, but a person can learn to have a peaceful existence with the disease and discover satisfactions through other dimensions of self. The focus exceeds the physical disease and expands to consider such aspects as the person's emotional comfort, quality of relationships, spiritual well-being, achievement of potential, and ability to discover purpose. The process and meaning of healing are highly individualized and unpredictable. Rather than being viewed as a failure to be resisted at all costs, death is considered a natural process that serves a purpose. And, although cure is not possible in every circumstance, healing always is. Working within a healing framework rather than the cure-oriented paradigm of the biomedical system is significant in rehabilitative care.

## HOLISTIC NURSING

Holistic nursing is about healing. Holistic nurses concern themselves with the interrelationship of the physical, psychological, social, and spiritual dimensions of a person as they facilitate healing. They assist an individual through doing and being, e.g., through interventions such as medications, dressing changes, instruction, and other caregiving tasks, as well as by serving as tools in the healing process through their therapeutic presence and interactions.

Although the term *holistic nursing* has become popular in the last few decades, the concept of holism in nursing practice is not new. More than a century ago, Florence Nightingale laid the foundation for holistic practice by demonstrating that providing emotional and interpersonal support are as essential to caring for the sick as cleaning hospital rooms and changing dressings. Her writings emphasized the role of nursing to create an environment in which natural healing could take place.[1] A century thereafter, as nursing theories began to proliferate, the holistic orientation of nursing was highlighted as nursing was defined as

- Activities that supported a person in becoming a whole, integrated, balanced individual[2]
- A process that demands interpersonal and interactive relationship with the client in an effort to help the client mobilize resources to adapt to stress[3]
- The study of human and environmental energy fields[4]
- A caring relationship that helps a person expand consciousness to move toward an integrated whole[5]

- A combination of scientific knowledge with caring interactions[6]

In addition to having a holistic orientation, these theories imply that interventions that fall within the complementary and alternative realm (e.g., guided imagery, therapeutic touch, hypnotherapy, environmental modification) are used by nurses to support the healing process.

Holistic nursing as a specialty emerged from the birth of the American Holistic Nurses Association (AHNA). Displeased and discouraged by the disease- and dollar-oriented healthcare industry in the United States that relegated nurses to the role of task-doer, a small group of nurses founded the AHNA in 1980 as a means to express a different view of nursing—or perhaps better stated, to reemphasize the healing role of the nurse upon which the profession was founded. The AHNA also wanted to influence new directions in healthcare using a holistic paradigm. Since its inception, AHNA has promoted a philosophy of nursing that

- Views health and disease as part of the human experience
- Considers health as the harmonious balance of the body, mind, and spirit in an everlasting environment
- Accepts disease and distress as opportunities for increased awareness of the interconnectiveness of the body, mind, and spirit
- Empowers clients for maximum self-care

In addition to educational programs and publications, the AHNA has developed standards for holistic nursing and a certification process for nurses who desire to demonstrate specialization in this area.

## THE HOLISTIC NURSE AS A HEALING TOOL

As mentioned earlier, holistic nursing is as much about being as doing. Presence is an important part of the caring process in holistic nursing and implies that the nurse is completely available to and connecting with the client. Not only are physical connections made, but psychological and spiritual ones as well. Therapeutic presence requires that nurses assist clients by becoming part of the healing process rather than just performing tasks. Some of the ways holistic nurses facilitate a therapeutic presence that fosters healing are described in Box 22-1.

BOX 22-1

*Measures That Promote a Therapeutic Presence*

- Confirming the intent to help, know, accept, and serve before interacting with client
- Identifying unique aspects of the individual client
- Centering and focusing on the present time
- Taking a deep breath before entering the client's space
- Offering undivided attention and full availability to the client
- Minimizing distractions
- Actively listening
- Communicating openly and honestly
- Accepting the client's communication without judgment
- Demonstrating a stable, grounded demeanor
- Supporting and comforting
- Viewing the caregiving experience as a special opportunity to participate in the healing of another human being
- Engaging in an ongoing personal process of self-discovery and healing

The foundation of all therapeutic activity is built on relationships and interactions. Three components of relationship-centered care that are essential within a holistic model of practice have been identified.[7]

1. *Patient-practitioner relationship:* Active collaboration with client and family; integrating elements of caring, healing, values, and ethics to enhance and preserve dignity of client and family
2. *Community-practitioner relationship:* Recognizing, understanding, and working collaboratively with the various communities (e.g., family, friends, co-workers, neighbors, religious and social groups) that interact with the client and family
3. *Practitioner-practitioner relationship:* Respecting, understanding, sharing, coordinating, and communicating with all practitioners involved in client's care

To foster relationship-centered care, the holistic nurse must be committed to learning as an ongoing process, open communication, self-reflection and awareness, conflict resolution, empowerment of others, collaboration, and cooperation.

## HOLISTIC NURSING ACTIVITIES IN REHABILITATION

The administration of medications and treatments, instruction, assistance with ADLs, and other types of conventional caregiving certainly are important activities of nurses engaged in rehabilitative care. Holistic nurses will complement these traditional nursing functions with additional activities to foster holism and healing; some of these additional activities include whole person assessment, touch and intention, coaching, promoting psychological hardiness, caring for the spirit, and weaving the pieces together.

## Whole Person Assessment

Often, the scales of rehabilitation are tipped more heavily on the side of the physical aspects of care rather than the psychological, social, and spiritual components. Although this emphasis is important to ensure that basic life-sustaining needs are met, the impact of disability on the multiple facets of an individual's life must be considered and addressed. Meaningful assessment of the body, mind, and spirit demands more than completing a checklist of symptoms. The client must be helped to peel through the layers of beliefs, attitudes, perceptions, and feelings to reveal strengths and needs that influence the rehabilitative process. The holistic nurse creates a sacred space where feelings can be openly and safely expressed. Active listening, focused presence, and touching facilitate this activity.

Carefully planned questions, in terms of substance and style, stimulate disclosure of relevant information. Examples of the types of questions a holistic nurse would use in this process of discovery are listed in Box 22-2.

Important insights can be gained by encouraging the sharing of stories. By helping a client reflect on his or her life story, holistic nurses help that client to see the unique role he or she plays in his or her family and community despite, or perhaps because of, his or her

BOX 22-2

## Examples of Questions That Facilitate Holistic Assessment in Rehabilitation

- What do you see as your strengths? Your weaknesses?
- How well did you care for yourself before you developed this condition?
- What was your view regarding your health and your body before you developed this condition? What is it now?
- What has given your life meaning?
- What goals have you set for yourself?
- Does this condition interfere with your life goals?
- How has this condition affected your life?
- Do you believe you have the ability to improve your function?
- Has there been a sense of balance in your life? Is there now?
- How successful do you think you can be in making the changes in your life to support your rehabilitation/recovery?

- Do you feel you have the capacity to achieve a meaningful life while living with a disability?
- What type of support do you have in achieving your rehabilitation goals?
- Who are the significant people in your life?
- What role does faith play in your life?
- Do you believe in God or a higher power?
- Do you pray?
- Do you want others to pray for you?
- In what way do you believe that you can influence your rehabilitation?
- To what extent do you believe that you have the inner resources to cope with and improve this situation?
- How do you find peace and comfort?
- Do you believe that there is a reason you are in this condition?
- Has anything positive come out of this disability?

disability. Sometimes a story can be elicited merely by asking a client to describe his or her life. For a client who needs more guidance, the nurse may ask the client to describe the chapter titles within the book of his or her life story. The following case study is an example.

 ## A Case Study

### Multiple Sclerosis

Sherry Winthrop is a 42-year-old high school teacher, wife, and mother of two children—a 15-year-old son and a 12-year-old daughter who has developmental disabilities. Sherry believed that she had balanced the demands of an active career and family quite well. Although her husband also was a teacher with similar job demands, Sherry bore most of the responsibilities for the management of their household and special needs of their daughter. Then, her life changed. A slight tingling in her legs progressed to numbness and then paralysis. Other symptoms quickly appeared and a diagnosis of multiple sclerosis was made. Within a few months Sherry went from being a highly active person who had control of her life, home, and family to one who was dependent on others for basic ADLs.

Initially, Sherry's family was significantly disrupted. Her husband, never having shopped for groceries, prepared meals, done laundry, cleaned the house, or man-

aged the activities of two active children, was overwhelmed and frustrated. Her son was angry about the added demands placed on him and the disruption to his life. Her daughter displayed some behavioral problems as she faced performing more tasks without her mother's help. In reflecting on this situation, Sherry commented, "Thank goodness I was too absorbed in my own problems to be concerned with rescuing them," because she discovered that as the months progressed, her family not only adjusted but demonstrated strengths not apparent before her illness. She offered the following outline of the chapters in the book of her life story.

- A humble beginning: oldest of four children in a poor family
- The childhood that never was: having to be responsible for the care of younger siblings, cook meals, and manage the house because parents worked
- Taking the reins: recognizing that I need to achieve academically so that I could win a scholarship and get away from home
- Breaking loose: going away to college and working hard to get all that my parents couldn't provide
- Love finds me: meeting Paul and being swept off my feet
- A new beginning: adjusting to a new marriage and my first teaching job
- Focus on achievement: gaining acclaim as a top educator
- Integrating motherhood: adapting our son into our lifestyle

- Unexpected kink in plans: birth of a daughter with disabilities causes the need to modify career plans
- Shining as superwoman: the need to prove I could do it all
- Trying to be indispensable: doing way too much for my husband and children
- Crash: my multiple sclerosis strikes, causing major changes
- The gift: my limitations enable my husband and children to develop and shine in new ways
- Unveiling a new me: shedding the superwoman facade and learning to discover the person within
- Future: uncertain, but an adventure we all are prepared to face

Sherry's chapter titles not only reveal her understanding of her life journey and her attitude toward her condition but also help her to understand the strengths she possesses, the impact of her choices, and the lessons that can serve her as she travels down new paths. ✎

Active listening and affirmation of the importance of sharing stories (e.g., "What you have shared with me has been very useful in helping me to learn about your unique situation and needs.") are strategies that foster the use of this approach to collecting holistic information about clients.

Exploration into clients' use of complementary and alternative therapies is a basic component of the assessment process of holistic nurses. The direct, intimate nature of the caregiving activities in which nurses engage with clients often facilitates clients' sharing information with nurses that may not have been shared with other healthcare providers. In addition to learning about the therapies and products used, the holistic nurse will probe into related factors, such as clients' motivation for using complementary and alternative approaches and how these therapies are used.

On completion of the assessment, the nurse will
- Analyze and validate data collected
- Identify care needs
- Coordinate the development of an interdisciplinary care plan
- Aid the client in linking with the conventional and complementary/alternative practitioners that could prove useful
- Support and educate the client in the use of various therapies, and track progress to evaluate the effectiveness of the care plan and care activities

BOX 22-3

*Basic Steps in Therapeutic Touch*

1. **Centering:** The nurse relaxes, quiets the mind, and focuses on the intention to help the client.
2. **Assessing:** With the hands several inches from the client's body surface, the nurse runs his or her hands from head to toe over the entire body to identify areas of altered energy flow. These areas can have different sensations (e.g., hot, dull).
3. **Mobilizing:** The nurse runs his or her hands from head to toe several times to promote energy flow. The nurse is directing his or her own energy to unblock the client's energy.
4. **Targeting:** The nurse places his or her hands above areas that have been identified to have different sensations from the rest of the body or over areas that have been symptomatic.
5. **Grounding:** Most treatments end with the nurse placing his or her hands directly on the client's feet to assist in grounding the client.

## Touch and Intention

Touch is a common occurrence in nursing practice. In addition to the performance of many procedures that require direct physical contact, touch is used to convey compassion, facilitate communication, and provide comfort. Nurses' historical use of touch as an integral part of their caregiving activities makes therapeutic touch (TT) a popularly used complementary modality among holistic nurses.

Although the use of touch for healing has existed since ancient times, TT became popular in nursing in the 1970s with the work and research of Delores Krieger.[8] Krieger advanced the theory that people are energy fields and that obstructed energy could be responsible for unhealthy states. She proposed that the nurse could draw on the universal field of energy and transfer this energy to the client. This incoming energy could help the client to mobilize his or her own inner resources for healing and help to unblock the client's obstructed energy.

The term *therapeutic touch* is almost a misnomer for this healing modality because there is little direct physical contact between the practitioner and the individual being treated. Rather, TT is an energy-based therapy; the nurse enters the client's energy field to assess and treat energy imbalances. Box 22-3 outlines the steps in TT.

The first step of TT is for the nurse to center himself or herself and focus on the intent to heal (this is sometimes referred to as healing meditation). During this step the nurse quiets the mind and prepares physically and psychologically to connect with the client. This is considered a crucial step in the process to enable the nurse to be fully present in the moment with the client.

TT is used to reduce anxiety, relieve pain, and enhance immune function.[9-11] Healing Touch is a form of TT that uses interventions that surpass basic TT. A multilevel educational program and certification in Healing Touch is offered throughout the country by the Colorado Center for Healing Touch. Information is provided at the end of this chapter on locating resources for Healing Touch and TT.

## Coaching

The long-term and sometimes frustrating course of rehabilitation can prove discouraging for some clients. They may become overwhelmed with the many changes they face and new skills they must learn. Being told or taught what to do in itself isn't enough to guarantee that clients will accept and comply with the rehabilitation program. Regular and frequent encouragement, support, and caring (in the form of concern) must be provided to ensure success. Coaching is an effective strategy for achieving this.

Coaching has long been used to help athletes, actors, musicians, and other performers master tasks and achieve peak performance. Teaching, motivating, guiding, encouraging, supporting, and offering feedback are core elements of the coaching process. Coaching has important implications in rehabilitation for[12]

- Teaching and reinforcing knowledge and skills required to regain and improve function
- Empowering clients for self-care
- Motivating clients to commit and adhere to rehabilitation goals and activities
- Establishing realistic, acceptable goals
- Helping clients reframe their problems into opportunities
- Providing positive reinforcement, inspiration, and hope

The following case study is an example of how a holistic nurse used coaching to assist a family in coping with the realities of a chronic condition.

## A Case Study

### Congestive Heart Failure

Mr. Akers is a 68-year-old man with a history of manic-depressive disorder, congestive heart failure, and severe bilateral edema in both lower extremities secondary to fluid imbalance. He was discharged to his daughter's home after a hospitalization for an acute episode of congestive heart failure. His daughter and her family are assisting Mr. Akers with his daily care, and a nurse is visiting to monitor his status and assist the family in managing his care.

Since his discharge, Mr. Akers has demonstrated behaviors that indicate that his manic episodes are not under control. He walks incessantly during the day and night, which is having a negative effect on his edema and on his caregivers. His daughter is attempting to make Mr. Akers sit with his legs elevated all day and take a 2-hour nap every afternoon to reduce his edema and hyperactivity. Mr. Akers has resisted this, which has caused frequent arguments between him and his daughter.

During a home visit the nurse identified the tension in the family, in addition to the symptoms displayed by Mr. Akers. Mr. Akers' daughter angrily stated that she could not keep "working herself to death to care for her father if he wasn't going to do whatever he could to help himself." Mr. Akers responded with equal anger that his daughter "is bossing him around and treating him like some kind of invalid." Mr. Akers' son-in-law, trying to be a peacemaker between his wife and her father, suggested that maybe additional medications could be prescribed to remedy the problems.

Through speaking with Mr. Akers, the nurse determined that he did understand that he was becoming more hyperactive, the importance of reducing the edema, and the relationship of the edema to his increasing agitation. However, Mr. Akers had strong feelings about the quality of his life, needed to protect his self-esteem, and wanted to be as independent as possible. Further, he did not want to be as immobile as his daughter demanded because he wanted to avoid having to place greater burdens on her.

Mr. Akers' daughter expressed an understanding of her father's desires and wanted him to have the highest quality of life that he could. She admitted that she became so focused on reducing her father's edema that she went to an extreme and overlooked the impact of her demands on her father's quality of life. She also acknowledged that she often forgot that many of her father's behaviors were the result of his psychiatric illness rather than his merely being stubborn.

The nurse guided the family members in expressing their concerns and feelings so that all issues were in the open. She then outlined the facts.

1. The edema was contributing to Mr. Akers' behavioral problems and vice versa.
2. Being active and having opportunities to enjoy "normal" activities were of utmost importance to Mr. Akers.
3. Mr. Akers' edema needed to be reduced to improve his physical and mental health and quality of life.
4. Family tensions needed to be resolved to protect the health of all family members and to preserve the integrity of their relationships.
5. Mr. Akers had a right to make informed decisions regarding his care, even if this meant he could shorten his life span. He also had a responsibility to comply with the caregiving decisions that he had agreed upon with his family.

The nurse verified with the family that these were the major issues that needed to be addressed and they concurred. She reinforced her observation that Mr. Akers and his family shared a desire for him to live the highest quality of life possible.

The nurse provided education regarding factors that could exacerbate Mr. Akers' symptoms and possible actions that could be taken to decrease them. In reference to the management of his edema, the nurse presented Mr. Akers with options on a scale of 1 to 10 in which

> 1 = No change in actions; symptoms would progressively and quickly worsen
> 10 = Legs elevated most of the time and activities severely limited; edema would decrease

The nurse asked Mr. Akers to tell her and the family where he would like to be on the scale. Mr. Akers thought for a minute and responded that he could commit "to something near a 5, where he knew he would have some symptoms but could still do some of the things he liked." After ensuring that Mr. Akers understood the consequences of his trade-offs, the nurse counseled the family on the importance of accepting Mr. Akers' less-than-perfect choices.

Under the nurse's guidance, the family developed a plan of care to which everyone agreed to commit. The plan provided that Mr. Akers would participate in regular ADLs, garden for 15 to 30 minutes each day, and elevate his feet for at least 10 minutes out of every hour that he was ambulatory or standing. Mr. Akers agreed to comply with the plan without having to be forced by his daughter; his daughter agreed not to attempt to restrict her father's activities any more than what was agreed upon. The nurse wrote a contract based on the agreed plan, which was signed by all family members.

The nurse emphasized that although the plan may not be perfect, it was realistic and something that everyone could live with, which would promote its potential success. She advised them that on her next visit she would check progress and discuss additional interventions that

could prove helpful, such as TT, massage, acupuncture, and yoga. As she left, she praised them for their commitment to developing a realistic plan and assured them of her belief that they could make it work. The nurse intended to telephone before the next visit and between future visits to check compliance and offer guidance, encouragement, and praise. ∾

## Promoting Psychological Hardiness

Adapting to a disability and adjusting to changes are common challenges for clients undergoing rehabilitation. The full potential for restoration of function is more likely to be achieved if clients possess a psychological predisposition that enables them to adapt and accept changes. Psychological hardiness is such a predisposition.

There are certain characteristics associated with psychological hardiness.[13,14]

- An openness to risk taking and change
- Seeing problems and challenges experienced as a normal part of life
- Commitment to family, friends, and goals
- A sense of personal power and control over one's life
- An understanding that body, mind, and spirit constitute an integrated whole

These characteristics are both contributors to and outcomes of a healthy state. Further, they can influence attitudes and behaviors that promote successful rehabilitation. Recognizing this, the holistic nurse reinforces and helps clients to strengthen psychological hardiness. Some ways in which this is accomplished are by helping clients to recognize poor health habits; learn new behaviors to develop positive health habits; practice risk taking; improve relationships with significant others; recognize and exercise personal power; discover purpose and meaning of health conditions; and reflect on the interconnection of body, mind, and spirit.

## Caring for the Spirit

Spirituality is a concept that is broader than religious practices. It is the essence of our being, the intangible breath of our soul that enables us to see more to our lives than a physical existence. The care and nurturing of the spirit can provide the motivation and hope that allows clients to face what initially can be viewed as the insurmountable task of restoring or adapting to lost physical function.

The holistic nurse understands the significance of the care of the spirit to the healing process and provides this spiritual care by

- Assessing the way in which clients express spirituality, connect with God or another higher power, experience relationships, view disease and disability, make sense of suffering, and express spirituality through prayer or other means
- Identifying blocks to spiritual expression
- Helping clients accept the mystery of illness and suffering
- Providing a loving, accepting presence
- Actively listening
- Using touch and encouraging others to share physical expressions of caring
- Respecting and supporting rituals that aid clients in establishing sacred time and space
- Encouraging forgiveness of self and others
- Supporting opportunities for prayer, meditation, centering; praying with and for as appropriate
- Affording opportunities for creative expression (e.g., art, music, cooking)
- Encouraging the sharing of stories

In addition to caring for the spirit of clients, holistic nurses understand that to be effective healers they also must care for their own spirits. They need to affirm their own strengths and weaknesses, satisfy their need for meaning and purpose, reflect on and share their stories, and establish their own sacred space and rituals. The practices of prayer, meditation, imagery, and relaxation are among the ways that awareness and centering can occur to facilitate the nourishment of the spirit.

## Weaving the Pieces Together

The process of rehabilitation is a multifaceted, complex one demanding that the client learn new skills, overcome obstacles to self-care independence, adjust to role changes, interact with various disciplines, and stay focused and motivated to reach goals. The expertise of many healthcare providers—both from conventional and alternative medicine—can facilitate this process; however, if not coordinated, monitored, and supported, the result can be loose threads that create

### Resources

American Holistic Nurses Association
PO Box 2130
Flagstaff, AZ 86003
(800) 278-AHNA
www.ahna.org

Healing Touch International
12477 W Cedar Drive, Suite 202
Lakewood, CO 80228
(303) 989-7982
www.healingtouch.net

Nurse Healers-Professional Associates
    International, Inc.
3760 South Highland Drive Suite 429
Salt Lake City, Utah 84106
(801) 273-3399
www.therapeutic-touch.org

more frustration and difficulties for the individual who already may be overwhelmed with the effects of the disability.

The holistic nurse, in addition to providing the direct care that has been traditionally associated with nursing, serves as the expert coordinator of care by

- Identifying helpful therapies and resources to assist with assessed needs
- Facilitating the location and use of services
- Communicating and coordinating activities with all therapists and providers
- Educating the client and family about care options and requirements
- Advocating for the client
- Monitoring the impact of all therapies and caregiving activities on the client's body, mind, and spirit

By assisting the client to weave the multiple threads of care together, the holistic nurse helps to create a strong fabric of coordinated care that creates a synergy among the interdisciplinary team and optimizes the client's potential for success.

## References

1. Nightingale F: *Notes on nursing,* London, 1860, Harrison.
2. Roy C: Future of the Roy model: challenges to redefine adaptation, *Nurs Sci Q* 10:42-48, 1997.

3. Erickson H: *Modeling and role modeling: a theory and paradigm for nursing,* Lexington, Ky, 1983, Pine Press.
4. Rogers M: *The theoretical basis for nursing,* Philadelphia, 1970, FA Davis.
5. Newman M: *Health as expanding consciousness,* ed 2, New York, 1994, National League for Nursing.
6. Watson J: *Human science and human care,* New York, 1988, National League for Nursing.
7. Pew Health Professions Commission: *Health professions education and relationship-centered care,* San Francisco, 1994, Center for the Health Professions, University of California.
8. Krieger D: *Therapeutic touch: how to use your hands to help or heal,* Englewood Cliffs, NJ, 1979, Prentice-Hall.
9. Daley B: Therapeutic touch, nursing practice and contemporary cutaneous wound healing research, *J Adv Nurs* 25:1123-1132, 1997.
10. Easter A: The state of research on the effects of therapeutic touch, *J Holist Nurs* 15(2):158-175, 1997.
11. Peck SDE: The effectiveness of therapeutic touch for decreasing pain in elders with degenerative arthritis, *J Holistic Nurs* 15(2):176-198, 1997.
12. Eliopoulos C: Chronic care coaches: helping people to help people, *Home Healthc Nurse* 15(3):185-188, 1997.
13. Kobasa S: Hardiness and health: a prospective study, *J Pers Soc Psychol* 42:168-177, 1982.
14. Wang JF: Verification of the health-related Hardiness Scale: cross-cultural analysis, *Holist Nurs Pract* 13(3):44-52, 1999.

# II

# SPECIFIC REHABILITATION CONDITIONS

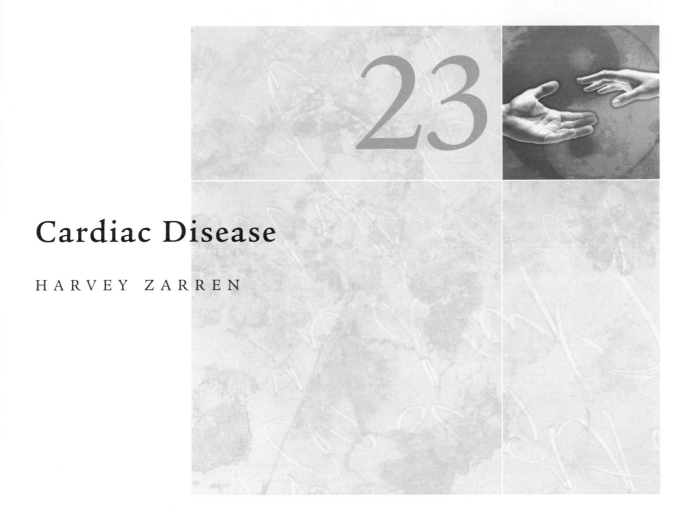

# 23

# Cardiac Disease

HARVEY ZARREN

Sharing one's expertise with compassion and love: this is the essence of relationship-centered medical care. In our technically based, scientifically focused, financially driven medical model, *compassion* and *love* are words that often seem out of place. However, at the level of the bedside, in the presence of a human being who has suffered a possibly life-threatening or disabling event, compassion and love are the essence of what is needed.

Rehabilitation can be defined as "restoring or bringing to a condition of good health, or useful and constructive activity."* Rehabilitative services—restorative help for sick or injured people—here is found a natural place for sharing knowledge and expertise with compassion and love.

By offering compassion and love, a caregiver can readily gain acceptance and credibility, even while soothing fear; overcoming avoidance, denial, or hostility; or bypassing resistance. Offering compassion and love is also useful while opening a patient to knowledge; reassuring someone confused, in pain, vulnerable, and guarded; or comforting someone at the end of life. Such a caregiver provides connection and relationship while offering knowledge, support, relief from suffering, and most importantly, hope.

In recovery efforts after illness, hope is a key, if not *the* key, ingredient: hope of recovery, hope of cessation of pain, hope of return to an active life, or hope at least of a death without suffering or loneliness. Hope is best fostered by human relationships and often by

*Merriam Webster's collegiate dictionary, ed 10, Springfield, Mass, 1999, Merriam-Webster, p 986.

belief in some higher power. In any acute situation with a given patient, a human relationship or connection that brings knowledge and support and is composed of expertise offered with compassion and love can most quickly provide hope.

Spiritual conviction or connection can provide enormous strength in the face of illness and disability. Those who come to an episode of illness with spiritual conviction or who gain it during or after an illness gain very valuable inner support.

In all cases, the most immediate need at the bedside or in the office or rehabilitation department is human caring. Respect, genuine listening, touch, humor, empathy, and nonmoralizing and nonjudgmental interactions all typify caregivers who most easily establish connection with sick and needy patients. These caregivers readily offer the hope that is an incredibly effective motivator for learning patience, courage, endurance, and persistence—all characteristics of the successfully rehabilitated patient.

## USING ALL THE TOOLS OF RECOVERY

Too often, the tools applied to rehabilitation are limited to technology and pharmaceuticals. Optimal rehabilitation efforts require that all tools of recovery must come together: science and technology, pharmaceuticals, exercise, educational classes, hope, motivation, humor, grieving, warmth, love, and compassion. All are essential parts of the recovery and rehabilitation process after illness. The human tools and the technical tools are more successful working in concert than they are working alone. If they cannot both be present, then the human tools are more likely to enlist, encourage, and stimulate a patient's own inner healing tools.[1]

Often the so-called alternative or complementary therapies are offered in more humane ways than are the rushed, financially scrutinized modalities of modern Western medicine. The nature of complementary therapies is to take time, to use repetition, and to open patients to inner growth. These are essential aspects of rehabilitative medicine.

## THE HEALING CONNECTION

In 1990, at Union Hospital (a member of The North Shore Medical Center) in Lynn, Massachusetts, the au-

BOX 23-1

*The Healing Connection*

The Healing Connection at Union Hospital connects patients, caregivers, families, friends, and administrators. We seek a greater vision that establishes respect for the healing qualities connected with interpersonal caring and interaction. Union Hospital provides educational, healing, and supportive experiences in a setting that recognizes and promotes the self-healing abilities of each individual. The Healing Connection ultimately places people and human interaction in the center of the healing process for the benefit of both patients and caregivers.

From the Healing Connection vision statement, Lynn, Massachusetts.

thor brought together a group of people to found an effort that would become The Healing Connection program. The vision statement of The Healing Connection declares respect for the healing qualities of interpersonal interaction, promotes the self-healing abilities of individuals, and places people and human interaction in the center of healing for the benefit of patients and caregivers (Box 23-1).

Once people are placed in the center of the healing process, then all therapeutic modalities become tools, and all useful tools can be applied. There then need not be competition between allopathic and complementary tools. All tools that suit a given patient in a given situation can be used by ethical, competent practitioners working together for the benefit of the patient. Integrated care can mean merely integrating tools; the people, both caregivers and patients, must be placed and must remain in the center of the healing process. The focus must always be on the people, not the tools! It is then that medical care in general and rehabilitative services in particular can apply any and all useful methods to assist patients in getting back to the greatest possible degree of wholeness.

## CARDIAC REHABILITATION

Cardiac rehabilitation is most often prescribed after an event such as a heart attack or after an intervention such as coronary bypass surgery. The goal of cardiac rehabilitation is to bring patients back to a condition of health or optimal activity. One goal might be to enable patients to return to work. Another might be to assist patients in understanding their illness and its treatments. Still others might be to help people improve their health to overcome disabilities and to help patients adjust to their illnesses and to any disabilities illness has conferred on them.

One goal of cardiac rehabilitation must be prevention. Primary prevention means preventing first cardiac illness episodes. Secondary prevention means preventing further events after an initial event. Cardiac rehabilitation is actually suited to both types of prevention, but it is generally used for secondary prevention after a cardiac event has occurred.

A goal commonly talked about for cardiac rehabilitation is to successfully prevent future events that are "costly" to the healthcare system. In reality, healthcare itself needs rehabilitation of its "heart" so that it might begin to become prevention oriented rather than intervention oriented.

Prevention is generally low cost (with the programs discussed in this chapter ranging from $800 to $5,000 in cost) and people oriented, emphasizing education, motivation, and personal responsibility. Technological interventions and pharmaceuticals are costly (with angioplasties costing about $18,000 and bypass surgery as much as $45,000). These expensive interventions are applied to people after they are sick. So far there has been little commercial interest in shifting healthcare to a prevention orientation. A commerce-centered, money-oriented culture might never make a shift toward prevention, regardless of the human cost resulting from an intervention-oriented system. Furthermore, the current system, based on intervention and managing money not wellness, is eroding the morale and wellness of caregivers as it seeks to do more technical care at a lower cost.

Cardiac rehabilitation is particularly suited to prevention, both primary and secondary, using all tools, both allopathic and complementary. Heart disease, by its very nature, lends itself particularly well to both prevention and the use of alternative and complementary tools.

## CARDIOVASCULAR DISEASE

Cardiovascular disease is the number one cause of death in the United States each year, killing more men and women than all cancers combined. In 1998,

949,619 persons in the United States died from cardiovascular disease. This amounted to 40.6% of all deaths.*

The major cause of cardiovascular illness in the United States is a condition called atherosclerosis. Atherosclerosis is a complicated process that ultimately narrows and occludes arteries, the blood vessels that carry oxygenated blood from the heart to all the organs and tissues of the body. Atherosclerosis also affects the function of arteries themselves, preventing the arteries from opening to carry more blood and oxygen when there is a demand, such as with exercise or excitement.

If the involved arteries are the coronary arteries to the heart muscle itself, then the result can be angina pectoris (pain), myocardial infarction (heart attack or death of heart muscle), arrhythmia (disruption of the regular, rhythmic beating of the heart), or congestive heart failure (weakening of each heartbeat, causing a backup of blood into the lungs or the body). In each case, the underlying disease is atherosclerosis.

Congestive heart failure is one of the major causes of hospital admissions in the United States. The major cause of congestive heart failure is coronary atherosclerosis. The major cause of atherosclerosis is the American lifestyle with its hurried consumption of vast amounts of saturated fat, primarily in the form of beef, dairy products, and eggs. This diet, coupled with a lifestyle of emotional isolation and loneliness and steadily decreasing exercise, results in an obese population with an enormous incidence of atherosclerosis. Other risk factors for atherosclerosis include smoking, hypertension (high blood pressure), diabetes mellitus, elevated homocysteine, sedentary lifestyle, aging, and family history. Cardiac rehabilitation using allopathic and complementary methods is a very effective way to work with all of the alterable risk factors.

Atherosclerosis is mostly preventable. Only 1 in 500 persons has a severe genetic form of the disease homozygous familial hypercholesterolemia. The other 499 persons determine by their diet and lifestyle whether they will get atherosclerotic cardiovascular disease.[2] Unfortunately our current medical efforts are geared almost exclusively toward intervening after atherosclerosis has already significantly damaged arteries, causing morbidity and mortality.

---

*Data from the American Heart Association.

## Results of Coronary Heart Disease

If patients survive the events resulting from coronary atherosclerosis, they are then left with a spectrum of physical, mental, and emotional conditions that can be addressed effectively by cardiac rehabilitation. Physically, patients might be limited to a greater or lesser degree in their ability to be active. They may be without symptoms, or they may have shortness of breath, fatigue, or chest pain on exertion. Mentally, they may have impaired functioning because of decreased blood flow to the brain. They may suffer mental fatigue or even strokes from clots traveling from the heart. Sometimes multiple small strokes result in dementia or confusion. Emotionally, it is common for people with heart disease to suffer from depression, fear, anger, and denial.

Some patients develop an enormous sense of gratitude and awareness after surviving a critical cardiac event such as a heart attack or after being resuscitated from cardiac arrest. Such people talk about "the gift" of a serious illness that has allowed them to open their eyes to the richness of being alive. More commonly, detrimental emotional effects occur after cardiac events. The concept of one's heart being vulnerable can lead to a wide range of feelings and stresses that can affect a person's life and ability to function. Work and leisure activities, thought processes, lifestyle, relationships, even day-to-day activities of living can all be affected.

The often magical interventions such as coronary bypass surgery, coronary angioplasty, implantable defibrillator and pacemaker therapy, and many medications can also cause disruptions of mental and emotional wellness. The therapies are remarkable for saving lives and improving physical function, but their other effects are often ignored by a rushed medical system seeking to be cost effective.

## Cardiovascular Regulatory Function

The function of the heart and blood vessels in the human body are under the influence of the central nervous system; therefore thoughts and feelings, even subconscious mental activity, can affect the heart and the opening and closing of blood vessels. Facial blushing during embarrassment is a good example of the effect of feelings on blood vessel tone. The blush is actually the opening or dilating of small blood vessels in the facial skin. The sympathetic branch of the nervous system raises heart rate, increases the active squeezing of the heart, and raises the blood pressure. The parasympathetic branch slows the heart rate and lowers blood pressure.

Hormones such as adrenaline (epinephrine), liberated from the adrenal glands, also affect the heart and blood vessels. Epinephrine speeds up the heart rate and causes the heart to squeeze harder. Norepinephrine, released by nerve endings, raises blood pressure and narrows blood vessels, increasing the resistance against which the heart beats. Goodman and Gilman's *The Pharmacological Basis of Therapeutics*[3] contains an in-depth discussion of the effects of nervous system mediators and various medications on the human cardiovascular system.

Treatment of cardiovascular disease and efforts at rehabilitation can affect the cardiovascular regulatory systems either in a supportive way to improve function, or in an adverse way, affecting function to the detriment of patients' wellness. Mechanically performed efforts at treatment, education, and therapy can promote fear, depression, anger, and frustration, all of which might affect the cardiovascular system adversely. Rushed, harassed caregivers can actually add to patients' burdens rather than helping alleviate symptoms and illness.

## COMPLEMENTARY AND ALTERNATIVE THERAPIES IN CARDIAC REHABILITATION

When patients have suffered a cardiac event or have undergone an intervention such as coronary artery bypass surgery and then enter a cardiac rehabilitation program, they need all the caring approaches associated with complementary therapies. They need time, and they need constant support and repetitious presentations of the knowledge needed for lifestyle change. They also need open-hearted attention by nonjudgmental advocates for their wellness. Patients also need opportunities and time for self-exploration.

To make and maintain the changes necessary for successful secondary prevention of further events, patients need approaches that will deal with physical, mental, emotional, spiritual, and tribal aspects of wellness. Programs that use all tools, including so-called complementary or alternative therapies, can do better at holistic approaches to patient change and evolution than programs that do not use all available tools.

Traditional cardiac rehabilitation programs provide graded exercise, often with monitoring; education about the cardiovascular system, medications, and testing; and classes on diet, blood pressure, smoking cessation, cholesterol, and exercise. Psychological support is also offered. Such programs can reduce mortality up to 25% after a heart attack.[4] With the addition of complementary and alternative methods, these programs could do even better.

The word *alternative* can mean "different from the usual or conventional."[*] Alternative medicine can be defined as "any of various systems of healing or treating disease not included in the traditional medical curricula taught in the United States."[†]

American medical education is defined by clinical and laboratory science. Certainly these fields have made major contributions to the care of sick patients through the use of high technology tools and pharmaceuticals, but the care of the patients' mental, emotional, spiritual, and tribal aspects of illness has often gone wanting.

Current managed care programs, with their focus almost entirely on the financial aspects of medical care, have further limited the ability of traditional Western medicine to care for "the whole patient." Harried physicians and nurses not only struggle to give adequate, humane care to patients but are themselves progressively becoming victims of stress and pressured lifestyles. It is no wonder that the number of applications is down for nursing and medical education programs.

It must be noted that so-called complementary therapies are often being westernized in their quest for a portion of the financial pie. As a result these therapies can become altered by the same pressures that have impacted traditional Western medicine. The result can be the deterioration of complementary methods and their ability to deal with the wholeness of patients.

## NUTRITION

One component in the complementary and alternative treatment and prevention of heart disease that has not yet reached anywhere near its full potential is nutrition. In traditional medical school education, nutrition is not taught as "frontline" information. Western physicians get little in the way of clinically useful nutrition information. Medical practice in general in the United States looks at nutrition as an afterthought. Patients with severe atherosclerotic vascular disease, even those on medication for cholesterol control, are often presented with a "house diet" in the doctor's orders. It is as if the patient's high cholesterol magically appears apart from what the patient eats! Furthermore, many physicians feel that patients won't adjust their nutritional behavior, so why bother? In fact, physicians often do not eat in a healthy fashion themselves.

Because of the education and behavior of physicians, nutrition can be looked at as a basic alternative therapy in the United States. Certainly, in cardiac rehabilitation, the energetic use of nutrition information and passionate support for nutritional change can be very useful.

The standard guideline that 30% of a person's calorie intake come from fat sources is not useful for the rehabilitation of cardiac patients. Many coronary disease reversal programs have used the 30% fat American Heart Association diet as part of control treatment, and the results are that over 10 years, 90% of coronary patients on a 30% fat diet will get clinically worse. In fact, this is the most likely reason for the usually stated limited duration of the benefits of coronary bypass surgery patients. Many bypass patients are taught the ineffective 30% fat diet; therefore their atherosclerosis progresses. A diet with a significantly lower percentage of fat is necessary to prevent, treat, and/or reverse coronary atherosclerosis.

Since 1992 the Healing Your Heart program at Union Hospital in Lynn, Massachusetts, has advocated diets very low in fat in an effort to treat, reverse, and prevent coronary atherosclerosis. Those patients using the information have been very successful at staying out of the hospital and at limiting clinical cardiac events. Although solid outcome data has not been compiled because of limited funding for research, I have witnessed a distinct difference in outcomes clinically in those who have persisted with very-low-fat, plant-based diets vs. those who have incorporated less rigorous dietary changes. It has been very uncommon for patients following the significant nutritional changes in the Healing Your Heart program, or in my private practice, to suffer recurrent hospitalization or to need recurrent procedures.

---

*Merriam Webster's collegiate dictionary, ed 10, Springfield, Mass, 1999, Merriam-Webster, p 34.
†Merriam Webster's collegiate dictionary, ed 10, Springfield, Mass, 1999, Merriam-Webster, p 34.

Not only do low-fat diets prevent progression of atherosclerosis, but a 1997 article entitled "Effect of a Single High-Fat Meal on Endothelial Function in Healthy Subjects"[5] has provided information that explains much of the symptom relief of very-low-fat diets. Blood vessels open more widely, or dilate, when the cuffs of muscle around the vessels relax, allowing the vessels to get bigger. The method of relaxation is the production of endothelial-derived relaxing factor (EDRF) by the vessel lining cells. A fatty meal can turn off relaxing factor production for 4 to 6 hours in a normal person, and clinically for up to 2 days in a person with atherosclerosis. A very-low-fat diet allows relaxing factor production to resume, thus angina and other symptoms improve, sometimes quite dramatically.

Truly good nutrition can be a major "alternative" therapy in cardiac rehabilitation. The Cardiac Rehabilitation Department at Union Hospital in Lynn, Massachusetts, has put to use nutrition information in its day-to-day practice. In fact, the hospital nutrition department provides low-fat vegetarian meals routinely to inpatients and in the cafeteria. The effect of appropriate nutrition to cardiovascular health cannot be overstated. A change in diet can provide significant immediate and long-term beneficial effects for cardiac patients. Proper nutrition can prevent the onset of atherosclerosis and its progression; can result in reversal of the process; and can restore normal vascular function, allowing arteries to open or dilate when necessary.

## DR. DEAN ORNISH

In 1990 a landmark book, *Dr. Dean Ornish's Program for Reversing Heart Disease,* was published, opening the door for a major change in thinking about the prevention and treatment of atherosclerotic heart disease.[6] Dr. Ornish has provided cardiac rehabilitation and the entire fields of cardiology and medicine with much useful information. One key to his program is his demonstration that a diet of 10% fat can indeed reverse and prevent progression of coronary atherosclerosis.[7] The medical profession's standard response to the Ornish program with its very-low-fat diet is, "No one will do it!" Not only is this not true, but it is a way to stay focused on high-tech interventions rather than working at a prevention system that can stop and reverse atherosclerosis.

Dr. Ornish's work has clearly demonstrated that lifestyle changes not only affect cardiac symptoms, but they can actually reverse the narrowing of coronary arteries caused by atherosclerosis. He demonstrated this with angiograms,[8] x-ray studies of arteries used in the past as the gold standard of research about atherosclerosis in coronary arteries. Dr. Ornish's program showed the effectiveness of combining good, evidence-based medicine with a multifaceted approach of proper nutrition, human interaction in support groups, exercise, efforts to stop harmful addictions such as smoking, and practices such as directed visualization and meditation. Patients got better, felt better, and had changes in their coronary arteries. We now know that some of their symptom relief was based on coronary artery function improvement.

Dr. Ornish's approach has used scientific methods,[9-11] but with a distinctly human, open attitude, looking at patients as whole persons, not just carriers of hearts with diseased vessels. His approach has enabled him to look at the field of heart disease with holistic eyes, in the fashion of physicians from days before the focus on high technology interventions and pharmaceuticals.

Dr. Ornish moved on from looking at coronary atherosclerosis to looking at the whole human condition and root causes of disease and foundations of wellness. His book *Love and Survival,* published in 1998,[12] looks at the evidence that love and intimacy are directly related to health and wellness. Here again, Dr. Ornish has manifested his extraordinarily wide vision of wholeness in human beings and the need to address more issues than just the physical when looking at healthcare.

The views and evidence in *Love and Survival* are applicable in the field of cardiac rehabilitation, in which human beings beset with heart disease with all its implications must be supplied with information and opportunities for lifestyle change, all of it offered with compassion and love. In this setting, major changes and effects on wellness can be seen. Dr. Ornish's promulgation of complementary therapies for the treatment and prevention of coronary heart disease has opened the door for major advances in the field of cardiology. Indeed, Western medicine owes Dr. Ornish a major debt for his work in restoring human approaches to disease prevention and treatment, and in proving the effectiveness of such approaches with standard medical testing such as arteriography and nuclear positron emission tomography (PET) scans.

Follow-up data from Dr. Ornish's work shows prolonged useful results from his approach.[13] Angina in the experimental group decreased 91% at 1 year and 72% at 5 years. In the control group angina increased 186% at 1 year and decreased 36% at 5 years (although three of the patients had angioplasty). Coronary narrowing by angiogram in the experimental group improved 4.5% at 1 year and 7.9% at 5 years. In the control group, narrowing worsened 5.4% at 1 year and 27.7% at 5 years. Looking at events, myocardial infarction, angioplasty, bypass surgery, cardiac hospitalization, and cardiac death, there were a total of 25 events for the 28 patients in the experimental group and 45 events for the 20 patients in the control group. These results were all statistically significant.

Dr. Ornish's work epitomizes the sharing of expertise with compassion and love.

## DR. HERBERT BENSON

In 1975, Dr. Herbert Benson published *The Relaxation Response*,[14] a book that delineated the physiological responses to stress and a method called *the relaxation response* as a useful tool for dealing with stress. The relaxation response as delineated by Dr. Benson requires four components: a quiet environment, a mental device for focusing (such as a repetitive word), a passive attitude, and a comfortable position.[14]

Dr. Benson opened up the world of meditation and quieting techniques for affecting physiology and dealing with stress. He and his colleagues have done extensive work on the use of meditative techniques in a variety of medical conditions.[15,16] Their work continues actively today.

In *Beyond the Relaxation Response*,[17] Dr. Benson discussed combining relaxation response techniques with one's personal belief system to create the "faith factor" that could be used to treat a variety of medical problems. Using belief and meditation techniques, Dr. Benson related methods to deal even with symptoms such as angina pectoris, the pain from coronary atherosclerosis.

Again, Dr. Benson, like Dr. Ornish, is a pioneer, making nontechnological interventions palatable to Western medical practitioners by supplying research studies and data. It is investigators such as Drs. Benson and Ornish who pave the way for the use of complementary practices in fields such as cardiac rehabilitation.

## HEALING YOUR HEART

At Union Hospital in Lynn, Massachusetts, under the auspices of the Department of Cardiac Rehabilitation, a program called Healing Your Heart[17] has been assisting patients since 1992 with major lifestyle changes using techniques such as facilitated group support, yoga, and guided imagery and meditation. The following description of this program is intended to give the flavor of one particular approach to holistic cardiac rehab. The group is not supported by insurance but charges only $15 per week per person. The fee is designed to make the program available to all socioeconomic levels of the population. Scholarship money is available to those in need, coming from donations and organized community benefits and fundraisers.

A pilot program for Healing your Heart was initiated after a cardiac rehabilitation evening experience called Holistic Healing for the Heart. During that evening, 50 patients and 3 staff members listened to a brief talk on the effects of the nervous system and stress on the heart, then had a series of experiences, including guided imagery, breathing techniques, centering exercises, and some group massage. In the middle of the evening a woman burst into tears and related that she had just found out about recurrent breast cancer. For the remainder of the evening, the 3 staff members and the other 49 patients carried on a healing experience focused on the woman.

The experience of that evening, coupled with Dr. Ornish's findings on lifestyle change, resulted in the organization of the Healing Your Heart pilot program by the author and the nursing director of Cardiac Rehabilitation at Union Hospital. The CEO of the hospital understood that there is a place for a program that gives service to the community without being a major revenue generator and provided funds for the pilot program which was carried out with 13 patients attending three sessions per week for 12 weeks. In addition to the rehab nurse and the cardiologist, the team included a yoga instructor, a meditation and guided imagery teacher, a group process facilitator, and a cooking/nutrition teacher.

Patients spent about 3 hours in each session. They learned about low-fat vegetarian diets; participated in facilitated group support; and learned yoga, guided imagery, and meditation techniques. The patients had coronary disease and significant other medical problems, such as diabetes mellitus, and most of them were not able to undergo any further surgery or interventions. Some had rapidly progressing atherosclerosis with multiple hospital admissions for pain or congestive heart failure. All were taking multiple medications. These were people who could not look to technology for improvement of their health. Instead, they found a way to mobilize their own healing resources. They learned the value of sharing; humor; crying; and stretching their bodies, minds, and spirits. They learned useful tools for coping with stress and tools for dealing with their illnesses. They learned that they were each not the only ones with their problems. They shared solutions. They shared the strengths and frailties of being human.

The program was as educational for the faculty as for the patients. We learned to share, to be more openly human, and to see the amazing strength and ability of the human spirit to overcome and heal illness. We watched dramatic changes in symptoms, and we saw improved activity levels in people whose medications were not changed. We came to see the possibilities for helping people with low-cost, human interventions that are enormously powerful. We came to understand in a deeper way the potential of programs such as cardiac rehabilitation.

After the profound experience of the pilot program, the Healing Your Heart program was established, meeting Tuesday afternoons or Thursday evenings each week. The program originally cost $10 a week. It continues to offer group-facilitated experience, yoga, and guided imagery and meditation. Most patients have already completed our usual cardiac rehabilitation program.

The human growth experiences learned from the pilot program and from Healing Your Heart have altered cardiac rehabilitation. The changes have been subtle, with staff members opening their already expansive hearts and with patients being exposed to the idea that no one is beyond help.

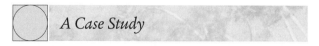

## A Case Study

### Coronary Artery Disease

Bill S. is a patient with severe coronary artery disease. He has been living on a few patent arteries and after two prior bypass operations is not a candidate for surgery or other interventions. He had an ejection fraction of 35% (50% is

low normal), and several portions of his circumflex artery were the only patent cardiac vessels. He had severe symptoms of recurrent angina that dramatically improved after his Healing Your Heart experience. He often meditates on a vision of the Isle of Capri. Using his Healing Your Heart skills, he has dealt successfully with heart failure and an emergency operation for a ruptured abdominal aortic aneurysm. He is active, travels, lives independently, and sometimes plays golf with his son.  ∾

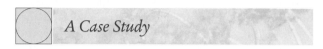

## A Case Study

### Triple-Vessel Disease

Marie S. was in her late 70s when she was told she needed coronary bypass surgery because of severely symptomatic angiographically proven triple-vessel disease. She elected to put off the surgery, in case she might die during it, so that she could attend an important family event. She joined Healing Your Heart and was able to go to the family event. About 2½ months later, Marie came back saying her symptoms were entirely gone! She decided with her physician to wait on the surgery, and she has never had it. Five years later she is an active woman, able to tolerate walking several miles at a time, living independently, and still having no symptoms.  ∾

How do these nontechnical interventions work? Why have so many people been able to avoid interventions such as coronary bypass surgery? Why are some people able to mobilize their own healing abilities? As mentioned before, cardiac function is intimately involved with the function of the central nervous system. Emotions such as fear and despair can profoundly stress a heart starving for oxygen-carrying blood because of narrowed blood vessels. Hope and love can soothe and quiet a threatened heart, decreasing symptoms. Feeling out of control causes stress; feeling in control alleviates stress. Those who have their optimistic, happy, in-control, hopeful attitudes strengthened are able to mobilize their own ability to heal. These people are able to enlist the help of their own nervous system. They can mobilize the healing resources of their body instead of just struggling with their illness and their own heightened, adversely affected sympathetic nervous system.

Feeling supported in a group can also enhance a person's own healing abilities. Sharing feelings often decreases internal emotional pressure, similar to draining an abscess. Sharing grief, disappointment, and fear, as well as joy, success, and fun, can enhance the body's ability to heal. Feeling at ease allows blood pressure and heart rate to drop and peripheral blood vessel resistance to go down, allowing the heart to beat easier, decreasing its need for oxygen and decreasing symptoms of coronary heart disease. Decreasing sympathetic nervous system tone also decreases the potential for rhythm disturbances of the heart.

In group, participants share solutions for solving relationship problems. They learn effective ways for sticking with dietary changes. Staying away from even a single fatty meal can allow normal function of arteries so that they can open on demand, preserving adequate blood flow to the heart and other muscles.

Constant reinforcement for using tools for wellness in group interaction allows participants to get what they need for control of risk factors such as cholesterol and homocysteine. It encourages them to discipline themselves to stop smoking and to stop other addictive, dangerous behaviors. Repetition of information in cardiac rehabilitation classes and group experiences allows participants to assimilate information and to find effective ways to put it to work. Standard exercise in cardiac rehabilitation allows people to find safe levels of exercise and to redevelop a feeling of security in exercising their bodies.

Groups are also good settings for bringing out and sharing tools for coping and for sharing the universality of stressful life events. Ask a question such as "What is one stressful thing that happened to you today and what tools did you use to cope with it?" Out pours the vast array of things that can happen to a person living in our culture. Out comes a multitude of personal tools and techniques that can be shared, offered, and learned. Joy, pathos, anger, outrage, astonishment, and revelation all ripple through the group, bringing laughter, tears, encouragement, and connection. Here people come out of their emotional shell; here they see others having the same problems; here they learn things that help them cope. They then come back later and share their experiences with the techniques they've learned. They can try all the experiences to heal and rehabilitate wounded hearts: all real, not theoretical, "all out there" in the lives of real people.

Exercising with yoga, qigong, tai chi, or other similar techniques not only allows increased conditioning with more effective heart functioning but also seems to improve personal energy, often improves flexibility, increases lymphatic flow, and seems to connect people. These forms of exercise also improve mental discipline and seem to create a meditative state that can be useful in stress reduction.[18,19]

## ADDITIONAL COMPLEMENTARY THERAPIES

Music therapy has been shown to be helpful, even immediately after acute myocardial infarction,[20] and is an integral part of healing for cardiac patients. Active music can facilitate aerobic exercise. Gentle music can still anxiety and quiet stress. Meditative music can help people enter meditative states and can be useful in teaching meditation tools.

Jonathan Goldman explores some of the information about sound and healing in his book *Healing Sounds*.[21] He discusses resonance, the basic vibratory rate of all objects including the human body and its parts. Using vocal harmonic techniques, Mr. Goldman suggests that proper vibration states can be restored, creating healing. The book is a wonderful reference for the use of sound in healing.

Another form of "alternative" therapy that has been studied around heart disease is the use of prayer. Patients can use prayer alone and in groups to help themselves and each other. There is evidence for its effectiveness and for that of other kinds of distant healing.[22-24] In his book *Prayer Is Good Medicine*,[25] Dr. Larry Dossey discusses the healing benefits of prayer and cites the extensive literature on this subject, which is extensive.

In the Healing Your Heart program, patients are taught and encouraged to make interpersonal connections and to feel connected to all of creation. Dr. Paul Pearsall has explored the energy attributes and connections of human hearts and brains and the nature and influence of cellular memory in his breathtaking book, *The Heart's Code*.[26] In this book, Dr. Pearsall talks about the need for a "gentle, balanced, caring, connected, and loving orientation to the world." This is the essence of what an awakened cardiac rehabilitation program seeks to impart to patients.

## ADDITIONAL ASPECTS OF HOLISTIC CARDIAC REHABILITATION

A major barrier to the incorporation of multifaceted programs for cardiac intervention, even standard cardiac rehabilitation, is the feeling of referring physicians that methods of care not based on technology or pharmaceuticals are not really useful or valid. Indeed, many physicians still feel that nutrition is not even an area that matters. Furthermore, capitated managed care systems that take cardiac rehabilitation funds out of physicians' reimbursements further limit patient access to rehabilitation programs.

One way to get past or to transform these physician barriers is for cardiac rehabilitation programs to actively offer experiential programs for physicians. Such programs could include nutritional programs with excellent plant-based diets; experiences with yoga, tai chi, qigong, or other exercise techniques; meditation skills; and groups that encourage physicians to share their own pain and frustration. Cardiac rehabilitation programs could use the actual cases of heart disease among physicians as opportunities for creating physician-focused programs that would enable physicians to open up to more human-centered, experiential interventions for their patients.

A holistic cardiac rehabilitation program can extend its activities into primary prevention, even out into the community. Screening can be recommended for children of patients with heart disease. Efforts can be carried out in schools and in youth organizations to teach young people how to decrease their risk for future heart disease. Using all the tools, a rehabilitation department can reach out to community agencies such as police and fire departments, lowering risks of atherosclerosis and decreasing sick time, illness, and disability. Screening for homocysteine and for traditional risk factors such as cholesterol can be carried out, and stress management tools can be taught. Nutritional education and exercise regimens and group support techniques can all be advocated under cardiac rehabilitation.

Such outreach efforts serve the community as well as individuals and can reach out to older persons and other groups such as business organizations. Outreach efforts by a cardiac rehabilitation department, especially one both using usual and complementary tools, will build support and recognition for a hospital, making it a more attractive and integral part of a community.

## SUMMARY

A whole range of complementary and alternative therapies is available for cardiac rehabilitation. Any patient-supportive technique is a natural fit for rehabilitation in general and cardiac rehabilitation in particular.

### Resources

Healing Your Heart
c/o Wellness and Rehabilitation Department
Union Hospital
500 Lynnfield Street
Lynn, MA 01904

Harvey Zarren, MD, FACC
Connected Healing Institute
33 Hawthorne Road
Swampscott, MA 01907

Preventive Medicine Research Institute
1001 Bridgeway
Box 305
Sausalito, CA 94965

Mind-Body Medical Institute
One Deaconess Road
Boston, MA 02215

Bill Feeney
The Yoga for Health Foundation
Ickwell Bury
Biggleswade, SG18 9EF
England

The physical, mental, emotional, spiritual, and tribal concepts of *heart* make cardiac rehabilitation a fertile field for the use of all healing tools, allopathic and complementary. The key is to share the techniques, knowledge, and expertise with compassion and love.

## References

1. Zarren H: Using all the tools, *Spirit of Change,* pp 26-29, Jan/Feb 1999.
2. Roberts WC: Preventing and arresting coronary atherosclerosis, *Am Heart J* 130:580-600, 1995.
3. Hardman JG, Limbird LE (eds): *Goodman & Gilman's the pharmacological basis of therapeutics,* ed 9, New York, 1996, McGraw-Hill, pp 199-248.
4. Oldridge NB et al: Cardiac rehabilitation after myocardial infarction: combined experience of randomized clinical trials, *JAMA* 260:945-950, 1988.

5. Vogel R, Corretti M, Plotnick G: Effect of a single high-fat meal on endothelial function in healthy subjects, *Am J Cardiol* 79:350-354, 1997.

6. Ornish D: *Dr. Dean Ornish's program for reversing heart disease,* New York, 1990, Random House.

7. Ornish D et al: Can lifestyle changes reverse coronary atherosclerosis? the Lifestyle Heart Trial, *Lancet* 336:129-133, 1990.

8. Gould KL et al: Improved stenosis geometry by quantitative coronary arteriography after vigorous risk factor modification, *Am J Cardiol* 69:845-853, 1992.

9. Gould KL et al: Changes in myocardial perfusion abnormalities by positron emission tomography after long term, intense risk factor modification, *JAMA* 274:894-901, 1995.

10. Scherwitz L, Ornish D: The impact of major lifestyle changes on coronary stenosis, CHD risk factors, and psychological status: results from the San Francisco Lifestyle Heart Trial, *Homeostasis* 35:190-204, 1994.

11. Ornish D: Can life-style changes reverse coronary atherosclerosis? *Hosp Pract* May 1991.

12. Ornish D: *Love & survival: the scientific basis for the healing power of intimacy,* New York, 1998, HarperCollins.

13. Ornish D: Intensive lifestyle changes for reversal of coronary heart disease, *JAMA* 280(23):2001-2007, 1998.

14. Benson H: *The relaxation response,* New York, 1975, Avon Books.

15. Benson H, Marzetta BR, Rosner BA: Decreased blood pressure associated with the regular elicitation of the relaxation response: a study of hypertensive subjects. In Eliot RS (ed): *Contemporary problems in cardiology, vol I, stress and the heart,* New York, 1974, Futura, pp 293-302.

16. Benson H, Klemchuj HP, Graham JR: The usefulness of the relaxation response in the therapy of headache, *Headache* 14:49-52, 1974.

17. Benson H: *Beyond the relaxation response,* New York, 1984, Times Books.

18. Jin P: Efficacy of tai chi, brisk walking, meditation, and reading in reducing mental and emotional stress, *J Psychosom Res* 36(4):361-371, 1992.

19. Jin P: Changes in heart rate, noradrenaline, cortisol and mood during tai chi, *J Psychosom Res* 33(2):197-206, 1989.

20. White JM: Effects of relaxing music on autonomic balance and anxiety after acute myocardial infarction, *Am J Crit Care* 8(4):220-230, 1999.

21. Goldman J: *Healing sounds,* ed 2, Rockport, Mass, 1996, Element Books.

22. Byrd RC: Positive therapeutic effects of intercessory prayer in a coronary care unit population, *South Med J* 81(7):826-829, 1988.

23. Harris WS et al: A randomized, controlled trial of the effects of remote, intercessory prayer on outcomes in patients admitted to the coronary care unit, *Arch Intern Med* 159:2273-2278, 1999.

24. Sicher F et al: A randomized double-blind study of the effect of distant healing in a population with advanced AIDS, *West J Med* 169:356-363, 1998.

25. Dossey L: *Prayer is good medicine,* San Francisco, 1996, HarperCollins.

26. Pearsall P: *The heart's code,* New York, 1998, Broadway Books.

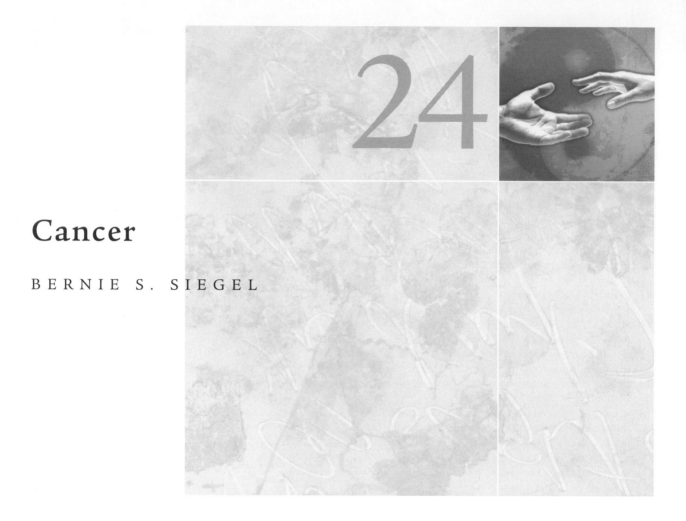

# Cancer

BERNIE S. SIEGEL

24

ollowing is an interview between the editor and Dr. Bernard S. Siegel, author of several self-help books for cancer patients. Dr. Siegel, who prefers to be called Bernie, was born in Brooklyn, New York. He attended Colgate University and Cornell University Medical College. He holds membership in two scholastic honor societies, Phi Beta Kappa and Alpha Omega Alpha, and graduated with honors. His surgical training took place at Yale New Haven Hospital, West Haven Veteran's Hospital, and the Children's Hospital of Pittsburgh. He retired from the practice of general and pediatric surgery in 1989 to speak to cancer patients and their caregivers.

### What is Most Helpful for Caregivers to Provide to Patients?

What is most helpful is hope. That does not mean lies and deceit, but sharing the truth with hope. People are not statistics, they are individuals. Let them know they can be an example to others. I see the qualities in those who out-perform the statistics. We need to pass this information on. I bring the survivors or natives together and let them coach each other.

They need a safe place to share their feelings so they are not stored within where they become destructive to the patient. I also let them know the only thing that is immortal is love.

A disease is not a punishment, but a loss of health. When you lose your car keys you look for them, rather than assume God wants you to walk home. So when you lose your health, search for it, too.

### What is the Most Important Idea About this Work That Caregivers Misunderstand?

They need to accept that it is the other person's experience, and they can only help them with their experience. Patients are the natives, and the caregivers are the tourists. Caregivers cannot fix everything, but they can be a resource in physical, psychological, and educational ways. Remember to ask, "What are you experiencing?" not "What is your diagnosis?" They are two very different things.

Caregivers can provide hope by reminding their loved ones that individuals are not statistics. One never knows the future, so encourage patients to live in the moment, fully aware of what feels right for them. I refer to that as living your chocolate ice cream. If one lives this way, the ability of the body to heal and reject illness is maximized. If one lives what is joyful, every cell knows that you appreciate life and works at keeping you alive. The innate process of self-healing is enhanced. This is not about failing to live forever, but reaping the benefits of living fully now. Guilt is not the issue, but participating in life is. So-called spontaneous remissions are not spontaneous and are not accidents. They are self-induced healings.

Caregivers are not there to create guilt if the patient is not doing what they think is best. Give them information through books and tapes so they know you care, but avoid the lectures and sermons. Caregivers are there to love and listen and help the patient define their path and way to healing. Remember and be willing to accept that healing at times may be related to leaving a body that is no longer a joy to inhabit.

When fear of the future arises again, remind them that one never knows the future. Help them to live in the moment and define their fears so that plans can be made, should any of the things they fear occur. The more specific they are, the less they will find they have to fear. Most of all, as the caregiver let them know that they shall never be alone. They then can live and die in the presence of loved ones, thus never failing anyone.

If caregivers are present and can listen, the patient will uncover his or her own needs and make the right choices. Always keep in mind Helen Keller's words: "Deafness is darker by far than blindness. If you don't listen, you become separated from people."

Also remember that you have needs too. One never knows who will die first, so caregivers should follow the same survival behavior that their patients do.

## What is Your Understanding of *Joie de Vivre*?

Animals and children understand this. It is living in the moment and not in the worrisome future. It is doing what makes you lose track of time. It is the most physiologic state there is. It is living the last 15 minutes of your life repeatedly. It is living your chocolate ice cream, and while you are doing that feeling too good to die.

The opposite is Monday morning, when we have more heart attacks, suicides, and illnesses. So don't let parents, teachers, and religions burden you with guilt, shame, and blame. Realize you are a child of God and go live the message. We are human beings, not doings. Go and create a life. Burn up, not out.

## What is the Will to Live?

The will to live is related to our ability to serve in the manner we choose, and not as others want us to. It is important to know that one's ability to love is not limited by physical disabilities. Once again, watch an animal after surgery awaken and lick and love its family. We need to know that as we go through life, we do give up certain things to enhance other features of our life. One is not truly disabled, but enabled. Attend the Special Olympics if you need to understand this better.

A 70-year-old landscaper I operated on refused treatment for his incurable stomach cancer because he wanted to go home and make the world beautiful before he died. He had no treatment for a cancer I couldn't completely resect because his lymph nodes were positive and the margins of his tumor resection contained cancer. He died at the age of 94 with no sign of cancer. The only thing he required of me was to repair a hernia he developed from lifting boulders in his landscape business. He never tried to avoid death. He went home to live and serve until he died.

I recommend that to all the caregivers and those they care for. I will add, "What is then left to fear?" This answer came from a 90-year-old cancer patient of mine: "Driving on the parkway at night." When that is all that life has left to fear, then you are truly alive and healed.

## Are There Certain Types of Patients Who Do Not Respond Well to Your Approaches, and What do You Say to Them?

I act as a coach. I don't judge people. I offer them inspiration, hope, empowerment, and love or survival behavior.

## Do You Believe There is a Cancer Personality?

Yes, and it has been shown in many studies, from Dr. Caroline Thomas' study of medical students to breast cancer patients.

## What is the Role of Teamwork in Cancer Rehabilitation?

As I said, it is up to the patient to provide the effort, but we are all coaches and team members who assist them. A good coach doesn't criticize individuals but shows them a better technique when they are not displaying the best form. We help people to live. Death is unavoidable, but many never really live before they die.

## How Do You Respond to Criticisms That Your Work has Never Been Subjected to Double-Blind Controlled Studies?

I am listed by the screwball who has the Quackwatch website because I have not done any original research to prove what I am saying. What they never tried to do in the 1970s was research. Who would give you money to do what no one believed in? And I'm practicing surgery, too, at that time. I sent letters to the American Cancer Society and the National Cancer Institute. Even medical journals refused my articles, saying they were interesting but inappropriate. Only Yale students did work with my patients for their graduate work theses. Medical journals where my work was appropriate said "We know this. It's not interesting." From them I got support, and from psychologists and psychiatrists like Karl Menninger and others. They'd already written about mind/body effects and documented it. Since then plenty of others have done research verifying my claims, and some were trying to prove I was wrong.

The only reason I founded Exceptional Cancer Patients (ECAP) is that the American Cancer Society wouldn't let me sit in on their groups to become a better doctor by learning from patients. It's more important when people who don't believe in you end up supporting you with experiments. It is more significant. Otherwise, the work is just dismissed as poorly controlled, printed in a lousy journal, etc.

David Spiegel was very angry about his results (ED: which showed that group therapy prolonged the life of patients with breast cancer) and the fact that our last names were alike. He wanted to prove it was nonsense, and look at him now (ED: Dr. Spiegel is one of America's most prominent mind/body medicine researchers).

Enough! When you have your experience, you don't need anything more. That, and my mother's and wife's love, and you can do anything and not worry about the response. It isn't about ego and inflation. I am criticized by my family, patients, and nurses. They polish my mirror better than any Quackwatch site on the Internet.

What follows now are excerpts from Dr. Siegel's book, *Peace, Love, and Healing,* which illustrate important aspects of living with cancer and cancer rehabilitation.

## FROM *PEACE, LOVE AND HEALING*

### The Five Questions

In my first book I suggested that readers ask themselves four questions about their illness. The list is now expanded to five, and because of what I have heard from participants in the workshops I've been giving around the country, I have also gotten additional insights into what can be learned from the first four. So read through them again, even if you've seen them before. By putting you in touch with what is happening at deep levels of consciousness, these questions can help direct you toward healing.

#### Do You Want to Live to Be a Hundred?

When I first asked this, I was trying to find out whether people felt enough in control of their lives to be able to look forward to the future without fear. How much ability did they have to confront pain and loss and use them as redirections? Only 15% to 20% said yes. Most just aren't willing to live that long unless they could get some guarantees—good health, enough money to live on, and so forth. I started to realize how much difficulty and pain there is in living to be a hundred.

What about all the phone calls you'll get telling you friends and loved ones have died? What can you do with all this suffering? I talked this problem over with God (we speak often—surgeons don't need an appointment), and now when I ask the question I tell people I have a bunch of cards in God's favorite colors, purple and gold, to give out to whomever wants them. They read, "The bearer of this card is guaranteed a life of one hundred years, with all the resources necessary." But God also said to me, "Bernie, don't forget to tell them to turn the card over and read the back before they take one, because on the back of the card it says, 'If not used properly you may outlive everyone you love.'" Think about what it's like to live to a hundred, watching a child die, a spouse die, friends die. Probably you're thinking you don't want to do that, that it would be less painful to be the first to go. But I know how to avoid the fate of outliving everyone you love.

Find some 95-year-olds. They know all the answers, because they've lived through everything that can happen. Whenever I have somebody who's 90 or 95 in my office, I introduce him or her to whichever medical student is being my shadow that month. I walk in and say, for the student's benefit, "I guess you've had a tough life." And the answer is always, "No, I haven't had a tough life. That's why I'm 95." "But," I say, "didn't your house burn down?" Yes. "Business go bankrupt?" Yes. "Child run away from home?" Yes. "Youngest son die?" Yes. "Husband die?" Yes. "Second husband die?" Yes. And then she'll say, "Gee, I guess I have had a tough life." But people like this have learned that the only way to make sure you never outlive all the people you love is to find new people to love. This is always possible, because God has given us a never-ending source of people to love. Through our pain we can find others to love and to heal. That's what groups like Alcoholics Anonymous and ECAP are all about. In fact, I always say that if you're fortunate enough to be an alcoholic or drug addict or have a disease, you can find a group to be a part of, and you'll have lots of people to love and be loved by. We need to start groups for people who just enjoy living.

## What Happened in the Year or Two Before Your Illness?

Originally this question was intended to get people to think about what traumatic events might have occurred in the years leading up to their illness that could have made them susceptible to it. In other words, if your organs are speaking to you, what events in your life might they be talking about? But many people criticized me for making them feel guilty over having caused their own illnesses, which was not at all the point. What I'm trying to do is to empower people, to give them ways to help them get well, not make them feel guilty for getting sick. I want people to realize that, although they may not be able to control all the events in their lives, they can control their response to those events. When people sit in my examining room and say things like, "I'll make this marriage work if it kills me," I want them to hear what they're saying, and see what kind of damage they are doing to themselves with these messages. The mind and body are a unit; they can't be separated. Look at what's happening in your life. Stop killing yourself.

## Why Do You Need Your Illness and What Benefits Do You Derive From It?

If I could change anything in my first book, it might be the wording of this question, which got so many people upset. It needs to be looked at together with the preceding question. Given what happened to you in the years leading up to your illness, what wishes do you think are being met by the illness, what benefits are you deriving from it? Freud long ago showed us the benefits of mental illnesses. The psychiatric literature is filled with case histories illustrating the erotic, self-punitive, and aggressive needs that illness can meet. The problem is that those of us in the body specialties have not been taught this and tend to concentrate on the body and act as though a person and a mind do not come with it. But they cannot be separated, and in order to understand a patient's illness we must always consider the possibility that it meets certain psychological needs that might not be met without it.

Our daughter Carolyn handed me a cartoon one day that showed a gentleman walking up and saying, "I feel great, what a beautiful day, I'll call in sick." Of course, we often think we have to get literally sick in order to get the rest or pleasure we need in our lives. Bobbie and I, therefore, taught our children when they were younger that if they needed a day off from school, they should take a health day, not a sick day. That made them look at life differently. I think all of us need to rethink our attitudes toward health and sickness.

Once you start looking at these issues, you see that there's often a reason why illnesses attack specific body parts or occur at particular times. The body can be very ingenious in getting what it needs. If you're an overworked television reporter and you want a day off, a broken ankle won't keep you off the set, so you get laryngitis. Sometimes the illness is so effective at getting the sick person the care and attention he needs that everyone around that person is exhausted by the effort of meeting those needs. In physical diagnosis there is something I call "Siegel's Sign." When a family comes into my office with everybody looking sick except for one individual, I know that the one who looks well is the one with the illness. That one person is manipulating and controlling everybody else.

A lady who lived in housing for the elderly came into my office one day complaining about how sick she was and how many troubles she was having. I told her that if she wanted to feel better she should go back to her housing project, find someone sicker and with more troubles than she, make that person feel better, and watch what that did for her. When she came back to my office 2 weeks later I asked her, "Well, what happened?" She said, "I went through the whole project, there's nobody sicker, with more troubles than me." People like her need their illness to relate to the world. It is too frightening for them to try connecting to others without it.

I'm not blaming anyone for using illness. Rather, I want you to look at how you might be benefiting from illness and then figure out how you can meet those same needs in a healthier way. Stop punishing yourself in order to get what you need from them, get out of that job you hate—then maybe you won't need an illness. You are mortal. Think of the value of your time.

## What Does the Illness Mean to You?

People who think their disease represents a failure were generally made to feel like failures by parents or other authority figures. But that doesn't mean that they are failures. One woman who described her disease as a failure was the daughter of parents who had both committed suicide. It's not hard to see where she got her feelings about herself.

Another answer people often give is that they see the disease as a punishment or crucifixion. One woman wrote me that she though her disease was tied to her guilt at not being able to be with her mother when *she* was sick. Her mother used to say to her "that she hoped I would suffer everything that she suffered." Parents can have this effect on us—but we can also escape their legacy by becoming aware of it, as this lady was also in the process of doing. She knew that she was entitled to resurrection and not continued persecution.

Of course, some parents give their kids a great legacy. People whose parents gave them the message that "F" is for feedback, not failure, understand that they can make use of the setbacks that occur in their lives to help them grow and be redirected. (Five F's, for example, while a bit heavy, will certainly serve to "redirect" a child toward another, more suitable course of study.) They understand the message of the *Book of Job*—that afflictions heal and adversity opens you up to a new reality. If you can see your illness in that light, you and your family can grow from the experience and be healed by it. The person with the illness can be the great healer in the family by showing everybody how to live and love despite an affliction. From that example, they can learn that life is full of challenges—challenges that represent an opportunity for heroism. When the individual is gone, the family will not forget those lessons.

However, for those of you who cannot forgive yourselves for the failure you think your disease represents, who feel that you shouldn't have been vulnerable to it in the first place or should have been able to defeat it if only you'd fought harder, visualized better, or prayed longer, there can be no such healing. Instead, the burden on everyone will be greater. The message you give your family is that anything short of a cure is a failure. When you do that, you leave behind a terrible emptiness—not just the sense of loss that we all feel when someone we love dies, but a feeling of hopelessness and meaninglessness. Don't pass on to your children the legacy of hopelessness that you received. Now is the time to say no to those feelings in your own life and to the people who created them in you so that your life and the lives of those around you will be different, no matter how short or long the span of time remaining to you.

Later in this chapter, you'll read that an illness may be your greatest dream trying to come true. I know this may be hard to believe when you are dealing with a serious illness, but when you hear one person after another say that their illness is the best thing that ever happened to them, you may start to believe. It's up to you, however, to decide how to interpret your illness—as a failure or as an opportunity for new direction.

## Describe Your Disease and What You Are Experiencing

Contrary to what Susan Sontag has written in her book *Illness as Metaphor,* there is always more to disease than the mere physical diagnosis. When you ask people to describe their disease, fewer than 5% say things like, "I have far-advanced ovarian cancer" or "carcinoma of the colon." Yes, a few intellectuals and physicians do respond that way, but those are the people it's hardest to help. I have to say to them that I know how to treat their diseases, but I don't know how to help them with what they are experiencing.

The people it is easier to help are the ones who describe their experience of the disease because as they talk about their illness, the words always apply to the life that gave rise to it. A friend of mine told me that she had a bad pain in her neck for several days, until she started talking about it and asking why it was there. Then she remembered that she had always called her brother a pain in the neck, but he had died quite suddenly a year before and she had been missing him terribly. Once she realized that she had brought him back to her in this form, she decided she could hold on to her memories of him without the pain—and it went away.

A couple came in to talk to me because the wife said she was having trouble communicating with her husband. When I asked the husband to describe his disease, he told me, "I'm in remission." But when I asked the wife to describe her experience of his disease she said, "I'm in hell." When one person is in hell and the other is in remission, you start to see why they can't communicate.

I talked to a woman who said, "My cancer is invisible, they can't even find the primary site." Her response made her realize that she was putting too much of her energy into hiding something. Then I asked her if she came from a home where she was taught never to reveal her feelings. My questions started her on a process of inner exploration that helped her heal her life.

When a lady hospitalized for abdominal pain described the pain as being like a basketball inside, I told the medical student who was with me to ask her what pressures existed in her life. It turned out that she was chauffeuring all three of her daughters to basketball practice every day and she was worn out. I told her that if she found another ride for the kids, I thought the basketball would be removed from her abdomen.

A gentleman and his daughter came in to see me and the daughter told me that her father just wasn't living. "What's going on inside of you?" I asked him. "Oh, I've got something wild and uncontrollable inside of me," he answered. Sometimes people who live very quiet, controlled lives have their body rebel against them in order to create some excitement, so I suggested to him that if he made a little more noise in his life, maybe he wouldn't need something wild inside of him. A few weeks later I got a wonderful call from his family: "Our father's alive again! He's speaking up and asserting himself and doing things he enjoys."

Thinking about what the disease metaphor means in your life can be very empowering. Jungian psychotherapist and author Arnold Mindell often shares a little myth in which a child is walking through the woods and in the roots of a tree sees a bottle with a cork in it. When he picks up the bottle and yanks the cork out, a genie appears. It says to him, "Aha, I've got you in my power now." But the boy is no dummy, and he looks at the genie and says, "Well, if you're so powerful and smart, let's see you get back in the bottle." The genie goes back in, and the boy slaps the cork in

so that the genie is now rebottled. When we turn toward our disease and ask, "Why are you threatening me, what do you want from me, why are you here?" even "Why do you want to kill me?" we can rebottle the symptoms and obtain their potential gifts. When we do that we also begin to see the positive side of our disease.

"I don't believe that a person actually creates disease, but that his soul is expressing an important message to him through the disease," says Mindell. This was common knowledge in other times and other cultures, but our own focus is so exclusively on the mechanics of the disease that we ignore the message. When you start looking for the message, however, you realize that there always is one.

I was in the hospital one night when I was stopped by a gentleman who wanted me to visit his wife in her room. Rachel had been an exceptional patient, he said, but now she was lying in a coma, close to death, and she was in the hospital to die. I walked in to see her, leaned down and whispered into her ear—because I know people can hear you in coma (as well as when they're asleep or under anesthesia)—"Your husband tells me you have been an exceptional lady. But if you're tired and sore and need to go, it's alright. Your love will remain with your family."

The next day when I walked into the room she was awake, and she said, "I don't want to die." So I asked her to describe her illness. "It's an obstruction," she told me, and I suggested to her that she needed to deal with all the obstructions in her life. It was 5 days before I had a chance to visit her again, but when I walked into her room there was no one in the bed. Instead there was an attractive lady sitting in the window seat. I asked her if she knew where Rachel was. "I'm Rachel," she said, "and I'm going home today." At least 9 months later she was still at home, and although I've lost track of her since, I feel sure that she did indeed deal with the obstructions in her life. Her story is just one of the many I've witnessed that show the truth of my belief that illness is symbolic of life's dilemmas. "The physical disorder," Jung says of such cases, "appears as a direct mimetic expression of the psychic situation."

A recent letter that moved me very deeply described another of these cases in which the disease was a direct expression of an inner dilemma. "Love and happiness surrounded Peter" during his life, his widow wrote, "but not a single day passed that he did not feel the pain endured by his people during the Holocaust." She went on to describe his experience:

In June of 1985, Peter underwent a 14-hour operation which not one of his many physicians expected him to survive. They were further astounded by the diagnosis—a large malignant tumor of the heart. What followed were 20 months of unbearable suffering for Peter and for us a frantic search for treatment, help, and answers. The first question we asked ourselves was how a man who led such a healthy life could be afflicted with cancer. But in this respect we were not unique, as many other cancer victims are puzzled by the same question. What made Peter's case so unusual was the site of his lesion. Our search led us to doctors researching psychological aspects of illness. . . .

Tragically it all became very clear; Peter's condition was the physical manifestation of the Holocaust. The cancer in his heart was the internal expression of the ugliness he witnessed and carried with him in his heart. Peter was just not able or willing to confront and "release" the past, although he was urged by therapists to do so. He was unable to translate his subconscious rage and pain into verbal expression. Although Peter was, by nature, a tolerant and nonjudgmental man, he vehemently opposed the suggestion that he "forgive the world" for allowing the Holocaust to happen.

There is such love, understanding, and wisdom in this letter that I am reminded once again not just of the meaningfulness of illness, but of the solace to be gained from acknowledging that meaning, rather than seeing our afflictions as random. If we see disease as an opportunity for the revelation and unfolding of our individual blueprint, we heal, inwardly and sometimes outwardly as well. As one workshop member said, "We need to heal from the inside out."

One of the most vivid and revealing disease descriptions I've ever seen came from a woman who wrote me about her experience of multiple sclerosis:

This disease could be described [as] an inactive volcano that suddenly goes crazy. At first it sits there blowing just enough smoke to be irritating. And I feel safe during these times. When the main eruption begins, I want to flee and get off the island. There is no place to escape to. I have to watch while the hot lava flows wherever it wants to in my body. I never know if flowers will be able to grow again in those damaged spots or if the trees will grow again to protect me from the painful burn of the sun. Will fruit trees grow on this barren land so that I can pass something on to others? The lava flow scares me. I don't know what areas to protect and I don't know when to protect them. The burns caused are so painful, and the healing is very slow. The losses caused

by the burns may never be replaced. But when the healing comes, it feels good. At first, I was very disappointed that the burns weren't healed in a way that returned me to me. I have been very angry over having no control over the lava flow. This volcano even causes some of my friends to flee the island when it becomes active. But for the friends who stay we share the burn and soothe each other. It is when we feel the pain and the healing together that it is really all right inside.

Writing that description was part of a journey of self-discovery that transformed the life of a woman who had been ill for many years. "When I stop to consider the inner healing that has taken place over the last 8 years," she wrote in a recent letter to me, "I can truly say that this disease has been a blessing that has allowed and is allowing me to make the inner changes that are necessary for me to become a healed person." Does that sound like guilt, fault, or blame?

Another description of a disease, perhaps less vivid but no less revealing in its way, came from a critically ill gentleman who was in my office one day. When I asked him to tell me about his disease, he said, "It's an inconvenience." I told him, "You could die of an inconvenience, you know." He was putting on an incredible performance for his neighbors and coworkers so that he could convince them that that's all it was. Every day he would leave the house, go to work, come home, and collapse the second he got there. Then his family would feed him and put him to bed, and the next day he would start the whole grueling act again. He was determined not to deal with the reality of his illness but to perform, and there was no time for sharing or communication with his family. The effort to deny his illness was draining them all. I worked with him and got him to take some time off to be with his family and to share love with them. This was a healing experience and a relief for everyone.

Some people think of their illness as a blockage or as something trying to manage their life, and I ask them what might be stopping the flow or taking over their life's energy. One woman said, "My tumors are barnacles." Her mother is hanging onto her. A man described his disease as an incredibly beautiful white light and I said, "It sounds as if your disease is too beautiful to give up," which forced him to see how dependent he was on it. The man who described his disease as "proliferating" felt that he was being crowded out by his family. The woman who described her disease as a prison resisted all the treatment options I offered: "Surgery hurts, radiation burns, chemotherapy makes your hair fall out," she said. When I finally asked her "Why don't you just eat vegetables," her answer was, "I don't like them." She couldn't see that she had any choices, hence her prison.

Once you start to use the questions to redirect your life, however, your experience of illness changes. You may have started out thinking of it as a volcano, a barnacle, or an obstruction, but you may move on to thinking of it as a gift, a challenge, a wake-up call, or a beauty mark.

By calling your attention to feelings and problems you may not have been aware of, the disease may be the first step in overcoming them. That's one of the reasons why I hope more doctors will use them in addition to the traditional review of systems. But doctors tend to be mechanics who focus only on defects in the physical mechanism because that's what their inadequate training has taught them to do.

In a study done at Ben-Gurion University in Israel by psychologist Dan Bar-On, 89 heart attack patients and their doctors were interviewed about why they thought the attack had occurred. The physician was much more likely than the patient to put the blame on strictly physiological factors like obesity or smoking, while many of the men tended to blame psychosocial circumstances like a bad work situation. Men who saw their own role in bringing on their heart attacks—for example, those who considered themselves "angry people" under a lot of pressure at work—planned to do something to change their circumstances, and these men made the best recoveries. But regardless of how much progress the patients made, they were better at predicting their degree of recovery than their doctors were, which Bar-On attributes to their greater understanding of what caused the attack in the first place. I agree with Bar-On and see this as yet another instance of the necessity for the doctor to understand the patient's disease as the patient does. Asking for a description of the illness is one step in that direction.

## FROM *PEACE, LOVE AND HEALING:* HEALING THE CHILD WITHIN

### Disease as Punishment

Another of our misconceptions about disease is that it is a punishment for our sins. Generally this guilt has no basis in reality but has been instilled in us by our parents, teachers, and other authority figures in our lives. As a result of the guilt, we long for the multiple crucifixions we think we deserve. My hope is that if we view disease this way, we can use it to open us to the possibility of resurrection.

Freud described this function of disease when he talked about symptoms expressing and gratifying a triple wish. One of the triple wishes has to do with the pleasure-seeking needs of the organism (and that's why I ask my patients to think about what needs of theirs are being met by the disease), the second with aggressive intent toward others (as when we use our illnesses to manipulate those around us), and the third with self-punitive measures as a means of atonement. Karl Menninger relates in *The Vital Balance* that at first he was dubious of this theory—who, after all, "would crave even a minor discomfort, to say nothing of a more serious one?" But his practice taught him the wisdom of Freud's theory, he says. Menniger illustrates the longing-for-atonement theme with the example of a man who had killed his child and then suffered a nervous breakdown. When the man later lost an arm in an accident, he became emotionally healthy again because he felt he had atoned for what he had done to his son. The loss of an arm meant that he had suffered enough.

This way of looking at disease is another of the things I wish we would teach in medical school because every doctor will encounter people who are sick for reasons that are not physical. People may go blind because there is something they do not wish to see, may lose the use of their limbs because they don't want to move, may become helpless because they don't know how else to get the help they need. We doctors need to be trained to look for the reasons behind illness, even when the reasons are psychological rather than physiological in nature.

In the Bible there is a gentleman whom Woody Allen called a very well-adjusted child. For those of you who don't recognize him from this description, his name was Jesus. Jesus was a healer, but he was a terrible doctor: When he saw a man who was paralyzed he said, "Your sins are forgiven," not "Rise and walk." Any good doctor would have tried to get the man back on his feet by applying braces or operating, or at least referring him to an orthopedic surgeon. When people asked Jesus why he took this other approach, he said, "Which is easier, and which would you rather have?" Jesus knew the importance of a healed life, and he knew that a cure is often the byproduct of healing. He healed and cured through forgiveness and faith.

By speaking of the need for forgiveness, I do not at all mean to imply that you are sinners, nor do I think that that was what Jesus meant. Before Jesus healed the blind man he was asked, "Who sinned, this fellow or his patient?" and he said, "Neither." The healing of the blind man was not an issue of sin but of manifesting God's healing gifts, which exist in us all. But many of you feel that you have brought your diseases on yourselves through sin, and Jesus knew that, which is why he knew the crippled man needed forgiveness.

Often this is what our patients need too—not our forgiveness but their own. If they can forgive themselves, they won't need sick minds and bodies. If they can't find enough self-love to grant themselves this forgiveness, then disease can be the atonement that finally releases them from guilt, after which they can finally allow themselves to get well.

I had a psychotherapist in my office one day who just couldn't accept what I was saying about people needing multiple crucifixions and using their disease as punishment. As often happens, God helped out by sending him a patient to explain it to him. She attributed her extraordinary survival to the release from guilt she achieved through illness:

The guilt was so overwhelming that I didn't know how I could continue living unless I found a way to suffer. I felt that I was a bad person and that I didn't deserve to continue living without some sort of suffering in my life. There was no forgiveness. I just couldn't overcome that until I had the cancer. Then, once I had the cancer I said to myself, it's OK, you've suffered enough. Now you can do something positive for yourself.

Her resurrection can now occur. The healer's role is to guide people into self-forgiveness so they will no longer feel that they need to atone, to get them to understand that they are not sinners, and to provide a path to self-healing and self-love.

## Self-Love

I've heard so many of these stories about self-punishment that I'm considering running for the presidency. My reason for wanting to be president is to enact two vital pieces of legislation. One is a law that will say you must love yourself, and my administration will enforce this by having love patrol officers in purple and yellow uniforms walking up and down the streets of every city asking each citizen, "Do you love yourself?" Any-

one answering no will be fined severely. It will be too expensive not to love yourself.

The other major item on my administration's agenda will be to set up a true social security system. You will be assigned a number that puts you in a group that meets for 2 hours every week. There you will receive love and discipline that your family does not provide. This is what our exceptional patient groups do now, and what groups like Adult Children of Alcoholics also do. But there are no "wellness" groups for people who love life and want to live to be a hundred. Until now, if you wanted to join a group, you had to have cancer, AIDS, scleroderma, or some other affliction, or be a drug addict, alcoholic, divorced, overweight, or fit into some other recognized problem category. Recently, however, someone gave me a flyer for something called the Radical Self-Love Group. Maybe this is the start of a new movement. Maybe we won't have to hurt before we begin to live.

I hope that the group membership will help with what I see as the biggest problem in my work—getting people to want to live and undertake the necessary changes in their life. It is all well and good to talk about the healing system and how to activate it, but when you realize what condition our society is in, you begin to understand that this information is not going to make a difference immediately. What is important is creating a society in which self-love and love of others are present. Recently, I read an article by Ushanda io Elima about the Efe Pygmies, who live that way. According to Jean-Pierre Hallet, who grew up among the Efes and administers The Pygmy Fund (Box 277, Malibu, CA 90265), which is dedicated to their physical and cultural survival, they are very expressive of their feelings for each other.

There is a great deal of touching and affection among all Pygmies. Babies and small children are held and often carried. Older children and adults often touch one another. They frequently hold hands or sit with an arm around a friend or place their head in another's lap. Anyone feeling the need for reassurance may touch someone briefly or go for a hug. There is also a great deal of cuddling.

The result of this upbringing is a society in which "Pygmies concentrate their attention on the betterment of their personal relations, which are based on trust." There is no crime, no infidelity, no stigma against sexuality, and great respect not only for each other, especially the elders among them, but for the forest in which they dwell. If we would love one generation of the world's children as the Pygmies love theirs, the planet would change, and our problems disappear.

If you doubt the damage caused by the lack of self-love in our lives, you have only to look around you. Notice how many people commit suicide, overtly or otherwise, with accidents and untreated illnesses. We're so self-destructive that there have to be laws—what I call please-love-yourself laws—even to get us to wear seatbelts or helmets. We poison and numb ourselves with cigarettes, tranquilizers, drugs, alcohol, and unhealthy diets, and we seek out relationships that can never work in a desperate attempt to convince ourselves of our own value. No relationship in the world can make us feel worthy if we don't know that we are.

Without self-love it's hard to fight for one's life. When we give advice to someone about how to live, it's fine if it falls on the ears of an individual who wants to live. But if it falls on the ears of someone who does not love life, there's no point to it. Why live longer if one does not enjoy living? I think the message needs to be, "I love you and I hope someday you will love yourself." Criticizing doesn't help; it will only destroy a relationship and create a feeling of failure.

If you have given love in your early years so that you know that you are lovable, it can be an incredibly difficult journey to try to find it within yourself. Don't think it can't be done. It can. You are capable of changing and finding your true self. That's what groups are for, what psychotherapy can help you do. Alternatively, a bit of what Martin Seligan would call "cognitive retraining" can be useful. That's what was needed by a woman with multiple sclerosis who first wrote to me several years ago. She admitted that many of her problems, physical as well as emotional, were related to her lack of self-love, but said she couldn't seem to stop the negative feelings. In one of her early letter she asks:

How can I love myself when there is one self-disappointment after another? If I were another person trying to love me, I would turn to greener pastures because of the "well today—sick tomorrow" characteristic of MS. How can you love someone so lacking in dependability? You trade in you car when it stops being reliable. You divorce your spouse when he keeps disappointing you. I'm locked up in here with this belligerent self that I would have ordered out, traded in, or divorced a long time ago, if I could have. Am I supposed to learn to love this?

In my reply, I told her about Evy McDonald sitting in front of her mirror and tried to get her to see that the limitations of our bodies need never limit our ability to be loved or to love ourselves. But change doesn't come overnight. It's hard work. In a letter written almost a year after the one quoted above, this lady compared the process of learning to self-love to that of acquiring any other skill, a subject she knows something about from her years as a schoolteacher. Reviewing her progress in what she calls "Loving and Accepting 101," she explains what it is that still holds her back: "I do have the cognitive capability. I am motivated. I am listening. But I'm having some problems getting my assignments completed."

Well, as the professor in this course of study she is pursuing, I feel sure that one of these days this hardworking lady will graduate, as she says she hopes to, "Magna cum love!" Self-love can be acquired, even late in life, no matter what your circumstances. If you read *The Velveteen Rabbit* you will learn what it is to be real and will understand that it doesn't matter if "most of your hair has been loved off, and your eyes drop out and you get loose in the joints and very shabby," because "once you are REAL you can't be ugly, except to people who don't understand."

## Disease As a Gift

We're used to the idea of disease as a punishment or failure—but a gift? Think about what I call spiritual flat tires, and you may begin to understand what I mean. Something that happened to a friend of mine recently reminded me once again that nothing is good or bad in and of itself.

This gentleman has a farm. He loves the old-fashioned way of doing things so he doesn't have any mechanical equipment and plows his fields with a horse. One day as he was plowing his field the horse dropped dead. Everyone in the village said. "Gee, what an awful thing to happen." He just responded, "We'll see." He was so at peace and calm that we all got together and, because we admired his attitude so much, gave him a new horse as a gift. Then everyone's reaction was, "What a lucky man." And he said, "We'll see." A few days later the horse, being strange to his farm, jumped a fence and ran off, and everyone said, "Oh, poor fellow." He said, "We'll see." A week later the horse returned with a dozen wild horses following it. Everyone said, "What a lucky man." And he said, "We'll see." The next day his son went out riding, because now they had more than one horse, but the boy fell off the horse and broke his leg. Everybody said, "Oh, poor boy," but my friend said, "We'll see." The next day the army came to town taking all the young men for service, but they left his son because of his broken leg. Everyone said, "What a lucky kid," and my friend said, "We'll see."

We, too, have to learn to step back and start saying, "We'll see." Instead of judging the events in our lives as good or bad, right or wrong, we must recognize that of itself nothing is good or bad, and everything has the potential to help us get back on the universe's schedule. This does not mean that we have to like what happens, simply that we must remain open to the uses even of adversity. A disease may serve as a redirection—or, as I often describe it, a reset button (which starts you up again the same way the reset button works on a jammed garbage disposal), which reminds me of something that a man at one of my exceptional patients groups meetings said: "I'm here because my 'We'll see' button got me through the night and my reset button is waiting to be pushed."

When you learn to live your life with a "We'll see" attitude, you will understand how it is that disease can be considered a gift. You will know why it is that people asked to describe their illness have called it a beauty mark, a wake-up call, a challenge and a new beginning. The beauty mark was a malignant melanoma, the wake-up call was breast cancer, the challenge and the new beginning can be anything from amyotrophic lateral sclerosis to lupus.

Now when I tell an audience of 500 people with AIDS that they have a gift, they don't throw shoes at me or get up and run out yelling, "What are you telling us?" because they know. They understand that illness can help heal their lives, that it can bring new meaning to relationships with lovers, family, and friends. In some cases it has enabled critically ill young men to find love in a home from which they had been rejected because they were gay. It has brought a community together to love and support each other. And so they do say, "My disease is a gift." That doesn't mean they don't wish to be well, but they wouldn't give up what they have achieved because of their illness.

Does it take courage to be open to this kind of healing? Sure. Do I have the right to tell you your disease is a gift? No, I do not. The gift is yours only if you choose to create it—as I've seen thousands of others do. Listen to the people who have lived the experience, and realize you are the source of your healing.

In the midst of chemotherapy and radiation treatments one woman took time to write me: "I consider my cancer to be such a blessing because through it we have learned so much about how to handle our lives, how to speak out our feelings to each other, how to throw away the junk forever and have more contentment in our lives."

Almost identical sentiments were expressed by a man in an AIDS group:

If I beat this disease, AIDS will be the best thing that ever happened to me because it has been a gigantic, cosmic kick in the ass. It has made me ask, Who are you? What is your life? Are you happy with who you are and what your life is? Sometimes when I say that, it comes out sounding like I reduced AIDS to an EST seminar or something. But however it sounds, that's how I feel.

A 22-year-old man who, with the aid of his doctors, is healing himself of brain cancer, says:

I've learned to live. I love living. I love my family, my friends, my job, everything. And everyone. Every day I wake up and I feel alive! At peace. . . . Please excuse this outburst. I get carried away sometimes.

I've been dealing with cancer for more than a year now. I'm almost glad I got it. It's changed my whole outlook on living. I *live* from day to day. I make the most out of every day.

Stephen Levine, author and counselor, who has worked with hundreds of sick and dying people, once met someone who told him that cancer is the gift for the person who has everything. She was a beautiful 50-year-old woman who had a double mastectomy and she got up at a workshop to explain what she meant.

Three years ago, I was graced with cancer. I looked my whole life for a teacher, and it wasn't until I got cancer that I really started to pay attention to the preciousness of each breath, to the momentum of each thought, until I saw that this moment is all. All my other teachers gave me ideas. This caused me to directly experience my life. When I got cancer, it was up to me to get born before I died.

Feelings like these may be hard to believe in if you haven't personally experienced a serious illness—or even if you have. A young medical student I had worked with was in an automobile accident that left her a paraplegic. She said in a letter to me that she now knows her paraplegia is a gift to her—but "I can't believe I'm really writing this." And yet it's the message I hear all the time. Why? Because the great lesson people learn from life-threatening illness is the difference between what is and is not important.

Love is high on everyone's list of the important things. In the face of illness, this can sometimes mean healing a marriage gone bad, at other times letting go of one that is beyond repair and going on to new things.

A woman who had cancer wrote me a letter describing how she arrived at the decision to seek a divorce after her diagnosis: "I felt, at the time I came down with breast cancer, that I could not live another moment without the love I had so craved my entire life. I felt that love was more important than my next breath of air." After her surgery, as she records in a diary she sent me, she committed herself to life and love:

**I am going to regain my positive attitude toward life, enjoy every day as if it is my last, and have a beautiful love affair. I need to make love and I'm going to do it. . . . In the oddest possible way, this experience has lifted me up out of my despair and isolation. . . . I only hope I can have the strength and will to walk with confidence into the new light that has been shed on my dark road. . . . Human love is the most important thing in life.**

Within the year she had a new husband and a horse—the latter "a present I have waited for every Christmas of my life since childhood. I finally got it! A person should never give up hope. . . . I find a difference in myself: I am not willing to settle for less than the life I desire. . . . I realize the value of living and incorporate that realization into my daily life. . . . I want to live!"

This letter reminded me of a woman at one of my workshops who said that when her doctor told her she had cancer and would have to have a mastectomy, she decided to get a divorce too—and give up a tit and an ass! This is much healthier than deciding you're going to make your marriage work if it kills you.

On the other hand, disease can be the catalyst that enables some couples to find the life and love they need within their marriages. A husband and wife came to my office and when I asked them each to describe his disease, the wife said she saw it as a blossom, an opportunity for growth, the husband said it was eating him up alive. Now when for one it is a blossom and for the other it's a destroyer, you know these are two people who need to communicate better—and the miracle was that from then on, in the time they had left together, they did.

He had been a man who never expressed his needs but kept everything inside of him where, as he said, it was devouring him. But after that conversation in my office things were different. As his wife explained when she told her story several years later at a workshop, this previously quiet, unassertive man started speaking up about his needs as they headed to the parking lot—and he didn't stop. First he told her exactly where he wanted her to bring the car to pick him up, then he told her what route he wanted her to take to get home, how fast she should go, and how to get him from the car into the house with the least possible discomfort to him.

That night they stayed up all night talking about their life together, going through a lot of garbage, as she put it, and a lot of wonderful things too. The next night he insisted that she sleep in the narrow hospital bed with him, even though his doctors had said he needed his rest and should sleep alone. Then he asked her to bring in all of his close friends so that he could pick one of them to mount what he called his halos—beautiful concentric mahogany rings he had carved and gilded in earlier years, as part of his work as an artist. Not long afterward he died beneath those golden rings, with the sun pouring in through the windows and his wife at his side, whispering to him that he would be with the angels. The days they had together after they finally learned to listen to each other were a gift to both of them, one that they might never have had without his illness.

The closing of a piece that appeared several years ago in the *New England Journal of Medicine* is typical of what I call "last paragraphs"—the place where you see the summing up of what a person has learned and accomplished through the experience of illness. These last paragraphs all sound alike, which says to me that the process of healing one's life is the same for all of us, in that we are all members of the same species. Surgeon Robert M. Mack, in his summation of what having cancer has meant to him, says:

**I am very grateful just to be alive. I am very glad to have been permitted to learn to live with, rather than simply die from, my cancer. Mostly, I am glad to measure my life not in terms of what it once was or what I might have wished it to be but in terms of how wonderful it is now.**

A woman in a self-created remission from ovarian cancer writes of the joy she too has discovered in the simplest daily activities.

What an experience having cancer is. My whole life will be different for it as long as I live, and, yes, I am one of those who wants to live to be a hundred. An exceptional nurse at the hospital told me to "live each day to the max." Do you know what the max turned out to be once I was up and around again after two surgeries in 5 weeks' time? It was hanging up laundry in the sun with a cat rubbing against my leg.

Finally there are the words of a woman who has done many years of self-healing. When I first met her about 8 years ago she had extensive breast cancer and was using a walker; now she is teaching school and running workshops: "I imagine someday I'll die of cancer. I don't know what I'll die of, whether it's cancer, a heart attack, or a car crash. I don't really think about it anymore. I'm busy living my life."

## Shopping List for Change: A Five-Part Therapeutic Program

Let me now present you with a list of things I would like to see you do every day to help you become an exceptional human being. In this way you will heal your life as well as the lives of others, and possibly cure any afflictions.

1. Keep a daily journal recording your feelings and dreams. In tests of college students and executives, those individuals who had been asked to keep journals were shown to have a more active immune system and to develop fewer colds and other illnesses during exam time and periods of work stress. Even after they stopped keeping the journals, the immune system remained more active for up to 6 months. Including periodic drawings may also help.
2. Join a therapy group that meets for 2 hours every week, where you will receive love, confrontation, and discipline. It should not be a victim group. If it is a group where everyone complains every week, then don't go back. If you can't find a group specific to your needs, go to an Adult Children of Alcoholics meeting or any other group you like. The affliction doesn't have to be the same as yours; it's the attitude that is important.
3. Meditate, visualize, pray, or listen to quiet music to interrupt your day 4 to 6 times with healing intervals that allow you to refocus, distress, and give your body "live" messages. These are to relax you, not to make you feel you have more work or are not doing it well. So pick what feels right for you.
4. Live one hour at a time, based on your feelings. If you are close to death, 10 minutes might be the time you have to focus on. What I mean by that is not to live as if you're going to die in 1 hour or 10 minutes but to ask yourself at the beginning of that period how you feel. If you do not like how you feel, then resolve those feelings or let go of them within the time limit. This teaches you that you are in charge of your feelings. When your time is significant to you, you will make a point of not wasting it in feelings that you don't like.
5. Twice a day for 15 minutes sit or stand naked in front of a mirror. Work with the feelings that come up—the negativity for most of us—and then learn to love what you see in the mirror just as Evy McDonald did, progressing from her image of herself as a "bowl of Jello" in a wheelchair to a part-by-part appreciation of herself, beginning with her smile, proceeding to her soft hair, and moving on to each of her body parts until she had put herself back together and could honestly say that she found the whole beautiful.

Now that you've read this list, you see why so many people prefer having operations. Only a truly exceptional human being will take on this work. Once you do all of these things, however, you find that you begin to live more and more in the moment, and life becomes a series of moments that you are in charge of. Then joy will enter your life and you will be in heaven without dying.

## FROM *PEACE, LOVE AND HEALING:* COMMUNICATING WITH YOUR BODY

### Edward's Credo

What I Know
1. I have a bad cancer. I read my protocol and know it may kill me.
2. I know how bad this cancer is—I used to be in hospital management.
3. I know all treatments involve risk, including death.
4. Many people die from what I have. I know the statistics.

Therefore
1. There is no need to repeat the above. I have heard it many times from well-meaning people

who feel it is the physician's duty to level with the patient on the dark side, particularly when I have appeared too hopeful at times.

2. Good thoughts, friendship, advice, encouragement, hope, love, energy, and smiles are all gratefully accepted. Please leave pessimism, downers, bitterness, pity, and negative preachiness at the door, without, of course, being dishonest.

Please Know

1. I know you can help me in a positive way if you want to. But please remember that my life belongs to me, those I love, and those who love me.

2. My wife and I are convinced that good medicine is more than highly important knowledge and skills, chemicals and protoplasm. We also believe in the body's mental powers and immunological abilities, as well as the spiritual. We need all the help we can get to bring all of these resources to bear on my problem and to help you help me.

3. I have much to live for and I am trying very hard to do whatever I can mentally and physically to make whatever you prescribe to do as effective as possible.

4. I personally know of people with what I have who have done well despite the poor odds. I intend to also, by buying as much good time as I can for me and those I love. Perhaps we can do even more. That is why I am here. Otherwise, I would not be.

5. There is hope in my heart. Do not do anything to encourage its replacement with pessimism or bitterness, for it will inevitably lessen my comfort level and worsen my conditions.

I wish both doctors and patients would read "Edwards' Credo"—doctors so they'll stop undoing the potential benefits of their medicines with the destructiveness of their words and patients so they'll be inspired to defy those doctors who persist in sentencing their patients to death.

# FROM *PEACE, MEDICINE, AND MIRACLES:* BEGINNING THE JOURNEY

## The Patient's Bill of Rights

A patient's effort to take responsibility and participate in medical choices must begin while he or she is still fighting the shock of the diagnosis and try-

ing to mobilize the will to live. It is the doctor's duty to try to immediately forge a bond of trust by learning about and accepting the patient's beliefs, conscious and unconscious. The quickest way to develop a patient's trust and independence is simply to be human, to share their pain, and avoid playing the role of a mechanic/lifesaver. But, because so many doctors are caught up in that role, patients often must help change them. Toward this end, I advise patients to insist on the following Patient's Bill of Rights, in the form of an open letter to physicians.

Dear Doctor:

Please don't conceal the diagnosis. We both know I came to you to learn if I have cancer or some other serious disease. If I know what I have, I know what I am fighting, and there is less to fear. If you hide the name and the facts, you deprive me of the chance to help myself. When you are questioning whether I should be told, I already know. You may feel better if you don't tell me, but your deception hurts me.

Do not tell me how long I have to live! I alone can decide how long I will live. It is my desires, my goals, my values, my strengths, and my will to live that will make the decision.

Teach me and my family about how and why my illness happened to me. Help me and my family to live now. Tell me about nutrition and my body's needs. Tell me how to handle the knowledge and how my mind and body can work together. Healing comes from within, but I want to combine my strength with yours. If you and I are a team, I will live a longer and better life.

Doctor, don't let your negative beliefs, your fears, and your prejudices affect my health. Don't stand in the way of my getting well and exceeding your expectations. Give me the chance to be the exception to your statistics.

Teach me about your beliefs and therapies and help me to incorporate them into mine. However, remember that my beliefs are the most important. What I don't believe in won't help me.

You must learn what my disease means to me—death, pain, or fear of the unknown. If my belief system accepts alternative therapy and not recognized therapy, do not desert me. Please try to convert my beliefs, and be patient and await my conversion. It may come at a time when I am desperately ill and in great need of your therapy.

Doctor, teach me and my family to live with my problem when I am not with you. Take time for our questions and give us your attention when we need it. It is important that I feel free to talk with you and question you. I will live a longer and more meaningful life if you and I can develop a significant relationship. I need you in my life to achieve my new goals.

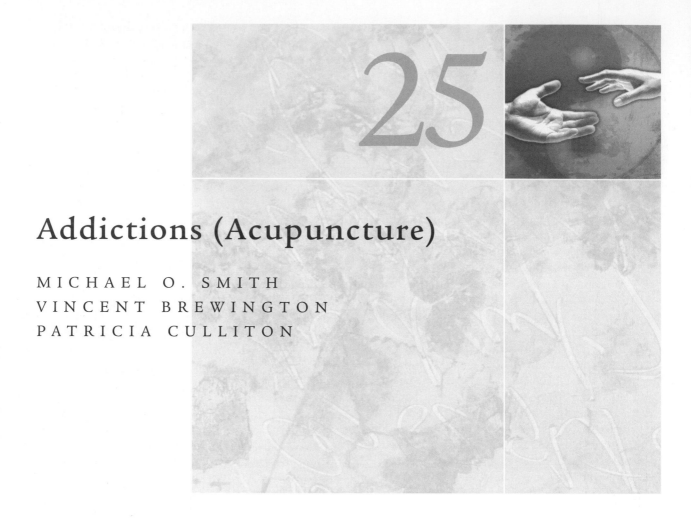

# Addictions (Acupuncture)

MICHAEL O. SMITH
VINCENT BREWINGTON
PATRICIA CULLITON

cupuncture is currently used in the treatment of addictions by approximately 600 substance abuse programs. Clinical evidence supports its effectiveness in ameliorating withdrawal and craving symptoms associated with alcohol, opiate, and cocaine dependence, as well as symptoms associated with most other commonly abused substances. Acupuncture for cocaine dependence has been recognized as a particularly important innovation because there are presently no established pharmaceutical treatments for it. Programs as a foundation for later psychosocial recovery use acupuncture because it is a nonverbal, nonthreatening "first step" intervention that has an immediate calming effect on patients. Initial participation with acupuncture has been found to improve patients' overall treatment retention and to facilitate their subsequent involvement in treatment.

In most programs patients receive treatment of 4 to 5 ear acupuncture points while seated in a large group room so that a substantial number of patients can be treated conveniently. This safe and cost-efficient procedure has gained increasing acceptance from agencies responsible for overseeing substance abuse treatment. This chapter describes the practical use of and research findings related to acupuncture for the treatment of addiction. Mechanisms of action that involve physiology and psychosocial process are covered.

## BACKGROUND

Acupuncture is a major component of the ancient tradition of Chinese Medicine. The principles and goals have remained constant throughout time. The textbook that is most often used today, the *Nei Jing*, was written 2,000 years ago. Numerous nineteenth century U.S. practitioners, including Sir William Osler, used acupuncture. In the early 1970s American interest was renewed when relations with China were opened.

Acupuncture consists of the stimulation of specified locations on the surface of the body that alters and improves bodily function. The Chinese term for a treatment location is *xue*, which means "opening." The traditional Chinese names for these locations often refer to flow on the surface of the earth, such as valley, marsh, crevice, or stream. In the West the term *point* is used. Acupuncture points are physiologically distinct from the immediate environment; they have less electrical resistance and therefore greater electrical conductivity. The points are warmer than the surrounding area by 0.1 to 0.2 degree. The difference in warmth and electrical activity can be detected both by the human hand and by instruments. A painful response to pressure may also be used as a point indicator. The precise location of these phenomena varies within a small area that corresponds to the acupuncture point as denoted on an acupuncture chart. Descriptions of the location and functions of these points have remained constant throughout the centuries.

Acupuncture points can be stimulated by various means: touch, movement, heat, electricity, and needling. Health-related procedures such as acupressure, shiatsu, reiki, and tai ji chuan work on the same principles as acupuncture even though no needles are used. However, needling is the most convenient and efficient means of stimulating acupuncture points.

## PHYSIOLOGICAL MECHANISMS OF ACTION

There have been many efforts made to determine the underlying physiological mechanisms of acupuncture. Acupuncture charts have a superficial resemblance to Western neuroanatomical charts. However, the functions of the meridian channels on acupuncture charts differ substantially from those of nearby peripheral nerve trunks. Ear acupuncture is a particularly clear example of this. The acupuncture chart of the external ear identifies more than 100 separate acupuncture points. These points relate primarily to different body locations and to various organic functions. One can easily verify some of these correlations by noting that the shoulder point on the ear shows abnormally low

electrical resistance in patients with shoulder injuries, as does the ureter point in patients who are passing a kidney stone. The simple innervation pattern of the external ear cannot be used to explain these effects.

Researchers have noted the following variety of specific physiological effects associated with acupuncture as cited in Brewingtion.[1] It has been reported that acupuncture at traditional points produced dramatic effects in electroencephalogram (EEG), galvanic skin response (GSR), blood flow, and breathing rate, while stimulation by needle placement in placebo points produced no appreciable effects. Various studies have linked acupuncture to the production of endogenous opiate peptides, such as beta-endorphins and metenkephalins, and this has been speculated to be a physiological mechanism behind the effects of the treatment on withdrawal discomfort. Acupuncture has also been linked to changes in other neurotransmitters, including adrenocorticotropic hormone (ACTH) and cortisol levels, serotonin and norepinephrine, and 5-HT. A review of research linking endogenous opiate peptide (EOP) production to optimal immune system functioning concluded that acupuncture appears to have beneficial effects on the immune system. A substantial collection of literature thus exists supporting the claim that acupuncture has a variety of neurochemical and other physiological effects.

It should be noted that certain medications—namely, methadone, corticosteroids, and benzodiazepines—seem to suppress part of the acupuncture effect. Patients taking these medications in substantial quantity clearly experience less relaxation during treatment and seem to have a slower response to treatment. Nevertheless, acupuncture is an effective treatment for secondary addiction in high-dose methadone patients. Acupuncture is also widely used to treat adrenal-suppressed patients who need to be weaned off corticosteroid medication. This may suggest that part of the initial relaxation response is endorphin and steroid dependent but that the more important mechanisms relate to a different type of process.

## THE LINCOLN HOSPITAL PROTOCOL

Acupuncture treatment for drug and alcohol problems was primarily developed at Lincoln Hospital, a city-owned facility in the impoverished South Bronx section of New York City. The Substance Abuse Division at Lincoln is a state-licensed treatment program that has provided more than 500,000 acupuncture treatments over the past 20 years. Dr. Yoshiaki Omura[2] was the consultant who began the program.

Initially, in 1974, Lincoln used Dr. H.L. Wen's method,[3] applying electrical stimulation to the lung point in the ear. Lincoln was a methadone detoxification program at that time; therefore acupuncture was used as an adjunctive treatment for prolonged withdrawal symptoms after the 10-day detoxification cycle. Patients reported less malaise and better relaxation in symptom surveys. Subsequently, twice-daily acupuncture was used concurrently with tapering methadone doses. Reduction in opiate withdrawal symptoms and prolonged program retention were noted.

It was accidentally discovered that electrical stimulation was not necessary to produce symptomatic relief. Simple manual needling produced a more prolonged effect. Patients were able to use acupuncture only once daily and still experience a suppression of their withdrawal symptoms. A reduction in craving for alcohol and heroin was described for the first time. This observation corresponds to the general rule in acupuncture that strong stimulation has primarily a symptom-suppression or sedation effect and that gen-

tle stimulation has more of a long-term, preventive, or tonification effect.

The addition of the *shen men* (spirit gate), a point known for producing relaxation, expanded the acupuncture protocol. Other ear points were tried on the basis of lower resistance, pain sensitivity, and clinical indication during a several-year developmental process. Dr. Michael Smith of Lincoln added the sympathetic, kidney, and liver points to create a basic five-point formula (Figure 25-1). Numerous other point formulas using body acupuncture points were tried on an individual basis without any significant improvement. Some programs omit the sympathetic point in pregnant patients; however, there is no basis in acupuncture texts for this precaution.

A standard acupuncture textbook[4] describes the functions of each of the five points in the basic formula as follows.

1. *Sympathetic:* Used for numerous diseases related to disruption in both sympathetic and parasympathetic nervous systems. It has a strong analgesic and relaxant effect on internal organs and dilates blood vessels.
2. *Shen men:* Regulates excitation and inhibition of the cerebral cortex and sedative and antial-

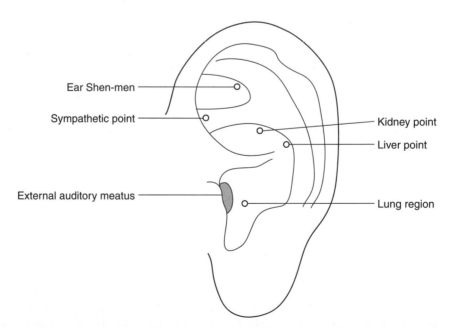

*Figure 25-1* Ear with five ear detoxification points marked. (Modified from Maoliang Q, ed: *Chinese acupuncture and moxibustion,* Edinburgh, 1993, Churchill Livingstone.)

lergy effects. Used for many neuropsychiatric disorders.

3. *Lung:* Used for analgesia, sweating, and various respiratory conditions.
4. *Liver:* Used for hepatitis, anemia, neuralgia, muscle spasms, and eye diseases.
5. *Kidney:* Conditions strengthening points for the cerebrum, hematopoietic system, and kidneys. Used for neurasthenia, lassitude, headache, and urogenital problems.

The value of using one standard group of acupuncture points became increasingly clear. The standard formula seemed to be equally effective for different drugs of abuse at different stages of treatment. Patients responded better when acupuncture treatment was administered quickly without a self-conscious, diagnostic prelude. Because acupuncture produces a homeostatic response, it was not necessary to adjust the formula for mood swings, agitation, or energy.

A group setting enhances the acupuncture effect. A group size of less than six members seems to diminish symptom relief and retention significantly. Patients receiving acupuncture in an individual setting are often self-conscious and easily distracted. These problems are more evident in the management of new patients. In general, acupuncture treatment sessions need to last 20 to 25 minutes. Because chemical dependency patients are more resistant and dysfunctional than others, they should be instructed to remain in the acupuncture group setting for 40 to 45 minutes so that a full effect is obtained. The atmosphere of the treatment room should be adjusted to fit varying clinical circumstances. Programs with a significant number of new intakes and/or socially isolated patients should use a well-lighted room and allow a moderate amount of conversation to minimize alienation and encourage social bonding. On the other hand, programs with relatively fixed clientele who relate to each other regularly in other group setting should dim the lights and not allow any conversation to minimize distracting cross-talk. Background music is often used in the latter circumstance.

## ACUPUNCTURE TECHNIQUE

Acupuncture needles are stainless steel shafts of varying length and thickness. Most Western facilities use the needles once and discard them. Acupuncture needles are provided in convenient sterile packages. Needles are inserted with a brief but steady movement. Ear needles penetrate ⅛ inch, contacting the cartilage if it is present in that location. Needles are twirled 180 degrees for smooth insertion. The patient may feel a momentary sensation similar to a pinch. Occasionally there is a brief sharper sensation that may cause the patient to complain. The procedure is nearly painless and causes the rapid onset of a gratifying sense of relaxation. On first exposure, most patients express fear of the pain of needle insertion and are confused by the idea that little needles can cope with their big problems. Letting prospective patients observe the actual process of treatment easily resolves this fear. It is a mistake to rely on leaflets and verbal explanations.

Patients may notice local paresthesia effects such as warmth and tingling. There may be sensations of warmth, electrical movement, or heaviness in other parts of the body, although these reactions are more typical of body acupuncture than ear acupuncture. Patients may feel quite sleepy after each of the first several treatments. This reaction is part of the quiet recovery process and passes readily. Some patients develop a headache at the end of a treatment session. Shortening the length of the session or reducing the number of needles resolves this problem. Rarely, a needling reaction occurs in which the patient feels dizzy and lightheaded and may actually faint. This reaction (postural hypotension) occurs in many medical and dental settings. When it occurs, one should remove the needles and help the patient to lie down on a flat surface. The syncope will resolve within a few minutes and the patient will exhibit relaxed behavior as though the full treatment had been given. Needling reactions occur more often in persons with a relatively labile autonomic nervous system. Fortunately these reactions are quite rare in the treatment of addiction. Patients should be told to eat before coming for treatment to reduce the possibility of a needling reaction.

The insertion of acupuncture needles never causes bleeding. Hence there is no need for special blood contact precautions during the application of treatment. Based on our experience, treatment sites in the ear bleed about 1% of time after the needles are removed. Thus 10% to 20% of patients will have such a reaction. There are several methods used to cope with this problem in terms of appropriate risk management precautions. Commonly, the patients are asked to remove their own needles and place them directly in a sharps container. Staff may remove needles by only touching the handle and giving the patient a cotton pad to use if bleeding is noted. A small hematoma may occur.

Staff members may press each location with a Q-tip as necessary. Those who are involved in removing needles usually wear gloves, although most gloves do not allow the dexterity needed to grasp small needles. It should be noted that ear needles are inserted so shallowly that about 10% fall out during treatment. Therefore many needles must be retrieved that have fallen on the patient's clothing. Even wearing gloves will not protect staff members who might try to search for such needles. Hence the patients must be instructed to located any fallen needles and discard them properly. Often programs use a needle count procedure. Patients place needles in a paper cup or bowl so that staff can verify that all needles are present before they are discarded in the sharps container. This procedure is particularly appropriate if acupuncture is conducted in a room that is used for other purposes.

## TRAINING PROGRAMS

The location of ear points and the technique of insertion can be taught effectively in a 70-hour apprenticeship-based program. A wide range of substance abuse clinicians can staff most acupuncture components. Training must include a clinical apprenticeship because coping with the individual distractions and group process is more important and more difficult than the technical skill of repetitive needle insertion. Each clinician can provide about 15 treatments per hour in a group setting. Licensed or certified acupuncturists should provide general supervision. This arrangement allows for acupuncture to be integrated with existing services in a flexible and cost-effective manner. Lincoln Hospital has trained more than 3,000 clinicians in the past 10 years. The National Acupuncture Detoxification Association (NADA) was established in 1985 to increase the use of the Lincoln model and to maintain quality and responsibility in the field.[5] More than 1,000 programs outside of the United States have implemented the Lincoln model of acupuncture addiction treatment. Most of this expansion has occurred in public institutions such as hospitals and correctional facilities, as well as in street outreach programs.[6,7]

Dr. Smith developed an herbal formula known as sleep mix, which is used in most acupuncture-for-addiction settings and many other healthcare settings as well. The formula includes camomile, peppermint, yarrow, skullcap, hops, and catnip. These are inexpensive herbs traditionally used in Europe and are reputed to calm and soothe the nervous system and tend to stimulate circulation and the elimination of waste products. The herbal formula is taken as a tea on a nightly basis or throughout the day as symptoms indicate. Sleep mix can be used for the treatment of conventional stress and insomnia and to provide an adjunctive support in addiction treatment settings. Sleep mix is particularly appropriate for the management of alcohol withdrawal symptoms. Patients receiving conventional benzodiazepine treatment will often voluntarily refuse this medication if sleep mix is available.[8,9]

The Lincoln Hospital model can be summarized and defined as follows.

1. Clinicians use three to five ear acupuncture points, including sympathetic, shen men, lung, kidney, and liver.
2. Treatment is provided in a group setting for the duration of 40 to 45 minutes.
3. Acupuncture treatment is integrated with all the conventional elements of psychosocial rehabilitation.
4. Several components of the Lincoln program are commonly combined with acupuncture in other treatment facilities. These include
   a. A supportive, nonconfrontational approach to individual counseling
   b. An emphasis on Narcotics Anonymous (NA) and other 12-step activities early in the treatment process
   c. A lack of screening for appropriate patients
   d. The use of herbal sleep mix
   e. The use of frequent toxicology screenings
   f. A willingness to work with court-related agencies
   g. A tolerant, informal, family-like atmosphere[10,11]

## CONTROLLED RESEARCH

H.L. Wen[3] of Hong Kong was the first physician to report successful treatment of addiction withdrawal symptoms. He observed that opium addicts receiving electro acupuncture (EA) as postsurgical analgesia experienced relief of withdrawal symptoms. The lung ear point was used. Subsequently Dr. Wen conducted several basic clinical pilot studies that formed the basis of subsequent research.

Results from available placebo-design studies support the conclusion that the effectiveness of acupuncture in facilitating abstinence with alcohol, opiate, and cocaine abusers is not due to a simple placebo effect.[1] Seven published studies involving animal subjects (i.e., mice or rats) indicate that EA reduces opiate withdrawal symptoms with morphine-addicted subjects. In these studies, experimental and control animals show behavioral differences with regard to rodent opiate withdrawal symptoms such as hyperactivity, wet dog shakes, and teeth chattering. Each of these studies notes significantly fewer withdrawal symptoms in subjects receiving EA compared with controls. Significantly different hormonal and beta-endorphin levels post-EA are noted between experimental and control subjects in several of these studies.[12]

A number of controlled studies have been conducted on human subjects using various modified versions of the Lincoln Hospital ear point formula. Washburn[13] reported that opiate-addicted individuals receiving correct site acupuncture showed significantly better program attendance compared with subjects receiving acupuncture on placebo sites. Two placebo-design studies provide strong support for the use of acupuncture as a treatment for alcoholics. Bullock[14] studied 54 chronic alcohol abusers randomly assigned to receive acupuncture either at points related to addiction or at nearby point locations not specifically related to addiction. Subjects were treated in an inpatient setting but were free to leave the program each day. Throughout the study, experimental subjects showed significantly better outcomes in attendance and self-reported need for alcohol. Significant differences favoring the experimental group were also found with regard to (1) the number self-reported drinking episodes, (2) self-reports concerning the effectiveness of acupuncture in affecting the desire to drink, and (3) the number of subjects admitted to a local detoxification unit for alcohol-related treatment.

Bullock[15] replicated Bullock[14] using a larger (n = 80) sample over a longer (6 months) follow-up period. Of patients in the treatment group, 21 of 40 completed the 8-week treatment as compared with 1 of 40 controls (Table 25-1). Significant differences favoring the experimental group were again noted. Placebo subjects self-reported over twice the number of drinking episodes reported by experimentals. Placebo subjects were also readmitted to the local hospital alcohol

TABLE 25-1

*Program Completion Rates in Hennepin Study*

| | No. in treatment group (%) | Control no. (%) | p Value |
|---|---|---|---|
| Phase I (daily acupuncture for 2 weeks) | 37 (92) | 21 (52) | 0.001 |
| Phase II (3 times weekly for 4 weeks) | 26 (65) | 3 (7) | 0.001 |
| Phase III (2 times weekly for 2 weeks) | 21 (52) | 1 (2.1) | 0.001 |

detoxification unit at over twice the rate of experimental subjects during the follow-up period. Worner[16] examined outpatient treatment outcomes for a sample (n = 56) of alcoholic subjects assigned to one of three conditions: acupuncture (n = 19), sham transdermal stimulation (n = 21), or control/standard care (n = 16). Acupuncture involved both ear and body points and was provided only 3 times weekly over a 3-month period. Subjects exposed to sham transdermal stimulation had ECG pads attached to their arms and legs and were told that the procedure was a needleless form of acupuncture. No significant between-group differences were noted on outcome measures (e.g., retention, Alcoholics Anonymous [AA] attendance, alcohol relapse). It was concluded that the purported effectiveness of acupuncture for treating alcohol withdrawal may be a placebo effect and that results were at variance with Bullock.[14] While statistically significant effects were not observed, it should be noted that the acupuncture group showed the best outcomes on seven of eight measures reported. Given this trend, it seems probable that results would have reached statistical significance if a larger sample were used.

Lipton[17] conducted a placebo-design experiment on the effectiveness of acupuncture treatment for chronic cocaine/crack abuse. Subjects (n = 150) were randomly assigned to receive either auricular acupuncture at correct sites or acupuncture at nearby ear points not related to detoxification. Self-report measures and urinalysis profiles showed a significant tendency in both groups toward decreased cocaine consumption. Pretreatment cocaine/crack usage averaged about 20 days per month with all subjects. Self-reported use was reduced to an average of 5 days per month with both groups. Urinalysis profiles indicated superior outcomes with the experimental group during treatment. Over the course of treatment, experimental subjects showed a significant tendency toward greater day-to-day decreases in cocaine metabolite levels. This result was particularly pronounced after 2 weeks of treatment. Placebo subjects who remained in treatment longer than 2 weeks showed cocaine metabolite levels that were on average slightly higher than those shown at baseline (i.e., on treatment day 1). Experimental subjects consistently showed lower than baseline metabolite levels throughout treatment.

Konefal[18] examined the efficacy of different acupuncture point protocols with patients with various substance abuse problems. Subjects (n = 321) were randomly assigned to one of three groups: a one-needle auricular treatment protocol using the shen men point, the five-needle Lincoln protocol, or the five-needle Lincoln protocol plus selected body points for self-reported symptoms. All groups showed an increase in the proportion of drug-free urine tests over the course of treatment. However, subjects with the single-needle protocol showed significantly less improvement compared with the other two groups.

During the trial and error search for a more effective ear acupuncture formula for addiction treatment, it was clear that a large number of points had some effect on acute withdrawal symptoms. Ear acupuncture charts indicate that all areas on the anterior surface of the ear are identified as active treatment locations. Using a placebo or sham acupuncture technique is actually an effort to use relatively ineffective points, in contrast to the conventional use of totally ineffective sugar pills in pharmaceutical trials. Sham points are usually located on the external helix or rim of the ear, although there is no consensus about the level of effectiveness of this procedure. Bullock's alcoholism studies[14] used highly failure-prone subjects and hence may have revealed the difference between active and sham points more effectively.

## CLINICAL APPLICATIONS
### Opiate Addictions

Opiate addiction was first treated by Dr. Wen in Hong Kong and has been treated at Lincoln Hospital since 1974. Acupuncture provides nearly complete relief of acute observable opiate withdrawal symptoms in 5 to 30 minutes. This effect lasts for 8 to 24 hours. The duration of this effect increases with the number of serial treatments provided. Patients often sleep during the session and may feel hungry afterward.[19] Patients who are acutely intoxicated at the time acupuncture is administered will behave in a much less intoxicated manner after the session. Surprisingly, these patients are gratified by this result, in contrast to patient reports of discomfort after Narcan administration.

Acupuncture for opiate addiction is typically administered 2 to 3 times daily in acute detoxification settings. Alternatively, it may be administered only once daily with Clonidine or Methadone on an outpatient basis. Many patients do well on once-daily acupuncture because they taper their illicit opiate usage over a 3 to 4 day period. The addition of an acupuncture component to an opiate detoxification program typically leads to a 50% increase in retention for completion of the recommend length of stay.

## Alcohol Addiction

Directors of the acupuncture social setting detoxification program conducted by the Tulalip Tribe at Marysville, Washington, estimate a yearly savings of $148,000 resulting from less frequent referrals to hospital programs. Inpatient alcohol detoxification units typically combine acupuncture and herbal sleep mix with a tapering benzodiazepine protocol. Patients report fewer symptoms and better sleep. Their vital signs indicate stability, and hence there is much less use of benzodiazepines. One residential program in Connecticut noted a 90% decrease in Valium use when only herbal sleep mix was added to its protocol.

Retention of alcohol detoxification patients generally increases by 50% when an acupuncture component is added to conventional settings. Some alcoholics who receive acupuncture actually report an aversion to alcohol. Woodhull Hospital in Brooklyn reported that 94% of the patients in the acupuncture supplement group remained abstinent as compared with 43% of the control group, which only received conventional outpatient services. The widely quoted controlled study by Bullock[15] showed a 52% retention of alcoholism patients as compared with a 2% sham acupuncture retention rate.

## Cocaine Addiction

Cocaine addiction has provided the most important challenge for acupuncture treatment because there are no significant pharmaceutical agents for this condition. Acupuncture patients report more calmness and reduced craving for cocaine even after the first treatment. The acute psychological indicators of cocaine toxicity are visibly reduced during the treatment session. This improvement is sustained for a variable period after the first acupuncture treatment. After three to seven sequential treatments the anticraving effect is more or less continuous as long as acupuncture is received on a regular basis.[8,14]

Researchers from the substance abuse treatment unit at Yale describe 32 cocaine-dependent methadone-maintained patients who received an 8-week course of auricular acupuncture for the treatment of cocaine dependence. Of these patients, 50% completed treatment, and 88% of those who completed treatment attained abstinence (defined as providing cocaine-free urine samples for the last 2 weeks of the study), yielding an overall abstinence rate of 44%. Abstainers reported decreased depression, a shift in self-definition, decreased craving, and increased aversion to cocaine-related cues. Post-hoc comparisons to pharmacotherapy with desipramine (DMI), amantadine (AMA), and placebo revealed a higher abstinence rate for acupuncture (44%) than for AMA (15%) or placebo (13%), but not significantly higher than for DMI (26%).[20]

Urinalysis outcomes were examined for Lincoln Hospital patients with cocaine or crack addictions who had more than 20 treatment visits and were active during the 1-week study period in March 1991. At Lincoln, patients typically provide urine samples for testing during each visit. Of the entire study group of 226 patients, 149 had more than 80% negative tests during their entire treatment involvement. Of the remaining patients, 39 had at least 80% negative tests during the 2 weeks before data collection (Table 25-2).

The beneficial effects of acupuncture in cocaine treatment often lead to dramatic increases in retention of cocaine patients. Women in Need, a program located near Times Square in New York City, reported the following outcome figures in its treatment of pregnant crack users: (1) Patients with conventional outpatient treatment averaged 3 visits per year; (2) patients who took acupuncture in addition to conventional treatment averaged 27 visits per year; (3) patients who participated in an educational component in addition to acupuncture and conventional treatment averaged 67 visits per

year. Because patients who average 3 visits per year would be unlikely to participate in an educational component, it seems possible that the increased retention correlated with acupuncture set a foundation for successful participation in the educational component.

## Methadone Maintenance

Methadone maintenance patients receive acupuncture in a number of different settings. Patients report a decrease in secondary symptoms of methadone use such as constipation, sweating, and sleep problems. Typically there is a substantial drop in requests for symptomatic medication. Treatment staff usually notice decreased hostility and increased compliance in methadone-acupuncture patients. The most important impact of acupuncture in maintenance programs is reduction of secondary substance abuse—primarily involving alcohol and cocaine, even in patients with minimal motivation.[20] Reductions in secondary alcohol use are also commonly described. Acupuncture is effective with patients in any dosage level of methadone.

Lincoln Hospital used methadone and acupuncture together from 1974 to 1978.[6,19] Several hundred methadone maintenance patients were detoxified during that period using tapered doses of methadone and acupuncture. Based on our previous non-acupuncture experience, we observed that patients were much more comfortable and confident in the acupuncture setting. Although patients regularly complained about withdrawal symptoms, there were very few requests for dosage increase. The large majority of patients completed the entire detoxification process and provided at least one negative toxicology screening after the cessation of methadone. Methadone dosages were decreased

TABLE 25-2

### Toxicology Test Results*

| | Number | Percentage (%) |
|---|---|---|
| More than 80% negative | 149 | 65 |
| At least 80% negative | 39 | 17 |
| Recent relapse | 26 | 12 |
| 30%-70% positive | 5 | 3 |
| More than 80% positive | 7 | 3 |

*All 226 patients who were active in the Lincoln Hospital Program in March 1991 and who had more than 20 total visits during this study. Chart shows cumulative totals of daily testing of all crack cocaine patients.

5 to 10 mg per week, with a slower schedule during the final 10 mg. Starting levels of methadone ranged from 20 mg to 90 mg, with a median of 60 mg. Acupuncture was provided 6 days per week and continued up to 2 months after the last methadone dose. Although many of these patients had been referred for administrative or mandatory detoxification resulting from secondary drug use, toxicology screenings were usually drug-free after the first 2 to 3 weeks of treatment.

Methadone withdrawal is notable for its unpredictable variations in symptoms and significant post-withdrawal malaise. Symptoms such as depression, anergy, and atypical insomnia are quite difficult to manage without acupuncture. Patients are usually fearful and have considerable difficulty participating in psychosocial therapy during the detoxification period. Acupuncture is particularly valuable in the methadone-to-abstinence (MTA) setting because the patient's future well-being depends on his or her ability to accept psychosocial support.

## Effects on Relapse

Acupuncture detoxification programs report substantial reduction in their recidivism rates. The Hooper Foundation in Portland, Oregon, cited a decrease in recidivism from 25% to 6% in comparison to the previous nonacupuncture year. Kent-Sussex in Delaware reported a decrease in recidivism from 87% to 18%.

Substance Abuse Recovery in Flint, Michigan, noted that 83% of a group of 100 General Motors employees were drug- and alcohol-free productive workers a year after entering acupuncture-based treatment. Most of these patients had repeated prior attempts at treatment and frequent relapse. The entire 17% failure group had less than five program visits. Of the success group, 74% continued to attend AA and NA meetings after completing the treatment program. Programs specifically designed for adolescents, such as the Alcohol Treatment Center in Chicago and a Job Corps–related program in Brooklyn, have shown retention rates comparable to adult programs.

Easy access and better retention encourage the outpatient management of difficult patients with less need for additional drugs or services. One can select times for hospitalization more appropriately. An outpatient continuum also facilitates primary healthcare management for AIDS, tuberculosis, and sexually transmitted diseases. Acupuncture is used in a large

proportion of AIDS prevention and outreach programs in New York and London, as well as in other cities. These facilities include needle exchange and harm reduction programs; recovery readiness, and pretreatment programs, as well as health service providers for HIV-positive and AIDS patients. In relationship to substance abuse treatment, each of these programs faces similar dilemmas. Their clients are likely to have ever-increasing addiction-related problems; however, these clients minimize their need for help. Furthermore these clients are often overwhelmed by problems relating to immune deficiency. Acupuncture is a uniquely appropriate entry-level treatment because it is convenient, relaxing, and not dependent on any mutually agreed upon diagnosis or treatment plan. Acupuncture also provides treatment for emotions such as fear and depression. Many of these clients may be ashamed and confused, not knowing how to describe their ever-changing feelings in a conventional therapeutic context.

## PSYCHOSOCIAL MECHANISMS OF ACTION

It is essential to understand the psychological and social mechanisms of action of acupuncture to use this modality effectively. Acupuncture has an impact on the patient's thoughts and feelings that is different from conventional pharmaceutical treatments. The use of acupuncture has a valuable and profound impact on the dynamics of the treatment processes as a whole. We should emphasize that substance abuse acupuncture is provided in a group setting. The new acupuncture patient is immediately introduced to a calm and supportive group process. Patients describe acupuncture as a unique kind of balancing experience. "I was relaxed but alert. I was able to relax without losing control." Patients who are depressed or tired say that they feel more energetic. This encouraging and balancing group experience becomes a critically important basis for the entire substance abuse treatment process.

The perception that a person can be both relaxed and alert is rather unusual in Western culture. We are used to associating relaxation with somewhat lazy or spacey behavior and alertness with a certain degree of anxiety. The relaxed and alert state is basic to the concept of health in all Asian cultures. Acupuncture encourages a centering, focusing process that is typical of meditation and yoga. Therapists report that patients are able to listen to and remember what we tell them, and restless impulsive behavior is greatly reduced. On the other hand, discouragement and apathy are reduced as well.

One of the striking characteristics of the acupuncture treatment setting is that each patient seems comfortable in his or her own space and in his or her own thinking process. One patient explained, "I sat and thought about things in a slow way like I did when I was 10 years old." Acupuncture treatment causes the perception of various relaxing bodily processes. Patients gradually gain confidence that their mind and body can function in a more balanced and autonomous manner. A hopeful process is developed on a private and personal basis, laying a foundation for the development of increasing self-awareness and self-responsibility.

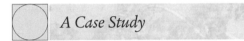

## A Case Study

### Facilitating Access to Treatment

A woman who was 6 months pregnant entered our clinic several years ago. She said, "I can't tell you much about myself because my husband is out in the street with a baseball bat. He'll hit me in my knees if I say too much." We provided an emergency acupuncture treatment and conducted a simplified intake interview. Two weeks later this patient told us, "This is my husband. He doesn't have a drug problem, but he is nervous. Can you help him?" Both of them received acupuncture that day. The woman needed nonverbal access to treatment because of real physical danger that made a standard intake problematic. Overprotective spouses often forcefully oppose all social contacts outside of the marriage. This patient was protected because there was no premature verbal bonding or disclosure of information that would have threatened the husband. The whole process was so supportive that the husband was able to trust his wife and seek help himself. Like many fearful people, he was literally unable to make any verbal approach on his own.

The nature of the recovery from addiction is such that patients often have quickly changing needs for crisis relief and wellness treatment. Many persons in recovery have relatively high levels of wellness functioning. Even so, a crisis of craving or past association may reappear at any time. Conventional treatment settings have trouble coping with such intense and confusing

behavioral swings. Often merely the fear of a possible crisis can sabotage clinical progress. Acupuncture provides either crisis or wellness treatment using the same ear point formula. The nonverbal, present-time aspects of the treatment make it easy to respond to a patient in whatever stage of crisis or denial may exist.

Acupuncture provides uniquely valuable assistance in coping with the challenge of internal redefinition. Patients often begin acupuncture treatment seeking external escape and sedation as they do when they use drugs. When there is a rapid calming effect, they often assume that there was some sort of chemical agent in the acupuncture needle. After a few treatments they come to the astonishing conclusion that acupuncture works by revealing and employing their internal capability to feel calm rather than by inserting an external chemical. Patients begin to realize that their mind is capable of calm focused thoughts on a regular basis. There seems to be no indication of permanent damage to their thinking and consciousness. On the contrary, their ability to listen, think, and learn seems to be growing steadily each day.[10,11]

Addiction patients often cannot tolerate intense interpersonal relationships. Using a conventional one-to-one approach often creates a brittle therapeutic connection that is easily broken by events or any stress. Patients have difficulty trusting a counselor's words when they can hardly trust themselves. Even after confiding to a counselor during an intake session, patients may feel frightened and confused about expanding that relationship. Many of their concerns are so complex and troublesome that talking honestly about their life could be difficult in the best of circumstances. The ambivalence typical of addicts makes it easy to develop misunderstandings. All of these factors support the usefulness of nonverbal techniques during early and critical relapse phases of treatment and critical periods of relapse.

## References

1. Brewington V, Smith M, Lipton D: Acupuncture as a detoxification treatment: an analysis of controlled research, *J Subst Abuse Treat* 11(4):298-307, 1994.
2. Omura Y, Smith M, Wong F, et al: Electroacupuncture for drug addiction withdrawal, *Acupunct Electrotherapeut Res Int J* 1:231-233, 1975.
3. Wen HL, Cheung SYC: Treatment of drug addiction by acupuncture and electrical stimulation, *Asian J Med* 9:139-141, 1973.

4. Bensky D, O'Connor G: *Acupuncture: a comprehensive text,* Seattle, 1985, Eastland Press.

5. Ackerman RW: *Acupuncture as treatment for substance abuse and its application during pregnancy,* nadaclear@aol.com, 1995, NADA Clearinghouse.

6. Mitchell ER: *Fighting drug abuse with acupuncture,* Berkeley, Calif, 1995, Pacific View Press.

7. *Guidepoints: Acupuncture in Recovery,* a monthly newsletter, 7402 NE 58th St, Vancouver, WA 98662.

8. Smith MO: Testimony presented to NIH Office of Alternative Medicine, May 21, 1993.

9. Smith MO, Khan I: An acupuncture programme for treatment of drug addicted persons, *Bull Narc* 40(1):35-41, 1988.

10. Brumbaugh A: *Transformation and recovery: a guide for the design and development of acupuncture based chemical dependency treatment programs,* Santa Barbara, Calif, 1993, Still Point Press.

11. Brumbaugh A: Acupuncture: new perspectives in chemical dependency treatment, *J Subst Abuse Treat* 10:35-43, 1993.

12. Culliton PD, Kiresuk TJ: Overview of substance abuse acupuncture treatment research, *J Altern Complement Med* 2(1):149-165, 1996.

13. Washburn AM, Fullilove RE, Fullilove MT, et al: Acupuncture heroin detoxification: a single-blind clinical trial, *J Subst Abuse Treat* 10:345-351, 1993.

14. Bullock ML, Umen AJ, Culliton PD, et al: Acupuncture treatment of alcoholic recidivism: a pilot study, *Alcohol Clin Exp Res* 11(3):292-295, 1987.

15. Bullock ML, Culliton PD, Olander RT: Controlled trial of acupuncture for severe recidivist alcoholism, *Lancet* 1(8652):1435-1439, 1989.

16. Worner TM, Zeller B, Schwartz H, et al: Acupuncture fails to improve treatment outcome in alcoholics, *Drug Alcohol Depend* 30:169-173, 1992.

17. Lipton DS, Brewington V, Smith MO: Acupuncture for crack cocaine detoxification: experimental evaluation of efficacy, *J Subst Abuse Treat* 11(3):205-215, 1994.

18. Konefal J, Duncan R, Clemence C: Comparison of three levels of auricular acupuncture in an outpatient substance abuse treatment program, *Altern Med J* 2(5):8-17, 1995.

19. Shakur M, Smith MO: The use of acupuncture in the treatment of drug addiction, *Am J Acupunct* 7(3):223-228, 1979.

20. Margolin A, Avants KS, Chang P: Acupuncture for the treatment of cocaine dependence in methadone patients, *Am J Addict* 2(3):194-201, 1993.

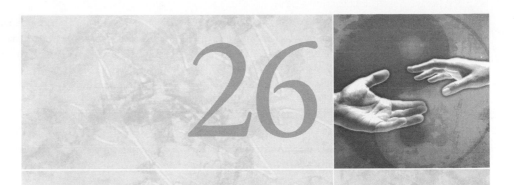

# 26

# Addictions (Alcoholics Anonymous)

## PRISCILLA IVIMEY

*Do not let any prejudice you may have against spiritual terms deter you from honestly asking yourself what they may mean to you.*

BILL W., Cofounder of Alcoholics Anonymous

As reflected in Bill W.'s quotation,[1] the mere mention of spirituality or religion evokes diverse and sometimes negative reactions that may well inhibit a true understanding of this profound concept and its potential benefits. Spirituality as discussed in this chapter refers to a sense of direction, meaning, and connectedness with self and others and with a Higher Being. Given increasing evidence of the efficacy of spirituality as a powerful strategy in treatment, the scientific community is beginning to stress the need for various disciplines to collaborate and further investigate the role of spirituality in rehabilitation and addiction recovery.

Scientific interest in the spiritual element has been demonstrated by several organizations, including the National Institute on Alcoholism and Alcohol Abuse (NIAAA) and the National Institute for the Integration of Health and Spirituality (NCIHS). "There is a need for open and honest dialogue among researchers studying spirituality and addictions. Indeed, communication . . . is crucial for researchers to break down suspicions and stereotypes, to stimulate collaboration on research projects, and to attract new scientists to this field."[2] It is important to note that the U.S. Joint Commission for Accreditation of Healthcare Organizations (JCAHO) now requires that accredited facilities assess patient spirituality as part of healthcare.

This chapter focuses on how and why spiritual issues play a vital role in the treatment and rehabilitation of addicted individuals. Emphasis will be placed on 12-step programs, particularly Alcoholics Anonymous (AA), whose program is the foundation of many 12-step programs. Because the spiritual component of AA is often misunderstood and even frowned upon by many, even by some AA members, the notion of a spiritual component in the treatment of addictions has been and continues to be a controversial issue. Through the course of this chapter, I explore the importance of spirituality in treatment programs and discuss the spiritual aspect of addictions, particularly the spiritual aspect of AA.

# SPIRITUAL ASPECTS OF THE DISEASE OF ADDICTION

## The Human Need for Connectedness

Addiction is a disease characterized by compulsion, loss of control, and continued use in spite of adverse consequences. Because addiction is a progressive disease, it is often fatal in the absence of appropriate treatment. Some researchers have suggested that the disease of addiction is a symptom of a spiritual illness.

To more fully understand how spirituality and addictions are related, it is necessary to examine some historical writings. Certain modern philosophers believe that the story of the Garden of Eden, as related in the Bible, might not refer to the physical act of Adam's taking a bite from the fruit of the Tree of Knowledge but rather to the development of self-awareness.[3] Upon taking the bite of the apple, Adam and Eve became aware of their humanness, their incompleteness, and their separateness from God. An unbearable feeling of isolation resulted, which compelled Adam and Eve, or future humanity, to seek relief from this intolerable pain and suffering. Today, many individuals seek relief through connectedness to something greater than self. Other individuals may turn to chemicals as a solution to these feelings of isolation.[4] That is, this chemical "solution" provides for the avoidance of the intolerable pain caused by social isolation.

In therapy sessions and daily conversations, individuals in varying stages of recovery from addictions often make statements about their feelings, their experiences, or their thoughts regarding their profound feelings of separateness. As one of my clients recently stated, "I tried to connect with Jack Daniels." Clients in treatment for addictions commonly report a tremendous feeling of emptiness, which they liken to a "black hole in space" that is impossible to fill or even to locate.

## Take Comfort in Suffering

Suffering and pain have received a very bad reputation in this part of the world. The television or radio cannot be on for more than 5 minutes without an advertiser informing you how to "get rid of your pain FAST, guaranteed or your money back." Billions of dollars have been spent on the research, development, marketing, and subsequent purchase of prescription and nonprescription products that are purported to relieve or eliminate pain.

Total abstinence from all substances or procedures for pain relief is not suggested, but it is important to note that pain and suffering, whether physical and/or emotional, can well be the vehicle that directs the recovery process toward surrender. "The blessing of suffering brings us deeper into our spiritual life. The word 'suffer' comes from the Latin *sufferre*, meaning 'to carry below,' . . . suffering brings us deeper. If we did not have suffering to carry us deeper, we would always stay just on the surface of life."[5] Helen Keller sums up the benefit of suffering with her words: "I thank God for my handicaps, for through them, I have found my self, my work, and my God."

Although suffering is a universal phenomenon, one's perception of pain and suffering is clearly not universal. My clients in the hospital-based addictions program where I worked often remarked on the profound influence and personal "meaning" they attribute to their own suffering. For example, many clients have made comments such as "If it weren't for the pain in my life, I never would have gotten into recovery." It is often the "sweet desperation" of their pain that helps catapult clients into taking an action. Some clients express an actual sense of gratitude for the suffering they endured as the result of their addictions. I am speaking of the suffering/action connection that I have witnessed so often in persons with addictions. As one client stated, "I got sick and tired of being sick and tired."

Clients often express a felt sense of gratitude for their suffering for it is the suffering that prompted the action or surrender into recovery. In this regard, the levels of stress have a role in increasing the motivation to change or search for a change strategy. Critical life events often stimulate the motivation to change. Milestones that prompt change range from spiritual inspiration or religious conversion to traumatic accidents or severe illnesses. It should be noted that, in relation to spiritual terminology, "the term gratitude refers to awareness or recognition of God's grace. . . . Cessation of problematic behavior is generally interpreted by members as divine intervention, and in this light, abstinence itself is a gift from God."[6]

## Forgiveness

The benefit of forgiveness in the treatment of depression, anxiety, anger, addictions, and other psychosocial challenges has received considerable attention in the literature. Forgiveness appears to be correlated with a decrease in depression, anxiety, and Type A hostility in men and women who formally practice a forgiveness protocol.[7] Forgiveness can be seen as an antidote to the resentment that robs the individual of a spiritual life.

## READINESS AND WILLINGNESS TO CHANGE

### Avoidance of Pain

Various psychiatric problems are thought to result from the avoidance of pain. A strong capacity to tolerate pain is not a hallmark characteristic of one suffering from addictions. While addicted individuals certainly do experience pain and suffering as the result of their addictive behavior, they often require assistance in making the connection between their pain and suffering and their use of substances. There are assets and deficits in substance use.

Depending on the client's stage of readiness to change, the benefits of continued substance use may very much outweigh the deficits of continued use. According to Varney,[8] "Helping clients see the connection between substance use and adverse consequences to themselves or others is an important motivational strategy" to enhance their willingness to change.

## Therapeutic Approaches and Recovery

One technique that has received widespread support in facilitating the movement of the client along the continuum of readiness and willingness to change is motivational interviewing. Developed by Miller and Rollnick,[9] motivational interviewing is a therapeutic style that can help addicted individuals resolve issues related to their ambivalence regarding usage. Clinicians are enthusiastically adapting the use of motivational interviewing not simply as a set of techniques for use in addictions treatment but also as a way of interacting with clients who are resistive to acknowledging their substance abuse.

To better understand motivational interviewing, the reader is encouraged to reflect on his or her own experience of trying to persuade someone to change, such as the fruitless task of trying to convince a smoker to stop smoking before he or she is ready to stop. Given the difficulty associated with change, Prochaska and DiClemente[10] presented a stage model of the process of change, which describes how people change their addictive behaviors. Individuals move through a series of stages of change as they progress in modifying the problem behavior. Each stage of readiness requires tasks to be accomplished and certain processes to be used to move through the stages and thus achieve change.

At first glance, motivational interviewing and AA may appear to be unlikely bedfellows in a scholarly discussion of addictions and spirituality. However, there are many similarities between the principles of motivational interviewing and the writings of Bill W, co-founder of AA, who years earlier advocated certain practices when interacting with individuals with substance use issues. In a chapter in the *Big Book of Alcoholics Anonymous*[1] entitled "Working with Others," specific suggestions are made as to how alcoholics can help one another maintain sobriety. These successful suggestions bear a striking resemblance to strategies used in motivational interviewing. Table 26-1 highlights some of these similarities.

In addition to motivational interviewing, there are many other approaches to the treatment of persons with addictions. One size clearly does not fit all. When used with mainstream medicine, alternative treatments such as acupuncture, Ayurveda, and meditation can offer a medically safe totality of treatment. The integration of spirituality into the rehabilitation of

TABLE 26-1

*Comparisons of Motivational Interviewing and AA Writings*

| Motivational Interviewing | Writings on AA by Bill W. |
| --- | --- |
| De-emphasis on label. Admission of alcoholism not seen as necessary for change to occur.<br><br>Motivation for change occurs when people perceive a discrepancy between where they are and where they want to be. To this end, motivational interviewing seeks to raise the clients' awareness of the personal consequences of their drinking. | "Be careful not to brand him (the alcoholic) as an alcoholic. Let him draw his own conclusion."<br><br>"If your talk has been sane, quiet, and full of human understanding . . . maybe you have disturbed him about the question of alcoholism. This is all to the good." |

From Alcoholics Anonymous World Service: *Alcoholics Anonymous,* ed 4, New York, 2001, Alcoholics Anonymous World Service.

a person with substance use disorder begins with the process of assessing both the individual's personality structure and his or her spiritual beliefs.[4]

## Spiritual Assessment

A number of authorities have stated that there is a need for spiritual assessment before any treatment can be effectively implemented. Religion and spirituality are often inversely related to the prevalence of substance use. "Understanding clients' spirituality can promote clearer communication, offering contextual information that is important to the process of treatment."[6] Conducting a spiritual assessment need not be a fearful, laborious task. Often clinicians are surprised at their clients' eagerness and relief when given the opportunity to speak of their spiritual beliefs and concerns.

Although there is no universally accepted way to conduct a spiritual assessment, asking the following questions can be helpful:

1. Do you believe in a Higher Power/God?
2. Describe your Higher Power.
3. Do you currently practice a specific religion?
4. What spiritual practices have you used in the past?
5. How important is your spirituality in your day-to-day functioning?
6. What gives your life purpose?
7. Tell me about a personal experience involving a Higher Power.

## Alcoholics Anonymous and 12-Step Programs

There are various treatment modalities for caring for persons with addictions. In the remainder of this chapter, the focus is on 12-step programs, especially AA, and how these programs address the spiritual issues identified earlier in this chapter. The term *12-step program* is a generic name typically used for programs based on the philosophy and traditions of AA, which was founded in 1935 and now has over 96,000 groups worldwide. Twelve-step programs now constitute the largest self-help system in the world. While they are not the only path to recovery, AA and other 12-step programs (e.g., Overeaters Anonymous, Narcotics Anonymous) are commonly used in the field of addictions treatment. The only requirement for membership to a 12-step program is a desire to stop drinking or using the designated substance.

Recent clinical trials with substance abusers have demonstrated that a 12-step treatment modal is as effective as cognitive-behavioral approaches.[11] Correlational research suggests that 12-step participation is associated with reductions in targeted behavior, such as drinking, illicit drug use, or overeating. Furthermore, membership in a 12-step program has been associated with improved psychosocial functioning and increased commitment to change. In addition, this participation may offset the influence of unsupportive social networks.[12]

A number of recent outcome studies have focused on the influence of spirituality in recovery, as demonstrated through 12-step and non–12-step program intervention. In one study, which compared clients who participated in a variety of outpatient programs, the majority of clients were found to have experienced a significant increase in spirituality, as measured by the Spiritual Well-Being Scale.[13] Sandoz[14] studied 57 members of AA and found that 82% of the participants claimed to have had a spiritual experience that was unrelated to religious denomination or church attendance.

The efficacy of including spirituality as a focus in addictions treatment has received considerable support in the literature. After extensively studying personal changes in recovering alcoholics with at least several years' sobriety, Turner[15] and Summer[16] concluded that spiritual changes were essential ingredients in the recovery process. A review of the literature from a variety of disciplines reveals that increased spiritual and/or religious involvement has consistently been positively related to physical well-being and inversely related to the manifestation of disorders.[6]

Spiritual exploration for the addicted individual often starts with a suggestion by a friend, family member, or clinician to attend an AA meeting. Unfortunately, many clinicians know very little about AA other than "It offers group support, it's free, and it looks good on the treatment plan." There is a crucial need for the therapist to have a basic understanding of 12-step programs if he or she is to either refer or support the client's participation in such a program.

## History of Alcoholics Anonymous

One of the defining moments in the development of AA occurred on a cold afternoon in November 1934, when two men sat at household kitchen table located at 182 Clinton Street in Brooklyn, New York. One of the men was unshaven, tattered, and drunk. The other man was clean shaven, articulate, and expressing to his inebriated friend his newfound discovery of religion, which had helped him to not drink anymore. As history tells us, this unkempt, disheveled drunk was Bill W., one of the cofounders of AA. What made this kitchen discussion crucial to the development of the AA program was the profound act of connectedness, of the kinship of common suffering—one alcoholic had been helping another. As a result of this act, Bill W. was inspired to devote a substantial part of his remaining adult life to the development of AA.

Few people are aware that Dr. Carl Jung, the famous psychoanalyst, had a substantial influence on the development of AA. In 1931, several years before Bill W.'s kitchen table discussion, Dr. Jung had been treating a patient named Roland H. for alcoholism. Roland had suffered yet another relapse and returned to the psychiatrist's care, looking to Jung for some avenue of hope. At that time, Jung informed Roland of the hopelessness of his recovery so far as any further medical or psychiatric treatment was concerned. He then spoke of a spiritual experience of a genuine conversion which, though infrequent, did bring recovery to alcoholics. Roland subsequently communicated this experience to Bill W. after being introduced by a mutual friend.

Years after this experience between Roland and Dr. Jung, Bill W. wrote Jung to inform him that "this candid and humble statement of yours was beyond a doubt the first foundation upon which our society (AA) has been built."[17] That is, as a result of Carl Jung's works, Bill W. became aware of the importance of the sense of hopelessness and the necessity for spiritual conversion in the recovery of alcoholics.

Bill W. was also greatly helped by Dr. William D. Silkworth, a physician who treated alcoholics in his practice. Struggling with his sobriety and exploring his own spirituality, Bill W. sought solace through discussions with Dr. Silkworth, who helped Bill W. to understand some of the medical ramifications of the disease. These discussions further assisted Bill W. to reflect and clarify his thinking, which largely formed the tenets of AA, while providing Bill W. with the support he required during these difficult times.

While tenuously sober and on a stressful business trip to Akron, Ohio, Bill W. sensed his closeness to relapse. "He suddenly realized that, in order to save himself, he must carry his message to another alcoholic."[17] Through various circumstances, he was directed to another alcoholic, a physician named Bob Smith, who would become a cofounder of AA. Upon hearing about some of Bill W.'s discussions with Dr. Silkworth and Bill W.'s own exploration with spirituality, Dr. Bob found renewed hope to secure his own spiritual path to recovery, which before had been fruitless. In addition to meeting with each other regularly, Bill W. and Dr. Bob proceeded to frantically seek out and help other suffering alcoholics.

## Spirituality Plus Pragmatism Equal "The Slogans"

Nowhere do we see the combination of spirituality and pragmatism more evident than in the slogans of

AA. The AA slogans are a compendium of short statements that convey specific messages about how to cope with potentially stressful situations or feelings (Table 26-2).

"Therapists should not only be familiar with AA slogans but should actively use them in therapy to promote AA involvement and advise patients on how to handle difficult situations."[18] I find it best to use slogans judiciously with my clients. I attempt to give meaning to the slogans by connecting them to clients' experience. Teaching clients to connect particular slogans to situations in their life that trigger risky emotions can be extremely helpful. For example, a client who often took on too much unnecessary work would put himself at high risk for relapse. The benefit of the slogan "Easy Does It" allowed him to slow down to a productive speed and not risk feeling overwhelmed, which could be a trigger feeling for relapse.

Table 26-2 illustrates how commonly used AA slogans provide immediate solutions to typical stressful situations encountered by all of us on a daily basis. The value of these slogans lies in their simplicity. These simple slogans are often described by members of AA as spiritual in their simplicity. Furthermore, they afford immediate relief from or resolution of a problem without the need for extensive processing of feelings or thoughts. To a certain extent, the use of slogans takes on a behavioral component in that specific slogans become paired with the reduction of anxiety, frustration, and other discomforting feelings when one is confronted with difficult experiences.

## Spiritual Values in Alcoholics Anonymous

The addict's sense of isolation and alienation is vast and profoundly experienced. Often cut off from family, friends, self, and spiritual purpose, the person with an addiction is deprived of sustaining connectedness and related energy. Let me be very clear! I am not writing about the unfortunate person you may see sleeping alone in the park with a brown paper bag securely snuggled to his or her chest. I am writing of those very unfortunate individuals who go home to their family, who have friends, yet who experience the total isolation of loneliness. As one of my clients described, "I was always alone in a crowd. I felt like an outsider, a stranger in my own family."

Isolation and alienation are equal opportunity employers who do not discriminate on the basis of race, education, wealth, or any other demographic variable. As therapists, we have a need to be cognizant of the universality of alienation because those in higher socioeconomic strata may appear to be connected outwardly but inwardly may well feel very disconnected. Conversely, the impact of poverty can never be minimized relative to opportunities for an individual to connect on a variety of levels.

TABLE 26-2

## AA Slogans and Interpretations

| AA Slogan | Possible Interpretations |
| --- | --- |
| "Easy Does It" | Don't go so fast—slow down. |
| | This addresses issues of over commitment. |
| "Live and Let Live" | Enjoy your life (LIVE!) and let others enjoy their life. |
| "Keep It Simple" | Keep it simple. |
| "HALT" | Acronym: STOP and don't let yourself get too *Hungry, Angry, Lonely* or *Tired*. |
| | Any one of these states can make one vulnerable to relapse. As such, halt what you are doing and take care of yourself to minimize vulnerable states. |
| "Let GO, Let GOD" | God is in charge, and because you are not God (as is established in Step Two), let God take charge. |
| | This slogan gives direction toward spiritual surrender. |
| "One Day at a Time" | Focus on today—some say a moment at a time. |
| | This helps one to stay in the day and not be overwhelmed by worry for the future or guilt over the past. |
| "First Things First" | The first priority is: Don't drink no matter the feeling state. |
| | This slogan also encourages logical thought as a coping strategy. |

## Forgiveness

Although Bill W. was not exposed to recent research, he found forgiveness and the "letting go of resentments" a major consideration for recovery. When writing about the importance of forgiveness and recovery, Bill W. wrote: "Resentments [are] the 'number one' offender. . . . We have been spiritually sick . . . for when harboring such feelings, we shut ourselves off from the sunlight of the Spirit."[1]

## Surrender

Similar to suffering, surrender is another spiritual aspect in the treatment of addictions that has unjustly received a negative connotation. It may be helpful to note here what is not meant by surrender as it relates to the treatment of persons with addictions. Surrender is not a practice of avoidance. Surrender is not "doing nothing." Surrender is not about being a "doormat" for an abusive spouse. Surrender is not about seeing self as a weak, hopeless individual with no inherent value or purpose.

"We perceive that only through utter defeat are we able to take our first steps toward liberation and strength. Our admissions of personal powerlessness finally turn out to be firm bedrock upon which happy and purposeful lives may be built."[19]

## The Twelve Steps of Alcoholics Anonymous

In the development of AA, Bill W. soon became aware of the need for a spiritual blueprint or framework for obtaining and maintaining sobriety. This awareness led him to develop what some would refer to as the "divinely inspired" 12 steps of AA. These 12 steps are listed in Table 26-3, along with recovery issues that are typically experienced or reflected in the respective step. The choice of pronouns used in writing these steps exemplifies one of the foundations of all 12 step programs. That is, the use of "we" and "us" reflects the

TABLE 26-3

## The 12-Steps of AA and Their Corresponding Recovery Issues

| The 12 Steps of AA | Recovery Issue |
| --- | --- |
| 1. We admitted we were powerless over alcohol—that our lives had become unmanageable. | Surrender to a Higher Power—an opportunity for one to realize that he or she is not God. This is the beginning of placing hope in a power greater that oneself—a Transcendent Power. This sense of Hope in a Transcendent Power is a cornerstone of recovery. |
| 2. We came to believe that a Power greater than ourselves could restore us to sanity. | Belief in a Higher Power and Hope in a Power other than self continues. The good news here is the realization that there is a God. The bad news is: I am not Him/Her. |
| 3. We made a decision to turn our will and our lives over to the care of God as we understood Him. | Surrender and develop a connected relationship with God. The Hope in a Higher Being continues. This step asks members to make the decision to surrender to the CARE of God. Seems like an easy request! Yet, self-will can make this surrender seem impossible. "Thy will be done, not mine." This is not about surrendering to the perpetrator, it is not about doing nothing, it is not about avoiding. It is about taking the action of surrendering to the CARE of God. |
| 4. We made a searching and fearless moral inventory of ourselves. | The beginning of self-examination. Like any inventory, the member takes stock of himself or herself and examines what is "there." |
| 5. We admitted to God, to ourselves, and to another human being the exact nature of our wrongs. | This "confession" is common in many spiritual practices. Such practice lessens one's sense of isolation, guilt, and "terminal" uniqueness. This step also gives one an exercise in developing trust and humility. |
| 6. We were entirely ready to have God remove all these defects of character. | For many in AA, the obsession with and the compulsion for substances is lifted. The belief here is that if God can and does lift the obsession for substance abuse, certainly He or She can remove one's character defects. Being ENTIRELY ready to have God remove ALL defects of character is another example of a spiritual surrender. |

*Continued*

TABLE 26-3

*The 12-Steps of AA and Recovery Issues—cont'd*

| The 12 Steps of AA | Recovery Issue |
|---|---|
| 7. We humbly asked Him to remove our shortcomings. | Allow for the spiritual experience of Humility. "The attainment of greater humility is the foundation principle of each of AA's Twelve Steps. For without some degree of humility, no alcoholic can stay sober at all."[19] |
| 8. We made a list of all persons we had harmed and became willing to make amends to them all. | Allows for increase of connectedness and a start in coping with deadly resentment. |
| 9. We made direct amends to such people wherever possible, except when to do so would injure them or others. | Promotes relational connectedness. Also, this step helps to promote the development of self-restraint. "We must avoid quick tempered criticism and furious, power driven argument. The same goes for sulking or silent scorn. These are emotional booby traps bated with pride and vengefulness."[19] These states are dangerous to one in recovery. |
| 10. We continued to take personal inventory and when we were wrong promptly admitted it. | Upon completion of Step 9, members found it necessary to continue, on a daily basis, to right wrongs ASAP. This spiritual practice of making amends assists in minimizing the accumulation of guilt. |
| 11. We sought through prayer and meditation to improve our conscious contact with God as we understood Him, praying only for knowledge of His will for us and the power to carry that out. | An act in seeking both God's knowledge of one's well-being and the ability to comply with and carry out God's desires. Prayer and meditation are used here to improve one's connection with God so that God will be become clearer to the individual. |
| 12. Having had a spiritual awakening as the result of these steps, we tried to carry this message to alcoholics, and to practice these principles in all our affairs. | There are many definitions of "spiritual awakening." AA writes about the person who has had a spiritual awakening ". . . in a very real sense he [sic] has been transformed, because he has laid hold of a source of strength which, in one way or another, he had denied himself. He finds himself in possession of a degree of honesty, tolerance, unselfishness, peace of mind and love."[19] |
| | Connectedness and service are seen as a safety line to continued sobriety. When in doubt, 12-Step members encourage doing service for another suffering addict. The benefit of the spiritual practice of service was made clear to Bill W. when he found himself close to relapse as described earlier in this chapter. |

power of connectedness as an antidote for the deadly experience of isolation and alienation.

As stated earlier, *12-step program* is the generic name for the many descendants of AA, which formulated the principles and traditions on which these groups are based. Overeaters Anonymous, Cocaine Anonymous, and Narcotics Anonymous are just a few of the descendants of AA. The name of each group denotes the drug of choice for its participants. All of these 12-step programs consider themselves a "fellowship," a gathering of people who have a common problem—the addictive use of a specific substance or behavior. As in AA, these 12-step programs strongly encourage group members to assist others and themselves to obtain and maintain abstinence from the identified substance or behavior.

**Prayer**

The use of prayer in recovery has been recognized by many authorities as a powerful vehicle for change and healing. While there is no "best way to pray," a number of my clients who are members of 12-step programs have reported to me the remarkable sense of relief they have received through the process of prayer.

As presented in step 11 (see Table 26-3), prayer is coupled with meditation as a vehicle for seeking to improve conscious contact with a higher power. The purpose of this contact is to be shown God's will and then to be granted the power to carry out that divine will. This step is further intended to highlight the need to seek God's will and not one's own: "Thy will, not mine." Another client of mine nicely distinguished the meaning of prayer from meditation by saying, "Prayer is talking to God, while meditation is listening to God."

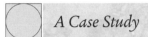

## A Case Study

### Alcoholism and Resentments

Anna was a 27-year-old stenographer with an 8-year history of recovery from alcoholism. She was suffering emotional and physical pain secondary to a long-standing resentment she held toward her ex–best friend. Anna held her former friend responsible for Anna's losing a substantial amount of money. Despite the use of cognitive-behavioral strategies to address the resentment, she still felt deep-seated anger. However, the understanding that resentment could pose a trigger for relapse, coupled with the pain of resentment, allowed Anna to have the willingness to try anything to rid herself of this resentment, no matter how difficult.

Several members from Anna's AA group suggested a rather daunting task for Anna. It was recommended that she pray for 10 consecutive days, asking her Higher Power to bestow divine providence and gifts on her former friend. Initially this task was very painful and appeared somewhat ludicrous to Anna because she felt nothing but ill will toward this woman. However, as Anna continued to pray daily, she began to feel less hatred and resentment for her former friend. At the end of 10 days, she expressed a remarkable sense of relief from the pain of her resentment. Anna was able to maintain her sobriety. ❧

### Meditation

Meditation can offer clients with addictions an opportunity to develop the skills needed to support sobriety. The benefit of being "present in the moment" can be an extremely helpful antidote to the anxieties of catastrophic thinking and negative self-talk. Being present in the moment offers one an opportunity to come to a deeper understanding of impermanence, or the passing of events. There is a beginning and an end to the wide spectrum of the human condition, including feelings, cravings, pain, and thoughts, to name

but a few. Addicted individuals often get "stuck" in the belief that their current pain and discomfort will never end, thus triggering a need for immediate relief through substance abuse. Meditation allows the AA member to see and experience desire and craving as something that passes. The resulting hope gives way to a spiritual comfort that lessens the need for substance use.

Meditation can also promote compassionate self-observation, which is critical for 12-step members, particularly when working on step 4 (see Table 26-3). This step encompasses taking a personal inventory of one's assets and deficits, a process that often evokes many feelings and startling self-revelations. Analogous to running a business, there is a need to periodically take inventory of one's collective assets and deficits before one knows how to proceed and improve.

"Meditation is something which can always be further developed. It has no boundaries, of width or of height.... Perhaps one of the greatest rewards of meditation and prayer is the sense of belonging that comes to us."[19] Because isolation and aloneness are often a trigger for substance abuse, this sense of belonging is critical to the person in recovery. The related self-regulation stategy of biofeedback has enabled many patients to experience this sense of connection to a Higher Power, especially during theta brainwave training (see Chapter 32).[20]

## CLINICAL CONSIDERATIONS AND QUESTIONS

As clinicians knowing the benefits of "the tool of spirituality," are we not ethically responsible to explore this tool with our patients? Can we withhold the discussion of a treatment that we know to be beneficial to so many others suffering from addictions? Clinicians must consider several salient points when exploring spirituality with their clients. What is the client's cultural background? Because there is a vast array of cultural and spiritual practices in this world, it is impossible for the clinician to possess complete knowledge of all such practices. The process of continuing education allows for us all to broaden our knowledge concerning such issues. This continuing education may include interprofessional collaboration with clergy. In addition, as with any cultural or counseling issues, the clinician must seek supervision with the purpose of gaining insights and information regarding clients' cultural or spiritual practices. That is, "Clients generally do not want to be understood just in parts but as a whole person and we believe (with JCAHO) that all healthcare providers should know something of their client's spirituality to develop a comprehensive understanding of their problem and design an appropriate treatment plan."[6]

The process of developing understanding and acceptance of the client's spiritual beliefs may not be as spontaneous as some of us "open-minded, spiritual, nonjudgmental, empathic" clinicians may imagine. Clinicians may benefit from giving serious and playful attention to their own spiritual values and practices. If there are differences in spiritual belief between client and clinician that pose a problem, a referral may be necessary.

Another significant area of clinical importance encompasses relapse prevention. Relapse is a state of mind that precedes actual use and is associated with some early warning signs such as irritability, hopelessness, lying, frustration, resentment, and anger. Spiritual bankruptcy can provide rich underpinnings to the growth of these possible feeling/thinking states, which precede relapse. Perhaps spiritual practice would provide a defense against their growth.

## SUMMARY

The importance of spirituality relative to general health and well-being is currently receiving increased media attention and scientific support. Spirituality relative to addictions was brought to the forefront in 1935 with the founding of AA. Through the process of their own recovery and the recovery of early members, the cofounders of AA saw that conscious contact with a Higher Power was imperative for recovery. This conscious contact not only supports relapse prevention but it may also provide one with an awareness of purpose in life. AA, with its 12 steps, offers one a practical yet spiritual path to seek this connectedness with a Higher Power. Clinicians may well benefit their clients as they increase their knowledge of the pragmatic and spiritual constructs of AA and other 12-step programs.

## References

1. Alcoholics Anonymous World Service: *Alcoholics Anonymous,* ed 3, New York, 1976, Alcoholics Anonymous World Services.

2. Larson DB, Sawyers JP, McCullough ME (eds): *Scientific research on spirituality and health: a consensus report,* Rockville, Md, 1998, National Institute for Healthcare Research.

3. Fromn E: *Escape from freedom,* New York, 1965, Avon Books.

4. Morgan O, Jordan M: *Addiction and spirituality,* Washington, DC, 1999, American Psychological Association.

5. Gerzon R: *Finding serenity in the age of anxiety,* New York, 1987, Macmillan.

6. Miller WR: *Integrating spirituality into treatment,* Washington DC, 1999, American Psychological Association.

7. Coyle CT, Enright RD: Forgiveness intervention with post abortion men, *J Consult Clin Psychol* 65:1042-1046, 1997.

8. Varney SM, Rohsenow DJ, Dey AN, et al: Factors associated with help seeking and perceived dependence among cocaine users, *Am J Drug Alcohol Abuse* 21(1):81-91, 1995.

9. Miller WR, Rollnick S: *Motivational interviewing: preparing people to change addictive behavior,* New York, 1991, Guilford Press.

10. Prochaska JO, DiClemente CC: Toward a comprehensive model of change. In Miller WR, Heather N: *Treating addictive behaviors: processes of change,* 1986.

11. Ouimette PC, Finney JW, Moos RH: Twelve-step and cognitive-behavioral treatment for substance abuse: a comparison of treatment effectiveness, *J Consult Clin Psychol* 65(2):230-240, 1997.

12. Emrick CD, Tonigan JS, Montgomery H, et al: Alcoholics Anonymous: what is currently known? In McCrady BS, Miller WR: *Research on Alcoholics Anonymous: opportunities and alternatives,* New Brunswick, NJ, 1993, Rutgers Center of Alcohol Studies.

13. Borman PD, Dixon DN: Spirituality and the 12 steps of substance abuse recovery, *J Psychol Theol* 26(3), 1998.

14. Sandoz C: Exploring the spiritual experiences of the twelve steps of Alcoholics Anonymous, *J Ministry Addiction Recovery* 6(1):99-107, 1999.

15. Turner C: Spiritual experiences of recovering alcoholics, *Dissertation Abstracts Int* 56(30):1128A (University Microfilms No. 9521866), 1993.

16. Sommer SM: A way of life: long-term recovery in alcoholics, *Dissertation Abstracts Int* 53(7):3795B, (University Microfilms No. 9236722), 1992.

17. Kurtz E: *Not-God: a history of Alcoholics Anonymous,* Center City, Minn, 1979, Hazelden Educational Materials.

18. Project MATCH Research Group: *Twelve step facilitation therapy manual,* Washington, DC, 1999, U.S. Department of Health and Human Services, National Institutes of Health.

19. Alcoholics Anonymous World Services: *Twelve steps and twelve traditions,* New York, 1978, Alcoholics Anonymous World Services.

20. Peniston E, Kulkoshy P: Alpha-theta brainwave training and β-endorphin levels in alcoholics, *Alc Clin Exp Res,* 13:271, 1989.

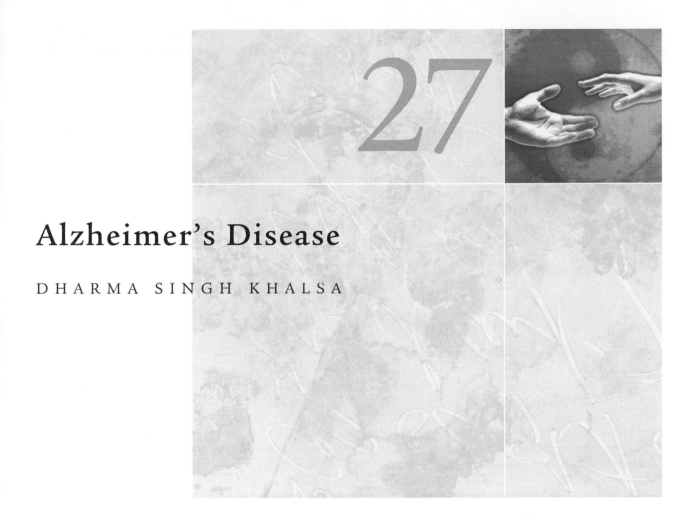

# 27

# Alzheimer's Disease

DHARMA SINGH KHALSA

The integrative medical model is based on good science and good sense. Conventionalists, who focus narrowly on this gene or that neurotransmitter, often overlook the fact that the brain is a flesh and blood organ. Because the brain is flesh and blood, like the heart, for example, it will respond to health-promoting interventions such as improved blood flow, good nutrition, stress reduction, and exercise. Because an integrative approach brings surviving neurons to their optimal potential, using it can reverse many of the symptoms of Alzheimer's disease (AD) and slow its progression.

Like many degenerative diseases associated with aging, memory loss spans a spectrum of signs, symptoms, etiologies, pathogeneses, and prognoses. Although the term *memory loss* does not imply a specific cause, it signifies a clinical syndrome characterized by the acquired loss of cognitive and emotional abilities severe enough to interfere with daily functioning and the quality of life.

The best known of the dementias is AD, which affects over 4 million Americans at an annual cost of $155 billion. These figures are expected to rise dramatically as the population ages: as many as 16 million people may suffer from the disease by the year 2025. AD is the third most expensive healthcare problem in the country.[1]

## PATHOPHYSIOLOGY

The term *age-associated memory impairment (AAMI)* was initially used to describe the minor memory difficulties that were previously believed to accompany the

*Warning Signs of Alzheimer's Disease*

According to the Alzheimer's Association the 10 warning signs for Alzheimer's disease are the following:
1. Recent memory loss that affects job skill
2. Difficulty performing familiar tasks
3. Problems with language
4. Disorientation to time and space
5. Poor or decreased judgment
6. Problems with abstract thinking
7. Misplacing objects of importance
8. Changes in mood or behavior
9. Changes in personality
10. Loss of initiative

Courtesy Alzheimer's Association.

aging process. This impairment is now known to exist in patients as young as 50 years of age. An at-risk population with mild cognitive impairment (MCI) that converts to AD at a rate of approximately 12% per year has been identified and is discussed later in this chapter.[2] Moreover, Lupien[3] has noted a conversion to AD in subjects with cortisol-induced stress-related memory loss. This emerging etiology for cognitive dysfunction is included in the discussion on chronic stress.

Neuroscientists now agree that memory loss is a disease that begins to attack the brain 30 to 40 years before symptoms appear. Snowden[4] showed that nuns who displayed linguistic difficulties in their twenties had a higher incidence of AD later in life. Using positron emission tomographic (PET) scans, Reiman et al[5] noted that patients can have lesions consistent with severe cognitive decline years before symptoms are seen. It is becoming increasingly clear therefore that AD is an insidious process similar to other chronic diseases such as heart disease and as such has lifestyle management implications.

## PLAQUES OR TANGLES?

For a century, scientists have wondered which of the brain lesions associated with AD is more important—the plaques that litter the empty spaces between nerve cells or the stringy tangles that erupt from within the cell. An enzyme called *secretase* on the surface of the brain cell makes a protein called beta-amyloid (BAP). Patients with AD have too much amyloid, which forms the so-called plaques on the outside of brain cells. These plaques grow so dense that they trigger an inflammatory reaction from the brain's immune system that kills nerve cells. Among the powerful weapons the immune system brings to bear are oxygen-based free radicals, which is one reason antioxidants such as vitamin E are helpful in treating AD.

A strong piece of evidence supports the beta-amyloid theory: a significant number of mice genetically engineered to develop plaques remain plaque free compared with controls when vaccinated with a fragment of beta-amyloid. Researchers then vaccinated 1-year-old mice whose brains were riddled with plaques. These mice became plaque free. Unfortunately, the preliminary studies testing this vaccine in humans proved unsuccessful and have been stopped.

The second major school of thought among neuroscientists concerns tau, a molecule that acts much like the ties on a railroad track. Tau assembles microtubules that support the structure of the nerve cell. Chemical changes in the nerve cell cause the tau molecules to change shape so that they no longer hold the microtubules in place. The "railroad ties" begin to twist and tangle, causing neuronal cell death.

Many questions remain. For one, are the plaques and tangles seen in AD causative or simply tombstones? Is there some still unknown biochemical event that precedes the formation of plaques and tangles and causes the inflammatory death knell? AD, no less than heart disease, certainly has multiple causes. Like aging itself, there are risk factors to the development of AD, which means that lifestyle choices, especially how we handle stress, are critically important.

## RISK FACTORS FOR MEMORY LOSS

### Hard Risk Factors

The following are the hard risk factors for the development of AD.

**Increased age.** Increased age is the most important risk factor. Of those aged 65 years, 10% will develop Alzheimer's disease. The incidence at age 85 years is 50%.

**Family history.** The risk of developing AD is increased three- to fourfold if a first-degree relative has the disease.

**Genetic factors.** Individuals with two APOE4 genes on chromosome 19 are at least 8 times more likely than others to develop AD. Gatz et al[6] noted that the APOE4 gene exerts its maximal effect on people in their sixties and is a strong predictor of AD. The APOE4 gene is also a strong predictor for heart disease.

**Head injury.** AD risk doubles in patients who have suffered traumatic brain injuries early in life. Moderate head injury increased the risk of AD by 2 to 3 times, whereas severe head injury more than quadrupled the risk of dementia.

**Gender.** Because women have longer life spans than men, they have a higher incidence of AD. Lower estrogen levels may also play an important role in AD.[7]

**Educational level.** The risk of developing AD decreases with the number of years of formal education. This highlights research suggesting that mental activity throughout life is neuroprotective.[8]

## Lifestyle Risk Factors That Can Be Influenced By Integrative Medicine

The following are the lifestyle risk factors for the development of AD that can be influenced by integrative medicine.

**Mild cognitive impairment.** MCI is characterized primarily by recent memory loss. It is the "transitional state" that can occur between normal aging, AAMI, and dementia. People with MCI are at an increased risk to develop AD at a rate of 12% to 15% per year. Symptoms of MCI are distinguished from normal aging by recent memory loss. For example, people with MCI commonly suffer from forgetfulness and may visibly have difficulty learning new information and recalling previously learned information. The primary distinction between people with MCI and AD appears to be in the areas of cognition outside of memory. Unlike people with AD, those with MCI are able to function normally in daily activities requiring other cognitive abilities such as thinking, understanding, and decision making.[9]

**Nutrition.** Americans who consume a high-calorie, high-fat diet have a much higher incidence of AD than persons living in countries where a relatively low-fat diet is eaten. A high-fat and high-calorie intake leads to oxidative stress, which contributes to the onset and progression of cognitive decline.

The dietary consumption of fish—especially salmon and tuna, which contain decosahexaenoic acid, an omega-3, long chain, polyunsaturated fatty acid—is considered beneficial to cognitive health.

Researchers at New York University's Nathan Kline Institute put transgenic mice on high-fat diets then observed an increase in the rate at which beta-amyloid built up in their brains. Cholesterol-lowering medication slowed the rate of plaque formation.[10,11]

**Mind/body factors.** Innovative neurobiological research has shown that chronic unbalanced stress exerts a powerful negative effect on the development and progression of cognitive decline. In response to chronic stress, the adrenal gland releases cortisol, which has an inhibitory effect on human learning and memory.[12]

Lupien has shown that subjects (median age 70 years) with the highest level of cortisol elevation at the end of a 4-year study period had a marked deficit in explicit memory loss, a hippocampal-dependent memory function. The group with the lowest cortisol levels displayed no deficit. In an extension of this work, Lupien observed that without intervention, subjects in the high-cortisol group can progress to AD. Magnetic resonance imaging (MRI) scans also disclosed hippocampal atrophy among this group. Subjects consistently reported morning stress, tension, and anxiety.

Cortisol produces memory dysfunction in three ways: (1) by preventing the uptake of glucose by the hippocampus, (2) by inhibiting synaptic transmission, and (3) by causing neuron injury and cellular death.[13] Because of these events, brain cells react abnormally with the excitatory neurotransmitter glutamic acid, creating an intracellular flood of calcium that leads to increased free radical production. Free radicals injure the mitochondria, the microtubules, and even the nucleus itself, resulting in dendritic atrophy and neuron death.[14] McEwen[15] has shown that this abortization of dendritic spines is reversible. In addition, stress-relieving techniques such as meditation have been shown to reduce cortisol levels and enhance cognitive function in patients with MCI and AD.[16]

This review suggests that lifestyle modification, including proper nutrition, stress management, and cardiovascular disease risk reduction, may play a strong role in the reversal of AD.

# AN INTEGRATIVE MODEL FOR BRAIN LONGEVITY

A true integrative medical model combines evidence-based therapies on nutrition, stress reduction, exercise, and pharmaceuticals into a total synergistic program. Gould et al[17] have shown that this type of program can reverse coronary artery disease, and I have had compelling success in my own practice involving patients with AD.

At this juncture there is a major difference of opinion between the conventionalist who only prescribes a cholinesterase inhibitor such as donepezil (Aricept) and perhaps vitamin E in the treatment of MCI or AD and the forward-thinking clinician who practices integrative medicine. The integrative medicine practitioner knows by virtue of experience and knowledge that there is much that can be done to slow the progression and in many cases reverse the symptoms of MCI and AD. What follows is an organized and scientific approach to the treatment of cognitive decline.

## Lifestyle Factors

The following lifestyle factors affect mental functioning and the development of AD.

**Physical and cognitive exercise.** Aerobic conditioning has been shown to improve some aspects of mental function by 20% to 30%. Smith et al[18] have demonstrated that physical exercise has a retardant effect on the development of AD. In a retrospective analysis of subjects aged 40 to 60 years, those who followed a regular exercise program had a lower incidence of AD than those who did not follow an exercise program. Exercise increases cerebral blood flow and the production of nerve growth factors.

Another type of exercise that is effective for promoting mental function is cognitive exercise. Based on research by Diamond et al,[19] an integrative medical program that includes cognitive stimulation such as discussing news headlines, working crossword puzzles, listening to or playing music, or creating art could help to maintain cognitive ability. Mental training increases dendritic sprouting and enhances central nervous system plasticity.[20] In addition to having positive medical benefits, cognitive exercise allows patients and their spouses to spend quality time together.

**Nutrition:** The four key points are to (1) reduce dietary fat, (2) reduce dietary cholesterol, (3) add omega-3–rich foods such as salmon or tuna to the diet, and (4) lower caloric consumption.

A number of studies have shown that a diet restricted in calories and consisting of 15% to 20% fat can help prevent and treat AD. This approach extends the life expectancy of animals and enhances the health and cognitive ability of humans. In my consultation practice, I have my nutritionist work with patients to create a 15% to 20% fat diet based on their preferences. Several studies have shown that this caloric restriction diet can be beneficial.[21-23] Results of the Biosphere II experiment on caloric restriction and reduced fat consumption show reductions in triglyceride and cholesterol levels, which is important when considering the treatment of AD.[24]

**Supplements:** The most important supplements to consider are the B-complex vitamins; antioxidants such as vitamin E; the nutrients phosphatidyl serine (PS) and coenzyme Q 10; and the botanicals ginkgo biloba, huperzine A and vinpocetine.

The B-complex vitamins are critical for neurotransmittal control and carbohydrate energy metabolism. Niacin (vitamin $B_3$) has been shown to have memory-improving benefits.[25] Folate reduces homocysteine, high levels of which have been implicated in heart disease and AD. An integrative brain program should also contain adequate antioxidants and vitamin C in the diet, as well as through supplementation.[26] Vitamin E at a dose of 2,000 IU daily has been shown to slow the progression of mid-stage AD, primarily because it protects cell membranes from oxidative damage.[27]

Additional brain-specific nutrients that play a part in the prevention and treatment of AD are
- Phosphatidyl serine (PS): intake of up to 300 mg/day
- Ubiquinone (coenzyme Q 10): intake of up to 100 mg/day
- Ginkgo biloba: intake of up to 240 mg/day
- The omega-3 fatty acid DHA: intake of  50 to 100 mg/day

Newer nutrients that hold great promise are
- Huperzine A: intake of 100 to 200 μg/day
- Vinpocetine: intake of 2.5 to 10 mg/day

PS is a negatively charged phospholipid that is almost exclusively located in cell membranes. It has a set of unique physiological properties that are important to neuronal functions, including stimulation of neurotransmitter release, activation of the ion-transport mechanism, and increase of glucose and cyclic adenosine monophosphate levels in the brain. In the aging brain, a decline in these functions is associated with memory impairment and deficits in cognitive abilities.

PS has been the subject of 23 studies, 12 of them double blind. The findings indicate that PS improves short-term memory, mood, concentration, and ADLs.[28] Although early research used bovine PS, concern over possible slow viral infection prompted the search for an alternative plant source. A novel PS product made by enzymatic conversion of soy lecithin has now been developed and shown to be beneficial in patients with memory loss, including those with AD.[29] It has been my experience that PS is highly effective, especially for improving the ability to recall the names of persons and objects. (A decrease in this ability is a symptom of AD.) For some reason, conventionalists have decided not to include PS in their armamentarium against AD.

Ubiquinone, a powerful neuroprotective agent, works as a dynamic antioxidant throughout the brain cell membrane and mitochondria, where it is involved in the production of high-energy phosphate compounds.[30]

**Botanicals.** Ginkgo biloba increases microvascular circulation, scavenges free radicals, and helps improve concentration and short-term memory in both patients with AAMI and AD. A recent 52-week, randomized double-blind, placebo-controlled, parallel-group, multi-centered study showed that in 309 patients with mild to severe AD or multi-infarct dementia, there were modest, although significant, improvements. These changes were equal to those of drugs with a higher side effect profile and were of a sufficient magnitude to be recognized by the patient's caregivers.[31] Recent reports in the medical and lay media have emphasized the need to exercise caution when combining vitamin E and ginkgo biloba, especially in patients taking anticoagulants. In patients taking Coumadin, for example, I would measure the appropriate coagulation parameters and perhaps lower the dose of all the compounds. I believe it is a disservice to the AD patient, however, to automatically withhold compounds with a proven benefit in fighting AD because of a purely theoretical concern. If the patient is not on Coumadin, I do not believe there is a danger of excessive bleeding. In my clinical experience I have not seen it, nor have I heard of it from any practitioner of integrative medicine.

Huperzine A is a natural anticholinesterase inhibitor derived from Chinese club moss. Many studies, mostly in China, show that huperzine surpassed Aricept in reversing memory deficits in aging animals. Huperzine's activity is also reportedly long lasting. What makes huperzine attractive is its apparent lack of serious side effects and low toxicity. I use 50 μg once or twice daily depending on the severity of symptoms.

Vinpocetine, a nutrient derived from the periwinkle plant, has been shown to increase cerebral blood flow and enhance neuronal metabolism. I find the dose of 2.5 to 5 mg twice daily less stimulating and hence more effective than the higher doses recommended by others.

**Mind/body factors.** Because of the effects of chronic unbalanced stress and cortisol secretion on memory, it is beneficial to suppress elevated glucocorticoid levels or normalize their release. Because age increases the vulnerability to stress and cortisol-induced hippocampal damage, stress-relieving meditation is highly recommended for patients of all ages to reduce cortisol levels and limit the loss of hippocampal neurons.

Meditation has consistently been found to decrease cortisol levels and promote normalization of adaptive mechanisms.[32] Practitioners of meditation also display lower levels of lipid peroxidase, a marker of free radical production, and higher levels of the hormone dehydroepiandrosterone (DHEA), which I consider important for optimal brain function. Researchers such as Wallace[33] have reviewed studies that note the positive health benefits of meditation on cognition. In a landmark study of older persons, it was found that meditators had a greater life expectancy than did nonmeditators.[34]

Specific brain exercises, called *kriyas,* are derived from the science of Kundalini Yoga as taught by Yogi Bhajan. They combine breathing, finger movements, and regenerating sound currents. The practice of these exercises serves a dual purpose: they induce a meditative state and stimulate the central nervous system. Kriyas have been clinically shown be very useful for increasing global brain energy. PET scans demonstrate that these types of exercises enhance regional cerebral blood flow, oxygen delivery, and glucose use. Beyond that, recent research at Harvard proved that what I call *Medical Meditation,* based on kriyas, is quite specific in increasing activity in the hippocampus when compared with basic meditation. Moreover, this same research group is studying the effect of meditation on cortisol levels and grades in school-age children.[35]

**Pharmaceuticals.** There are currently three drugs approved by the FDA to treat early AD. All three are

## Mind/Body Exercise for Mild Cognitive Impairment and Alzheimer's Disease

The following exercise is called *kirtan kriya*. This kriya involves the chanting of the primal sounds.

Say each of these words repeatedly, in order: *Sa Ta Na Ma*. The *a* in these words is pronounced as a soft *a*, or *ah*.

Repeat this mantra while sitting with your spine straight, and your mental energy focused on the area of your brow, or forebrain. Yogis believe that this stimulates your pituitary. You can find this spot by rolling your eyes to the top, or root of your nose.

For 2 minutes, chant in your normal voice. For the next 2 minutes, chant in a whisper. For the middle 3 minutes, chant silently, while still touching the fingertips. Then reverse the order, whispering for 2 minutes and chanting the mantra out loud for the last 2 minutes. The total time is 11 minutes.

The *mudras,* or finger positions, are very important in this kriya. On *Sa,* touch the index fingers of each hand to your thumbs. On *Ta,* touch your middle fingers to your thumbs. On *Na,* touch your ring fingers to your thumbs. On *Ma,* touch your little fingers to your thumbs (Figure 27-1).

At the end, inhale very deeply, stretch your hands above your head, and then bring them down in a sweeping motion as you exhale.

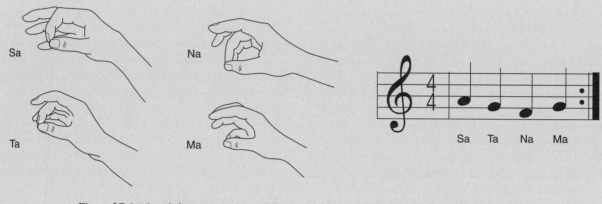

*Figure 27-1* Visual demonstration of the mind/body exercise for mild cognitive impairment and Alzheimer's disease.

acetylcholinesterase inhibitors and therefore act to increase the level of the neurotransmitter acetylcholine (ACh). ACh is critically important for memory formation and retrieval.

The first, tacrine (Cognex), is minimally effective and has poor patient compliance because of its side effects. It is no longer used. The second, donepezil HCl (Aricept), is moderately effective at improving short-term memory in patients with early AD. Neither have any effect on the progression of the disease. Rivastigmine (Exelon) is slightly more effective than the others and has the best side effect profile of the available cholinesterase-inhibiting drugs.[36] Others are in production and will be available soon.

Deprenyl, an MAO-B inhibitor, was shown to limit degeneration of patients with AD in a 5-year double-blind study with a dose of 10 mg/day.[37] The drug also slowed the progression of AD as part of a large-scale, multi-center trial. Deprenyl acts to increase the level of important catecholamines, especially dopamine, which are decreased in AD. It also inhibits oxidative deamination, thereby reducing neuronal damage.

DHEA and/or pregnenolone, both neurospecific hormones and precursors to estrogen, are also useful. A recent animal study demonstrated that DHEA effects excitability in the hippocampus, thereby enhancing memory function at dosages of 50 mg/day. Another study showed that DHEA enhances ACh release from hippocampal neurons in the rat brain. DHEA levels have been shown to be consistently low in patients with AD.[38] Pregnenolone has been the subject of research in both animals and humans. It is found to be a powerful memory enhancer. A recent study has demonstrated improved memory with pregnenolone use in older persons.[39]

As noted, estrogen deficiency in postmenopausal women is a factor in the development of AD. Observational studies indicate that estrogen replacement delays the expression of AD by 40% to 70%. It enhances hippocampal plasticity and increases nerve growth factor. Estrogen has antioxidant properties that protect the neuron from oxidative stress. Estrogen also enhances glucose transport in neurotissue, which may be impaired in AD. Finally, estrogen stimulates the production of several neurotransmitters, of which deficiency characterizes AD.[40]

Use of the hormone melatonin is a reasonable alternative to the use of benzodiazepines in patients with AD. Melatonin restores circadian rhythm and may help to prevent wandering. A good starting dose is 3 mg at bedtime.

**Spirituality.** Beyond reported improvements in memory, concentration, learning ability, and ADLs, patients enrolled in an integrative medical program will also note positive changes in what can be described as personal awareness. This awareness sometimes manifests as a sense of increased self-knowledge or spirituality and leads to a feeling of connectedness. Some patients report that this spiritual connection leads to a profound level of wisdom—the combination of age, intelligence, and experience. This wisdom or maturity brings greater life satisfaction. These changes are consistent with the work of Benson, Larson, and McCullough,[41] who established that following an integrative medical program, including mind/body interactions, enhances spirituality. Spirituality was expressed as experiencing the presence of a higher power close to that person. Furthermore, spirituality, faith, belief, and religiosity are now well known to be associated with fewer medical symptoms and better outcomes when medical interventions are needed.

With the aging of the population, both the incidence and prevalence of cognitive decline, including AAMI, MCI, and AD, is expected to rise. An integrative medical program can have a powerful impact on these diseases.

## Therapeutic Review

### Diagnosis

1. *Patient history:* Family history is important because of the correlation between AD in patients and their first-degree relatives. A personal history of illnesses, especially cardiovascular disease, and metabolic disorders is also useful. Other areas of concern include medication usage and a history of head trauma. In general, the diagnosis of MCI can be made if an individual has a memory complaint and has an abnormal memory for his or her age and level of education. Moreover, the person will demonstrate normal ADLs and a normal level of general cognitive function. The patient with MCI is not demented.

2. *Cognitive assessment:* I have found the Mini-Mental State examination (MMSE) to be valuable in an office setting. It offers a relatively rapid and reliable means of assessing cognitive function, memory, and visual/spatial skills (Figure 27-2). People with low levels of education, however, tend to do poorly on this test, independent of any effects of cognitive function. Moreover, the test is less sensitive in individuals with higher educational levels: they may have a normal score on the MMSE yet have early signs of dementia. Repeated MMSE testing offers a good means of tracking disease progression and monitoring the effects of treatment.

3. *Physical examination and laboratory tests:* The physical examination and standard neurological evaluation may reveal evidence of a stroke. Focal findings of hemiparesis, sensory loss, cranial nerve deficits, and ataxia are not consistent with a diagnosis of AD. Conventional laboratory testing should include a complete blood count, electrolyte and metabolic panels, thyroid function tests, assessment of vitamin $B_{12}$ level, homocysteine, and tests for syphilis and HIV. Beyond that, the integrative medical practitioner will also test for certain hormone levels. Measuring DHEA has proven clinically useful. In my experience, patients with AD have markedly low levels of DHEA. I also measure levels of free testosterone in males and estrogen in females. And although full hormone replacement therapy is not a regular part of my work, I do order an insulin-like growth factor (IGF-1) level. Urinalysis, electrocardiogram, chest x-ray examination, and determination of folate levels are no longer recommended.

**Mini-Mental State Examination**

**Orientation to Time**

"What is the date?"

**Registration**

"Listen carefully, I am going to say three words. You say them back after I stop.
Ready? Here they are...
HOUSE (pause), CAR (pause), LAKE (pause).
Now repeat those words back to me."
(Repeat up to 5 times, but score only the first trial.)

**Naming**

"What is this?" [Point to a pencil or pen.]

**Reading**

"Please read this and do what it says." [Show examinee the words on the stimulus form.]
CLOSE YOUR EYES

*Figure 27-2* Sample items from the Mini-Mental State Examination (MMSE). The complete MMSE can be purchased from PAR, Inc, at 800-331-8378 or 813-968-3003. (From Mini Mental, LLC: 1975, 1998, 2001, Odessa, Fla, Psychological Assessment Resources.)

4. *Neuroimaging:* Although when to use it is somewhat controversial, I have found neuroimaging to be useful for identifying lesions such as hippocampal and cerebral atrophy that are consistent with AD. I believe neuroimaging can help determine the stage of dementia and the patient's prognosis.

Some experts suggest computed tomography (CT) or MRI for all patients with suspected AD. Others consider PET more useful when the diagnosis is uncertain. PET can be used to identify a declining metabolic rate in the parietal/temporal lobe, which is characteristic of AD.

5. *Genetic testing:* Determining APOE4 status can contribute to diagnostic accuracy in patients who already have a clinical diagnosis of AD. Genetic testing is most commonly used in academic medicine.

## Treatment

1. *Diet:* 15% to 20% fat diet based on patient preferences. Include organic fruits and vegetables and fish rich in omega-3 fatty acids such as salmon and flax seed oil.
2. *Supplements*
   a. Vitamin E: 2,000 IU/day
   b. Coenzyme Q 10: 100 to 300 mg/day
   c. Ginkgo biloba: 240 mg/day
   d. Phosphatidyl serine: 100 to 300 mg/day
   e. DHA: 500 to 1,000 mg/day
   f. Huperzine A: 100 to 200 μg/day
   g. Vinpocetine: 5 to 10 mg/day
   NOTE: Watch out for the rare potential of clotting abnormalities in patients on Coumadin. Also, there is a very rare possibility of increased clotting time in patients taking maximum doses of ginkgo biloba, vitamin E, and DHA, especially with ASA.
3. *Stress management:* Morning meditation for at least 15 minutes daily.
4. *Exercise:* Physical, mental, and mind/body exercise should be part of integrative prescription.
5. *Pharmaceuticals:* Deprenyl 5 mg twice daily does slow progression. Exelon is the most effective conventional drug available, and others are in the pipeline. Start with 2.5 mg twice daily and work up as per package insert. CAUTION: *Do not use Deprenyl with antidepressant medications—fatal reactions can occur.* Deprenyl can be used in conjunction with anticholinesterase drugs.
6. *Hormone replacement therapy*
   a. DHEA 25 to 100 mg/day, depending on sex and blood level

### Resource

Alzheimer's Prevention Foundation
Dharma Signh Khalsa, MD, President and Medical Director
2420 N Pantano Road
Tucson, AZ  85715
Phone: 520-749-8374
Fax: 520-296-6640
www.alzheimersprevention.org

   b. Pregnenolone 10-100 mg/day
   c. Melatonin 3 mg/day at bedtime; proper dose allows complete nights sleep without AM grogginess
   NOTE: When using DHEA, measure and follow PSA level. If elevated, do not use DHEA. Also consider using the herb saw palmetto with DHEA.

## SUMMARY

An integrative approach to Mild Cognitive Impairment and Alzheimer's disease utilizes physical and cognitive exercises, nutritional review, and use of appropriate supplements and botanicals, mind/body exercises, and spiritual practices, as well as pharmaceuticals, holds great promise for preventing and treating these widespread health problems.

## References

1. Ernst R, Hay J: The U.S. economic and social cost of Alzheimer's disease revisited, *Am J Pub Health* 84:1261-1264, 1991.
2. Thal LJ: Trials to prevent Alzheimer's disease in a population at risk. Abstracts of the Fourth International Nice/Springfield Symposium on Advances in Alzheimer Therapy, p 86, 1996.
3. Lupien S: Personal communication, 1999.
4. Snowdon DA, Kemper SJ, Mortimer JA, et al: Linguistic ability in early life and cognitive function and Alzheimer's disease in late life: findings form the nun study, *JAMA* 275(7):528-532, 1996.
5. Reimen EM, Caselli RJ, Yun L, et al: Preclinical evidence of Alzheimer's disease in persons homozygous for the 4-allele for apolipoprotein E, *N Engl J Med* 334:752-758, 1996.
6. Gatz M, Lowe B, Berg S, et al: Dementia: not just a search for the gene, *Gerontologist* 34:251-255, 1994.

7. Birge SJ, Mortel KF: Estrogen and the treatment of Alzheimer's disease, *Am J Med* 103:36S-45S, 1997.

8. Katzman R, Kawas C: The epidemiology of dementia and Alzheimer's disease. In Katzman JR, Bich KL (eds): *Alzheimer disease,* New York, 1994, Raven Press, pp 105-122.

9. Shah Y, Tangalos E, Petersen R: Mild cognitive impairment: when is it a precursor to Alzheimer's disease? *Geriatrics* 55(9):62-68, 2000.

10. Grant WB: Dietary links to Alzheimer's disease, *Alz Dis Rev* 2:42-45, 1997.

11. Hendrie HC, Ogunniyi A, Hall KS, et al: Incidence of dementia and Alzheimer disease in 2 communities: Yoruba residing in Ibadan, Nigeria, and African Americans residing in Indianapolis, Indiana, *JAMA* 285:739-747, 2001.

12. Lupiens S, Lecour SA, Lussier I, et al: Basal cerebral cortisol levels and cognitive deficits in human aging, *J Neurosci* 14(5):2983-2993, 1994.

13. Stein-Behrens BA, Sapolsky RM: Stress, glucocorticoids, and aging, *Aging* 4(3):197-210, 1992.

14. Sapolsky RM, McEwen BS: Stress, glucocorticoids and their role in degenerative changes in the aging hippocampus. In Crook T, Bartus R (eds): *Treatment development strategies for Alzheimer's disease,* Madison, Conn, 1986, MPA Press.

15. McEwen BS, Sapolsky RM: Stress and cognitive functions, *Curr Opin Neurobiol* 5:205-206, 1995.

16. Khalsa DS, Stauth C: *In meditation as medicine: activate the power of your natural healing force,* New York, 2001, Pocket Books.

17. Gould LK, Ornish D, Scherwitz L, et al: Changes in myocardial perfusion abnormalities by positron emission tomography after long-term, intense risk factor modification, *JAMA* 274:894-901, 1995.

18. Smith AL, Fredlund R, et al: The protective effects of physical exercise on the development of Alzheimer's disease, *Neurology* 50:A89-A90, 1998.

19. Diamond MC, Lindner B, Johnson R, et al: Differences in occipital corticol synapses from environmentally enriched, impoverished and standard colony rats, *J Neurosci Res* 1:109-119, 1975.

20. Cotman C: Synaptic plasticity, neurotrophic factors and transplantation in the aged brain. In *Handbook of the biology of aging,* San Diego, 1990, Academic Press, pp 255-274.

21. Walford RL, Spindler SR: The response to calorie restriction in mammals shows features also common to hibernation: a cross-adaptation hypothesis, *J Gerontol A Biol Sci Med Sci* 52(4):B179-183, 1997.

22. Weindruch R: Caloric restriction and aging, *Sci Am* 274:46-52, 1996.

23. Weindruch R, Walford RL: *The retardation of aging and disease by dietary restriction,* Springfield, Ill, 1998, Charles C Thomas.

24. Verdery R, Walford R: *Caloric restriction in Biosphere II: effects of energy restriction on lipid and lipoprotein levels and HDL subfractions,* American Aging Association Annual Meeting, abstract no. 75, p 37, 1996.

25. Zhang X, Zhand BZ, Zhang WW: Protective effects of nicotinic acid on disturbance of memory induced by cerebral ischemia-reperfusion in rats, *Clin J Pharm Tox* 10:178-180, 1996.

26. Peetot GJ, Cole R, Conaway C, et al: *Adult lifetime dietary patterns of antioxidant vitamin and carotenoid consumption in a case control study of risk factors for Alzheimer's disease,* American Aging Association Annual Meeting, abstract no. 78, p 38, 1996.

27. Sano M et al: A controlled trial of selegiline, alpha-tocopherol, or both as treatment for Alzheimer's disease, *N Engl J Med* 336:1216-1222, 1997.

28. Crook TN et al: Effects of phosphatidylserine in Alzheimer's disease, *Psychopharmacol Bull* 28:61-66, 1992.

29. Gindin J, Nouikov D, Kedar A, et al: *The effect of plant phosphatidyl serine on age-associated memory impairment and mood in the functional elderly,* an unpublished paper from The Geriatric Institute for education and research, and Department of Geriatrics, Kaplan Hospital, Revohat, Israel, 1995.

30. Beal FM: Cell death by oxidants: neuroprotective antioxidant therapies. Presented at the Fourth International Nice /Springfield Symposium on Advances in Alzheimer's Therapy, April 1996.

31. LeBars PL, Katz MM, et al: A placebo-controlled, double-blind, randomized trial of an extract of ginkgo biloba for dementia, *JAMA* 278:1327-1332, 1997.

32. Jevning R, Wilson AF, Davidson JM: Adrenocortical activity during meditation, *Horm Behav* 10:54-60, 1978.

33. Wallace RR: *The physiology of consciousness,* a joint publication of the Institute of Science, Technology and Public Policy and Maharishi International University Press.

34. Alexander CN, Langer EJ, Newman RI, et al: Transcendental meditation: mindfulness and longevity in experimental studies in the elderly, *J Pers Soc Psychol* 6:950-964, 1989.

35. Khalsa DS, Stauth C: *In meditation as medicine,* New York, 2001, Pocket Books.

36. Khalsa DS: Exelon: a new drug for Alzheimer's disease, *Int J Antiaging Med* 1:10-12, 1998.

37. Riekhman P: Rationale to treat AD with selegiline. Presented at the Fourth International Nice/Springfield Symposium on Advances in Alzheimer Therapy, April 1996.

38. Rhodes ME, Li PK, Flood JF, et al: Enhancement of hippocampal acetylcholine release by the neurosteroid: dehydroepiandrosterone sulfate—an in vivo microdialysis study, *Brain Res* 733:284-286, 1996.

39. Flood JF, Morley JE, Roberts E: Memory-enhancing effects in male mice of pregnenolone and steroids metabolically derived from it, *Proc Natl Acad Sci* 89(5):1567-1571, 1992.

40. Berge SJ, Mortel KF: Estrogen and the treatment of Alzheimer's disease, *Am J Med* 103:36S-45S, 1997.

41. Larson DB, Sawyers JP, McCullough ME (eds): *Scientific research on spirituality and health: a consensus report,* Rockville, Md, 1998, National Institute for Healthcare Research.

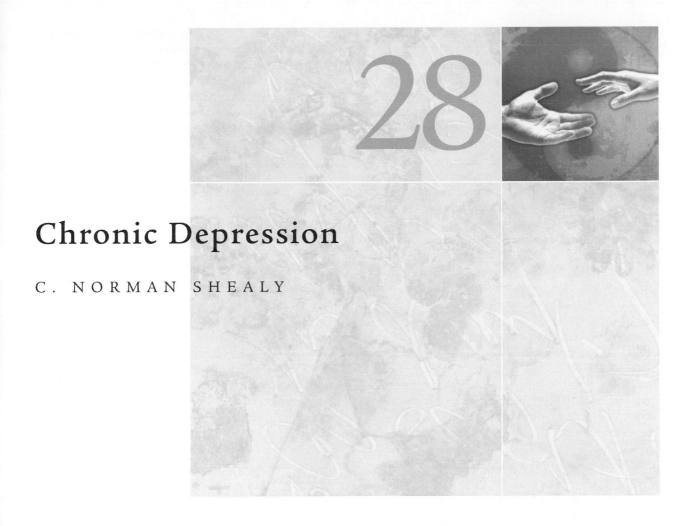

# Chronic Depression

## C. NORMAN SHEALY

## BACKGROUND

For 30 years, our work at the Shealy Wellness Center has focused primarily on treating individuals with chronic pain, virtually all of whom are also suffering from chronic depression, a finding others have also reported.[1] Given that depression so often coexists with other rehabilitation conditions such as stroke or spinal cord injury, effective treatment of depression is a cornerstone of the rehabilitation process. Indeed, in the past 13 years our major research has been directed toward elucidating the neurochemical basis of depression and developing nonpharmacological methods for treating it.

## CLINICAL INTERVENTION

### Psychotherapy

In contrast, in 1993 the Agency for Health Care Policy and Research (AHCPR) published clinical practice guidelines focusing on treatment of depression in primary care. The guidelines encouraged primary care physicians to provide pharmacotherapy to depressed patients as the first line of treatment.[2]

In the 1960's and up until about 1974, we used tricyclic antidepressants, gradually tried some of the newer ones such as Desyrel, and actually twice prescribed Prozac before realizing just how serious the complications of Prozac are, with severe anxiety,

343

agitation, and insomnia in all too many patients. In the *Physician's Desk Reference*[3] we find with Prozac 36% of patients very much improved or much improved at 20 mg/day, 39% at 40 mg/day and 47% at 60 mg/day. Prozac has had perhaps more publicity and a greater public education of its use than any other antidepressant drug. When we look at the complication rate with Prozac, 9% report asthenia, 21% nausea, 11% anorexia, 10% dry mouth, 16% insomnia, 12% anxiety, 14% nervousness (that suggests to me significant anxiety in 26%), and a variety of other complications.

With Celexa, another selective serotonin reuptake inhibitor, I find little evidence that it is any more effective than Prozac, and it includes complications or "side effects" of dry mouth in 20% of patients, increased sweating in 11%, tremor in 8%, nausea in 21%, somnolence in 18%, insomnia in 15%, and even ejaculation disorder in 6%, along with a wide variety of other symptoms.

Extensive literature review gives no evidence of any antidepressant drug that has a highly successful outcome even of 50%. "Minimal" improvement is of no clinical significance; and even at 60 mg there are only an additional 24% of individuals "minimally improved" with Prozac. Thus after a very careful review of many antidepressant drugs, I conclude that the average very much improved or much improved result is somewhere between 36% and, at best, 47%, with significant complications or undesirable side effects in a minimum of 25% of patients.

Psychotherapy alone does not seem to fare much better. Thus we set about in the early 1970's to look for safe, effective, alternative approaches to the management of depression.[4,5,6] Virtually all of the neurochemistry related to depression has revolved around serotonin and catecholamines, primarily norepinephrine.

## Electrical Stimulation via TENS

In 1975, Saul Liss presented me with the Pain Suppressor, a transcutaneous electrical nerve stimulation (TENS) unit that delivers 1 mA (milliampere) transcranially at ultra high frequency (15,000 Hz). I serendipitously placed one of the leads on my forehead and saw a flickering light. Testing it in a variety of ways around the body but with one electrode on the cranium for about 40 minutes one evening, I fell asleep at 11:30 PM but woke up 3 hours later unable to fall back asleep. Some weeks later I applied the stimulator trans-

cranially at just over 2 mA of current for 1 hour both to myself and to my medical colleague. We found a doubling of serotonin level in my colleague and an increase to 5 times the upper limit of normal in my own blood about an hour after such stimulation. This was the beginning of a look at the last 26 years at both the Liss TENS device, as well as a variety of other alternative approaches for managing pain.

Our first clinical study involved a look at 24-hour output of 5HIAA, 5-hydroxyindoleacetic acid, the excretion by-product of serotonin, in 27 patients.[7] We found that 40% of the chronically depressed patients had serotonin levels below the lower limit and 40% had levels above the upper limit of normal. After 2 weeks of transcranial stimulation using 1 to 2 mA of current at 15,000 cycles per second, all of the patients who had low levels of serotonin had their levels brought up to the normal range and all of those who had elevated levels of serotonin initially had their levels fall to within the normal range. There was no change in the 20% of patients who had had a normal range at the beginning and, interestingly, that group of patients with normal levels of serotonin was recalcitrant to treatment of all types for both their pain and depression.[2] These initial observations have influenced our work with depression since that time.

The next study, which has never before been published, was a simple trial of the Liss stimulator in 24 patients with chronic depression. As in all such studies, the majority of subjects (14) were women, with only 10 men. Subjects ranged in age from 30 to 64 years, and all of them had failed one or more antidepressant drugs and had moderate to severe depression as measured by the Zung screening test for depression. They were instructed in the use of the cranial stimulator, which was to be used for 1 hour each morning at home for 2 weeks. At the end of the 2 weeks, 12 of the patients were very much improved or much improved. All patients had Zung scores of 55 or above before treatment. Twelve of them were improved down to 40 or below after treatment the cut-off score for mild depression. No further treatment was done and gradually, as one might expect, over the next several months most of them drifted back into depression.

## Neurochemical Markers

Recognizing that depression is certainly a much more complicated problem than either a lack of production or excess production of serotonin and/or norepinephrine, we began investigating a broader neuro-chemical profile. For a number of years, the dexamethasone suppression test and the thyroid releasing hormone stimulation test were thought to be useful in diagnosing depression, but they were never widely accepted.[8-15] There also was great argument about their accuracy for bipolar depression, which represents no more than 10% of depressed patients. Our earliest study looked at total catecholamine production, where we found elevations of catecholamines in 55% of chronically depressed patients at rest and 77% after standing for 5 minutes.[16]

Coupled with our earlier work on serotonin, we then began to look at other potentially important neurochemicals, eventually evaluating baseline fasting levels of serotonin, melatonin, beta-endorphins, norepinephrine, and cholinesterase, as well as the ratios between norepinephrine and serotonin, norepinephrine and beta endorphins, norepinephrine and cholinesterase, serotonin and beta endorphins, and norepinephrine divided by the serotonin and beta endorphin ratio. We found that a serotonin-to-beta endorphin ratio of less than 5 leads to an 88% chance of the individual's being clinically depressed. Interestingly, a low norepinephrine level in itself was not suggestive of depression unless the cholinesterase was relatively high. High beta endorphin levels were found in about 10% of persons who had an agitated depression; therefore low serotonin, low beta endorphin, and high cholinesterase all are suggestive of depression.[17]

## DHEA

In 1992, we learned of the critical importance of dehydroepiandrosterone (DHEA). DHEA is the single most abundant hormone in the human body but, interestingly, it has been reported that the vast majority of people over 30 years of age have incremental decreases so that by age 80 years they have less than 10% of the level of a healthy 30-year-old. Furthermore, it has been demonstrated that most illnesses (except schizophrenia) are associated with low or deficient levels of DHEA. We found DHEA levels in about 50% of depressed patients to be well below the mean of the normal range and 50% to be in the deficient range by standard laboratory tests. The normal ranges are males 180 to 1,250 ng/dL and females 130-980 ng/dL. Incidentally, the only accurate laboratory that we have found for measuring DHEA is what was originally Nichols Lab in San Juan Capistrano, California—now part of Quest Diagnostics, with only the laboratory in San Juan Capistrano being accurate.[18]

Of individuals with chronic long-standing depression, 92% had abnormalities in serotonin, beta endorphin, norepinephrine, melatonin, or cholinesterase or their ratio, and 100% had low or deficient levels of DHEA. In addition, later studies have shown that 86% of depressed patients have deficient levels of blood taurine, which is now considered by most scientists to be an essential amino acid, and of the significantly depressed individuals, 100% are found to be deficient in magnesium, either by the magnesium load test or intracellular magnesium testing.[19] It has been well demonstrated that testing for serum magnesium is useless because it is deficient only in patients with acute alcoholism or severe starvation. Thus in clinical practice with neurochemical and biochemical testing in nearly 1,000 patients, we see a broad spectrum of abnormalities.

We have also looked at individual techniques that might raise DHEA back into the normal range or stabilize serotonin and beta endorphin levels, as well as reduce catecholamine or norepinephrine levels. Our interventions have included transcranial stimulation. The Liss stimulator is a later derivation of the original Pain Suppressor mentioned earlier. This particular device puts out 1 to 4 mA of current at 15,000 Hz, modified both 15 and 500 times per second. We have demonstrated that it significantly raises both cerebral spinal fluid level and blood levels of serotonin and beta endorphins.

## Photostimulation

Photostimulation has been used since the early 1950s to induce a state of relaxation. We have worked with it using frequencies between 1 Hz and 12 Hz. It is important to remain below 15 Hz because 1 person in 10,000 may have photo-induced epilepsy, but there has never been a report of an epileptic seizure induced at a frequency below 12 Hz. Photostimulation significantly increases DHEA and beta endorphin levels (Figure 28-1).

Other interventions have included relaxing music, which increases DHEA and beta endorphin levels; physical exercise, which increases DHEA and beta endorphin levels; a combination of vitamin C, methylsulphonylmethane, and beta 1,3 glucan, which increases DHEA; electrical stimulation of 12 specific acupuncture points that we call the Ring of Fire,

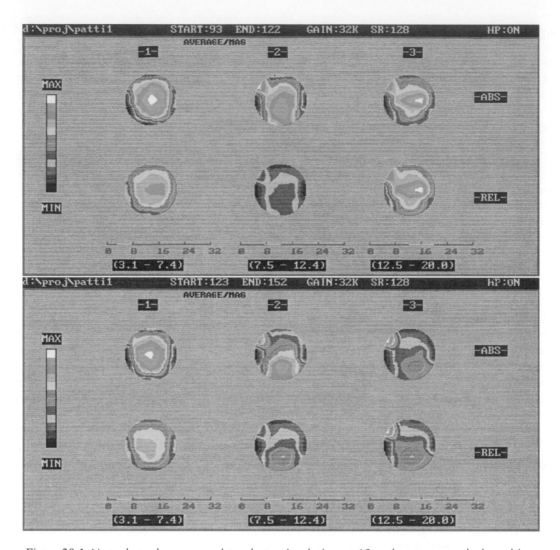

*Figure 28-1* Note that when exposed to photostimulation at 12 cycles per second, the subject has a marked increase in beta activity in the right central hemisphere. There is a marked increase in theta activity centrally and in the right central area and a marked increase in alpha frequency in the central and right occipital area. Again, this is an inappropriate response to photostimulation.

which significantly increases DHEA; soaks in an unusual substance called Yinergy oil, which has a content of 25% magnesium chloride that significantly raises both DHEA and intracellular magnesium; and natural progesterone cream, which raises DHEA.[20,21] Intracellular magnesium levels may be raised by taking magnesium taurate 375 mg daily, but our experience suggests that it takes up to 1 year to adequately replenish magnesium when used orally. Almost all magnesium supplements have the possibility of a laxative effect, and even if the level does not cause diarrhea, a rapid gut transit time of less than 12 hours impedes the absorption of magnesium orally.

In addition to these neurochemical abnormalities, we have done computerized EEG brain mapping in over 600 patients with chronic depression and have found three types of abnormality. First, these individuals routinely demonstrate striking EEG abnormalities (Figure 28-2). Sixty percent of the time there is a focus of increased activity in the right frontal lobe brain map, of any frequency—delta, theta, alpha, or beta. Forty percent of the time the increased frequency may occur in another lobe of the brain. Second, these patients do not follow photostimulation. When presented with photostimulation of 10 cycles per second, for example, their EEG frequency may increase to 20 cycles per second or a decrease to 3 cycles per second but do not follow the appropriate stimulation. Third, these patients are usually hypersensitive to electromagnetic influences. A radio, not turned on but plugged in, emits 50 milligauss of electromagnetic energy; when placed within 6 inches of the vertex of the head, it causes significant further increases in the abnormality of the EEG. Over time, with therapy, the EEG begins to be symmetrical, and after about 3 months, the EEG begins to follow photostimulation appropriately.[22]

## SUMMARY OF FINDINGS

In working with some 15,000 patients with chronic depression, two thirds of whom also had chronic pain, we have found neurochemical abnormalities, including levels both above the upper limit and below the lower limit of normal and in some 92% of patients in relation to serotonin, melatonin, beta endorphin, norepinephrine, cholinesterase, or their ratio, with levels below the mean or below the lower limit of normal in 100% of patients in relation to DHEA, with 86% of

them having low levels of taurine, and 100% having deficiencies in one to seven amino acids.

Based on the work of the past 30 years, summarized previously, depression presents a pattern of common features.

1. Depression is a multifactorial disease, resulting from cumulative physical, emotional, chemical, and electromagnetic stress.
2. Depression is invariably associated with one or more biochemical abnormalities.
   a. DHEA levels in the lower 2 quartiles in 50% of patients and below "normal" in 50% of patients
   b. Excess or deficiency of one or more of the following:
      (1) Norepinephrine
      (2) Serotonin
      (3) Melatonin
      (4) Beta endorphin
      (5) Cholinesterase and/or the ratios of serotonin to melatonin and norepinephrine to serotonin
      (6) Deficiencies of one to seven essential amino acids, most often taurine
      (7) Deficiency of magnesium
3. There is an electrical imbalance of the brain electroencephalograph, including
   a. Focal excess activity in one lobe of the brain, most often right frontal
   b. Failure to follow photostimulation appropriately
   c. Increased asymmetry produced by exposure to moderate electromagnetic stress (radio, plugged in but not turned on)

Therapy should be directed at correcting these abnormalities through five major approaches.

1. Liss TENS to rebalance serotonin and beta endorphin levels.
2. Photostimulation to increase beta endorphin and EEG symmetry.
3. Vibratory music consisting of the use of a bed in which are imbedded sound transducers so that the patient both feels as well as hears the music. We have found that this increases the beta endorphin level and gives an experience of peaceful deep relaxation.
4. Education to improve knowledge of the psychology and physiology of depression.
5. Nutritional guidelines, especially in relation to magnesium and amino acids.

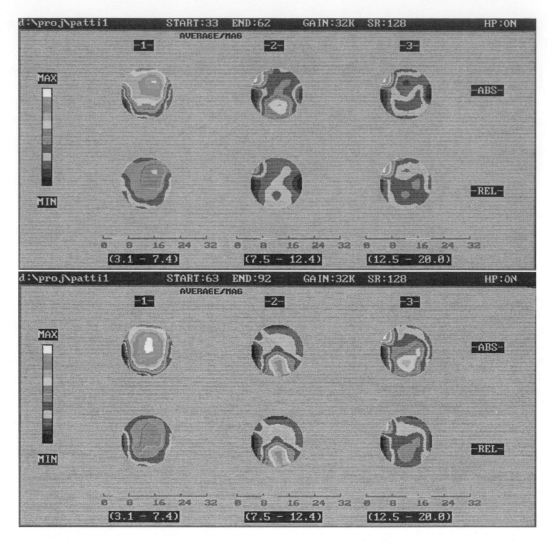

*Figure 28-2* This is an EEG of one of our chronically depressed patients who also has chronic pain. Note that there is a very strong theta activity, particularly dominant in the right frontal area with some dominant theta and beta in the left frontal temporal area. This is typical of the asymmetry seen in depressed patients.

If this 5-step treatment protocol is used, a significant majority of depressed patients will improve without pharmaceutical intervention.

# CLINICAL TREATMENT PROGRAM

Some 12 years ago we began refining experiments with various components that have been shown to have some effect on depression and/or neurochemical homeostasis. As noted earlier, we had demonstrated that cranial electrical stimulation with a Liss TENS device brought 50% of patients out of depression safely without side effects and without any other intervention. We then added to that basic treatment vibratory music in which the patient spent 1 hour a day for 10 days over a 2-week period lying on a music bed with vibratory speakers so that the patient could sense both a kinetic and an audio awareness of the music. We already knew that this helped raise at least the beta endorphin level.

We also added photostimulation because it had been shown to raise DHEA and beta endorphin levels. In photostimulation we use from 1 to a maximum of 12 cycles per second of either red light reflected against a blue background or a white light, most often not above 7.5 Hz. (There has never been a report of an epileptic seizure induced by photostimulation below 15 Hz.) At the present time, this is best accomplished by the use of a strobe light available at most home electronics stores. Although we have tried various colored lights, I cannot be certain that it makes any difference whether one uses a simple plain white light or various colors such as green, violet, red, or yellow.

We added a basic 10-hour educational program to give patients an understanding of our philosophy and the physiology of stress and depression. Numerous variations on this approach have been used. And with over 400 patients, we have demonstrated that this combination of cranial electrical stimulation, education, vibratory music, and photostimulation leads to a marked improvement in 85% of patients within 2 weeks. In a later study we looked at just education, photostimulation, and vibratory music and found that 58% of depressed patients improved markedly. In many of our studies we have used not only the Zung test as a screen but, in a majority of studies, also the Minnesota Multiphasic Personality Inventory (MMPI). In general, the Zung has been a very satisfactory test for us and although one does determine other psychopathology with

the MMPI, we do not feel that it adds a great deal of clinical usefulness when one is studying only chronically depressed individuals with moderate levels of dysthymia.

We also routinely advise patients on good nutritional practices, especially to improve their intake of amino acids. The most common amino acid deficiency is taurine. The easiest way to replenish amino acids is to prepare a "meat broth" using 1 quart of water, 8 ounces of cubed meat of any kind (fish, chicken, turkey, beef, etc.), cooking for 8 to 12 hours on low heat or in a slow cooker with 2 tablespoons of vinegar and seasonings. This helps dissolve the amino acids out of the meat so that they are easily available. We also recommend taking a good broad-spectrum multivitamin/mineral and participating in a progressive exercise program. We have given hundreds of patients up to 10 shots of magnesium chloride intravenously, 2 gm per dose, and although it seems to help, we do not find it any better than soaking the feet in the 25% magnesium chloride oil or Yinergy oil, which is much simpler.

When the patients go home, they are given a workbook *(90 Days to Stress Free Living)*, which contains a 3-month program of daily physical, mental, emotional, and spiritual exercises. Consistently, without any further intervention, at 3- and 6-month follow-ups 70% of the patients who enter our program remain very improved or very much improved. Approximately 25% of patients need either continuing photostimulation or intermittent use of the Liss stimulator to maintain their improvement. The 15% who regress often benefit from further treatment with one or more of the elements of the essential protocol.

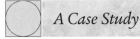

*A Case Study*

### Endogenous Depression

R.B., a 41-year-old man with lifelong depression, had been unsuccessfully treated with appropriate dosages of Desyrel and amitriptyline and had made numerous attempts at psychotherapy, which had been of no value to him. He had no medical problems. On the entry into our treatment program, he had a Zung score of 69, which is moderately to severely depressed. Mild depression is generally considered 50 to 59, moderate 60 to 69, and severe above 69. On the MMPI his depression scale was over 2 standard deviations above the mean, with similar elevations on hysteria and hypochondriasis. This triad is present in at least 75% of the patients we have seen with chronic depression, often with one or more elevations as well. He entered a 2-week intensive program, 4 hours per day, with 1 hour of education, 1 hour of vibratory music, 1 hour of cranial stimulation with a Liss TENS, and 1 hour of photostimulation. On day 12, his Zung score was 48, his MMPI now was totally normal, and he reported being the happiest he could remember. On the last day of a 2-week intensive program, he put on a very humorous skit for the rest of the patients. This man has been followed for another 10 years. He has had occasional counseling sessions and sometimes has used photostimulation. Although he had no known precipitating basis for depression, his remarkable improvement emphasizes the rehabilitative effect of the treatment protocol. ∾

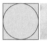

### A Case Study

*Depression and Physical Abuse*

M.B., 45-year-old woman with a history of marked physical abuse as a child and depression for at least 30 years, had seen many psychotherapists and had been tried on appropriate dosages of Prozac, amitriptyline, and Zoloft without improvement in her depression. On entry into the program, she had a Zung score of 63, and on the MMPI her depression scale was 2.5 standard deviations above the mean. She was treated initially with the same approach used with R.B. (see previous case study), and at the end of the treatment program, her Zung test was 35, the MMPI depression scale was at the mean, and she was almost euphoric at the change in her mood. She has been followed for some 8 years. During this time she has required the use of the cranial stimulator for 1 week about 4 times per year and some ongoing counseling, but she has remained free of depression and has had no further antidepressant drug therapy. M.B. feels fully rehabilitated. ∾

### A Case Study

*Post-Stroke Depression*

C.S., a 68-year-old man, had suffered a relatively mild right hemispheric stroke 1 year earlier. He was left with a slight spasticity of the left side but no intractable pain and no other major deficit. However, he entered a deep depression and remained depressed for 3 years. He had been tried on several antidepressant drugs before therapy. On entry into the 2-week intensive program, he had a Zung score of 68. He received the standard protocol, and at completion of the treatment program his Zung was 48. He has been followed for over 2 years and has remained out of depression. ∾

### A Case Study

*Spinal Cord Injury*

F.J., a 40-year-old ski instructor, was coming down a steep slope, swerved to avoid hitting another skier, and hit a post. He was instantly rendered paraplegic from T8 down; had been through extensive rehabilitation; and was self-sufficient, although wheelchair bound. He entered the program because of significant depression related to his physical condition. His Zung score was 58 on admission to the program. Following the 2-week intensive, his Zung score was 45. He has been followed for some 5 years and has become productive and continues with a sedentary job. ∾

## SUMMARY

The basic treatment program consists of the Liss TENS device transcranially for 40 to 60 minutes each morning. This alone will relieve depression in 50% of chronic patients. It is better than any known antidepressant drug without complications or side effects. Alterna-

### Resources

Shealy Wellness Center
1328 E Evergreen
Springfield, MO 65803
www.shealyhealthnet.com

Medi Consultants
265 Vreeland Avenue
Paterson, NJ 07504
(973) 278-0200
(Liss TENS)

Self-Health Systems
5607 S 222nd Road
Fair Grove, MO 65648
www.selfhealthsystems.com
(Yinergy Oil)

Holos University Graduate Seminary
Doctoral Degrees in Energy Medicine
5607 S 222nd Road
Fair Grove, MO 65648
(888) 272-6109

tively, with photostimulation (primarily with 1 to 7.5 cycles per second), vibratory music, and education, 58% of patients are markedly improved. This also is better than any known drug and is without complications.

When we combine the Liss stimulator with the other three modalities, 85% of patients are markedly or very markedly improved within 2 weeks, and a minimum of 70% maintain this when followed for many months thereafter. We also recommend nutritional changes and exercise, which are followed to a greater or lesser extent by most patients.

Approximately 25% of patients require intermittent use of the Liss stimulator, and a similar number continue to use photostimulation at home. Our results in managing moderate to severe dysthymia are almost twice as good as those of any drug without any of the complications seen with pharmacotherapy.

## References

1. Von Korff M, Le Resche L, Dworkin SF: First onset of common pain symptoms: a prospective study of depression as a risk factor, *Pain* 55:251-258, 1993.
2. Winslow R: U.S. agency urges early diagnosis of depression, *Wall Street Journal* April 15, 1993.
3. *Physicians' desk reference,* ed 55, Mount Dale, NJ, 2001, Medical Economics.
4. Johnson J, Weissman M, Klerman GL: Service utilization and social morbidity associated with depressive symptoms in the community, *JAMA* 267(11):1478, 1992.
5. Meredith LS et al: Counseling typically provided for depression, *Arch Gen Psychiatry* 53:905, 1996.
6. Keller MB et al: A comparison of nefazodone, the cognitive behavioral-analysis system of psychotherapy, and their combination for the treatment of chronic depression, *N Engl J Med* 342(20):1462, 2000.
7. Shealy CN, Kwako J, Hughes S: Effects of transcranial neurostimulation upon mood and serotonin production: a preliminary report, *Il dolore* 1(1):13-16, 1979.
8. Lieber AL: *The use of biological markers in diagnosing depression: clinical advances in the treatment of depression,* New York, undated article.
9. Atkinson JH et al: Basal and post-dexamethasone cortisol and prolactin concentrations in depressed and nondepressed patients with chronic pain syndromes, New York, 1985, Elseiver Science.
10. Bates HM: The dexamethasone suppression test: a psychiatric monitor, *Lab Manage* pp 19-21, Jan 1982.
11. Meltzer HY et al: Serotonin uptake in blood platelets and the dexamethasone suppression test in depressed patients, *Psychiatry Res* 8:41-47, 1983.
12. Sachar EJ et al: *Recent studies in the neuroendocrinology of major depressive disorders: advances in psychoneuroendocrinology,* NY State Psych Inst 5:314-325, 1980.
13. Rothschild AJ: Biology of depression, *Med Clin North Am* 72(4):765, 1988.
14. Extein I, Pottash ALC, Gold MS: The thyrotropin-releasing hormone test in the diagnosis of unipolar depression, *Psychiatry Res* 5:311-316, 1981.
15. Hirschfeld RM, Koslow SH, Kupfer DJ: The clinical utility of the dexamethasone suppression test in psychiatry, *JAMA* 250(16):2172, 1983.
16. Shealy CN et al: Depression a diagnostic, neurochemical profile and therapy with cranial electrical stimulation (CES), *J Neuro Ortho Med Surg* 10(4):319, 1989.
17. Shealy CN et al: The neurochemistry of depression, *Am J Pain Manage* 2(1):13, 1992.
18. Shealy CN, Cady RK, Cox RH: Pain, stress and depression: psychoneurophysiology and therapy, *Stress Med* 11:75-77, 1995.
19. Cox RII et al: Significant magnesium deficiency in depression, *J Neuro Ortho Med Surg* 17:709, 1996.
20. Shealy CN: *DHEA: the youth and health hormone,* New Canaan, Conn, 1996, Keats Publishing.
21. Shealy CN et al: Cerebrospinal fluid and plasma neurochemicals: response to cranial electrical stimulation, *J Neuro Ortho Med Surg* 18(21):94, 1998.
22. Shealy CN: Electromagnetic dysthymia, *J Neuro Ortho Med Surg* 17(3):193, 1997.

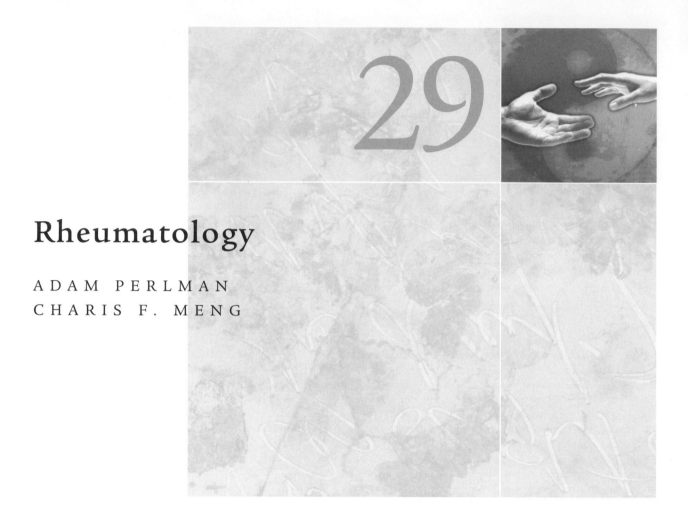

# 29

# Rheumatology

ADAM PERLMAN
CHARIS F. MENG

Over the last decade there has been a growing recognition that increasing numbers of patients in the United States and abroad are using complementary and alternative medicine (CAM) as an adjunct to their conventional medical care. Although the reasons for this trend are multiple, one contributing factor is the continued inability of modern medicine to adequately treat many chronic and debilitating diseases. The scope of rheumatic diseases is broad; however, a common characteristic is the tendency to be chronic and associated with significant morbidity and potential disability. It should therefore not be surprising that patients with rheumatological conditions commonly use CAM.

In a study conducted at a university hospital rheumatology clinic in the United States, 94% of patients interviewed reported that they have used CAM or visited a CAM practitioner. In 1992 Visser et al[1] reported that from 68% to 94% of patients with rheumatoid arthritis surveyed had used alternative methods of treatment at least once. The percentage of patients who had ever visited an alternative practitioner for rheumatic disease ranged from 25% to 54%. More recently Rao et al[2] found in a telephone survey conducted at three university and three private rheumatology practices that approximately two thirds of respondents had used CAM. Of the respondents, 56% currently used CAM and 90% regularly used CAM or had done so in the past.

With chronic musculoskeletal conditions being a leading indication for the use of CAM, clinicians who routinely treat patients with rheumatic disease must become proficient at talking with patients and advising them about the use or avoidance or various CAM therapies.

# OSTEOARTHRITIS

Osteoarthritis (OA) is the most common form of arthritis and the second most common cause of long-term disability among adults in the United States. OA is a complex disease affecting millions of people and is without a known cure. Although multiple risk factors such as history of trauma, inflammatory arthritis, genetics, diet, estrogen use, and some metabolic disorders are associated with the development of OA, the most prevalent risk factor in the United States is obesity.

The pathophysiology of OA is not fully understood; however, it involves degeneration of bone and soft tissue structure in and around the joint, including synovium, ligaments, and bridging muscles. Current conventional management of patients with OA involves nonpharmacological, pharmacological, and surgical therapies. However, despite recent advances, the mainstay of management of the patient with OA remains control of pain and improvement in function, as well as health-related quality of life with avoidance of therapeutic toxicity if possible. The less than optimum response to available therapies and common intolerance to or toxicity from available medications often lead to frustration on the part of both patients and clinicians. This frustration has led to a growing interest in various CAM therapies as an adjunct to conventional care in the management of patients with OA.

## Complementary and Alternative Treatments

### Glucosamine and Chondroitin Sulfate

Two popular dietary supplements used for the treatment of OA and often sold in combination are glucosamine and chondroitin sulfate. Glucosamine sulfate is the sulfate derivative of the monosaccharide glucosamine. Glucosamine is the principle component of glycosaminoglycans in cartilage matrix and synovial fluids. Chondroitin sulfate is also a glycosaminoglycan and is required for the formation of proteoglycans in cartilage.

What is particularly intriguing about glucosamine and chondroitin sulfate is that unlike nonsteroidal antiinflammatory drugs (NSAIDs), which are symptom modifying, glucosamine and chondroitin are potentially structure-modifying drugs. Thus these compounds might alter joint structure favorably and interfere with the progression of disease. This is contrary to what has been observed with some NSAIDs, which have been shown to worsen disease progression. Glucosamine and chondroitin sulfate may enable the syntheses of glycosaminoglycans to keep up with the rate of degeneration that accrues in OA, thus allowing increased amounts of healthy cartilage matrix to form. Numerous short- to medium-term clinical trials have evaluated glucosamine and chondroitin sulfate, many of which have demonstrated favorable effects. A recent meta-analysis of 15 double-blind randomized placebo-controlled trials found a moderate to large effect on OA symptoms; however, methodological problems may have lead to exaggerated estimates of benefit. In a recent long-term study, administration of glucosamine sulfate over 3 years was shown to prevent joint structure changes in patients with OA of the knee and to lead to significant improvement in symptoms.

Glucosamine and chondroitin sulfate are sold as dietary supplements in most health and nutrition stores, as well as pharmacies. The recommended dosage for glucosamine is 500 mg 3 times daily, and the usual dosage of chondroitin is 400 mg 3 times daily. Both glucosamine and chondroitin sulfate are well tolerated, although occasional side effects such as dyspepsia, nausea, or headache have being reported. There are currently no reported drug interactions.

Glucosamine and chondroitin sulfate are often sold in combination; however, it is unclear whether the combination is superior to either treatment alone. In December 1999 and January 2000, consumerlab.com purchased 25 brands of glucosamine sulfate, chondroitin sulfate, and glucosamine/chondroitin combination products to test whether the products contained the amounts listed on their respective labels. It was found that almost 33% of the products did not contain the stated amount.

### S-Adenosyl-L-Methionine

S-Adenosyl-L-Methionine (SAM-e) is a physiological molecule formed in the body from the essential amino acid methionine. It is metabolized from protein-rich food in combination with adenosine triphosphate

(ATP). SAM-e was approved for sale as a dietary supplement in 1999 by the U.S. Food and Drug Administration; however, it has been in use since the mid-1970s, primarily in Europe, to treat depression and arthritis.

SAM-e was first observed to have beneficial effects on OA while it was being used to treat patients for mood disorders. Since that time, multiple randomized controlled trials (RCTs) suggest that SAM-e may be an effective treatment for OA. In a randomized double-blind study, 36 patients with OA of the knee, hip, and/or spine received 1,200 mg/day of SAM-e or 1,200 mg/day of ibuprofen for 4 weeks. Clinical parameters such as morning stiffness, pain at rest, pain on motion, crepitus, swelling, and limitation of affected joints showed similar improvement in both treatment groups. Both treatments were well tolerated, with no patients withdrawing from the study. In a large, long-term open trial, 108 patients with OA of the knee, hip, and spine were started on 600 mg/day of SAM-e for 2 weeks, followed by 400 mg/day for 2 years. Morning stiffness and pain parameters were noted to have improved after the first week of treatment and this continued to the end of the 2-year period. Although the mechanism of action of SAM-e in OA is not fully understood, it may be related to the ability of SAM-e to stimulate proteoglycan synthesis in OA cartilage by increasing levels of ATP. The optimal dosage for SAM-e has not being determined. Oral doses used in human study on SAM-e and OA have ranged from 400 to 1,600 mg/day, with very few adverse affects. The Arthritis Foundation's *Guide to Alternative Therapies* notes that although SAM-e is a promising treatment worth trying for pain relief, more scientific evidence is needed to prove it supports cartilage repair.

## Methyl Sulfonyl Methane

Methyl sulfonyl methane (MSM) is a dietary supplement commonly sold for the treatment of OA. The MSM metabolite dimethyl sulfoxide is found naturally in the human body. Sulfur is necessary for the formation of connective tissue; therefore MSM is thought to be useful in the treatment of OA because it can function as a sulfur donor. Animal studies have suggested that MSM may help decrease inflammatory joint disease. Unfortunately there are no published human trials. Although MSM is promoted as being nontoxic, clinical data are lacking and further scientific study is needed to define the efficacy and safety of this supplement.

## Acupuncture

Acupuncture may be beneficial for the treatment of various rheumatological conditions, including OA. Acupuncture is a component of Traditional Chinese Medicine (TCM), which dates back at least 2,500 years. Acupuncture is based on identifying certain patterns of signs and symptoms that reflect an imbalance in or disharmony of internal organs or chi energy, leading to disease. Acupuncture practitioners seek to correct the imbalance through the superficial insertion of sterile disposable needles at specific points throughout the body.

Although no direct relationship between acupuncture and biological structure has been found, studies indicate that acupuncture points are physiologically unique areas of the body. Investigations employing contemporary Western scientific method have sought to determine whether the magnitude of the analgesic effect of acupuncture may be mediated through neurohormonal, spinal cord, midbrain, or other pathways. Acupuncture analgesia is believed to work through the release of endorphins, which has been demonstrated by both animal and human studies. Specifically, acupuncture stimulates the release of beta-endorphins into the cerebrospinal fluid, and its analgesic effect can be reversed by naloxone and antiserum against endorphins.[3] High-frequency acupuncture stimulation can activate the release of monoamines, serotonin, and norepinephrine.[4]

Numerous randomized controlled trials have been undertaken to assess the efficacy of acupuncture for OA. Although many trials have found significant improvement in pain and functional outcome measures compared with sham acupuncture or standard care, the effectiveness of acupuncture for OA has not been proven. A recent systematic review of 11 RCTs of acupuncture for OA concluded that the most rigorously conducted studies suggest that acupuncture is not superior to sham needling in reducing pain from OA; however, future studies are needed. A 1997 National Institutes of Health (NIH) consensus panel concluded that acupuncture may be useful for OA and other rheumatological conditions such as low back and carpal tunnel syndrome. The panel also concluded that acupuncture is safe compared with many standard therapies.

Acupuncture may serve as a good adjunct to a conventional medical regimen by allowing a reduction in NSAID dosage, therefore potentially decreasing side effects occasionally seen with long-term NSAID use.

Each state has its own requirements for acupuncture licensure and certification. Patients should be referred only to a licensed or certified practitioner. The National Certification Commission for Acupuncture and Oriental Medicine publishes a directory of practitioners (www.nccaom.org). For chronic painful conditions, acupuncture often requires four or more treatments before efficacy can truly be assessed. Although acupuncture is generally safe and adverse reactions are uncommon, transient dizziness, temporary exacerbation of pain, occasional bruising, or rare swelling may occur.

At the Siegler Center for Integrative Medicine at Saint Barnabas Medical Center in Livingston, New Jersey, we have treated a number of patients with OA. By combining exercise at our wellness center with acupuncture and appropriate dietary supplement use (most commonly glucosamine and chondroitin sulfate), many patients have noted decreased pain and improved quality of life. Medical centers across the country either have or are currently developing CAM centers to provide these services.

# FIBROMYALGIA

Fibromyalgia is a chronic, noninflammatory syndrome of widespread pain and tenderness that affects between 1% and 4% of the population in primarily industrialized nations.[5] Women are 1.5 times more likely than men to be diagnosed with fibromyalgia. Commonly associated symptoms include depression, fatigue, sleep disturbances, and headache. Fibromyalgia belongs to a spectrum of overlapping conditions that share as their common feature pain (widespread or regional), fatigue, and organ dysfunction. These conditions include chronic fatigue syndrome, migraine headaches, irritable bowel syndrome, and mitral valve prolapse syndrome.

The American College of Rheumatology (ACR) criteria for the diagnosis of fibromyalgia includes a history of widespread pain in all four quadrants of the body plus the axial skeleton and the presence of 11 of 18 tender points on examination.[6] Only about half of the patients diagnosed with fibromyalgia in clinical practice meet the ACR criteria; the rest of patients often have more localized pain. Regional myofascial disorder is diagnosed when the patient's pain is confined to one quadrant of the body.

Fibromyalgia is a generalized disturbance of sensory processing in the central nervous system.[7] Genetic causes and environmental stressors including trauma, viral infection, and autoimmune and endocrine disorders have been identified as possible triggers of this condition. Elevated substance P and decreased serotonin and norepinephrine metabolites in the cerebrospinal fluid have been found,[8] and there are abnormalities in the pain processing areas of the brain on photon emission testing.[9] A nonrestorative sleep disorder associated with alpha-EEG sleep anomalies has also been described.[10]

Conventional medical therapy for fibromyalgia includes medications, exercise, and behavioral therapy. Tricyclic agents such as amitriptyline can be used to treat both the pain and sleep disturbances. Other antidepressive agents such as selective serotonin reuptake inhibitors (SSRIs) are also used. Low-dose NSAIDs, acetaminophen, and tramadol may be of benefit. An aerobic exercise program is integral to treatment. Treatment goals are directed toward physical tolerance and long-term compliance. The exercise program should also be low-impact (e.g., stationary bike, walking, aquatic exercises).

## Complementary and Alternative Treatments

### Cognitive Behavioral Therapy

Cognitive behavioral therapy (CBT) is often discussed as both a conventional and a CAM treatment, generally considered a part of mind-body medicine. Regardless of its category, it is beneficial in the multidisciplinary approach to the fibromyalgia patient, improving both pain and mood symptoms. CBT teaches patients new thought and behavior patterns for coping with chronic illness. Techniques used in CBT include goal setting, guided imagery, relaxation training, appropriate scheduling, and problem solving.

Nielson et al[11] conducted an uncontrolled study of 30 fibromyalgia patients who underwent a 3-week program of CBT. The CBT techniques were combined with exercise, physical therapy, biofeedback, and relaxation training. There were significant improvements in pain, affective distress, and dysfunction, which were maintained up to 30 months after treatment. Another study evaluated an eight-session program of CBT (meditation and qigong) for 20 fibromyalgia patients and found significant reductions in pain, anxiety, and depression, all maintained at 6-month follow-up.[12]

When counseling a patient about CBT, let the patient know that treatment takes time and commitment and that some of the techniques may be learned in a private setting while others may be learned in a group setting. CBT should be part of a comprehensive management program.

## Biofeedback

Another mind-body therapy that has been studied in fibromyalgia is biofeedback. One study of 119 fibromyalgia subjects studied biofeedback/relaxation training in comparison to exercise, combination treatment, and education/attention control.[13] All three treatment groups showed improvement in function compared with the control group. Smaller controlled studies of electromyographic (EMG) biofeedback also had positive results.[13,15]

As mentioned with CBT, biofeedback requires time and patience to learn properly. It should be combined with other mind/body techniques and conventional management. There are no side effects to biofeedback, and once learned it can be practiced independently by the patient.

## Acupuncture

Among CAM therapies, acupuncture is commonly used by fibromyalgia patients. As mentioned earlier, acupuncture is a method of stimulating specific points on the body surface with fine needles to treat various medical conditions. Commonly electroacupuncture—acupuncture with electrical stimulation—is used to enhance results. In TCM, acupuncture is one modality of many treatments that include the use of Chinese herbs, moxibustion (the burning of the dried herb *Artemisia vulgaris*), and massage therapy. Through its long history of migration from China to the rest of Asia, Europe, and North America, acupuncture has evolved into several different systems. These distinct forms of acupuncture include traditional Chinese, Japanese, Korean, and French acupuncture.

The clinical studies of acupuncture on fibromyalgia have been largely positive, but most of these trials were small, were uncontrolled, or had other methodological limitations. One methodologically rigorous RCT compared a 3-week program of electroacupuncture with a sham control in 70 fibromyalgia patients.[16] Statistically significant improvements in visual analog pain scores, pain threshold, analgesic tablet use, sleep quality, and global assessment scores occurred in the acupuncture group. Similarly, a NIH consensus development panel concluded that acupuncture may be a useful adjunctive or alternative treatment or may be part of a comprehensive management program for fibromyalgia.[17]

The standard course of acupuncture treatment for a chronic pain condition is twice a week for 4 to 6 weeks.[18] Typically one treatment lasts 20 minutes. If by 3 to 4 weeks no appreciable improvement is noted, the patient should consider discontinuing treatment. Possible side effects include local bruising, aching, and skin rash.[18] Older patients may feel lightheaded afterward, and some experience nausea. Very few serious side effects, such as internal organ or nerve injury, have been reported.[19] Patients with bleeding disorders or on anticoagulant medications have a higher risk of bleeding, and, while this is not an absolute contraindication to acupuncture, these patients may be advised to try noninvasive treatments. Patients with cardiac pacemakers, cardiac arrhythmias, or epilepsy should not receive electroacupuncture.[17] Pregnant patients should avoid acupuncture in the abdominal, pelvic, and lumbosacral areas.[18]

Of note: Some studies showed worsening of fibromyalgia after acupuncture.[20] Because of the heightened pain state in the condition, fibromyalgia patients may also be more reluctant to be needled. In such cases, it may be prudent to avoid electrical stimulation of the needles in sensitive patients, particularly in the beginning. The potential for exacerbation of symptoms should be included in counseling the fibromyalgia patient about acupuncture.

## Massage

There are many different forms of massage: acupressure, rolfing, neuromuscular massage, myofascial release, soft tissue massage, deep tissue massage, and Swedish massage. Swedish massage emphasizes the physical manipulation of muscles and joints to improve function. The Asian forms of massage, such as acupressure, concentrate on promoting the flow of vital energy.

There is very little literature on the role of massage therapy for fibromyalgia. A small controlled trial randomized 23 fibromyalgia patients to connective tissue massage and 25 patients to a control group.[21] Massage was found to reduce pain, depression, and analgesic use and to improve quality of life.

If your fibromyalgia patient is interested in massage, recommend the gentler forms of massage because he or she is probably pain sensitive. Also, have your patient avoid the more vigorous therapies such as deep tissue massage if he or she has metastatic cancer, hypertension, varicose veins, or phlebitis or is pregnant.[22]

# RHEUMATOID ARTHRITIS

Rheumatoid arthritis (RA) is a chronic autoimmune inflammatory disorder that affects primarily the joints but that may be extraarticular as well. RA has a prevalence of 1% of the population, typically affecting women, with a female-to-male ratio of 3:1.[23] This ratio becomes more equal between the sexes when the onset of disease is later in life. Most commonly RA strikes persons in their fifth to seventh decades of life.

RA classically presents as an inflammatory, symmetrical polyarthritis of the proximal small joints of the hands, feet, elbows, knees, shoulders, and ankles. Bursitis, tenosynovitis, and cervical spine disease are also common. Acutely affected joints are erythematous, painful, swollen, and warm to the touch. Ongoing inflammation leads to deformities such as ulnar deviation at the wrists, boutonnière and swan neck deformities, and restricted range of motion (ROM).

Systemic features of RA include morning stiffness, fatigue, serositis, vasculitis, and subcutaneous nodules. Ocular, cardiac, pulmonary, and hematological involvement may occur. These extraarticular manifestations signal a worse disease prognosis. Laboratory studies detect rheumatoid factor in up to 80% of patients with RA. Other markers of inflammation, such as an erythrocyte sedimentation rate (ESR) and C-reactive protein (CRP), are often elevated during disease activity. Radiographically, soft tissue swelling, periarticular osteopenia bony erosions, and joint deformities reflect the chronic inflammatory nature of the disease.

Conventional treatments for RA are tailored to the severity of disease presentation. Treatment goals are to control the inflammation, prevent joint damage, relieve symptoms, and restore function. In milder cases, these goals may be accomplished by physical therapy, education, and use of NSAIDs and disease-modifying agents such as hydroxychloroquine or Azulfidine. More severe presentations often require adding methotrexate, systemic corticosteroids, and/or anti-tumor necrosis factor (TNF) agents. Cyclophospha-mide is reserved for the most serious or refractory cases. Treatment may sometimes be limited by adverse effects because NSAIDs are associated with an increased risk of gastrointestinal (GI), renal, central nervous system, and cardiovascular complications. The primary side effect resulting from the use of corticosteroids and immunosuppressive medications is infection. Methotrexate may result in liver disease, and cyclophosphamide can cause hemorrhagic cystitis.

## Complementary and Alternative Therapies

### Acupuncture

The data on acupuncture for the treatment of rheumatoid arthritis have been largely derived from uncontrolled studies reporting positive results. One small placebo-controlled RCT treated 10 patients with RA who had symmetrical knee arthritis. One knee was given true acupuncture and the other knee sham acupuncture. There was significant pain reduction in the knee treated with true acupuncture, which lasted on average 1 to 3 months, compared with the knee treated with sham acupuncture, which had less than 10 hours of pain relief.[24]

If a patient is interested in acupuncture for RA, he or she should receive the same counseling about the standard course of treatment and adverse effects as described for OA and fibromyalgia. Because a RA patient may be on prednisone and other treatments that suppress immunity and thin the blood, careful technique is mandatory.

### Overall Nutrition

There has been a longstanding interest in the possible relationship between diet and RA. The data, however, have not been consistent in showing that a specific diet, fasting, vitamins, or minerals can benefit RA. Currently there is no proven role for these dietary modifications in the management of RA. However, several promising studies on dietary supplements for RA are reviewed next. These studies warrant further research; however, if your patients are interested, the dietary supplements that follow are probably safe to try in the context of a balanced diet.

### Fish Oil

Fish oil supplementation has been fairly well studied in RA. Coldwater fish such as salmon, mackerel, and herring are rich in omega-3 polyunsaturated fatty acids. The omega-3 polyunsaturated fatty acids, among other lipids, are incorporated into cell membranes and suppress arachidonic acid–derived prostaglandin and leukotriene synthesis. Animal studies showed that omega-3 fatty acid–rich fish oil and vitamin E lowered cytokine levels in a mouse model for RA, including IL-6, IL-10 and TNF-alpha.[25]

A small, uncontrolled study of 39 RA patients described decreased levels of eicosapentaenoic acid and total n-3 polyunsaturated fatty acids in the plasma and synovial fluid, respectively, compared with control subjects.[26] Another study examined the effects of gammalinolenic acid, another omega-3 fatty acid, on IL-1 and TNF in both in vitro and in vivo studies of RA patients. They found that the secretion of both cytokines was reduced compared with the control group, which received safflower oil.

A number of RCTs have been conducted on fish oil supplementation for RA.[27] Most studies examine eicosapentaenoic acid (EPA) and docosahexaenoic acid (DHA), both omega-3 fatty acids. These studies show consistent evidence that dietary n-3 fatty acids supplied as fish oil can provide at least modest benefit for RA, reducing joint pain, stiffness, and occasionally swelling.[28-30] Plant seed oils such as evening primrose oil, borage, and flaxseed oil also contain omega fatty acids and have been studied, with variable results.[31,32]

If your patient is interested in fish oil supplements, the usual dose is 3,000 mg total of EPA/DHA.[33] The patient should be cautioned about GI side effects such as nausea, dyspepsia, and diarrhea. Blood-thinning effects are also a concern, particularly if the patient is on NSAIDs. Because these supplements are unregulated products, patients should be counseled about variation in product quality. Increasing dietary intake of salmon, mackerel, herring, anchovies, and lake trout is another option.

### Vitamins

Several vitamins have been suggested as having potential analgesic and immunomodulatory effects in RA. The vitamin D analog, alphacalcidiol, was studied in a small, uncontrolled open-label trial for the treatment of acute RA.[34] Of the patients who received 2 μg/day of oral alphacalcidiol, 89% had either complete remission or satisfactory improvement defined by ESR, CRP, morning stiffness, Richie index, and Lee index. No side effects were observed.

Vitamin D or calciferol is found in cod liver oil, salmon, mackerel, eel, and fortified foods such as milk. Sunlight exposure is another important source of vitamin D. No published clinical trials on vitamin D as a treatment for RA have been conducted. The adequate intake (AI) of vitamin D recommended for healthy adults ranges from 200 to 600 international units (IU) daily. High-dose vitamin D above 2,000 IU daily may increase the risk of adverse effects such as nausea, vomiting, anorexia, constipation, and weight loss. It can also elevate calcium levels, which may in turn cause cardiac arrhythmias.

Vitamin E, an antioxidant vitamin, has been studied in RA. A randomized trial in Germany compared vitamin E 400 mg 3 times daily to diclofenac for chronic RA.[35] There were similar improvements in grip strength, Richie index, and pain after 3 weeks of treatment in both groups. Vitamin E was also studied in a placebo-controlled double-blinded trial in which RA patients were given 600 mg twice daily of vitamin E or placebo for 12 weeks.[36] Pain measures decreased significantly in the vitamin E treatment group, but measures of inflammation and oxidative modification of proteins and lipids did not.

Patients who take vitamin E supplements should be made aware of the blood-thinning effects of vitamin E, particularly if they are on concomitant therapy with aspirin and/or NSAIDs. While there is no recommended daily allowance (RDA) for vitamin E, its upper tolerable intake level has been set at 1,000 mg (1,500 IU) by the Institute of Medicine. Dietary sources of vitamin E include vegetable oils, nuts, and leafy green vegetables.

## CHRONIC LOW BACK PAIN

Chronic low back pain (CLBP) is a prevalent disorder causing significant disability and economic burden for the nation.[37] Of the general population, 80% experience back pain at some point, with onset most often between the ages of 30 and 50 years. The majority of cases resolve spontaneously. However, up to 10% of back pain sufferers continue to suffer from low back pain for longer than 3 months and are classified as CLBP sufferers.

CLBP encompasses a wide spectrum of etiologies and presentations of back pain. It is often helpful to classify back pain as resulting from mechanical, nonmechanical, or visceral etiologies.[9] The vast majority of back pain (97% of cases seen in the primary care setting) results from mechanical causes such as lumbar strain or sprain, degenerative disease of the disks and facet joints, herniated disk, compression fractures, or spinal stenosis. Nonmechanical conditions such as tumor, infection, or inflammatory disease cause back pain in about 1% of patients. Referred pain from visceral disease of the pelvic organs or kidneys or aortic aneurysm make up the remaining 2% of cases. The diagnostic evaluation therefore is directed toward identifying risk factors (heavy lifting or obesity), systemic symptoms, or neurological compromise (sciatica or pseudoclaudication).

Conventional treatments for mechanical back pain include avoidance of heavy lifting and other exacerbating activities, weight loss, and exercises to strengthen the lower back and abdominal muscles.[11] Analgesic agents, NSAIDs, and muscle relaxants are most commonly prescribed. If there is a herniated disk or spinal stenosis, epidural steroid injections may offer temporary relief. Lumbar diskectomy, decompressive laminectomy, and spinal fusion are reserved for pain that is refractory to conservative management or the occurrence of neurological complications.

# Complementary and Alternative Treatments

## Spinal Manipulation

Manipulation and manual medicine can be categorized into high-velocity and low-force therapies. Of the two, chiropractors are more likely to practice high-velocity therapy. The premise behind manipulation therapies is that injury and inflammation to a joint can cause an increase in muscle tone and joint immobilization for protection against further injury.[38] The limitation in ROM may continue beyond the acute injury period, and pain afferents become sensitized by joint movement. Manipulation of a joint may increase the ROM and decrease pain through a reflexive relaxation mechanism. Similarly, ligamentous injury leading to muscle spasm may also be treated by manipulation, which can cause reflex relaxation of the muscle.[39] For back pain, adjusting of the lumbar spine to open the space between zygapophysial joints also has been performed and evaluated by MRI studies.[40]

Several systematic reviews on the efficacy of spinal manipulation for back pain have found varying results. The most recent review examined eight RCTs on low back pain in which subjects were treated by chiropractors.[41] The reviewers found that all RCTs were limited by methodological flaws and therefore their results did not provide convincing evidence for the effectiveness of chiropractic treatment for acute or chronic low back pain. An earlier review by the same authors assessed 35 RCTs, comparing spinal manipulation with other treatments for the treatment of back and neck pain.[42] Their conclusion was similar, stating that although there were some promising results, the efficacy of manipulation was not convincingly shown. A third review studied 21 RCTs of manipulative therapy for low back pain. The conclusion was that there was some indication that manipulative therapy had short-term results. Long-term effects of the treatment were not adequately evaluated.[43]

No systematic reports on the rate of serious complications of spinal manipulation such as cauda equina syndrome and death have been conducted in the United Sates. However, there have been case reports, which probably underestimate the true incidence of adverse events. Based on these reports, the rate of occurrence of cauda equina syndrome is about 1 case per 100 million manipulations.[44]

If your patient is interested in spinal manipulation for relief of back pain, he or she should be told to expect more frequent in-office interventions, ranging from 2 to 5 sessions per week for the first 1 to 2 weeks. Decreasing frequency of visits should follow. For chronic disorders, repeated use of passive care should be avoided so that the patient's own sense of responsibility for his or her health is not diminished. Contraindications to high-velocity thrust procedures include acute RA flare, acute fracture or dislocation, malignancy, bone or joint infection, spondylolisthesis with progressive slippage, and bleeding disorders.[45]

## Acupuncture

Low back pain is one of the most common conditions for which acupuncture is used. The NIH consensus panel of 1997 concluded that acupuncture is an acceptable treatment for low back pain. As mentioned earlier, acupuncture analgesia is believed to work through the release of endorphins.

The literature on acupuncture for the treatment of CLBP has yielded conflicting results. Two systematic reviews have reached similar conclusions. Ernst and White[46] analyzed 12 RCTs of acupuncture for back pain. The odds ratio of improvement with acupuncture compared with control interventions was 2.30 (95% confidence intervals 1.28 to 4.13). For sham-controlled studies, the odds ratio was 1.37 (95% confidence interval 0.84 to 2.25). They concluded that acupuncture was superior to various control interventions but that there was insufficient evidence to state whether it was superior to placebo. A systematic review in the same year analyzed 11 RCTs for back pain. Because the overall methodological quality of these studies was judged to be low, the results of the trials were inconclusive.[47]

Counseling a patient with CLBP about acupuncture is the same as that described for spinal manipulation. A trial of 4 to 6 weeks of biweekly treatments is commonly prescribed.

### Massage

Most of the literature on massage has focused on back pain. A systematic review examined 4 RCTs that compared massage therapy as a monotherapy for back pain with various control interventions.[48] All trials were judged to have major methodological flaws. The massage therapies included light effleurage, soft tissue, or underwater massage 2 to 3 times per week. Massage therapy was found to be as effective as spinal manipulation, transcutaneous electric nerve stimulation (TENS), or no treatment. One trial found massage therapy to be less effective than spinal manipulation immediately after therapy.

Counseling your patient with CLBP about massage is similar to that described for fibromyalgia. Patients with RA, ankylosing spondylitis, or osteoporosis should be advised to avoid the more vigorous therapies such as deep tissue massage. Massage should be avoided if the joints are inflamed or infection is present. Broken skin should not be massaged.

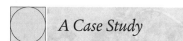

### A Case Study

#### Chronic Low Back Pain

M.W. is a 54-year-old male with a history of hypertension, peptic ulcer disease, and CLBP and knee pain secondary to OA. He complained of frequent pain and early morning stiffness in his lower back and bilateral knees. He had tried multiple NSAIDs in the past; however, he was unable to tolerate them secondary to GI discomfort. He currently takes Tylenol prn, and exercises 3 times per week. He has felt that he is significantly limited secondary to pain.

M.W. was encouraged to maintain his exercise program and was started on glucosamine 500 mg twice daily with chondroitin sulfate 400 mg twice daily in combination, in addition to a trial of eight acupuncture treatments. He returned for follow-up in 8 weeks noting significant subjective improvement in pain and function. ∾

## SUMMARY

Rheumatological disorders are among the leading reasons for the use of CAM therapies. OA, RA, fibromyalgia, and CLBP are chronic conditions associated with pain and disability. Conventional management may not offer adequate pain relief, leading patients to seek CAM options. The most commonly used CAM therapies, including their efficacy, safety, and recommendations, have been reviewed in this chapter. Acupuncture, mind-body techniques, massage therapy, and dietary modifications and/or supplements may have a role in the management of rheumatological disorders; however, it is important that patients seek treatment from qualified providers, that an adequate trial of treatment is undertaken, and that these therapies are part of a comprehensive management program. For many of these CAM therapies, more research studies evaluating the mechanism, long-term efficacy, and safety are needed.

## References

1. Visser GJ, Peters L, Rasker JJ: Rheumatologists and their patients who seek alternative care, *Br J Rheumatol* 31:485-490, 1992.
2. Rao JK, Mihaliak K, Kroenke K: Use of complementary therapies for arthritis among patients of rheumatologists, *Ann Intern Med* 131:409-416, 1999.
3. Ulett G, Han S, Han J: Electroacupuncture: mechanisms and clinical application, *Biol Psychiatry* 44(2):129-138, 1998.
4. Takeshige C, Sato T, Mera T, et al: Descending pain inhibitory system involved in acupuncture analgesia, *Brain Res Bull* 29(5):617-634, 1992.
5. Clauw D: Fibromyalgia syndrome: an update on current understanding and medical management, *Rheumatol Grand Rounds* 3(4):1-8, 2000.
6. Wolfe F, Smythe HA, Yunus MB, et al: The ACR 1990 criteria for the classification of fibromyalgia report of the multicenter criteria committee. *Arthritis Rheum* 33:160, 1993.

7. Yunus MB: Towards a model of pathophysiology of fibromyalgia, aberrant central pain mechanisms with peripheral modulation. *J Rheumatol* 19:846, 1993.

8. Russell IJ, Orr MD, Littman B, Vipraio G, et al: Elevated cerebrospinal fluid levels of substance P in patients with the fibromyalgia syndrome, *Arthritis Rheum* 37:1593, 1994.

9. Mountz J, Bradley L, Modell J, et al: Fibromyalgia in women: abnormalities of regional cerebral blood flow in the thalamus and the caudate nucleus are associated with low pain thresholds, *Arthritis Rheum* 38:926-938, 1995.

10. Dauvilliers Y, Touchon J: Sleep in fibromyalgia: review of clinical and polysomnographic data, *Neurophysiol Clin* 31(1):18-33, 2001.

11. Nielson WR, Walker C, McCain G: Cognitive behavioral treatment of fibromyalgia syndrome: preliminary findings, *J Rheumatol* 19:98-103, 1992.

12. Creamer P, Singh B, Berman B, et al: Evidence of sustained improvement from a mind-body intervention in patients with fibromyalgia (FM). Abstract presented at the American College of Rheumatology 62nd Annual Scientific Meeting, San Diego, Calif, Nov 1998.

13. Buchelew SP, Conway R, Parker J, et al: Biofeedback/relaxation training and exercise interventions for fibromyalgia: a prospective trial, *Arthritis Care Res* 11(3):196-209, 1998.

14. Ferraccioli G, Ghirelli L, Scita F, et al: EMG-biofeedback training in fibromyalgia syndrome, *J Rheumatol* 14(4):820-825, 1987.

15. Sarnoch H, Adler F, Scholz OB: Relevance of muscular sensitivity, muscular activity and cognitive variables for pain reduction associated with EMG biofeedback in fibromyalgia, *Percept Mot Skills* 84(3):1043-1050, 1997.

16. Deluze C, Bosia L, Zirbs A, et al: Electroacupuncture in fibromyalgia: results of a controlled trial, *BMJ* 305:1249-1252, 1992.

17. NIH Consensus Conference: Acupuncture, *JAMA* 280(17):1518-1524, 1998.

18. Stux G, Pomeranz B: *Acupuncture: a textbook and atlas,* Berlin, Germany, 1987, Springer-Verlag.

19. Ernst E, White A: Life-threatening adverse reactions after acupuncture? a systematic review, *Pain* 71:123-126, 1997.

20. Waylonis GW: Long-term follow-up on patients with fibrositis treated with acupuncture, *Ohio State Med J* 73:299-302, 1977.

21. Brattberg G: Connective tissue massage in the treatment of fibromyalgia, *Eur J Pain* 3(3):235-244, 1999.

22. Horstman J: *The Arthritis Foundation's guide to alternative therapies,* Atlanta, 1999, Arthritis Foundation.

23. Goronzy J, Weyand C: Rheumatoid arthritis: epidemiology, pathology and pathogenesis. In Klippel J (ed): *Primer on the rheumatic diseases,* ed 11, Atlanta, 1997, Arthritis Foundation.

24. David J, Townsend S, Sathanathan R, et al: The effect of acupuncture on patients with rheumatoid arthritis: a randomized, placebo-controlled cross-over study, *Rheumatology* (Oxford) 38(9):864-869, 1999.

25. Venkatraman JT, Chu WC: Effects of dietary omega-3 and omega-6 lipids and vitamin E on serum cytokines, lipid mediators and anti-DNA antibodies in a mouse model for rheumatoid arthritis, *J Am Coll Nutr* 18(6):602-613, 1999.

26. Navarro E, Esteve M, Olive A, et al: Abnormal fatty acid pattern in rheumatoid arthritis: a rationale for treatment with marine and botanical lipids, *J Rheumatol* 27(2):298-303, 2000.

27. James MJ, Cleland LG: Dietary n-3 fatty acids and therapy for rheumatoid arthritis, *Semin Arthritis Rheum* 27(2):85-97, 1997.

28. Kremer JM, Jubiz W, Rynes RI, et al: Fish-oil fatty supplementation in patients with active rheumatoid arthritis, a double-blind controlled crossover study, *Ann Intern Med* 106:797-803, 1987.

29. Geusens P, Wouters C, Nijs J, et al: Long term effect of omega-3 fatty acid supplementation in active rheumatoid arthritis, *Arthritis Rheum* 37:824-829, 1994.

30. Skoldstam L, Borjesson O, Kjallman A, et al: Effect of six months of fish oil supplementation in stable rheumatoid arthritis, a double-blind controlled study, *Scand J Rheumatol* 21:178-185, 1992.

31. Brzeski M, Madhok R, Capell H: Preliminary report: evening primrose oil in patients with rheumatoid arthritis and side-effects of non-steroidal anti-inflammatory drugs, *Br J Rheumatol* 30:370-372, 1991.

32. Gemmell HA, Jacobson B: Effectiveness of flaxseed oil in the symptomatic treatment of rheumatoid arthritis: a single subject design, *Am J Clin Med* pp 151-154, 1989.

33. Horstman J: *The Arthritis Foundation's guide to alternative therapies,* Atlanta, 1999, Arthritis Foundation.

34. Andjelkovic Z, Vojinovic J, Pejnovic N, et al: Disease modifying and immunomodulatory effects of high dose 1 alpha (OH) D3 in rheumatoid arthritis patients, *Clin Exper Rheumatol* 17(4):453-456, 1999.

35. Wittenborg A, Petersen G, Lorkowski G, et al: Effectiveness of vitamin E in comparison with diclofenac sodium in the treatment of patients with chronic polyarthritis, *Z Rheumatol* 57(4):215-221, 1998.

36. Edmonds SE, Winyard PG, Guo R, et al: Putative analgesic activity of repeated oral doses of vitamin E in the treatment of rheumatoid arthritis: results of a prospective placebo controlled double blind trial, *Ann Rheum Dis* 56(11):649-655, 1997.

37. Deyo R, Weinstein J: Low back pain, *N Engl J Med* 344(5):363-370, 2001.

38. Fiechtner JJ, Brodeur RR: Manual and manipulation techniques for rheumatic disease: complementary and alternative therapies for rheumatic diseases, *Rheum Dis Clin North Am* 26(1):83-96, 2000.

39. Solomonow M, Zhou B, Harris M: The ligamento-muscular stabilizing system of the spine, *Spine* 23:2552-2562, 1988.

40. Cramer GD, Tuck NR, Knudsen JT, et al: Effects of side-posture positioning and side-posture adjusting on the lumbar zygapophysial joints as evaluated by magnetic resonance imaging: a before and after study with randomization, *J Manipulative Physiol Ther* 23(6):380-394, 2000.

41. Assendelft WJ, Koes BW, van der Heijden GJ, et al: The effectiveness of chiropractic for treatment of low back pain: an update and attempt at statistical pooling, *J Manipulative Physiol Ther* 19(8):499-507, 1996.

42. Koes BW, Assendelft WJ, van der Heijden GJ, et al: Spinal manipulation and mobilisation for back and neck pain: a blinded review, *BMJ* 303(6813):1298-303, 1991.

43. Abenhaim L, Bergeron AM: Twenty years of randomized clinical trials of manipulative therapy for back pain: a review, *Clin Invest Med* 15(6):527-535, 1992.

44. Shekelle PG, Adams AH, Chassin MR, et al: Spinal manipulation for low back pain, *Ann Int Med* 117(7):590-598, 1992.

45. Haldeman S, Rubinstein SM: The precipitation or aggravation of musculoskeletal pain in patients receiving spinal manipulative therapy, *J Manipulative Physiol Ther* 16(1):47-50, 1993.

46. Ernst E, White A: Acupuncture for back pain: a meta-analysis of randomized, controlled trials, *Arch Int Med* 158:2235-2241, 1998.

47. Van Tulder M, Cherkin D, Berman B, et al: The effectiveness of acupuncture in the management of acute and chronic low back pain, *Spine* 24(11):1113-1123, 1999.

48. Ernst E: Massage therapy for low back pain: a systematic review, *J Pain Symptom Manage* 17(1):65-69, 1999.

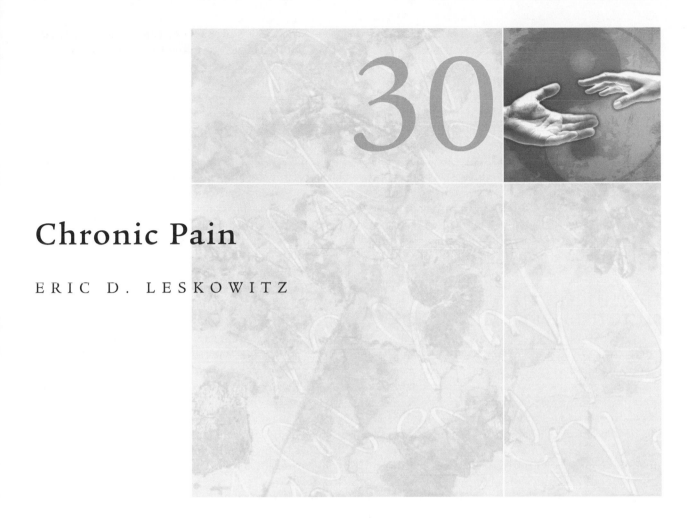

# Chronic Pain

ERIC D. LESKOWITZ

$\mathcal{P}$ain is the most common symptom reported by patients to their physicians and is the presenting symptom in over 80 million office visits to physicians each year. Although acute pain usually responds to supportive measures such as heat and rest, mild antiinflammatory medications, invasive interventions like surgery, on just the tincture of time, it often persists. Even after the application of nerve blocks and opiate medications, a large number of patients still report pain lasting longer than 6 months. These patients suffer from what is known as *chronic pain* and they can be challenging to treat, draining a disproportionate share of the American healthcare dollar. In this chapter we first review some relevant statistics about the inefficiency of the standard medical approach to the treatment of chronic pain and then briefly discuss the evo-

lution of medicine's view of the chronic pain syndrome (CPS). Finally, we move into the main focus of this chapter—the role of complementary and alternative medicine (CAM) modalities in the integrated multidisciplinary team approach that has become the practice standard in the management of chronic pain.

## OVERVIEW OF CHRONIC PAIN

Chronic pain is defined by the American Pain Society[1] as pain of nonmalignant (i.e., noncancerous) origin that persists for longer than 6 months despite appropriate conventional treatment. By some estimates, more than 80 million Americans have either chronic pain or recurrent acute pain syndromes.[2] Back pain alone was the third most common reason for surgery (over 270,000 procedures) and the fifth most common reason for hospitalization in the United States in 1997.[2] In 1994 over 2.9 million Americans were treated at pain treatment facilities or by pain management specialists,[3] and in the year before admission to a multidisciplinary pain treatment program, these patients each used on average $22,000 of healthcare resources.[4] If in addition to these medical costs we add the cost of disability compensation payments, lost workforce productivity, and the cost of associated legal services, the annual costs of chronic pain in America are estimated at well over $50 billion dollars.[4] The most important cost—human suffering—is, of course, simply impossible to calculate.

## EVOLUTION OF THE MULTIDISCIPLINARY PAIN CENTER

Against this daunting background of rising costs and stagnant outcomes came the multidisciplinary pain center (MPC) movement. In part patient driven (out of frustration at multiple caregivers who rarely communicated amongst themselves, leaving patients to juggle a bewildering and often contradictory array of therapies and medications) and in part physician driven (out of the understanding that the usual medical model of symptom suppression was not working), the era of MPCs began in the 1970s.

The MPC concept has evolved through several phases, with the current wide embrace of CAM being only the latest incarnation. Chronic pain was only first conceptualized as a discrete entity by psychologist Wilbert Fordyce[5] and anesthesiologist John Bonica[6] in the late 1960s and early 1970s. Using the techniques of behavioral psychology, Fordyce and Bonica were able to alter the "pain behaviors" that accompanied chronic pain—the helplessness, the need for attention, the faith in medicine as a cure-all, the all-encompassing focus on eliminating unpleasant bodily sensations. They believed that what doctors referred to as chronic pain was in fact a behavioral adaptation to a medical event, an adaptation that was primarily psychosocial in nature.

Thus many medical diagnoses are included under the CPS rubric because CPS refers more to a behavioral syndrome than to a specific pathophysiological process. For example, specific pain etiologies under-

lying the development of CPS can include myofascial pain, fibromyalgia, peripheral neuropathy, rheumatoid arthritis, osteoarthritis, and others. This difficulty in pinning down the physiological origins of CPS in part triggered the conceptual shift in chronic pain treatment over the past 30 years.

Fordyce and Bonica established the first pain management program in Seattle in 1968, with the emphasis on using operant conditioning to extinguish rather than reinforce pain behaviors. The goal was to cultivate self-efficacy behaviors whenever possible. The underlying physiology wasn't the primary focus (as long as a treatable medical illness was not involved), and the psychological meaning or origin of the pain was not psychoanalyzed, despite the prevailing psychodynamic theories of psychological medicine at that time. To illustrate this shift in clinical focus away from meaning-driven psychodynamics, consider this situation I encountered when I first began work at the Spaulding Rehabilitation Hospital (SRH) Pain Unit. I was not familiar with the practice of operant behavior conditioning or of cognitive behavioral therapy in general; therefore when a patient I was interviewing dropped her notebook and asked me to pick it up for her, my initial reflex was simply to bend over and get it. However, I was gently scolded by the treatment team for rewarding this dependent patient-role pain behavior. Instead, I soon learned that praising a patient's own efforts to pick the notebook up would reinforce autonomous behaviors at the same time that maladaptive pain behaviors were being extinguished by the treatment team's benign neglect of the moaning and grimacing that often accompany chronic pain. The so-called secondary gains that patients experienced at home—of reduced responsibilities and increased attention while in the patient role—would now be replaced by the higher rewards of increased autonomy and a more effective and fulfilling lifestyle.

This emerging clinical emphasis on psychological rather than physiological or nociceptive factors in chronic pain dovetailed nicely with the growing understanding in the 1970s and 1980s of the connection between stress and illness. The field of stress medicine grew rapidly by building on the work of its pioneers: Walter Cannon's study of the self-healing "wisdom of the body,"[7] Hans Selye's elucidation of the adrenal fight-or-flight reflex,[8] George Engel's development of the biopsychosocial model,[9] and Herbert Benson's description of an innate relaxation reflex[10] were all important pieces in the emerging field that was originally called psychosomatic medicine but which has now evolved into mind/body medicine, also known as psychoneuroimmunology (PNI). Chronic pain has been a fertile ground for implementing these mind/body therapies. Stress management techniques soon became a hallmark of most pain management programs because the stress/pain connection can become readily apparent, even to skeptics of mind/body interactions. For example, the onset of chronic headaches can often be traced to an increase in psychosocial stress levels in the patient's life, while muscle tension levels often clearly reflect external stressors. Learning to manage this stress can create dramatic psychophysiologically mediated changes in pain perception, which then translate into increased function and enjoyment of life. The role of such centrally mediated involvement was outlined in Melzack and Wall's famous gate-control theory of pain,[11] which provided the first anatomic rationale for including mental or psychological events in the analysis of the phenomenon of pain by showing how cortical and limbic events such as thoughts and emotions can literally close the synaptic gate on pain pathways lower down in the spinal cord and periphery.

Another key addition to the treatment protocols for chronic pain was the integration of standard rehabilitation treatments such as physical therapy (PT) and occupational therapy (OT) into the management of chronic pain.[12] Again, the focus was not on curing the pain but on helping the patient maximize his or her functional abilities while performing the activities that compose a normal lifestyle. This development meant that chronic pain would ideally be treated by integrated teams of collaborating practitioners rather than by a succession of individual clinicians. Whereas the standard clinical story for most chronic pain patients had been one of bouncing from doctor to doctor, receiving multiple prescriptions (which often contradicted the intent of each other, or produced unintended adverse reactions and interactions), now care was to be coordinated under one conductor's baton.[13]

Although these so-called MPCs have been organized along various lines and expertise models (with directors at different centers who are anesthesiologists, neurologists, psychologists, and psychiatrists), the most widely accepted model falls into the rehabilitation paradigm. Because the disability accompanying chronic pain is the most striking symptom of this disorder, it is appropriate that its treatment reflect the core values of rehabilitation medicine rather than acute care medicine. The focus is on improved function and enhanced enjoyment of life rather than symptom elimination or suppression, and it is this contrast with the philosophy of acute pain treatment—where pain is the enemy, against which is arrayed a wide range of medications and surgical interventions—that accounts for the unique perspective of chronic pain treatment. The focus is no longer on the symptom but on the person experiencing the symptom, and the goal is to learn how to manage the pain so that life can go on productively. As the title of one of the best current handbooks of pain management[14] puts it, the challenge is in learning *How to Manage Your Pain Before it Manages You.*

By its very nature chronic pain is ideally suited for the application of the philosophies and techniques of rehabilitation medicine. This also makes CPS prime territory for the application of CAM techniques. The focus of rehabilitation on patient empowerment and self-management, on clinical teamwork rather than hierarchical pyramids of power, on accepting and trying to understand symptoms rather than reflexively trying to eliminate them, and on working with the whole person—these rehabilitation values, as articulated by the American Association of Physical Medicine and Rehabilitation,[15] also reflect the core values of holistic medicine as articulated by the American Holistic Medical Association.[16] Therefore CAM and rehabilitation, and CAM and chronic pain, are natural partners, and as CAM has flourished in the last decade, chronic pain centers have been magnets for these approaches and have begun to routinely incorporate such modalities as biofeedback, acupuncture, and meditation in their regimens. Let us look now at how that integration works.

## COMPLEMENTARY AND ALTERNATIVE MEDICINE IN CHRONIC PAIN

Several hundred treatment techniques fall under the umbrella of CAM, and it is safe to say that all have been applied to the treatment of chronic pain! It would be quite easy to devote an entire book to the application of CAM modalities to chronic pain and, in fact, there is a growing need for such a book because the scientific literature on CAM and pain is exploding. Taylor's 1999 review article of CAM in CPS[17] alone lists 249 recent references to CAM as it relates to pain; Mauskop's text[18] is devoted exclusively to the even more focused topic of CAM and headache, while Lewith's text[19] is the earlier European precursor to more recent American work. Already in print are textbooks that cover such CAM/CPS overlaps as hypnosis,[20] biofeedback,[21] and acupuncture,[22] although the definitive CAM/CPS text has not yet appeared. This is just another way of saying that it is no longer possible to provide a comprehensive review of the topic of CAM and chronic pain in one chapter; therefore I will not even pretend to try.

Rather than pursue the strategy of briefly touching on the utility of many of the best-known CAM treatments in CPS or focusing in more detail on a handful of key interventions (as has been done elsewhere for hypnosis, meditation, herbs, and Therapeutic Touch[23]; references for which are included in this chapter's bibliography), we take a different route here. I remind readers that the preceding chapters of this textbook already contain a wealth of information on CAM and chronic pain because the technique-oriented chapters in Part I of this book all include sections on their applicability to the treatment of CPS. Any reader interested in the role of a particular CAM technique in treating chronic pain is referred to the relevant chapter in Part I for more details. In addition, almost half of the 60 plus case vignettes scattered throughout this book relate to the treatment of pain in some of its forms and can be similarly consulted. Therefore the focus of this chapter now shifts away from specific treatment techniques and onto the role of an overall guiding philosophy in integrating the various treatment modalities into one coherent program or approach to chronic pain.

## INTEGRATED TREATMENT PROGRAMS

Discussions of CAM techniques in chronic pain can easily leave the reader with the impression that pain is like any other symptom—it can be attacked by a vast array of modalities. In fact, there is a tendency for even the most holistically oriented pain practitioners to simply adopt the symptom-focused mentality of allopathic medicine practitioners and move from one treatment technique to another in the hopes of eventually eliminating the evil symptom of pain. However, what is important about holistic approaches to pain is not the use of novel or unique modalities but the

coordination and integration of care among various providers on the treatment team, all guided by the overarching philosophy of patient self-management and self-empowerment.

It is important to highlight the multidisciplinary nature of good chronic pain management because it is in teamwork that synergism occurs—the whole becomes greater than the sum of its parts. To illustrate this potentially abstract ideal, I provide a concrete description of this process in action by describing the structure and function of one hospital-based inpatient pain management program. This program serves as a typical example of the sort of integrative approach to chronic pain management that is found in many centers in America today.

The program I discuss is the one where I work—the Pain Management Program at SRH in Boston. It exemplifies many of the key features of MPCs, but it is also unusual in several respects. Our 18-bed inpatient pain unit is one of numerous traditional rehabilitation programs (stroke, amputee, spinal cord injury) in our 290-bed not-for-profit Harvard Medical School–affiliated hospital. It is one of the oldest such programs in America, having been started in 1976, early in the history of MPCs. This relatively long history (most of the existence of this relatively new field) has provided a solid foundation in the institutional culture of SRH. The credibility of the Pain Management Unit has made it easier for newer CAM treatments to be installed in more recent years because the core values shared by CAM and by rehabilitation—of teamwork, self-management, and innovation—are no longer controversial.

## COST-BENEFIT ASPECTS OF MULTIDISCIPLINARY PAIN CENTERS

Ours is the only remaining inpatient pain program in New England, a testament to the profound impact health maintenance organizations (HMOs) have had on the field of pain management. The trend among insurers has been to move the treatment of chronic pain to the outpatient setting, or to deny coverage altogether, to minimize costs. For example, outpatient PT and OT for pain must often be delivered within 60 days of the initial clinic evaluation because after 60 days the syndrome is deemed to be chronic and is no longer covered by many large insurance companies. However, behavioral retraining takes time and costs money, and the intensity and structure of an inpatient program are crucial to many patients. Numerous outcome studies have shown that MPCs are clearly more cost effective than straight medical or surgical interventionism.[24,25]

In part because of the reluctance of insurance companies to invest in expensive inpatient treatment unless and until absolutely necessary, the patient who finally comes to an MPC is usually profoundly impaired by pain. Ironically, he or she has usually accrued far higher medical costs through repeated failed surgeries, multiple medication trials, regular visits to the local emergency room, and fruitless diagnostic tests than the actual expense of the average inpatient stay ($30,000 for 4 weeks). Dr. Dennis Turk, former president of the American Pain Society, has documented the dramatic cost savings that would be available to insurers if they routinely funded this apparently expensive form of intervention,[26] especially in comparison with conservative treatments or surgical interventions, which do not produce cost savings commensurate with their significant upfront costs.

# A TYPICAL MULTIDISCIPLINARY PAIN CENTER

The typical SRH inpatient has numerous psychosocial symptoms on admission. He or she will often have developed a secondary drug dependence problem, having become addicted to the painkillers or tranquilizers prescribed by the primary care doctor. Social isolation and marital estrangement are common, and psychiatric comorbidity is the norm rather than the exception. Depression secondary to the pain is common,[27] as is posttraumatic stress disorder (PTSD) from either the inciting accident or injury or from an earlier pattern of childhood abuse and trauma.[28] The average Beck Depression Scale score of our inpatients is 25, indicating a moderate to severe degree of symptomatology; as Shealy demonstrates in Chapter 28 of this book,[29] chronic depression is a common but often unaddressed aspect of chronic pain.

By its very structure, this program and others like it counter the reductionist and fragmenting tendencies of allopathic medicine because all of the interventions and the treatment providers are interacting together under the same roof. To be semantically precise, such a program should be called *interdisciplinary* rather than *multidisciplinary* (where the multiple practitioners may never actually talk to one another but only provide sequential, and uncoordinated, treatments). All treatment strategies at SRH are developed at regular team meetings based on daily feedback from the patients. Most important, the patients join a community of more than a dozen other pain patients to discover that they are not alone in their experience of this invisible disease. Many program graduates have reported that the most profound experience for them was the discovery that other people exist who truly understand their situation (they were referring to the other patients, not to the staff!).

The basic philosophy of the program is one of self-management: to manage pain, to optimize function despite pain, to manage one's life by shifting the focus away from the elimination of pain itself and onto creating a more fulfilling lifestyle. Happiness despite pain is the paradoxical goal of most MPCs. There are three main tiers of intervention—medical, physical, and emotional/psychological. Each patient will be pursuing all three levels concurrently, and each level is amenable to the concurrent use of both traditional and CAM approaches.

- *Medical:* Among the most commonly addressed medical situations are implementation of long-acting opiate regimens when appropriate,[30] administration of trigger point (TrP) injections (especially for myofascial pain[31]), supervision of detoxification or medication tapering protocols, and treatment of concurrent medical illnesses. Diagnostic workups are not usually pursued with inpatients because exhaustive testing usually has been completed before entry and because focus on an often elusive surgical cure distracts from rehabilitation priorities and from the commitment to managing, rather than eliminating, pain.
- *Physical:* Chronic pain patients are often profoundly deconditioned, having spent months being inactive; it is not uncommon for patients to report spending literally 24 hours a day in bed for months, if not years. Hence PT to regain physical function and conditioning is a matter of crucial importance. Graded exercises stressing increased aerobic capacity, flexibility, and strength are the cornerstone of the PT approach to CPS.[32] Our PTs are the guides here, working with each patient individually for an

hour each day, as well as in a daily group setting (the morning stretch routine to start the day). Treadmills, exercycles, and upper-body exercises are used with the more fit patients, while for the more deconditioned simple unassisted walking or graduating from a wheelchair to a rolling walker may be an appropriate challenge.

These approaches are supplemented with biofeedback and postural analysis to overcome ingrained patterns of muscle tension. Dramatic improvements are common, in part because baseline fitness levels are so appallingly low, with secondary improvements in mood, sense of self-efficacy, and overall vitality commonly reported. A videotape showing the changes from pre- to post-program gait patterns and postural alignment is a dramatic form of undeniable positive feedback for many patients.

- *Emotional/psychological:* Emotional needs are addressed in several direct ways. The team psychologist works with general stress management training to help patients learn to observe and understand the stress/pain cycle in action.[33] Cognitive behavioral interventions help correct negativistic thought patterns—for example, the tendency to "catastrophize" or view every minor twinge as a medical emergency. This cognitive behavioral component, though developed by traditional academic psychologists, is in fact a mind/body intervention: Patients discover how their thoughts and feelings affect their pain.[34] The tool of biofeedback is invaluable in making this connection concrete and visible, and OTs provide instruction in this modality[35] so that patients can directly experience how their thoughts and emotions create changes in muscle tension (via electromyogram [EMG] biofeedback) or in their blood flow (via thermal biofeedback).

  The team psychiatrist is routinely consulted to address issues such as insomnia, depression, and PTSD. Behavioral measures are often sufficient to deal with the insomnia: establishment of regular circadian schedule, limitation of total daily caffeine intake, regular practice of relaxation techniques at bedtime. But occasional judicious use of such nonaddictive hypnotic agents as trazodone, zolpidem, melatonin, or a tricyclic antidepressant is sometimes necessary. Chronically depressed mood often responds dramatically to the resocialization, physical re-

conditioning, and supportive milieu of the program, but standard antidepressants are also regularly used when indicated. No one subtype of antidepressant is demonstrably more effective for pain-related depression; therefore side effect profiles often determine prescribing patterns. Because the hospital pharmacy does not yet include herbal preparations or nutritional supplements in its formulary, we have not been able to assess the effects of St. John's wort, for example, on our depressed patients. In consultation with staff physicians, patients are allowed to continue nutraceutical regimens begun on the outside, and the initiation of new supplements is often possible if family members can bring in the recommended substances (most commonly gingko biloba to help improve alertness, chondroitin and glucosamine to help with osteoarthritic pain, and flaxseed oil for certain inflammatory conditions).

The team social worker is a key player because chronic pain is a disease that affects the entire family system.[36] All family relationships, whether functional or dysfunctional to start with, become skewed by the longstanding patterns of pain and illness, and family interventions require more than simple supportive listening. Massive reeducation is often necessary to shift ingrained family behavioral patterns; patients must sign an initial treatment contract in which they agree that key family members will participate in a weekly family educational group focused on the nature of chronic pain, as well as individualized family counseling sessions to uncover key dynamics in each specific family.

Several common dynamic patterns in families with CPS include the following:

- The family that has inadvertently fostered the helpless patient role in their member with pain by being overly solicitous or helpful. Performing simple tasks for the patient can block any move to more autonomy by the patient.
- A lack of understanding of the nature of the CPS by other family members has led to estrangement and mistrust of the patient because his or her symptoms are invisible and impossible to validate and the degree of disability does not match the apparently normal appearance of the patient.
- Judgmental attitudes of family members regarding the need for psychiatric medications;

these medications are often seen as a shameful sign of weakness and therefore mental health services are often undermined or avoided because of family pressures.

- Unjustly concluding that the family member is malingering or a drug addict because opiate medications are prescribed; this is especially problematic given our society's current "black and white" attitude toward drugs today.

The spiritual dimension of chronic pain is not addressed by a specific team member or intervention, but patients are of course encouraged to pursue their own religious practices or to request consultation with our hospital's pastoral care providers. Training in mindfulness meditation is provided to all patients, but in a secular rather than spiritual context. However, patients are encouraged to link these practices and experiences to their own religious training and previous spiritual experiences. Patients with a dual diagnosis of alcohol or narcotic abuse can participate in our in-house Alcoholics Anonymous or Narcotics Anonymous meetings to work with their Higher Power more directly.

## Case Example

A composite case example is presented as a way of highlighting the various ways in which patients may respond to a multifaceted pain program. The story of Mary that follows is actually composed of elements from several different patient histories, but for simplicity of presentation they have been melded into one composite example. No one patient ever responds positively to all aspects of the program, but each modality has been helpful for a large subgroup of patients (although not all patients leave the program in better shape than when they started). Despite these caveats, the story of Mary is not unusual.

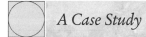 *A Case Study*

### Myofascial Pain Disorder

Mary was a married 47-year-old mother of three teenagers when she entered the SRH Pain Program. She had initially petitioned her insurer 15 months earlier for inpatient admission to help her deal with a 5-year history of headaches that began when Mary was involved in a motor vehicle ac-

cident at work. She had resumed work shortly after the accident and had dealt adequately with mild headaches, but the headaches began to worsen in frequency and intensity to the point where she had been unable to work for the past 1½ years. Her cognitive function had been so impaired by the regimen of opiates prescribed to her by her primary care provider that she could no longer handle her responsibilities as an administrative assistant at a small personnel agency. She was on short-term disability, but she had also filed suit against her employer because it had terminated her medical coverage and contested her Workers' Compensation claim. Her condition had deteriorated even further before admission while waiting for authorization of treatment. After 15 months of legal maneuvering with the State Department of Industrial Accidents, Mary succeeded in obtaining a court order that required her insurer to provide full coverage for inpatient pain rehabilitation.

When she arrived at SRH, she was emotionally drained from her legal ordeal and was in such poor physical condition that she could walk on a low-speed treadmill for only 2 minutes before attaining maximal heart rate and complaining of exhaustion. On the medical front, Mary was diagnosed with myofascial pain syndrome in her cervical spine triggered by the whiplash from her automobile accident but never previously diagnosed by providers who had been more focused on symptom suppression than on accurate diagnosis. This underlying primary syndrome had been indirectly triggering her chronic headaches. She had adapted to chronic discomfort by altering her body mechanics in a way that set up muscle strain patterns and TrPs in her cervical muscles, and these myofascial TrPs produced her referred occipital headaches.

The attending physiatrist recognized that the correct primary diagnosis of Mary's condition—myofascial pain disorder—was not appropriately treated with opiates but with a combination of behavioral and interventional approaches to help her relax muscle tension. She was successfully tapered off opiates over a 2-week period (the rapid acupuncture detoxification protocol described by Smith in Chapter 25 of this book[37] is not available at SRH). In tandem with this tapering, her short-term memory and concentration improved dramatically. Although the herb ginkgo biloba might have been helpful on theoretical grounds in reversing her opiate-induced cognitive problems,[33] in Mary's case it was felt that discontinuing opiates would suffice to eliminate these problems. A course of three TrP injections helped to break the cycle of tension/muscle spasm/headaches and created a window of opportunity during which she could initiate a new and more aggressive muscle stretching program. These injections did not use any local anesthetics or steroids but involved so-called dry needling, which is essentially indistinguishable from acupuncture[31] but is an acceptable procedure code for billing most insurance companies.

Several specific treatment modalities helped her to further minimize the muscle spasm that was contributing to her myofascial pain/headache syndrome. In PT she learned a series of stretching exercises, modified from classic yoga postures, that were to become part of her daily morning routine. Continuous self-monitoring during the day helped her to become aware of the dynamic changes in her own internal body state as she moved from situation to situation. In psychology, she learned to use EMG biofeedback to relax the specific cervical muscles that were triggering her headaches. Biofeedback also provided vivid proof that thinking about certain family issues caused an immediate surge in muscle tension levels. These family dynamics exacerbated her stress-responsive symptoms in a way that she had never noticed until she was afforded the luxury of spending several weeks away from the family system. Her first clue was a pattern noted by her treatment team. Mary had a strong tendency to try to please everyone on her treatment team and to try to take care of the other patients in the program. During discussions with the social worker she was able to relate this tendency to some family of origin issues. As the oldest sibling, she had taken on the responsibility of caring for younger siblings when her parents were incapacitated by their uncontrolled alcoholism. In her current nuclear family she had recreated these same patterns and was essentially burning her candle at both ends by attending to the needs of other family members even at the expense of her own health.

It was not easy to release this ingrained pattern. Guided self-hypnosis imagery helped her to give comfort to the ego state that seemed to motivate this behavior: the wounded inner child[38] who had never been loved unconditionally and could only gain love in exchange for performing household tasks. Mary was able to eliminate the nightmares that caused her chronic insomnia when she learned to self-administer an acupressure desensitization protocol[39] that, in her words, "took the fear out of the memories" of the traumatic automobile accident that had been replaying every night in her dreams.

OT further helped with Mary's stress management by showing her how to reorganize her days in accordance with the concepts of pacing and energy conservation. This practice helped her to diminish her tendency to overdo and eventually enabled her to return to work half-time. She instituted a home practice plan of pain self-management modalities that took 45 minutes daily and involved yoga stretches, mindfulness meditation, acupressure, and affirmation/prayer. She came to see occasional mild pain flare-ups as signals from her body that she had been overlooking her own emotional needs. A time-limited course of outpatient psychotherapy helped reinforce and maintain these positive behavioral changes, and when she was seen at 6-month follow-up, she was medication free and happier and more functional than she had been in years. ✌

## SUMMARY

As I hope this chapter illustrates, the applications of CAM to the field of pain management are rapidly growing and almost unlimited in potential. Despite continued reluctance by insurers to cover CAM treatments adequately in chronic pain, it seems likely that new outcome studies and continued consumer pressure will change the availability of CAM services in treating chronic pain. Even as we wait for these new research findings, at least one conclusion can be definitively made now: CAM interventions will be a routine aspect of chronic pain management in the twenty-first century.

## References

1. APS defintion: American Pain Foundation, www.painfoundation.org. Go to chronic pain: Pain Info Center.
2. Andersson G: The epidemiology of spinal disorders, In Frymoyer J (ed): *The adult spine,* Philadelphia, 1997, Lippincott-Raven, pp 93-142.
3. Marketdata Enterprises: *Chronic pain management programs: a market analysis,* Valley Stream, NY, 1995, Marketdata Enterprises.
4. Frymoyer J, Durett C: The economics of spinal disorders. In Frymoyer J (ed): *The adult spine,* Philadelphia, 1997, Lippincott-Raven.
5. Fordyce W: *Behavioral methods for chronic pain and illness,* St Louis, 1976, Mosby.
6. Bonica J: *The management of pain,* Philadelphia, 1990, Lea & Febiger.
7. Cannon W: *The wisdom of the body,* New York, 1932, WW Norton.
8. Selye H: *The stress of life,* New York, 1978, McGraw Hill.
9. Engel G: From biomedical to biopsychosocial: being scientific in the human domain, *Psychosomatics* 38(6):521-528, 1997.
10. Benson H: *The relaxation response,* New York, 1975, Avon Books.
11. Melzack R, Wall P: *The challenge of pain,* New York, 1983, Basic Books.
12. Wittink H, Michel TH: *Chronic pain management for physical therapists,* Woburn, Mass, 1997, Butterworth-Heinemann.
13. Bonica J: Evolution and current status of pain programs, *J Pain Symptom Manage* 5:368-374, 1990.
14. Caudill M: *Managing your pain before it manages you,* New York, 1995, Guilford Press.
15. American Holistic Medical Association: www.ahma.org
16. American Association of Physical Medicine & Rehabilitation: www.aapmr.org/about/mission.htm

17. Taylor AG: Complementary/alternative therapies in the treatment of pain. In Spencer JW, Jacobs JJ (eds): *Complementary and alternative medicine: an evidence-based approach,* St Louis, 1999, Mosby.

18. Mauskop A, Brill MA: *The headache alternative: a neurologist's guide to drug-free relief,* Salt Lake City, 1997, Science News Books.

19. Lewith G, Horn S: *Drug-free pain relief,* Rochester, Vt, 1987, Thorson.

20. Barber J (ed): *Hypnosis and suggestion in the treatment of pain: a clinical guide,* New York, 1996, WW Norton.

21. Scwartz M (ed): Biofeedback: a practitioner's guide, New York, 1995, Guilford Press.

22. Seem M: *A new American acupuncture: the myofascial release of the bodymind's holding patterns,* Boulder, Colo, 1993, Blue Poppy Press.

23. Leskowitz E: Complementary and alternative medicine for chronic pain. In Warfield C (ed): *Principles and practice of pain medicine,* ed 2, New York, 2002, McGraw Hill.

24. Malec J, Cayner J, Harvey R, et al: Pain management: long-term follow-up of an inpatient program, *Arch Phys Med Rehabil* 62:369-372, 1981.

25. Meilman P, Skultety F, Guck T, et al: Benign chronic pain: 18 month to ten year followup of a multidisciplinary program, *Clin J Pain* 1:131-137, 1985.

26. Turk D, Okifuji A: Treatment of chronic pain patients: clinical outcomes, cost-effectiveness, and cost-benefits of multidisciplinary pain centers, *Crit Rev Phys Rehabil Med* 10(2):181-208, 1998.

27. Blumer D, Heilbronn M: Chronic pain as a variant of depressive diseases: the pain-prone disorder, *J Nerv Ment Dis* 170:381-406, 1982.

28. Goldberg R, Goldstein R: Comparison of chronic pain patients and controls on traumatic events in childhood, *Disabil Rehabil* 27(17):756-763, 2000.

29. Shealy CN: Chronic depression in rehabilitation. In Leskowitz E (ed): *Complementary and alternative medicine in rehabilitation,* St Louis, 2002, Mosby.

30. Parrott T: Using opioid analgesics to manage chronic non-cancer pain in primary care, *J Am Board Fam Pract* 12(4):293-306, 1999.

31. Travell J, Simon D: *Myofascial pain and dysfunction: the trigger point manual,* Baltimore, 1992, Williams and Wilkins.

32. Iverson MD, Liang M, Bae SC: Selected arthritides. In Frontera W (ed): *Exercise in rehabilitation medicine,* Champaign, Ill, 2000, Human Kinetics.

33. Turk D: Biopsychosocial perspectives on chronic pain. In Getchel R, Turk D (eds): *Psychological approaches to pain management: a practitioner's guidebook,* New York, 1996, Guilford Press.

34. Turk D, Meichenbaum D, Genest M: *Pain and behavioral medicine: a cognitive-behavioral approach,* New York, 1983, Guilford Press.

35. Sherman R: Biofeedback for low back pain. In Basmajian J, Nyberg R (eds): *Rational manual therapies,* Baltimore, 1992, Williams & Wilkins.

36. Kerns R, Payne A: Treating families of chronic pain patients. In Getchel R, Turk D (eds), *Psychological approaches to pain management: a practitioner's guidebook,* New York, 1996, Guilford Press.

37. Smith M: Acupuncture detoxification. In Leskowitz E (ed): *Complementary and alternative medicine in rehabilitation,* St Louis, 2002, Mosby.

38. Frederick C, McNeal S: *Inner strengths: contemporary psychotherapy and hypnosis for ego strength,* New York, 1998, Lawrence Erlbaum Associates.

39. Gallo F: *Energy psychology,* Boca Raton, Fla, 1999, CRC Press.

## Selected Modality–Specific Bibliography

### Herbal Medicine

Blumenthal M (ed): *The German Commission E monographs: therapeutic guide to herbal medicine,* Austin, Tex, 1998, American Botanical Council.

Doyle E, Spence M: Cannabis as a medicine? *Br J Anaesth* 74:3359-3361, 1995.

Haustkappe M, Roizen M, Toledano A, et al: Review of the effectiveness of capsaicin for painful cutaneous disorders and neural dysfunction, *Clin J Pain* 14(2):97-106, 1998.

Murphy JJ, Heptinstall S, Mitchell JR: Randomised double-blind placebo-controlled trial of feverfew in migraine prevention, *Lancet* 2(8604):189-192, 1988.

Schmid G, Carita F, Bonanno G, et al: NK-3 receptors mediate enhancement of substance P release from capsaicin-sensitive spinal cord afferent terminals, *Br J Pharmacol* 125(4):621-626, 1998.

Srivastava MD, Mustafa T: Ginger *(Zingiber officinalis)* in rheumatism and other musculoskeletal disorders, *Med Hypotheses* 39(4):342, 1992.

### Homeopathy

Hart O, Mullee MA, Lewith G, et al: Double-blind, placebo-controlled, randomized clinical trial of homoeopathic arnica C30 for pain and infection after total abdominal hysterectomy, *J R Soc Med* 90(4):239-240, 1997.

Lokken P, Straumshein PA, Tveiten D, et al: Effect of homoeopathy on pain and other events after acute trauma: placebo controlled trial with bilateral oral surgery, *BMJ* 310(6992):1439-1442, 1995.

Vickers AJ, Fisher P, Smith C, et al: Homeopathic Arnica 30x is ineffective for muscle soreness after long-distance running: a randomized, double-blind, placebo-controlled trial, *Clin J Pain* 14:227-231, 1998.

Whitmarsh T: Evidence in complementary and alternative therapies: lessons from clinical trials of homeopathy in headache, *J Altern Complement Med* 3(4):307-310, 1997.

Whitmarsh TE, Coleston-Shields DM, Steiner TJ: Double-blind randomized placebo-controlled study of homoeopathic prophylaxis of migraine, *Cephalalgia* 17(5):600-604, 1997.

*Hypnosis*

Crawford HJ, Gur RC, Skolnick B, et al: Effects of hypnosis on regional cerebral blood flow during ischemic pain with and without suggested hypnotic analgesia, *Int J Psychophysiol* 15(3):181-195, 1993.

Crawford HJ, Knebel T, Kaplan L, et al: Hypnotic analgesia: 1. somatosensory event-related potential changes to noxious stimuli, and 2. transfer learning to reduce chronic low back pain, *Int J Clin Exp Hypn* 46(1):92-132, 1998.

Egbert LD, Battit GE, Welch CE, et al: Reduction of postoperative pain by encouragement and instruction of patients: a study of doctor-patient rapport, *N Engl J Med* (270):825-827, 1964.

Enqvist B, von Konow L, Bystedt T: Pre- and peri-operative suggestion in maxillofacial surgery: effects on blood loss and recovery, *Int J Clin Exp Hypn* 43(3):284-294, 1995.

Ewin DM: Emergency room hypnosis for the burned patient, *Am J Clin Hypnosis* 29(1):7-12, 1986.

Gainter M: Hypnotherapy for reflex sympathetic dystrophy, *Am J Clin Hypnosis* 34(4):227-232, 1992.

Huddleston P: *Prepare for surgery, heal faster: a guide to mind/body techniques,* Cambridge, Mass, 1996, Angel River Press.

Ochoa JD, Verdugo JD: Reflex sympathetic dystrophy: a common clinical avenue for somatoform expression, *Neurol Clin* 13(2):351-363, 1995.

Patterson DR, Questad KA, deLateur BJ: Hypnotherapy as an adjunct to narcotic analgesia for the treatment of pain for burn débridement, *Am J Clin Hypnosis* 31(3):156-163, 1989.

Spiegel D, Barabasz A: Effects of hypnotic instructions of P300 event-related-potential amplitudes: research and clinical applications, *Am J Clin Hypn* 31(1):11-17, 1988.

*Meditation*

Benson H: *The relaxation response,* New York, 1975, Avon Books.

Caudill M, Schnable R, Suttermeister P, et al: Decreased clinic use by chronic pain patients: response to behavioral medicine interventions, *Clin J Pain* (7):305-310, 1991.

Caudill M: *Managing pain before it manages you,* New York, 1995, Guilford Press.

Kabat-Zinn J: *Full catastrophe living: using the wisdom of your body and mind to face stress, pain, and illness,* New York, 1990, Delacorte Press.

Kabat-Zinn J, Lipworth L, Burney R, et al: Four-year follow-up of a meditation-based program for the self-regulation of chronic pain: treatment outcomes and compliance, *Clin J Pain* (2):159-173, 1987.

Kaplin KH, Goldenberg DL, Galvine-Nadeau M: The impact of a meditation-based stress reduction program on fibromyalgia, *Gen Hosp Psychiatry* (15):284-289, 1993.

*Therapeutic Touch*

Keller E, Bzdek B: Effects of Therapeutic Touch on tension headache pain, *Nurs Res* 35(2):68-74, 1986.

Leskowitz E: Phantom limb pain: subtle energy perspectives, *Subtle Energy and Energy Med* 7(4):1-27, 1998.

Leskowitz E: Current controversies in Therapeutic Touch. In Micozzi M (ed): *Current review of alternative medicine,* St Louis, 1999, Mosby.

Meehan T: Therapeutic Touch as a nursing intervention, *J Adv Nurs* 28(1):117-125, 1998.

Mulloney S, Wells-Federman C: Therapeutic Touch: a healing modality, *J Cardiovasc Nurs* 10(3):27-49, 1996.

Redner R, Briner B, Snellman L: Effects of a bioenergy healing technique on chronic pain, *Subtle Energies* 2(3):43-68, 1991.

Rosa L, Rosa E, Sarner L, et al: A close look at Therapeutic Touch, *JAMA* 279(13):1005-1010, 1998.

Schlitz M, Braud W: Distant intentionality and healing: assessing the evidence, *Altern Ther Health Med* 3(6):62-73, 1997.

Turner J: The effect of Therapeutic Touch on pain and anxiety in burn patients, *J Adv Nurs* 28(1):10-20, 1998.

Wu WH, Bandilla E, Ciccone D, et al: Effects of qigong on late-stage complex regional pain syndrome, *Altern Ther Health Med* 5(1):45-54, 1999.

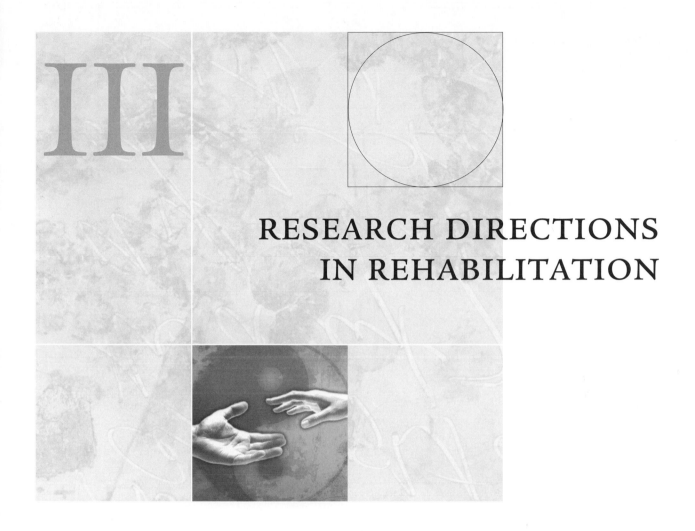

# III

# RESEARCH DIRECTIONS
# IN REHABILITATION

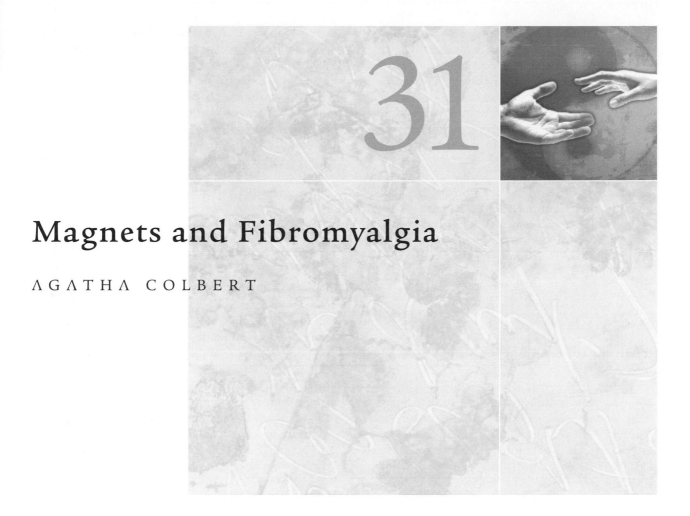

# Magnets and Fibromyalgia

ΛGΛTHΛ COLBERT

## ABSTRACT*

The objective of this double-blind, randomized controlled trial was to determine if the chronic pain and sleep disturbances experienced by patients with fibromyalgia can be improved by sleeping on a magnetic mattress pad. The study was performed in patients' homes and the private practice office of the principal investigator. The patients recruited were thirty-five female subjects diagnosed with fibromyalgia syndrome. Thirty met inclusion/exclusion criteria and entered the study. Twenty-five completed it. One was lost to follow-up. Three were withdrawn for protocol violations and one because of a recurrent hospitalization.

**Intervention.** The patients slept on an experimental (magnetized at a magnet surface field strength of 1100 ± 50 gauss (G) and delivering 200 to 600 G to the skin surface) or a sham (non-magnetized) mattress pad over a 16-week period.

**Outcome measures.** The outcome measures used were the Visual Analog Scales (VAS) for global well being, pain, sleep, fatigue, and tiredness on awakening; Total Myalgic Score; Pain Distribution Drawings; and a modified Fibromyalgia Impact Questionnaire.

**Results.** Subjects sleeping on the experimental mattress pad experienced a significant decrease in pain ($p < .006$), Total Myalgic Score ($p < .03$), and Pain Distribution Drawing ($p < .02$). Additionally, these subjects showed significant improvement in reported

*Colbert AP, Markov MS, Banerji M, et al: Magnetic mattress pad use in patients with fibromyalgia: a randomized double-blind pilot study, *J Back Musculoskel Rehab* 13:19-31, 1999.

sleep ($p$ <.01) and physical functioning as evidenced from the modified Fibromyalgia Impact Questionnaire ($p$ <.04). Subjects sleeping on the sham mattress pad experienced no significant change in these same outcome measures. Subjects in both the control and experimental groups showed improvement in tiredness on wakening, demonstrating a placebo effect in this parameter. Neither group showed any effect on global well being.

**Conclusions.** Patients sleeping on a magnetic mattress pad, with a magnetic surface field strength of 1100 ± 50 G delivering 200 to 600 G at the skin surface, provides statistically significant and clinically relevant pain relief and sleep improvement in subjects with fibromyalgia. No adverse reactions were noted during the 16-week trial period.

# COMMENTARY

## Scientific Foundation

Skeptics claim that magnetic therapy lacks a theoretical foundation and is wanting in empirical evidence. This is untrue. The worldwide basic science literature exploring the mechanisms of action on biological tissue of extremely low frequency electromagnetic fields (EMF) and magnetic fields (MF) is substantial.[1] Furthermore, a cohesive and comprehensive theoretical explanation for the mechanism of action energy healing through the piezoelectric effect in myofascial tissues, has been elegantly elucidated by Oschmann.[2] Compared to the wealth of literature documenting the influences of EMF and MF at the cellular and biochemical levels, there is a scarcity of published research on the clinical use of static or permanent magnets. A lack of understanding of the subtle energy modalities studied and an inherent bias against complementary and alternative therapies (CAM) by reviewers may account for the failure to accept original research for publication by Western medical journals.

## Static Magnetic Application Studies

To date, only eight peer-reviewed articles evaluating the effects of static magnet application to various body parts appear in the English literature. In all eight studies, magnets were used in the management of pain syndromes, including chronic neck and shoulder pain,[3] myofascial pain associated with post-polio syndrome,[4] heel pain,[5] peripheral neuropathy,[6] fibromyalgia,[7] chronic low pack pain,[8] wound healing after liposuction,[9] and chronic pelvic pain. Half of these studies found significant improvement in the experimental subjects when compared with the control groups. In the other four studies, there was either no significant difference in effect between the placebo and experimental groups or the study lacked sufficient power to document a marginal beneficial effect.

## Fibromyalgia Study

Our study[7] on magnetic mattress pads for treating patients with fibromyalgia (FM) provides a springboard for discussion of some of the obstacles a researcher in the field of therapeutic magnetism faces. The roadblocks encountered in bringing this work to publication appear to be shared by other CAM researchers. A brief preview of the study will precede some comments on these common editorial misconceptions.

The study, which was completed in the setting of a clinical practice, was approved by the Tufts University School of Medicine Investigational Review Board through the Department of Rehabilitation Medicine. The goal of the trial was to determine if sleeping on a magnetic mattress pad would in any way influence the pain and sleep problems associated with fibromyalgia. Our research design was a standard double-blind, randomized controlled trial. Twenty-five female patients meeting the American College of Rheumatology's diagnostic criteria for FM completed the study: 13 in the experimental group and 13 in the control group. The intervention consisted of sleeping nightly on either an experimental (magnetized at a magnetic surface field strength of 1100 ± 50 G and delivering 200 to 600 G to the skin surface) or a sham (non-magnetized) mattress pad over a 16-week period.

### Outcomes
Outcome measures included a Visual Analog Scale assessing pain, sleep, fatigue, tiredness on waking and general well being; a documentation of trigger point tenderness; a functional assessment of activities of daily living; and a pain drawing.

The results showed that those patients who slept on the magnetized pad experienced statistically significant improvement in their pain, sleep, fatigue, trigger point tenderness, and activities of daily living. Those patients sleeping on the non-magnetized pads showed no significant changes in these parameters. We concluded that the pain and sleep symptoms of patients with FM who slept on this particular magnetic mattress pad for 16 weeks were improved in a statistically significant and clinically relevant way. When this apparently simple and straightforward study was critiqued for publication, three misunderstandings came to light by the reviewers regarding energy medicine in general and magnetic therapy specifically.

First, the clinical condition to be treated was FM. Several peer reviewers stated that FM is a "controversial diagnosis" with no objective diagnostic findings and therefore no quantifiable outcome measures. The findings in FM as in several other chronic painful conditions, such as low back pain syndrome, irritable bowel syndrome, interstitial cystitis, phantom limb pain and chronic headaches, are almost entirely subjective. Paradoxically, patients with chronic symptomatology unresponsive to standard western medical regimens are those most likely to seek CAM interventions. The challenge therefore entails treating a refractory, poorly defined condition with a modality (subtle energy manipulation) that is most effective at the preorganic stage of the disease process and then attempting to measure changes for which there are no standardized laboratory tests. Although physiological changes cannot be documented, other objective parameters, such as decreased hospitalizations or physician visits, and decreased health care cost, for that particular individual should be considered for use as valid outcome measures.

Second, the gold standard for methodology in drug investigations and currently required in CAM research studies is the double-blind, randomized controlled trial. When evaluating the potential therapeutic benefits of a permanent magnet it is impossible to blind the participants unless they remain under 24-hour surveillance. Subjects can easily apply ferromagnetic objects, such as paper clips or nails, to test whether they have the sham or experimental magnetic product. The only research protocol in which investigators could be assured that the participants were absolutely blinded was the Valbona study[4] during which subjects were visually supervised for the 45-minute ap-

plication of magnetic disks. These authors reported that patients had a decreased point tenderness after a limited time period but could give no indication of whether 45 minutes was adequate for a long-term effect. In addition, the eight clinical trials previously mentioned have all been termed "pilot studies" involving 50 or fewer patients. The criticism is raised that the number of subjects are too few for the trials to be truly randomized. This is a "catch 22." We are at the nascent stages of biomagnetic research, and it is essential to collect pilot data. This data must then be published in peer-reviewed journals to gather enough preliminary information to warrant initiation of a large-scale study.

The third and perhaps most fundamental obstacle to researching the efficacy of magnets is that the optimum therapeutic magnetic field dosage and polarity have yet to be defined for specific conditions. Magnetic fields penetrate all tissues, including epidermis, dermis, subcutaneous tissue, dense connective tissue, and solid organs and bone, equally and in the same way as magnetic fields penetrate air. The dosage of magnetic energy that reaches the target organ therefore is primarily dependent on the size and strength of the magnet and the distance it is placed from that organ. The surface field strength of the applied magnets in the eight studies varied from 150 to 1300 G. In the FM study, it was estimated that an effective dosage of 200 to 600 G was delivered to the skin surface with the particular configuration of magnets embedded in the mattress pad and the approximate distance the magnets were from the body.

The duration and frequency of application of the magnets also varied enormously in the eight studies, from a single 45-minute utilization to nightly use for 16 weeks to continuous use for 4 months. If magnets have their effect via the body's signal transduction systems and act as electromagnetic triggers initiating the biochemical cascade of events that facilitate tissue healing, it would seem reasonable that an intermittent application is more appropriate than continuous use. The question then becomes "How intermittent?" and "Does the most effective dosage vary for different clinical conditions?"

Conventional wisdom among practitioners of magnetic therapy strongly suggests that there is an opposite therapeutic response when applying the negative vs. the positive poles of the magnet. Biophysicists, on the other hand, intuitively disagree with this premise saying it should make no difference which pole is applied. Clinical trials have not yet addressed this potentially critical issue.

## SUMMARY

People using magnetic therapy (it is estimated that 10% of the Japanese population and several million Americans are in this group) testify that these devices have positively influenced their previous pain problems with no adverse effects. Further scientific study, along the lines suggested by the pilot study, is clearly worth pursuing.

## *References*

1. Markov MS, Colbert AP: Magnetic and electromagnetic fields, *J Back Musculoskel Rehab* 2001.
2. Oschmann JL: *Energy medicine: the scientific basis,* Churchill Livingston, 2000, London.
3. Hong CZ, Lin JC, Bender LF, et al: Magnetic necklace: its therapeutic effectiveness on neck and shoulder pain, *Arch Phys Med Rehabil* 63:462-467, 1982.
4. Valbona C, Hazlewood CF, Jurida G: Response of pain to static magnetic fields in post-polio patients: a double-blind pilot study, *Arch Phys Med Rehabil* 78:1200-1203, 1997.
5. Caselli MA, Clark N, Lazarus S, et al: Evaluation of magnetic foil and PPT insoles in the treatment of heel pain, *J Am Podiatr Med Assoc* 87:11-16, 1997.
6. Weintraub MI: Magnetic bio-stimulation in painful diabetic neuropathy: a novel intervention—a randomized, double-placebo crossover study, *Am J Pain Man* 9:8-17, 1999.
7. Colbert AP, Markov MS, Banerji M, et al: Magnetic mattress pad use in patients with fibromyalgia: a randomized double-blind pilot study, *J Back Musculoskel Rehab* 13:19-31, 1999.
8. Collacott EA, Zimmerman JT, White DW, et al: Bipolar permanent magnets for the treatment of low back pain: a pilot study, *JAMA* 283:1322-1235, 2000.
9. Man D, Man B, Plosker H: The influence of permanent magnetic field therapy on wound healing in suction lipectomy patients, *Plast Reconstr Surg* 104(7):2261-2266, 1999.

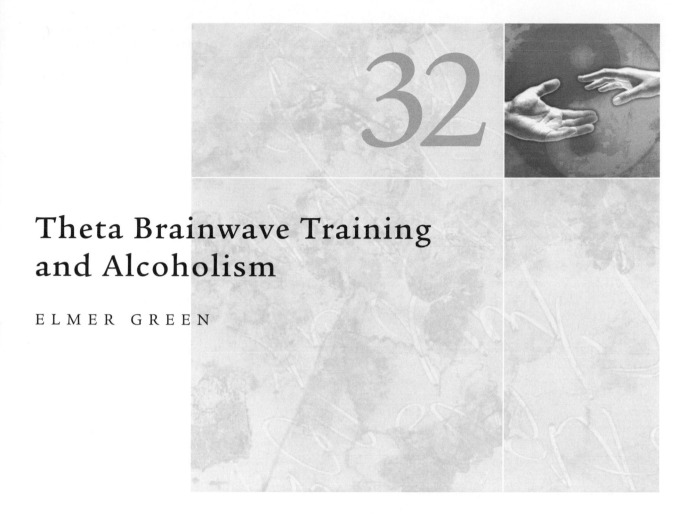

# Theta Brainwave Training and Alcoholism

ELMER GREEN

## ABSTRACT*

An alpha-theta brainwave biofeedback training program was applied as a novel treatment technique for chronic alcoholics. Following a temperature biofeedback pretraining phase, experimental subjects completed 15 30-minute sessions of alpha-theta biofeedback training. Compared with a nonalcoholic control group and a traditionally treated alcoholic control group, alcoholics receiving brainwave training (BWT) showed significant increases in percentages of electroencephalogram (EEG) records in alpha and theta rhythms and increased alpha rhythm amplitudes. Alcoholics receiving BWT showed a gradual increase in alpha and theta brain rhythms across the 15 experimental sessions. These experimentally treated alcoholics showed sharp reductions in self-assessed depression (Beck Depression Inventory) compared with the control groups. Alcoholics receiving standard medical treatment (abstinence, group psychotherapy, antidepressants) showed a significant elevation in serum beta-endorphin levels at the conclusion of the experiment. This neuropeptide is an index of stress and a stimulant of caloric (e.g., ethanol) intake. Application of BWT, a relaxation therapy, appears to counteract the increase in circulating beta-endorphin levels seen in the control group of alcoholics. Follow-up data at 13 months indicate

*From Peniston EG, Kulkosky PJ: Alpha-theta brainwave training and beta-endorphin levels in alcoholics, *Alcohol Clin Exp Res* 13:271-279, 1989.

sustained prevention of relapse in alcoholics that completed alpha-theta BWT.

## COMMENTARY

### Background

The psychologist Eugene (Gene) Peniston originated theta brainwave training (TBT) for addictions. He got his breakthrough idea for biofeedback-assisted control of alcoholism from his own hypnagogic imagery, which surfaced during a theta-training workshop in the Voluntary Controls Program of the Menninger Foundation in July 1987. Gene had "interrogated the unconscious" and asked for information on how best to work with alcoholics. He was rewarded with detailed procedures, which worked when he tried them at the Veterans Administration Hospital in Fort Lyons, Colorado.[1,2]

Interestingly, a few of our theta students (Dr. Green refers to his patients as "students" and "trainees"—Ed), after becoming deeply quiet and focusing attention inward, had full-blown "tunnel experiences," and contacted their High Self, similar to well-authenticated near-death experiences—but fortunately they didn't have to nearly die to get the body, emotions, and mind to quiet down enough to allow hypnagogic imagery to surface. In other words, without spending years meditating, some students reached one of the goals of meditation in a few days. They "discovered" their own High Self via auditory or visual hypnagogic imagery, and a new life opened up for them.

### Methodology

We use 24-channel multielectrode brainwave machines for research in the Life Sciences Institute and for analysis of unusual EEG problems, but we have found that 90% or more of what we wish to accomplish in theta training with addicts can be done with one active electrode placed over the left visual cortex. Placing the electrode on the left occiput is essential for most students because when the eyes are closed and that area is persuaded to "go into theta," the trainee's normal visual and auditory imagery shuts down and the mental monitor goes blank, ready to receive projections of hypnagogic imagery from a normally unconscious section of the psyche, the High Self.

In "wiring up" for a session, a circular electrode about ½ inch in diameter is positioned approximately 1 inch to the left of center at the back of the head and is held in place against the scalp by a Velcro headband. Electrical contact with the scalp is made with a salt gel, then, because trainees have skulls and scalps of different thickness, we adjust three "thresholds" for simultaneous feedback of beta, alpha, and theta rhythms, indicated by high, midrange, and low tones in earphones.

After a few minutes of eyes-closed relaxation, students begin to detect the way in which their thought processes affect the electrical rhythms of the left visual cortex and start learning how to turn on and off the various tones. First they practice physical heaviness and warmth, as in autogenic training. Then, as minutes pass, the three tones of the EEG machine signal an elimination of beta, then a reduction of alpha, and finally bursts of theta rhythm. What is important here is that the body, emotions, and mind become simultaneously quiet. If anything twitches—muscles, emotions, or thoughts—the theta tone goes away.

### Theory

There are two additional options in theta training other than (a) going through the tunnel and contacting the High Self or (b) backing out of the program: namely, (c) turning to the side to begin exploring the bardo (the astral realm described by Tibetans in their *Book of the Dead*), i.e., becoming a psychic traveler on the astral planes, or (d) focusing attention downward into the personality to modify mind, emotions, and physical body according to the will of the ego. The latter option, modifying the physical body without High-Self guidance, is what many Indian yogis do to demonstrate their "spiritual" powers, especially when they publicly display remarkable autonomic control, such as "regurgitating" the stomach itself.

Aside from obvious distortions, psychological dangers are often ignored in following (c) or (d). Egoistic self-importance and willpower can become so inflated that the student begins to believe that he or she is a spiritual power and refuses to sacrifice the ego at the entrance to the tunnel that leads to the transpersonal psyche. This can become a personality disaster, at least for the present lifetime.

Fortunately, alcoholics and other addicts have already suffered enough ego loss to be willing to accept hypnagogic advice from their own High Self, the "Being of Light" on the other side of the tunnel. Consequently option (a), going through "the door" during theta training, leads to insight and self-empowerment and sets back to "normal" the satiety center in the brain, whose homeostatic balance point has been chronically shoved aside by the self-indulgence of substance abuse.

## Final Points

TBT allows one to "logon" to the transpersonal mind-net that has also been called the Transpersonal Collective Unconscious, á la Carl Jung. At the same time the trainee comes face to face with his or her subconscious and superconscious "selves" and begins to recognize, communicate with, and negotiate with them.

However useful TBT may be as a rehabilitation therapy, it must be realized that it is merely a mindfulness training technique. It can take you to the inner door, the entrance to the "tunnel" of the average near-death experience, but then you must decide what to do. The theta brainwave teacher, like the leader Morpheus in the 1998 movie *The Matrix,* can guide you, much like the student Neo, to the Oracle's "door," to the "secret place within," but after that you are on your own.

When Morpheus took Neo to visit the Oracle, his exact words were, "I told you I can only show you the door. You have to walk through it." In theta training the EEG feedback machine is the doorknob, and intention and self-reliance open the door. When the door is open, hypnagogic dream-like imagery floods into consciousness. This imagery is discussed with students at the end of sessions, of course, but is never interpreted for them. This is the time-tested Rogerian method of Client-Centered Therapy. Socrates and Plato taught in the same way.

Learning to interpret one's own hypnagogic imagery is part of the student's task in theta training. This particular skill helps a person communicate with every part of his or her composite psyche. Incidentally, the main virtue needed in the theta instructor, we have found, is humility, i.e., elimination (as much as possible) of pride as a teacher. As a result, whatever progress is made builds the student's self-respect, self-esteem, and self-reliance—major goals of theta training for alcoholics.

Interestingly, we have observed during 30 years of biofeedback training that a number of students get full theta-state effects from standard thermal and muscle-tension training, without EEG feedback, and I learned to go into the theta state at will by practicing Mindfulness Meditation under a teacher's guidance. Therefore it is safe to say that theta training, along with all other forms of biofeedback, merely accelerate progress in contacting the High Self.

Of all the techniques I have investigated, though, TBT has proven to be the speediest, and, fortunately, as with every other type of biofeedback training used in rehabilitation, it needs no metaphysical explanation to make it work.

## References

1. Peniston EG, Kulkosky PJ: Alpha-theta brainwave training and beta-endorphin levels in alcoholics, *Alcohol Clin Exp Res* 13:271, 1989.
2. Fahrion SL: Human potential and personal transformation, *Subtle Energies* 6(1):55, 1995.

# Laser Acupuncture and Carpal Tunnel Syndrome

MARGARET A. NAESER

## ABSTRACT*

**Objective.** To access outcome of carpal tunnel syndrome (CTS) patients who previously failed standard medical/surgical treatments treated primarily with a painless, noninvasive technique using red-beam, low-level laser acupuncture and microamps transcutaneous electrical nerve stimulation (TENS) on the affected hand and secondarily with other alternative therapies.

**Design.** Open treatment protocol—patients diagnosed with CTS by their physicians.

**Setting.** Treatments performed by licensed acupuncturist in a private practice office.

**Subjects.** Total of 36 hands from 22 women and 9 men, ages 24 to 84 years, median pain duration 24 months; 14 hands failed 1 to 2 surgical release procedures.

**Intervention/treatment.** Primary treatment: red-beam, 670-nm, continuous wave, 5-mW diode laser pointer (1 to 7 joules [J] per point), and microamps TENS (<900 μA) on affected hands. Secondary treatment: infrared low-level laser (904 nm, pulsed, 10 W) and/or needle acupuncture on deeper acupuncture points; Chinese herbal medicine formulas and supplements on case-by-case basis; three treatments per week, 4 to 5 weeks.

**Outcome measures.** Pretreatment and posttreatment Melzack pain scores; profession and employment status recorded.

**Results.** Posttreatment, pain significantly reduced (p <0.0001), and 33 of 36 hands (91.6%) showed no

*From Branco K, Naeser MA: Carpal tunnel syndrome: clinical outcome after low-level laser acupuncture, microamps transcutaneous electrical nerve stimulation, and other alternative therapies—an open protocol study, *J Altern Complement Med* 5(1):5-26, 1999.

pain or pain reduced by >50%. All 14 hands that failed surgical release were successfully treated. Patients remained employed, if not retired. After 1 to 2 years, only 2 of 23 hands (8.3%) in patients <60 years of age had pain return; pain retreated within a few weeks.

**Conclusions.** Possible mechanisms for effectiveness include increased adenosine triphosphate (ATP) on cellular level, decreased inflammation, temporary increase in serotonin. There are potential cost savings with this treatment (current estimated cost per case = $12,000; this treatment = $1,000). Safe when applied by licensed acupuncturist trained in laser acupuncture; supplemental home treatments may be performed by patient under supervision of acupuncturist.

## COMMENTARY

### Potential Cost Savings

Surgery is performed in approximately 40% to 45% of CTS cases, with estimates of more than 460,000 procedures performed each year and a direct medical cost of over $1.9 billion.[7] A new conservative treatment for CTS is needed that would be applicable in the earlier stages of the disorder to permit continued employment, prevent disability, and reduce the need for surgery. LLLT plus microamps TENS applied to acupuncture points is one new conservative treatment. Our results suggest that mild or moderate CTS cases who have median nerve motor latencies that are <7 msec (sensory latencies may be absent) and who have no abnormality on EMG are excellent candidates for this type of treatment.[5,6,8]

The estimated cost to treat one case of CTS without surgical intervention in the United States is approximately $5,246.[9] The cost to provide treatment for one case of CTS with LLLT and microamps TENS is approximately $1,000 ($65 per office visit × 15 visits = $975). Thus there is a potential savings of at least $4,000 per mild to moderate CTS case who is treated with this new conservative method. Supplemental home treatments[10] are also possible with a current equipment cost of approximately $550. (The cost of a 5-mW red-beam laser diode is about $150, and the cost of the microamps TENS device used here is $400.)

In his study with LLLT to treat CTS, Weintraub[6] concluded that LLLT appears to be an attractive substitute for surgery. Our results support that conclusion, especially when this new conservative treatment is applied at the appropriate time (earlier stages, preferably within 1 year of symptom onset) and with the appropriate CTS cases (mild to moderate cases, as defined with nerve conduction studies, who have no abnormality on needle EMG). Based on these initial positive results, further research with LLLT and microamps TENS to treat a large number of CTS cases who meet these criteria would be appropriate. A range of 12 to 15 treatments is recommended.[8]

## FDA Regulations

LLLT is considered investigational by the FDA. No medical claims of cures are permitted in the United States at this time. The Naeser and Wei[3] laser acupuncture introductory textbook has a 48-page addendum that explains the FDA regulations from written materials from the 1980s. However, current understanding is that if low-level lasers are defined as coming within a state's scope of medical practice (as they are in Massachusetts for licensed acupuncturists), the FDA will not interfere if the acupuncturist does not make any medical claims of cures with LLLT.

There is an independent institutional review board (IIRB) for laser acupuncture research in Massachusetts with which the licensed acupuncturist may register his or her laser and laser acupuncture treatment protocols for specific disorders. This board is limited to acupuncturists in Massachusetts. The acupuncturist also obtains informed consent from each patient. There have been no problems or patient complaints in Massachusetts since the laser acupuncture IIRB has been in effect (1994). If more controlled research studies with LLLT are presented to the FDA, perhaps LLLT could be removed from the "Class III, Investigational Use" category in the United States.

## FUTURE AREAS FOR RESEARCH

There are multiple areas in which LLLT and laser acupuncture have promising application. In the area of neurological rehabilitation, these areas were reviewed in part in the report for the National Institutes of Health (NIH) Consensus Development Conference on Acupuncture.[11] The areas reviewed include treatment of paralysis in stroke,[12] spasticity in babies and children with cerebral palsy,[13] spinal cord injury,[14] Bell's palsy,[13] and pain in CTS.[3-6,8]

One advantage of LLLT is that it has the potential for daily treatment, and even for home treatment. Neurological conditions often require long-term treatment, and the advantage of supplemental home treatments cannot be underestimated. While TENS devices have long been used for self-administered home treatments, the use of LLLT for home treatment is new. This may take some time for medical staff, patients, and family members to accept. However, my experience has been uniformly positive when home treatments have been performed in a consistent, responsible manner.

While Mester's original work with red-beam LLLT[16] focused on wound healing, over the past 2 decades LLLT has also been used successfully to treat acute and chronic pain associated with musculoskeletal injuries, arthritic conditions, and postherpetic neuralgia.[17-24] In addition, LLLT has been used to treat a wide variety of other disorders. For example, LLLT has been used to significantly reduce postoperative vomiting in children. A 660-nm, 10-mW laser was used to stimulate acupuncture point PC 6 for 30 seconds, beginning 15 minutes before induction of anesthesia and 15 minutes after surgery.[25] Also, postoperative pain and the need for analgesia was significantly reduced for adults undergoing cholecystectomy if the surgical wound was treated for 6 to 8 minutes with a 830-nm, 60-mW laser immediately following skin closure before emergence from general anesthesia.[26] Red-beam LLLT has also been observed to significantly reduce allergic rhinitis if intranasal illumination is applied for 4.4 minutes, 3 times per day (6 J per day).[27] The beneficial antiinflammatory effect of LLLT has also been observed in alopecia areata cases who were treated within the first 2 years of onset. The usual dose is 4 to 8 J/cm² of red-beam LLLT applied to the bald patches 3 times per week (every other day) for 4 to 5 weeks.[2,28] Another promising use of LLLT is for the treatment of inner ear disorders, including tinnitus.[29] Improvement has been observed in over 800 cases treated with a combination of red-beam laser (630 to 700 nm) and near infrared laser (830 nm) applied into and surrounding the ear, with a total dosage of at least 4,000 J per 60-minute session. The patient is treated for 10 days as an outpatient, and supplemental home treatments are performed as necessary.

Future research with laser acupuncture should include early intervention with neurological disorders including stroke cases (within hours of onset), babies and children with cerebral palsy and/or delayed motor and speech development (preferably within 2 weeks post-birth for those hypoxic at birth—otherwise, before

---

## Websites and E-Mail Addresses

*General LLLT Information*
Extensive references and excellent information on worldwide LLLT research. Prepared by the Swedish Laser Society: www.laser.nu

*General Laser Acupuncture Information*
Web page (prepared by M. Naeser) helps answer questions from acupuncturists interested in laser acupuncture: www.Acupuncture.com/Acup/laser.htm

*Laser Acupuncture for Carpal Tunnel Syndrome and Repetitive Strain Injury*
Photographs demonstrating how therapy is performed (prepared by M. Naeser) help answer questions regarding laser acupuncture research to treat CTS and RSI: www.Acupuncture.com/Acup/Naeser.htm

*LLLT on Acupuncture Points for Spinal Cord Injury*
Prepared by Albert Bohbot, MD, France. Contains case histories and videotapes of patients before and after a series of treatments: www.laserponcture.net

*Low-Level Laser Acupuncture*
Prepared by Dr. Anu Makela, Finland, who conducts low-level laser acupuncture research in many areas, including diabetes mellitus and neurological disorders: anu.makela@icon.fi

*Laser Calculation Program for J/cm²*
Program (prepared by Scott Deuel, DC, Castle Rock, Colorado) calculates the number of seconds required to = 1 J, or the number of seconds required to = 1 J/cm² (continuous wave or pulsed wave) for a specific laser when provided with the mW output power and the diameter of the laser beam for that laser: LLLTDC@aol.com

*North American Association for Laser Therapy*
NAALT is a non-profit organization for practitioners interested in LLLT in the United States: www.naalt.org

1 or 2 years of age in those where development is slow), Bell's palsy cases (within 3 days of onset), spinal cord injury cases (within hours of the accident), herpes zoster cases (within the first few days, thus preventing development of postherpetic neuralgia), and rheumatoid arthritis cases (acute phase). LLLT is painless, noninvasive, and with-out negative side effects. This intervention may be considered complementary to many of the current treatments. However, in some cases stronger antiinflammatory agents may not always be necessary in conditions in which they would otherwise be a primary treatment.

## References

1. Seitz LM, Kleinkort JA: Low-power laser: its applications in physical therapy. In Michlovitz SL, Wolf SL, (eds): *Thermal agents in rehabilitation,* Philadelphia, 1986, FA Davis, pp 217-238.
2. Naeser MA, Wei XB: *Laser acupuncture: an introductory textbook for treatment of pain, paralysis, spasticity and other disorders,* Boston, 1994, Boston Chinese Medicine.
3. Wong E, Lee G, Zucherman J, et al: Successful management of female office workers with "repetitive stress injury" or "carpal tunnel syndrome" by a new treatment modality: application of low level laser, *Int J Clin Pharmacol Ther* 33(4):208-211, 1995.
4. Weintraub MI: Noninvasive laser neurolysis in carpal tunnel syndrome, *Muscle Nerve* 20:1029-1031, 1997.
5. Naeser MA, Hahn KK, Lieberman B: Real vs. sham laser acupuncture and microamps TENS to treat carpal tunnel syndrome and worksite wrist pain: pilot study, *Lasers Surg Med Suppl* 8:7, 1996.
6. Naeser MA, Hahn K, Lieberman B, et al: Carpal tunnel syndrome pain treated with laser acupuncture and microamps TENS, *Arch Phys Med Rehabil* In Press.
7. Vennix MJ, Hirsh DD, Faye YCT, et al: Predicting acute denervation in carpal tunnel syndrome, *Arch Phys Med Rehabil* 78:306-312, 1998.
8. Branco K, Naeser MA: Carpal tunnel syndrome: clinical outcome after low-level laser acupuncture, microamps transcutaneous electrical nerve stimulation, and other alternative therapies—an open protocol study, *J Altern Complement Med* 5(1):5-26, 1999.
9. Clairmont A: Economic aspects of carpal tunnel syndrome, *Arch Phys Med Rehabil* 8(3):571-576, 1997.
10. Naeser MA, Hahn C, Lieberman BE: *Naeser Laser Home Treatment Program for the Hand: an alternative therapy to treat painful symptoms of carpal tunnel syndrome and repetitive strain injury,* Catasauqua, Penn, 1997, The American Association of Oriental Medicine.
11. Naeser MA: Neurological rehabilitation: acupuncture and laser acupuncture to treat paralysis in stroke and other paralytic conditions and pain in carpal tunnel syndrome.
12. Naeser MA, Alexander MP, Stiassny-Eder D, et al: Laser acupuncture in the treatment of paralysis in stroke patients: a CT scan lesion site study, *Am J Acupunct* 23(l):13-28, 1995.
13. Asagai Y, Kianai H, Miura Y, et al: Application of low reactive-level laser therapy (LLLT) in the functional training of cerebral palsy patients, *Laser Ther* 6:195-202, 1994.
14. Rochkind S: Laser therapy in neuroscience, neurosurgery and neurorehabilitation. In Tuner J, Hode L, (eds): *Low level laser therapy: clinical practice and scientific background,* Grangesberg, Sweden, 1999, Prima Books, pp 276-279.
15. Wu XB: 100 Cases of facial paralysis treated with He-Ne laser irradiation on acupoints, *J Tradit Chin Med* 10(3):300, 1990.
16. Mester E, Mester AF, Mester A: The biomedical effects of laser application, *Lasers Surg Med* 5:31-39, 1985.
17. Fukuuchi A, Suzuki H, Inoue K: A double-blind trial of low reactive-level laser therapy in the treatment of chronic pain, *Laser Ther* 10:59-64, 1998.
18. Goldman JA, Chiapella J, Casey H, et al: Laser therapy of rheumatoid arthritis, *Lasers Surg Med* 1:93-101, 1980.
19. Kemmotsu O, Sato K, Furumido H, et al: Efficacy of low reactive-level laser therapy for pain attenuation of postherpetic neuralgia, *Laser Ther* 3:71-75, 1991.
20. Kleinkort JA, Foley RA: Laser acupuncture: its use in physical therapy, *Am J Acupunct* 12(1):51-56, 1984.
21. McKibben LS, Downie R: Treatment of postherpetic pain using a 904 nm low-energy infrared laser, *Laser Ther* 2:20, 1990.
22. Palmgren N, Jensen GF, Kaae K, et al: Low-power laser therapy in rheumatoid arthritis, *Lasers Med Sci* 4:193-196, 1989.
23. Soriano F, Rios R: Gallium arsenide laser treatment of chronic low back pain, *Laser Ther* 10:175-180, 1998.
24. Walker J: Relief from chronic pain by low power laser irradiation, *Neurosci Lett* 43:339-344, 1983.
25. Schlager A, Offer T, Baldissera I: Laser stimulation of acupuncture point P6 reduces postoperative vomiting in children undergoing strabismus surgery, *Br J Anaesth* 81:529-532, 1998.
26. Moore KC, Hira N, Broome IJ, et al: The effect of infrared diode laser irradiation on the duration and severity of postoperative pain, *Laser Ther* 4:145-149.
27. Neuman I, Finkelstein Y: Narrow-band red light phototherapy in perennial allergic rhinitis and nasal polyposis, *Ann Allergy Asthma Immunol* 78:399-406, 1997.
28. Trelles MA, Mayayo E, Cisneros JL: Alopecia areata treated by He/Ne laser, *Invest Clin Laser* 1(84):15-17, 1984.
29. Wilden L: The effect of low level laser light on inner ear diseases. In Tuner J, Hode L, (eds): *Low level laser therapy,* Grangesberg, Sweden, 1999, Prima Books.

In NIH Consensus Development Conference on Acupuncture, Office of Alternative Medicine and Office of Medical Applications of Research, Bethesda, Md, Nov 3-5, 1997, pp 93-109.

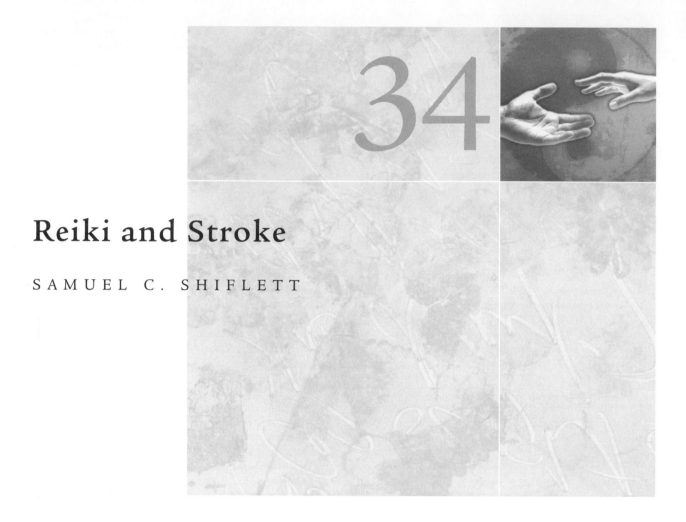

# Reiki and Stroke

SAMUEL C. SHIFLETT

## ABSTRACT*

**Objectives.** There were three objectives in this study: (1) to evaluate the effectiveness of Reiki as an adjunctive treatment for subacute stroke inpatients receiving standard rehabilitation, (2) to evaluate a double-blind procedure for training Reiki practitioners, (3) to determine whether double-blinded Reiki and sham practitioners could determine which condition they were in.

**Design and setting.** The design was a modified double-blind placebo controlled clinical trial with an additional historical control condition. The setting was a stroke unit of a major rehabilitation hospital. Fifty patients (31 male and 19 female) with subacute ischemic stroke were in this study.

**Interventions.** There were four conditions: Reiki master, Reiki practitioner, sham Reiki, and no treatment (historical control). Subjects received up to 10 treatments over a 2½ week period, in addition to standard rehabilitation.

**Outcome measures.** Functional Independence Measure (FIM) and the Center for Epidemiologic Studies Depression (CES-D) Scale were used.

**Results.** No effects due to Reiki were found on the FIM or CES-D, although typical effects due to age, gender, and time in rehabilitation were detected. Blinded practitioners (sham or Reiki) were unable to determine which condition they were in. Sham-Reiki

*This research was supported by National Institutes of Health Grant U24-HD32994. Material presented here is based on a manuscript by SC Shiflett, S Nayak, C Bid, P Miles, S Agostinelli, under review.

practitioners reported greater frequency of feeling heat in the hands compared to Reiki practitioners. There was no reported difference between the sham and the real Reiki practitioners in their ability to feel energy flowing through their hands. Post hoc analyses suggested that Reiki may have had limited effects on mood and energy levels.

Conclusion. Reiki did not have any clinically useful effect on stroke recovery in subacute hospitalized patients receiving standard-of-care rehabilitation therapy. Selective positive effects on mood and energy were not due to attentional or placebo effects.

## COMMENTARY

Healing touch, or laying on of hands, has been used for thousands of years for healing by manipulating nonphysical energy that supposedly permeates the physical body. Reiki (pronounced *ray-kee*), a form of energy healing that originated in Japan in the 1800's, has become an increasingly popular and accessible alternative healing technique throughout the West. It usually involves a practitioner's laying his or her hands lightly on specific locations on the head and torso of the person being treated.[1,2] Despite anecdotal reports of the effectiveness of Reiki for various health problems, research on this technique is very limited. Conditions studied include hemoglobin and hematocrit values[3,4] and dental surgery pain.[5] Other research suggests that Reiki, as with other touch therapies, has its primary effect on relaxation and stress reduction, sometimes accompanied by changes in immune indicators.[6]

While no formal research has been located that involves treatment of stroke, several informal claims by Reiki practitioners of improvement after stroke and brain injury were encouraging enough to consider further investigation of the technique in a controlled research design. Other interventions that involve subtle energy, or *chi,* as an explanatory model, specifically acupuncture, have shown some success in improving the speed and degree of functional recovery after stroke.[7-10] As limited as it is, this body of evidence suggests that it would be important to test the effectiveness of Reiki as a subtle energy intervention supporting standard rehabilitation in patients who had recently suffered a stroke.

The research design consisted of a randomized, placebo-controlled, double-blind procedure involving three treatment arms and a no-treatment historical control arm. Outcome measures included the Functional Independence Measure (FIM)[11] and the Center for Epidemiologic Studies Depression Scale (CES-D) measure of depressed mood.[12] Subjects were 38 inpatients at Kessler Institute for Rehabilitation, admitted as a result of an ischemic stroke. An initial average FIM item score of 4 or less was required to ensure that a patient's condition was at least moderately severe so as to reduce a possible ceiling effect on improvement in the patient's condition.

There were three treatment conditions: Reiki master, Reiki practitioner, and sham Reiki. The treatment protocol was the same in all conditions and involved lightly placing the hands on 12 locations on the patient's head and torso over a period of 30 minutes per treatment. Each patient received up to 10 treatments over a 2½-week period.

The Reiki master was a fully trained and initiated Reiki practitioner in the Usui system (Reiki Alliance) and had been practicing Reiki for over 10 years. She trained a total of 14 Kessler healthcare deliverers (nurses, physical therapists, and occupational therapists), who served as treaters. Half of the treaters received the full first-degree training (including initiation, or attunement, which is required to be a true Reiki practitioner); the other half learned the same techniques, but without initiation, and served as practitioners in the sham-Reiki control condition. Because initiation was the only aspect of training that distinguished Reiki training from non-Reiki training, the trainees were blinded to the condition they were in by the use of a special initiation procedure that did not involve the usual practice of the master touching them in a ritualistic manner. This procedure was explained to all trainees before they agreed to participate, and all were debriefed and sham Reiki practitioners were initiated into Reiki upon completion of the study.

## SELECTED RESULTS

In addition to the main factor of treatment group for the FIM, patient gender was included as a factor when preliminary analyses indicated that this was a potential moderator of functional independence. The main effect for treatment group, which is the primary test of our hypothesis, was not significant ($p > 0.50$) and thus did not confirm the hypothesis that Reiki would help in functional recovery during subacute stroke rehabilitation. However, the gender main effect was significant (F = 4.24; $p$ <0.05) and indicated that, regardless of treatment condition, males had a better recovery FIM than females. Although it does not achieve statistical significance, the gender x group interaction suggests that this finding may reflect a tendency for males to respond to Reiki whereas women do not, possibly because they appear to naturally improve more than do males, as happened in this study. CES-D post-treatment scores were analyzed using analysis of covariance (ANCOVA) with age; initial FIM score (as a correction for severity of impairment) and initial CES-D score entered as covariates. As expected, posttreatment depression was associated with pretreatment depression (F = 26.87; $p$ <0.001). There was a slight tendency for age to be related to depression at discharge from hospital, indicating that younger patients were more depressed than older patients (F = 3.89; $p$ <0.08). There were no other effects that even approached significance. The main effect for the treatment group did not reach statistical significance; thus the hypothesis that Reiki would help with mood was not supported. Using a Bonferroni procedure to correct for multiple tests, the analyses of the CES-D yielded a significant result on one item: "I can't get going," with the same pattern also present in several other items but not at the statistically significant level. Subjects in both the Reiki master and the Reiki practitioner conditions show a substantial increase in the ability to "get going," while the sham practitioner subjects actually report being less able to "get going."

When asked about their own perceptions, sham-Reiki practitioners unexpectedly reported greater frequency of feeling heat in the hands compared to Reiki practitioners. There was no reported difference between the sham and the real Reiki practitioners in their ability to feel energy flowing through their hands.

## SUMMARY

The lack of a detectable effect resulting from Reiki casts doubt on its ability to have a clinically meaningful effect in a medical condition where there is rapid natural improvement accompanied by rehabilitation-based improvement. Despite a number of successes, even the more invasive intervention of acupuncture has had some failures in showing positive results under these circumstances.[13,14] The finding of a possible gender interaction is certainly unexpected, but it con-

firms a similar finding from our laboratory involving post-stroke dysphagia patients receiving acupuncture (unpublished data). The possibility of gender effects in energy healing must be controlled for and possibly explored as a previously unrecognized phenomenon.

## References

1. Rand WL: *Reiki: the healing touch,* Southfield, Mich, 1991, Vision Publications.
2. Borang KK: *Thorson's principles of Reiki,* London, 1997, Thorson.
3. Wetzel WS. Reiki healing: a physiologic perspective, *J Holist Nurs* 7:47-53, 1989.
4. Wirth DP, Chang RJ, Eidelman WS, et al: Haematological indicators of complementary healing intervention, *Complement Ther Med* 4:14-20, 1996.
5. Wirth DP, Brenlan DR, Levine RJ, et al: The effect of complementary healing therapy on postoperative pain after surgical removal of impacted third molar teeth, *Complement Ther Med* 1:133-138, 1993.
6. Wardell DW, Engebretson J: Evaluation of Reiki touch healing, *J Adv Nurs* 33:439-445, 2001.
7. Johansson K, Lindgren I, Widner H, et al: Can sensory stimulation improve the functional outcome in stroke patients? *Neurology* 43:2189-2192, 1993.
8. Magnusson M, Johansson K, Johansson BB. Sensory stimulation promotes normalization of postural control after stroke, *Stroke* 25:1176-1180, 1994.
9. Wong AM, Su TY, Tang FT, et al: Clinical trial of electrical acupuncture on hemiplegic stroke patients, *Am J Phys Med Rehabil* 78(2):117-122, 1999.
10. Kjendahl A, Sallstrom S, Osten PE, et al: A one year follow-up study on the effects of acupuncture in the treatment of stroke patients in the subacute stage: a randomized, controlled study, *Clin Rehabil* 11(3):192-200, 1997.
11. Deutsch A, Braun S, Granger CV: The Functional Independence Measure and the Functional Independence Measure for Children: ten years of development, *Crit Rev Phys Med Rehabil* 8:267-281, 1996.
12. Shinar D, Gross CR, Price TR, et al: Screening for depression in stroke patients: the reliability and validity of the Center for Epidemiologic Studies Depression Scale, *Stroke* 17:241-245, 1986.
13. Johansson BB, Haker E, von Arbin M, et al: Acupuncture and transcutaneous nerve stimulation in stroke rehabilitation: a randomized, controlled trial, *Stroke* 32(3):707-713, 2001.
14. Gosman-Hedstrom G, Claesson L, Klingenstierna U, et al: Effects of acupuncture treatment on daily life activities and quality of life: a controlled, prospective, and randomized study of acute stroke patients, *Stroke* 29(10):2100-2108, 1998.

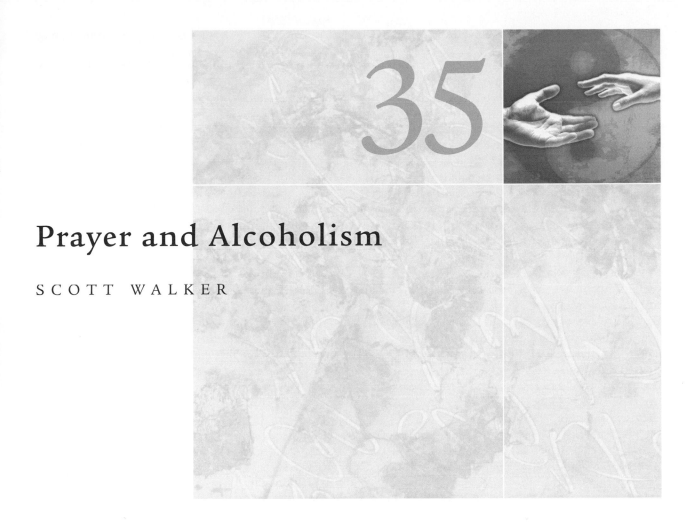

# Prayer and Alcoholism

SCOTT WALKER

## ABSTRACT*

**Objective.** To conduct a pilot study of the effect of intercessory prayer on patients entering treatment for alcohol abuse or dependence.

**Design.** In addition to standard treatment, 40 patients admitted to a public substance abuse treatment facility for treatment of alcohol problems who consented to participate were randomized to receive or not receive intercessory prayer (double blind) by outside volunteers. Assessments were conducted at baseline, 3 months, and 6 months.

**Results.** No differences were found between prayer intervention and nonintervention groups on alcohol consumption. Compared with a normative group of patients treated at the same facility, participants in the prayer study experienced a delay in drinking reduction. Those who reported at baseline that a family member or friend was already praying for them were found to be drinking significantly more at 6 months than were those who reported being unaware of anyone praying for them. Greater frequency of prayer by the participants themselves was associated with less drinking, but only at months 2 and 3.

**Conclusion.** Intercessory prayer did not demonstrate clinical benefit in the treatment of alcohol abuse and dependence under these study conditions. Prayer

*From Walker SR, Tonigan JS, Miller WR, et al: Intercessory prayer in the treatment of alcohol abuse and dependence: a pilot investigation, *Altern Ther Health Med* 3(6).79-86, 1997.

may be a complex phenomenon with many interacting variables.

## COMMENTARY

Funded by the newly formed National Institutes of Health Office of Alternative Medicine, I and many volunteers completed a research study of intercessory prayer (prayer offered on behalf of someone else) in the treatment of alcoholism. Prayers were offered by experienced volunteers from the community for one half of consenting, randomly assigned clients entering a public substance abuse treatment program. The study was designed in a prospective, randomized, double-blind, intent-to-treat protocol. The methods and results have been published elsewhere.[1]

On average, as expected when entering treatment, over time the clients reduced their consumption of alcohol. Although we did not have the statistical power to demonstrate a clear benefit for those receiving the outside intercessory prayers, there were other interesting and challenging findings deserving further investigation.

Those clients who reported that they were saying prayers for themselves with greater frequency drank less than the others, although only at months 2 and 3 of the follow-up. In future research, evaluation of prayer for oneself needs to assess qualitative dimensions of prayer in addition to frequency.

Step 11 of Alcoholics Anonymous[2] condones seeking "through prayer and meditation improved conscious contact with God as we understand Him." Research has found that different types of prayer are associated with different experiences.[3,4] Intuitive, meditative, or contemplative prayer (depending on whose system of nomenclature one is using) is most associated with the experience of contact with God. Twelve-step or religiously oriented treatment programs might enhance their clients' experience by teaching different types and methods of prayer. Research could evaluate acceptance and use of different types of prayer and subsequent outcomes.

We also found that clients involved in the study took longer to reduce their alcohol consumption compared with a normative group of clients also entering the treatment program. This delay in reducing alcohol consumption (regardless of whether a client was assigned to the prayer intervention group) suggests that even the expectation of a spiritual intervention may influence outcomes.

Three-armed studies are rare in medical research, but rigorous design may be needed to ferret out complex interactions and perhaps at times negative or unexpected influences. Innovative control groups may be necessary. Past experience with religion, prayer, and spirituality that affects attitude and receptiveness may be a key factor in whether a client responds to such interventions. Spiritual interventions likely require a multidimensional assessment of interactions between, and effects on, the "giver" and the "receiver." Indeed one study found more benefit for the "givers" of intercessory prayer.[5]

Of particular importance was the finding that at the beginning of the study about half of the clients were so socially disconnected that they were unaware of anyone offering prayers on their behalf. The other half reported that they knew of at least one family member praying for them. Surprisingly, those receiving prayer from family members did significantly less well over time (were drinking more at follow-up) than those who reported that they were not aware of anyone praying for them. Given that 90% of the U.S. population prays,[6] the possibility of negative effects from prayer needs thoughtful consideration by researchers and practitioners of prayer. Indeed one national survey found that one in five persons surveyed admitted to intentionally praying for harm to others.[7] Such "imprecatory" prayer has been explored elsewhere.[8]

Unconscious and conscious attitudes may be important in intercessory prayer. It is not only stigmatized members of our culture who need to be concerned. Our "loved ones" for whom we have personal resentments, fears, judgments, and control agendas may also be influenced by our prayers.

After the publication of this study, I heard surprisingly little response to the implied possibility that prayer by family could be associated with harm. It was as if an embarrassing topic were being publicly aired. One irate response I received stated, "My God is good and would never harm anyone." This is certainly my experience; therefore I had to explore the implications: What is happening when we pray?

The ubiquitous practice of cursing, hexing, and prayer to harm others speaks to a belief (consciously acknowledged or not) that prayers can be answered by beings other than a loving Higher Power, (perhaps one's Lower Power[s]). Most religions throughout history posit a dualistic (or more complex) structure to creation.

They encompass creative and destructive forces and beings (good, evil, and otherwise). Rather than ignore the wisdom of saints and seers, modern researchers need to consider the possibility that prayer may invoke destructive forces in addition to beneficent ones.

Apart from invoking third-party spiritual beings (God, saints, angels, demons, etc.) is the likelihood that much of what we call prayer involves direct psychic influence. That is to say, our directed will, wishes, or intent have potency to influence others in their own right. The extensive body of research into our psychic connection and mutual influence is becoming more accessible to the public.[9,10]

I believe that the spiritual and psychic realms are distinct, although interactive with each other. The lack of conceptual differentiation is problematic. Intuitive awareness and psychic potency can be confused with advanced spirituality. A metaphor would be the relationship between air and lungs. They interpenetrate and transform each other—each provides meaning and form for the other—yet each retains its own distinct properties and essence.

Those who practice energy medicine are aware that "energy follows thought." I suggest that Spirit rides on thoughts, emotions, and intentions that are aligned with a higher wisdom and intent ("Thy will be done"). In my experience, Spirit does not violate free will and does not participate in prayer that has judgment or the intent to violate the free will of another (even "for their own good"). When prayer intentions involve control, revenge, self-righteousness, spiritual pride, or similar motivations, perhaps they act with their own psychic force, or they may also engage other, less beneficent influences.

When examining psychic and spiritual influences one discovers that there are many currently known and unknown subtleties that may not be detectable by standard questionnaires and measuring instruments. Future research may need to examine the "immeasurable" by including individuals with a high degree of awareness beyond the usual five senses. We must develop novel methods of bringing the best of scientific method into such intuitive investigation. Tools of systematic examination to reduce illusion, deception, and wish fulfillment and to account for observer effects need to be adapted to the nonphysical realms. The benefit of scientific rigor was demonstrated by this study in findings that challenge basic assumptions such as the belief that all prayer is good.

## References

1. Walker SR et al: Intercessory prayer in the treatment of alcohol abuse and dependence: a pilot investigation, *Altern Ther Health Med* 3(6):79-86, 1997.
2. *Alcoholics Anonymous,* ed 3, New York, 1976, Alcoholics Anonymous World Services.
3. Hood RW, Spilka B, Hunsberger B, et al: *The psychology of religion: an empirical approach,* ed 2, New York, 1996, The Guilford Press.
4. Poloma MM, Gallup GH: *Varieties of prayer: a survey report,* Philadelphia, 1991, Trinity Press International.
5. O'Laoire S: An experimental study of the effects of distant, intercessory prayer on self-esteem, anxiety, and depression, *Altern Ther Health Med* 3(6):38-53, 1997.
6. Gallup GD: *Fifty years of Gallup surveys on religion,* The Gallup Report, Report No. 236, 1985.
7. Gallup Poll published in *Life,* March 1994.
8. Dossey L: *Be careful what you pray for . . . you just might get it: what we can do about the unintentional effects of our thoughts, prayer, and wishes,* San Francisco, 1997, HarperSanFrancisco.
9. Radin D: *The conscious universe: the scientific truth of psychic phenomena,* San Francisco, 1997, HarperEdge.
10. Targ R, Katra J: *Miracles of the mind,* Novato, Calif, 1998, New World Library.

# 36

# Functional Brain Imaging and Meditation

SARA LAZAR

HERBERT BENSON

## ABSTRACT*

Meditation is a conscious mental process that induces a set of integrated physiological changes termed the *relaxation response*. Functional magnetic resonance imaging (fMRI) was used to identify and characterize the brain regions that are active during a simple form of meditation. Significant (p $<10^{-7}$) signal increases were observed in the group-averaged data in the dorsolateral prefrontal and parietal cortices, hippocampus/parahippocampus, temporal lobe, pregenual anterior cingulate cortex, striatum, and pre- and post-central gyri during meditation.

Global fMRI signal decreases were also noted, although these were probably secondary to cardiorespiratory charges that often accompany meditation. The results indicate that the practice of meditation activates neural structures involved in attention and control of the autonomic nervous system.

## COMMENTARY

As their name implies, mind-body techniques consist of conscious mental exercises that bring about changes in both the mind and the body. Relaxation techniques such as meditation, hypnosis, and biofeedback can result in widespread changes in autonomic measures despite the fact that the subject is sitting quietly throughout the treatment. The integrated changes in autonomic activity have been termed the relaxation response and are thought to be the opposite of the stress response.[1]

Although numerous studies have documented the ability of relaxation response techniques to change

*From Lazar SW, Bush G, Gollub RL, et al: Functional brain mapping of the relaxation response and meditation, *Neuroreport* 11(7):1581-1585, 2000.

peripheral measures, the inability to observe direct brain activity elicited by these activities has limited our understanding of this half of the dynamic. Two neuroimaging techniques (fMRI and positron emission tomography [PET]) have been developed over the last 10 to 15 years that allow scientists to watch the activity of the brain while it executes a variety of tasks. These imaging techniques are now being used to explore what happens in the brain during mind-body interventions.

The use of neuroimaging techniques has provided several important contributions to the understanding of mind-body interventions. First, there has been some debate in the literature concerning whether meditation induces a discrete state distinct from simple rest or early stages of sleep. The neuroimaging results unambiguously resolve this dispute by clearly demonstrating that the patterns of brain activity that occur during meditation are different than the patterns that occur during sleep or simple rest.

Intriguingly, these first studies also indicate that there is not one unique "meditative state" but rather that practice of different styles of meditation (e.g., Kundalini or Buddhist meditation or yoga relaxation) lead to different patterns of brain activity. This is in line with subjective reports of meditation practitioners, who describe qualitatively different mental states after practicing these different styles of meditation.

Efforts are now being made to better define these states, both relative to each other and in comparison with more traditional states of consciousness. Meditation styles are now sometimes classified as either "mindfulness" or "concentration," based on the overall subjective effects of the practice. Some researchers have used comparisons of different styles of meditation to shed some light on the neural basis of consciousness.[2]

We have employed fMRI to study the neural activity generated during the practice of Kundalini meditation. Our studies show that multiple neural regions throughout the entire brain are used during the practice of meditation. Areas involved in attention and arousal such as the anterior cingulate and frontoparietal cortices, as well as regions involved in emotion processing such as the amygdala and basal ganglia, are recruited during meditation. Interestingly, although the conscious mental task the subjects perform i.e., observation of the breath and repetition of a mantra, during Kundalini meditation does not change, neural activity in these brain regions do change over time. This suggests that a change in mental state is occurring slowly during the meditation session. This is consistent with the subjective reports of experienced meditators, who claim their meditative state will gradually change and deepen throughout a regular practice session. In addition, the data indicate that regions involved in autonomic control, such as pontine respiratory centers and the hypothalamus, are activated during meditation as well.[3,4]

Efforts are now underway to understand how changes in the mind are related to changes in the body. Using fMRI, which records changes in neural activity on the time scale of a few seconds, we can identify spontaneous changes in brain activity that occur simultaneously with changes in peripheral measures. Such an understanding will begin to shed light on how thoughts and feelings in the mind can modulate the autonomic nervous system and influence health and well-being.

## SUMMARY

These experiments show that the mind cannot be separated from the body. Here, the mind was performing a task (i.e., repeating a sound or prayer). As documented by fMRI, this repetition led to specific reproducible changes in the brain in areas dealing with the autonomic nervous system and with attention. These changes in the brain led to changes in the body because mind and body are inseparably connected.

Medicine must evolve to a more balanced approach, viewing health and well-being as a three-legged stool: the first leg composed of pharmaceutical products, the second leg composed of surgery and interventional procedures, and the third leg one of self-care. A crucial component of self-care, along with lifestyle changes such as diet and exercise, will be the wide range of mind/body therapies.

## References

1. Benson H, Beary JF, Carol MP: The relaxation response, *Psychiatry* 37:37-46, 1974.
2. Lou HC, Kjaer TW, Friberg L, et al: A 150-H20 PET study of meditation and the resting state of normal consciousness, *Hum Brain Map* 7:98-105, 1999.
3. Lazar SW, Bush G, Gollub RL, et al: Functional brain mapping of the relaxation response and meditation, *Neuro Rep* 11(7):1581-1585, 2000.
4. Newberg A, Alavi A, Baime M, et al: The measurement of regional cerebral blood flow during the complex cognitive task of meditation: a preliminary SPECT study, *Psychiatry Res* 106(2):113-122, 2001.

# Therapeutic Touch and Phantom Limb Pain

ERIC D. LESKOWITZ

## ABSTRACT*

Phantom limb pain (PLP) is a widespread condition that responds poorly to conventional medical and surgical treatments. A case report is presented of the successful treatment of phantom leg pain in a 62-year-old man with peripheral vascular disease using the complementary medical technique of Therapeutic Touch (TT). The clinical and research literature of TT is briefly reviewed with regard to subjective outcome measures such as pain and anxiety, as well as to several objective measures of physiological function.

The possible role of nonspecific factors such as placebo responsiveness or hypnotic dissociation in this case are considered, as are the applicability of complementary and alternative medicine (CAM) to PLP, the neurological mechanisms that generate phantom sensations, and the possible mechanism of action of TT.

## COMMENTARY

The article summarized in the abstract is in fact only a very preliminary piece of work. While its findings are striking and suggestive, they require much confirmatory work before they can be considered conclusive. To

---

*From Leskowitz ED: Phantom limb pain treated with therapeutic touch: a case report, *Arch Phys Med Rehabil* 81:522-524, 2000.

summarize the work briefly, several cases of PLP—a notoriously difficult-to-treat form of chronic pain that occurs after a limb has been amputated—responded well to an energy-based therapy called *Therapeutic Touch (TT)*. This positive outcome might have been due to the power of suggestion or to nonspecific placebo effects, but there are two particular aspects of this treatment that force us to look beyond simplistic explanations and that hold great promise for new uses of CAM in rehabilitation. That potential is the focus of this commentary.

PLP patients have had limbs amputated for various medical or traumatic reasons, yet they feel severe pain in the empty space where their limb used to be. In TT, nurses smooth out their patient's purported energy field by moving their hands in a stroking motion near the surface of the patient's body, never making actual physical contact. Yet, improbably, both the patient and the therapist can feel a palpable sensation whenever the therapist's physical hands come close to the patient's phantom limb. This happens often enough and has been reported by enough other hands-on energy therapists that I no longer believe it to be a coincidental event. I doubt it is due to the power of suggestion because in my treatment sessions I intentionally avoid making leading comments about what the patient is likely to feel, and over the years I have developed a pretty good sense of when I am kidding myself.

Obviously the biomedical model of reality has no way of accounting for these unusual perceptions. According to this view, phantom pain is caused by the activity of the cerebral cortex, which in effect creates a hallucinatory sensation stemming from baseline nerve activity in the amputation stump. Remember that no nerves even exist in the painful phantom limb to generate these distal pain impulses. Of course this also means that no nerves exist out there in the apparently empty space where the phantom limb lies that might relay sensory signals from my hand to the patient's central nervous system (CNS).

So how can patients feel TT in their phantom limb, and what is it that the TT practitioner is feeling? I think these two phenomena can only be explained by a dramatic paradigm shift: Both anomalous sensations are mediated by the subtle energy field, not by the CNS. The TT practitioner feels the energy field of the patient, the electromagnetic template that underlies our physiology, while the patient's phantom limb is an active energy template that can also register perceptions from the field of the therapist's hand.

An exact analogy exists in physics: When iron filings outline the lines of force from a hidden bar magnet, they reveal the existence of an otherwise invisible level of subtle energy organization. The human body has a similar underlying organizational template, and phantom limbs offer a unique opportunity to visualize this subtle field without the distraction of the denser physical "glove" that usually covers the energetic "hand." I think it is only a matter of time before an imaging technology is developed (perhaps related to so-called Kirlian photography) that can actually picture this energy phantom in a more objectively verifiable manner than when my hands subjectively perceive the nonphysical domain.

Because our culture today places more faith in technology than in human subjective experience, I think we need to await this technological breakthrough before the full significance of PLP is recognized. Similarly, I believe that this energy field can transmit sensations and perceptions to the patient's awareness, even in the absence of neurons. That is because it is a matter of subtle, rather than gross, anatomy and physiology at work. When it is finally produced, this high-quality photographic image of the energy pattern underlying a phantom limb will constitute definitive proof of the validity of the subtle energy model of human anatomy and physiology. It will confirm what the mystics have been saying for thousands of years in a way that can be heard and accepted by the medical mainstream, not just by the initiates to the inner world of CAM. This will then open the door to full acceptance of man's multidimensional nature, of body, mind, and spirit. Because this energy matrix is felt to be only the densest level of a whole range of subtle energies, and because there are more refined layers that have a more spiritual quality to them, I think that the study of these layers will also help to explain many of the phenomena of distant healing.

It is not just in science fiction that one can talk about treating PLP by regenerating the missing limb. A biomagnetic researcher, Robert Becker, who was the orthopedic surgeon who developed transcutaneous electrical nerve stimulation (TENS) units to treat chronic pain, has actually induced the regeneration of amputated limbs in rats, a species that normally does not have the capacity to regenerate, by applying an altered magnetic field around the amputation stump. Perhaps it will someday be possible to couple molecular biology and DNA technology with novel electromagnetic devices to create a suitable energetic template for the regrowth of human structures like amputated limbs.

Perhaps it will someday become possible to bridge this physical gap in spinal cord transected patients, using energetic rather than structural connectors. If nerve connections are too infinitely complex to rewire, then perhaps a "short-circuiting" via subtle energy bonding may do the trick. This is one possible explanation for Dr. Chow's findings in Chapter 16 that Qigong therapy can restore movement after paralysis and it may be applicable in a wider range of spinal cord injury patients.

## SUMMARY

The scope of rehabilitation could expand greatly if we learn to shift our focus away from simply rearranging the iron filings atop the ailing magnetic field and focus instead on recharging, strengthening, and rebalancing the underlying biomagnetic field itself. When we are able to do this, then the iron filings—the cells of our body—can effortlessly reorient themselves in alignment with the newly healthy organizational energy matrix. Seen from this energy field perspective, rehabilitation's potential is unlimited.

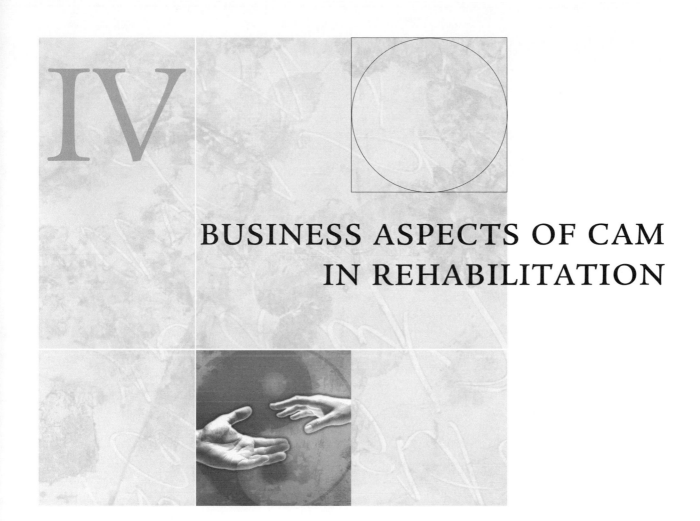

# BUSINESS ASPECTS OF CAM IN REHABILITATION

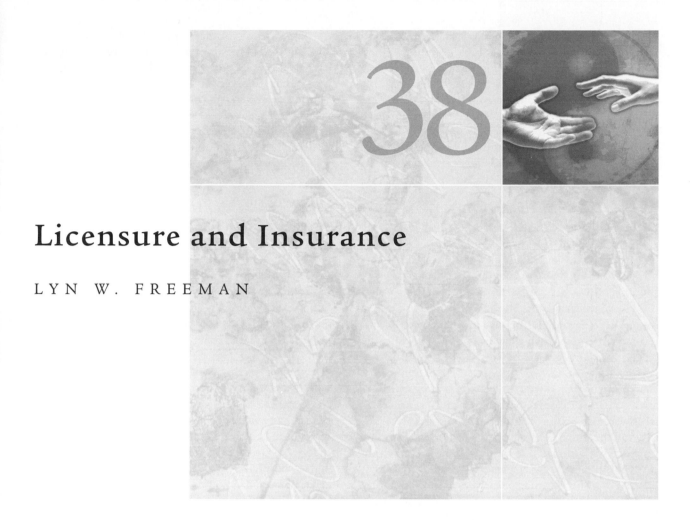

# Licensure and Insurance

LYN W. FREEMAN

The issues, law, and politics (public and governmental) surrounding licensure and insurance in complementary and alternative medicine (CAM) are complex and ever changing. This chapter is not intended to educate the reader in every aspect of CAM licensure and insurance. Instead, it provides an overview of these two important areas and points the reader to sources and websites that provide specific, state-by-state data on CAM licensure.

## HOW PREVALENT IS CAM?

In 1997 Eisenberg and colleagues performed a random household telephone survey of 1,539 adults in the United States. The question at issue was the individual and public use of CAM. More than 42% of individuals interviewed said that they had used an alter-native therapy within the last year. Of persons using an alternative therapy, 46% had visited an alternative practitioner for their care.

Eisenberg et al[1] had performed a similar study in 1990. Between 1990 and 1997, the reported public use of alternative therapies increased by more than 47%, making the use of complementary medicine one of the fastest growing healthcare trends in the United States.[2] The estimated number of visits to alternative practitioners in 1997 was more than 629 million, exceeding the total visits to all U.S. primary care physicians.

Individuals were not replacing allopathic medical care with CAM but were more typically using both at the same time. More than 15 million individuals, representing 18.4% of all prescription users, reported taking prescription medications during the same period they were taking herbal remedies or high-dose vitamins. InterActive Solutions' 1997 survey[3] of 1,500 persons confirmed Eisenberg's findings. They concluded that 42% of the population had used alternative care in the past year. Of those using CAM, 74% used those therapies in conjunction with conventional care. These two surveys confirmed that CAM is most commonly used by persons suffering from chronic conditions, including back pain, anxiety, depression, and headaches.

## CHRONIC DISEASE AND CAM USE

Other studies have also confirmed that patients suffering from chronic conditions turn to alternative therapies for additional care. Krauss et al[4] surveyed individuals with physical disabilities and discovered that a disabled population was more likely to use alternative therapies than a general population not suffering from physical disabilities. Astin's national survey[5] asked patients why they used CAM. He found that poor health status and chronic conditions of anxiety, back problems, pain, and urinary tract problems were predictors of alternative medical use. A variety of chronic diseases have been demonstrated to improve with alternative therapy use. They include cardiovascular disease; hypertension; asthma; ulcers; HIV/AIDS; the chronic pain caused by cancer, fibromyalgia, back pain, neck pain, headache, arthritis, and severe burns; epilepsy; anxiety; depression; and drug and alcohol addiction.[6]

In October 2000 at the Harvard/Stanford conference "Complementary and Alternative Medicine: Practice Applications and Evaluations," preliminary findings of an ongoing study were presented. Daniel Cherkin of the Seattle-based Group Health Cooperative Center for Health Studies summarized representative data on four major types of CAM providers and their patients. He discovered that roughly 75% of naturopathic and acupuncture patients and 50% of chiropractic and massage therapy patients receive treatment for chronic conditions. John Weeks,[7] editor of *The Integrator for the Business of Alternative Medicine,* commented on the implications of these findings for the delivery of medical care. It is generally accepted that allopathic medicine is less effective for treatment of chronic than acute conditions. However, CAM produces its best results for treatment of chronic disease states.

Research outcomes support the public's belief in CAM as a beneficial rehabilitative intervention for chronic medical conditions. In fact, 67% of the public report that availability of alternative care is an important factor in determining what healthcare plan they will select.[3] The public has wielded substantial power in determining whether insurance companies and health maintenance organizations (HMOs) will pay for CAM therapies.

## INSURANCE, HEALTH MAINTENANCE ORGANIZATIONS, AND CAM

In 1995, Washington was the first state in the nation to require health insurers to cover alternative therapies as part of their healthcare plans. The legislature added a new section to the state code regulating insurance that stated that all healthcare plans regulated by the insurance commissioner should be required to "Permit every category of health care provider to provide health care services or care for conditions included in the basic health plan services to the extent that the provision of such health services or care is within the health care provider's permitted scope of practice."[8] Despite ongoing litigation, there is considerable compliance with the law, no doubt in part because of public demand.

In 1996, west coast HMOs and insurance companies began to offer some type of CAM coverage as an optional plan. Those companies included Group Health Cooperative of Puget Sound in Washington State, Blue Cross of Washington and Alaska, PacifiCare and Regents' Blue Cross/Blue Shield of Oregon, and Health Net in California. The majority of larger HMOs in California also offer optional acupuncture and chiropractic care.

In 1997, the HMO organization Oxford Health Plans began providing its members access to CAM therapies that included acupuncture; chiropractic; yoga; massage therapy; nutritional counseling; and, in Connecticut, naturopathy. Patients could be referred by their primary care physician or seek out CAM treatment directly without referral.[8] Many insurance companies and HMOs have been concerned that the addition of CAM therapies would be costly. James Dillard, Oxford's medical director of complementary medicine, states that offering alternative therapies raised Oxford's employee premiums by only 3%.

In 1998 and 1999, National Market Measures conducted a study for Landmark Healthcare, Inc.,[9] to examine alternative care from the viewpoint of HMOs. Surveyed were 114 senior executives from 449 HMOs. The survey sample represented 25% of the entire universe of HMOs in the United States, and the survey revealed that two-thirds of the HMOs (67%) already offered at least one form of alternative care, usually chiropractic (65%) or acupuncture (31%). HMOs considering future offerings of CAM stated that they were most likely to add acupuncture, acupressure, massage therapy, or vitamin therapy over the next 2 to 3 years.

HMO executives offering CAM said that they did so primarily because their members, employers, and groups asked for it (38%); because it was required by law or mandate (38%); because it was clinically effective (8%); to differentiate themselves from their competitors (7%); to meet the competition (5%); or to attract new members (4%). Of HMO executives surveyed, 21% believed that CAM offerings would reduce total healthcare costs; 30% believed that CAM would have a neutral impact on total healthcare costs; and 49% believed that CAM offerings would increase their healthcare costs. In addition, 85% of HMO executives stated that the relationship between allopathic and alternative medical care providers would grow closer, and 47% perceived the relationship between the two medical approaches as "complementary."[6]

HMO executives believed that consumer demand will continue; 40% viewed the growth of demand as moderate, 34% viewed it as strong, and 27% viewed it as mild. No HMO executive believed that there would be no future public demand for CAM therapies.

It is inevitable that practicing health professionals will need to adapt to the integration of conventional and complementary medicine. Marla Orth, CEO of Landmark, stated, "With nearly 70% [of insurance companies and HMOs] offering some CAM, we have a good indication of where the industry is going to go."[10] HMO executives identified one primary motivator driving them to offer CAM: "Demand, demand, demand, demand, demand." Qualifications and credentials are considered to be more important when choosing CAM providers than when choosing allopathic providers. Insurance companies continue to broaden their coverage. While discount products dominate recent Blue Cross offerings, several pilot programs are underway that cover acupuncture and chiropractic and, in one case, even allow a CAM practitioner to serve as primary care provider.[11]

Innovative inroads have been created for HMO coverage of CAM. Simultaneously, research is being conducted on the outcomes of true integrative care. The prime example is the negotiated relationship being forged between HMOs and research organizations. Oxford Health Plans and the Integrative Medicine Center, jointly sponsored by Yale University and Griffin Health System, are piloting "the most integrative medicine-friendly and financially valuable relationship between an HMO and an integrative clinic to date."[12] Oxford pays for an initial coevaluation by an MD and naturopathic physician team. This joint visit is a distinctive feature of this model. Oxford additionally pays for two to three follow-up visits, patients pay their customary copayments, and the clinic shares annual reporting and clinical outcomes data with Oxford. The extended benefits were actively advertised via direct mailing to HMO members. James Dillard, Oxford's medical director, feels that the program has been successful so far. Data and analysis on this 12-month venture will be complete sometime in 2002.

Preliminary data presented by Daniel Cherkin (Group Health Cooperative Center for Health Studies) found that roughly 8% to 30% of patients seeing massage therapists or licensed acupuncturists were currently covered by insurance for their treatments while 50% to 70% of patients seeing chiropractors and naturopaths had some coverage for their CAM care.[13] Although the research was skewed toward coverage by the inclusion of Washington State providers who operate under the state's 1995 "every category of provider" mandate, the findings are still significant. They demonstrate the continuing movement by insurance companies to cover complementary treatments, and Cherkin's study revealed a significant source of data on CAM use, with the potential for future analysis of CAM treatment outcomes. This information, sitting in the computers of many large health plans, can be analyzed to assess the most cost-effective uses for CAM therapies. Cherkin also discovered that while between 18% and 53% of patients in all provider categories were also seeing an MD or an osteopath for simultaneous care, only 5% to 13% of the cases studied demonstrated any form of communication between the allopathic and complementary care provider. This suggests that integration has not yet resulted in provider cross-communication. Organizational policies that foster or require cross-communication between providers may be required to break the historical barriers that prevent communication between allopathic and complementary care providers.

## FEAR AND OTHER BARRIERS TO CAM

### Federation of State Medical Boards and CAM

Historically the Federation of State Medical Boards (FSMD) has been antagonistic toward MD involvement with CAM. Until 2 years ago, FSMD investigated CAM practices via the Special Commission on Health Care Fraud. In 1999, the group was renamed as Special Committee on Questionable and Deceptive Health Care Practices. Although the name change was meant to imply that there was some possible value in CAM interventions, the recommended CAM literature in the FSMB handout was dominated by the writings of William Jarvis, PhD; Victor Herbert, MD, JD; and Stephen Barrett, PhD. These three authors have been referred to as the "triumvirate who have made a living for two decades as quack busters, generally attacking all CAM, regardless of evidence."[14] Recently, James Winn, executive Vice President of FSMB, announced that David Eisenberg, MD (Harvard University's Center for Complementary and Alternative Medicine); Ken Pelletier, PhD (head of Stanford's CAM program); and Russell Greenfield, MD (a fellow at the Integrative Medicine Program, University of Arizona Health Sciences Center) have been named special consultants to FSMB. Winn further stated that physician fears of persecution if they employ alternative treatments are probably overstated. Indeed, only 5 of 4,500 FSMB action reports in 1999 involved CAM use by MDs.

Recently Tennessee, Texas, Illinois, and Kentucky all added position statements regarding CAM practice by physicians. These positions statements clarified which practices violate the state's medical practice acts. Tennessee came out against the practice of chelation except in the case of heavy metal poisoning or as part of a controlled trial; Texas required MDs to use an informed consent form with patients when practicing unconventional treatments; and Illinois and Kentucky list treatments as invalidated, nonvalidated, and validated. *Nonvalidated* refers to therapies having a basis in scientific theory but as yet unproven. Winn ex-

pects that more states will develop CAM guidelines and that valuable CAM research will come from MD practice of CAM.

### Physician Fear of Liability From Patient Referral to CAM Practitioners

Physicians or organizations may be unduly concerned with liability related to referral of patients to alternative medicine practitioners, especially if those practitioners are licensed and accredited.[15] When considering referral, the physician should ask four questions to determine if a referral or the use of alternative therapies poses potential liability. Those questions are

1. Is there good evidence to suggest that the therapy under question will offer no benefit to the patient in question or will subject the patient to unreasonable risk?
2. Does the physician have any special knowledge or experience that leads him or her to be concerned about the competency or practices of the particular practitioner under consideration for referral or use? For example, does the physician or organization already know of some conduct on the part of the practitioner that points to incompetence?
3. Is the alternative professional licensed in the state in which he or she will practice? Does the alternative professional carry his or her own liability insurance? (Although this is not typically a requirement, this would be an added benefit.)
4. Will this be a typical referral (i.e., will the referral constitute "arm's length" involvement, without ongoing supervision of the alternative practitioner as he or she manages patient care?).

If the referring medical provider can answer no to the first two questions, and yes to the last two, the likelihood is that the alternative professional alone would bear the burden of any harm should it occur.[2,16]

## CREDENTIALING OF CAM PROVIDERS

Depending on the category of care, CAM providers can be credentialed through a process of licensure, certification, or registration. Licensure is the most rigorous level of regulation and restricts the scope of practice so that it is illegal for unlicensed individuals to provide specific services. Certification is less restrictive and requires the practitioner to meet standards set by a stage agency that may designate a title, suggesting certification. Registration means the practitioner files his or her name and address with a state agency. Registration is considered appropriate only when there is little possibility of consumer harm from the intervention. Insurance companies typically only reimburse and HMOs only provide the services of CAM professionals who are licensed or certified.

## Developing a Model for Credentialing and Quality Assurance

Alternative Paths to Health was developed by Harvard Vanguard Medical Associates in November of 1997 and offers acupuncture, chiropractic care, and massage therapy at eight locations.[16] Although the CAM professionals providing care are not Harvard Vanguard employees, criteria for provider selection and credentialing has been strictly established. CAM providers are identified by referral from staff and alternative clinicians and by resume. Potential providers respond to a request for proposal (RFP) explaining Harvard Vanguard's practice guidelines. Interested applicants must provide information on their clinical practice, experience, and ability to meet expectations.

Promising candidates take part in a series of interviews to assess clinical and patient interaction skills, and candidates are asked to demonstrate their skills. When a candidate is tentatively selected, professional references are explored, including references from experts in the candidate's field. Selected providers sign a provider contract and a lease or fee agreement.[2]

In the Harvard Vanguard program, chiropractors and acupuncturists must be licensed in the state where they practice. Chiropractors are expected to be members of the American Chiropractic Association (ACA); acupuncturists, members of the National Commission for the Certification of Acupuncturists (NCCA); and massage therapists, members of the American Massage Therapists Association (AMTA) or the National Certification Board for Therapeutic Massage and Bodywork (NCBTMB.)

## Quality Assurance

Quality assurance is assessed by (1) patient satisfaction surveys; (2) interviews at program sites with conventional medical staff who share patients with the alternative providers; (3) alternative practitioner satisfaction surveys to determine the adequacy of staff support and practitioner satisfaction with program management, space, and practices; and (4) medical record audits. Universal precaution and confidentiality training is required of all Harvard Vanguard medical professionals. Peer review is also a component of quality assurance.

## Credentialing Standards

The credentialing program includes the components of (1) licensure, certification, or registration; (2) minimum malpractice and general liability insurance coverage; (3) investigation into previous state or local authority disciplinary actions; (4) membership in professional organizations; and (5) examination of continuing education efforts.

## Scope of Practice for Major Categories of CAM

In the United States, alternative medicine care is legislated in three ways: (1) provider acts that regulate a CAM practice by requiring licensure, registration, or certification; (2) single references in a statute that define the scope of practice; and (3) provisions of medical practice or disciplinary acts that authorize physicians or other providers to use alternative medicine modalities.[17]

State laws requiring licensure confer practice rights and detail the scope of practice and the academic or other qualifications required to receive licensure. However, in some states, laws conferring certification or registration may not significantly differ in language from licensure requirements. In the following pages we review the provider practice acts related to specific categories of CAM. Those categories include acupuncture, chiropractic, homeopathy, massage, naturopathy, Therapeutic Touch (TT), hypnosis, meditation, and imagery. For each category, information will be broken down by definition, scope of practice, regulation and authority, and sources of additional information.

# ACUPUNCTURE

## Definition

Acupuncture is described as the stimulation of acupuncture points in the body with needles for therapeutic purposes. The purpose of this therapy is to modify the perception of pain, normalize physiological functions, and treat bodily disease. Acupuncture works by correcting the balance of chi, the vital energy or life force that flows through 12 major energy pathways called meridians. The meridians are linked to specific internal organs or organ systems and to 361 acupuncture points.[18,19]

## Scope of Practice

Acupuncture is currently regulated by practice acts in 31 states and the District of Columbia.[20] Most states enacted laws after James Reston's favorable 1971 account of acupuncture in the *New York Times*.[21] In states where acupuncture practice acts have not been enacted, acupuncture practice rights may be limited to designated medical professions or granted to nonphysician acupuncturists who are under medical supervision. State enactments allow acupuncturists to use a variety of therapies. Although therapies vary from state to state, they may include the use of herbs, vitamins, and minerals; infrared treatments; oriental medical therapies; dietary guidelines and lifestyle counseling; mechanical, thermal, electrical, and electromagnetic treatment; cupping; moxibustion; exercise therapies; acupressure; breathing techniques; laser acupuncture; point injection therapy; and dermal friction.

## Regulation and Authority

The administrative structure for acupuncture varies state to state. Some states maintain regulatory authority via acupuncture boards composed of nonphysician acupuncturists. In those states, acupuncture may be regulated under a broader board authority for "acupuncture and oriental medicine" or just "oriental medicine." In other states, acupuncture is regulated under the auspices of a medical board that relies on a secondary acupuncture board or committee. Still other states regulate acupuncture within a state agency and with the assistance of an acupuncture unit.

Licensure is the most common method of acupuncture authorization, although some states may use registration or certification forms. Acupuncture registration or certification requirements are often similar in structure and law to the requirements of states that invoke acupuncture licensure. In some states, provider practice acts rely on mixed forms of authorization by requiring licensure and registration or by mandating a choice of registration or certification.[22] Some states have required nonphysician acupuncturists to be under the supervision of a licensed physician or some other medical provider. The right to practice acupuncture may be extended to other health providers. Practice rights may be extended to MDs, osteopaths, chiropractors, physician assistants, naturopaths, homeopaths, podiatrists, nurses, veterinarians, and dentists.

An interesting use of acupuncture is for the treatment of substance abuse. Authority to use acupuncture as part of substance abuse treatment is formally recognized in the statutory law of several states. In these states, individuals who do not meet the state qualifications of a licensed acupuncturist can still administer acupuncture as treatment for substance abuse (alcohol or chemical dependence). The individuals must be properly trained for this limited use of acupuncture and treatment must be administered through an approved hospital or clinical program. Those administering acupuncture in this limited form must still be under the supervision of a physician, dentist, or licensed acupuncturist.[23]

# CHIROPRACTIC

## Definition

Chiropractors work on the musculoskeletal system of the body (i.e., bones, joints, muscles, ligaments, and tendons). The focus of chiropractic is the spine and nervous system, and the hallmark of chiropractic care is the spinal adjustment. Chiropractic spinal adjustments may be delivered with high or low velocity (speed), as short or long lever (direct application to spinous processes vs. using arms and legs as fulcrums), high or low amplitude (force), and with or without recoil. Procedures are directed at specific joints or anatomical regions and may involve cavitation or gapping of a joint that produces an audible "pop" sound. The intent of the chiropractic adjustment is the cor-

*Sources of Additional Information*

Accreditation Commission for Acupuncture and
   Oriental Medicine (ACAOM)
1010 Wayne Avenue, Suite 1270
Silver Spring, MD 20910
(301) 608-9680
(301) 608-9576 FAX

The American Association of Acupuncture and
   Oriental Medicine (AAAOM)
433 Front Street
Catasauqua, PA 18032
(610) 266-1433
(610) 264-2768 FAX
aaom1@aol.com
www.aaom.org/

   AAAOM assisted in the formation of both the National Commission for the Certification of Acupuncturists (NCCA, now NCCAOM) and the National Council of Acupuncture Schools and Colleges (NCASC, now CCAOM) and administers a stringent national certification process based on recognized standards of competence and education.

The American Academy of Medical Acupuncture
   (AAMA)
4929 Wilshire Blvd, Suite 428
Los Angeles, CA 90010
(323) 937-5514
(323) 937-0959 FAX
E-mail: jdowden@prodigy.net
www.medicalacupuncture.org

Acupuncture and Oriental Medicine Alliance
14637 Starr Road SE
Olalla, WA 98359
(253) 851-6896
(253) 851-6883 FAX
www.AcupunctureAlliance.org

   This website contains a wealth of information, including a list of states with statutes, regulations, and bills in progress; an overview of state laws and regulations; a summary of eligibility and examination requirements for licensure; and state licensing boards. It also contains information on upcoming conferences and workshops, as well as publications of interest.

National Certification Commission for Acupuncture
   and Oriental Medicine (NCCOAM)
11 Canal Center Plaza, Suite 300
Alexandria, VA 22314
(703) 548-9004
(703) 548-9079 FAX
www.nccaom.org

   This website contains information on certification and state regulations, certification programs, and professional development activities.

rection of subluxation, i.e., the structural dysfunction of joints and muscles.[24] Another way to describe a chiropractic adjustment is a very fast but highly controlled thrust of specific force applied directly to the bony processes. Chiropractors are trained to thrust into a spinal joint with an exact amount of force and speed, producing correct realignment of the spine.

## Scope of Practice

Practice acts provide for a broad range of therapeutic techniques and vary from state to state. Practice laws may authorize chiropractors to incorporate di-
etary advice and nutritional care (including vitamins and herbal recommendations) as part of their care. Some states forbid chiropractors from prescribing or profiting from the recommendation of specific vitamins and food supplements. Colonic irrigation may be ruled within the scope of practice for chiropractors, or chiropractors may be required to obtain additional certification before offering this ancillary procedure. In Arizona and Colorado chiropractors are permitted to practice acupuncture as part of their practice. In Louisiana and Ohio they are prohibited from practicing acupuncture. The general physical exam is considered an integral part of chiropractic care in some states and not within the chiropractic

## Sources of Additional Information

American Chiropractic Association
1701 Clarendon Blvd.
Arlington, VA 22209
(800) 986-4636
(703) 243-2593 FAX
www.amerchiro.org

Federation of Chiropractic Licensing Boards
901 54th Avenue, Suite 101
Greeley, CO 80634
(970) 356-3500
(970) 356-3599 FAX
www.fclb.org

International Chiropractors Association
1110 N Glebe Road, Suite 1000
Arlington, VA 22201
(800) 423-4690
(703) 528-5023 FAX
E-mail: chiro@chiropractic.org
www.chiropractic.org

National Association for Chiropractic Medicine (NACM)
15427 Baybrook Drive
Houston, TX 77062
(281) 280-8262
(281) 280-8262 FAX
www.chiromed.org

NACM is a consumer advocacy association of chiropractors who confine their scope of practice to scientific parameters and seek to make legitimate the use of professional manipulative procedures in mainstream healthcare delivery. It offers consumer assistance in finding member practitioners.

National Board of Chiropractic Examiners (NBCE)
901 54th Avenue
Greeley, CO 80634
(970) 356-9100
(970) 356-6134 FAX
E-mail: nbce@nbce.org
www.nbce.org

NBCE is the principal testing agency for the chiropractic profession. Established in 1963, it develops and administers standardized national examinations according to established guidelines.

scope of practice in others. The argument that chiropractors are limited to spinal manipulation has arisen in a variety of contexts. In other states (Alaska, for example) the scope of practice includes "counseling on dietary regimen, sanitary measures, physical and mental attitudes affecting health, personal hygiene, occupational safety, lifestyle habits, posture, rest, and work habits that enhance the effects of chiropractic adjustment."[23] Some states include x-ray examination, urine analysis, taking or ordering blood tests and other routine laboratory tests, and the performance of physical exams.

## Regulation and Authority

Chiropractors have well-established practice acts in every state. However, chiropractic boards have different requirements for education, scope of practice, and continuing education requirements. It is important to review the criteria for the jurisdictions in which the

chiropractor is licensed. Many chiropractors hold licenses in more than one jurisdiction. The Federation of Chiropractic Licensing Boards website (see the box above) displays the practice acts for all states.

## HOMEOPATHY

## Definition

Homeopathy is a system of medicine based on the use of infinitesimal doses of medicines capable of producing symptoms similar to those of the disease treated.[25]

## Scope of Practice

Homeopathic practice acts currently exist in only three states: Arizona, Connecticut, and Nevada. In states that do not have homeopathic practice acts, the right to practice may still be recognized under the

## Sources of Additional Information

The Foundation for Homeopathic Education and
    Research
2124 Kittredge Street
Berkeley, CA 94704
(510) 649-0294 (inquiries/catalog requests)
(800) 359-9051 (orders within the U.S.)
(510) 649-1955 FAX
E-mail: mail@homeopathic.com
www.homeopathic.com

Educational Resources
Homeopathic Education Services
2124 Kittredge Street
Berkeley, CA 94705
(510) 649-0294
(510) 649-1955 FAX
www.homeopathic.com

National Center for Homeopathy (NCH)
801 N Fairfax Street, Suite 306
Alexandria, VA 22314
(703) 548-7790
(703) 548-7792 FAX
www.homeopathic.org

*Certification Bodies and Degrees*
American Board of Homeotherapeutics
801 N Fairfax Street, Suite 306
Alexandria, VA 22314
(703) 548-7790
(703) 548-7792 FAX
www.homeopathyusa.org/specialtyboard/

Diplomate Certification Contact: George Guess, MD,
    DHt, President
2776 Hydraulic Road #5
Charlottesville, VA 22903
    The certifying body for MDs and osteopaths that can
issue a doctorate in homeotherapeutics (DHt)

Homeopathic Academy of Naturopathic Physicians
    (HANP)
Susan Wolfer, Executive Director
12132 SE Foster Place
Portland, OR 97266
(503) 761-3298
(503) 762-1929 FAX
E-mail: hanp@igc.apc.org
www.healthy.net/HANP/
    Provides doctoral certification (DHANP) in home-
opathy for naturopaths.

Council for Homeopathic Certification (CHC)
PO Box 12180
La Crescenta, CA 91224-0880
(866) 242-3399
(818) 541-9173 FAX
E-mail: hswope@igc.org
www.homeopathicdirectory.com
    Has the strictest certification standards of any
body; can issue a Certificate of Classical Homeopathy
(CCH) to licensed health professionals and nonli-
censed individuals.

National Board of Homeopathic Examiners (NBHE)
5663 NW 29th Street
Margate, FL 33063
(954) 420-0669
www.nbhe.org
    NBHE was started for and by chiropractic physi-
cians but now certifies any graduate of an accredited
homeopathic training program. A DNBHE, or diplomate with the board, is awarded to MDs, osteopaths,
dentists, and chiropractors. A RNBHE, or registrant
with the board, is awarded for nonphysician health
professionals such as nurses, nurse practitioners,
physician assistants, and acupuncturists. A CPHT,
or certified practitioner of homeotherapeutics, is
awarded to laypersons.

North American Society of Homeopaths (NASH)
1122 East Pike Street #1122
Seattle, WA 98122
(206) 720-7000
(208) 248-1942 FAX
E-mail: nashinfo@aol.com
www.homeopathy.org

British Homeopathic Site With Worldwide Links
www.homeopathyhome.com

scope of practice acts for other healthcare and medical professions.

## Regulation and Authority

Arizona and Nevada have independent homeopathy boards, while Connecticut used the state Homeopathic Medical Examining Board as an advisory unit to the State Department of Public Health and Addiction Services. All three states authorize the practice of homeopathy through licensure. In states where no licensing boards exist, homeopathy is sometimes granted under the practice acts of other alternative practices such as naturopathy, oriental medicine, or chiropractic. Some states authorize the use of homeopathic treatments by physicians.[22]

## MASSAGE

## Definition

Massage is defined as the intentional and systematic manipulation of the soft tissues of the body to enhance health and healing. The primary characteristics

---

### Sources of Additional Information

American Massage Therapy Association (AMTA)
820 Davis Street, Suite 100
Evanston, IL 60201-4444
(847) 864-0123
(847) 864-1178 FAX
www.amtamassage.org

AMTA represents more than 40,000 massage therapists in 30 countries and seeks to advance the profession through the development of ethics and standards, certification, school accreditation, continuing education, professional publications, legislation, public education, and member support.

Associated Bodywork & Massage Professionals
(ABMP)
1271 Sugarbush Drive
Evergreen, CO 80439-9766
(800) 458-2267
(303) 674-0859 FAX
E-mail: expectmore@abmp.com
www.abmp.com

ABMP is a professional membership association providing services and information, promoting ethical practices, protecting the rights of practitioners, and educating the public.

*Educational Resources*
Touch Research Institutes
Department of Pediatrics
University of Miami School of Medicine
PO Box 016820 (Dept. 820)
1601 NW 12th Avenue

7th floor, Suite 7037
Miami, FL 33101
(305) 243-6781
(305) 243-4872 (TRI Wellness)
(305) 243-6488 FAX
E-mail: field@nsu.acast.nova.edu *or*
tfield@med.miami.edu
www.miami.edu/touch-research

*Certification Bodies*
The National Certification Board for Therapeutic
Massage and Bodywork (NCBTMB)
8201 Greensboro Drive, Suite 300
McLean, VA 22102
(800) 296-0664
(703) 610-9015
(703) 610-9005 FAX
E-mail: smcmahon@ncbtmb.com
www.ncbtmb.com

NCBTMB is a credentialing body that delivers the only nationally accredited exam for the field of massage and bodywork therapies. It was accredited in 1993 by the National Commission for Certifying Agencies (NCCA), and the accrediting body of the National Organization for Competency Assurance (NOCA). To be certified by NCBTMB, practitioners must complete a minimum of 500 class clock hours of supervised education and training, pass a rigorous exam, comply with a code of ethics, complete 50 hours of continuing education, and perform at least 200 therapeutic massages during the 4-year certification period.

of massage are the applications of touch and movement. Massage includes a variety of manual techniques, including the application of fixed or movable pressure. Massage is primarily delivered with the hands, but the forearms, elbows, and feet may also be used for the delivery of massage.[26,27]

## Scope of Practice

The legislative definition of massage varies considerably from state to state and may include reference to manipulation or treatment of the soft or superficial tissues or muscles by manual or mechanical means; the use of hands, feet, arms, and elbows for delivery of massage; and the use of friction, stroking, percussion, kneading, or vibration. Massage procedures may include the use of topical oils or lotions; chemical or herbal body applications; heat lamp or infrared heat; salts; hot or cold packs or ice; tub, shower, steam, dry heat, cabinet bath, whirlpool, sauna bath, or sitz bath; and hydrotherapy, heliotherapy, or electrotherapy. In some states, Swedish gymnastics, reflexology, shiatsu, stretching, passive joint movement, and rehabilitative procedures may be employed.[23]

## Regulation and Authority

Currently 23 states have practice acts for massage therapists.[28] Some states employ massage boards with independent regulatory authority. In other states, the profession is regulated within a state department and usually with the assistance of a massage board or committee. One state (Ohio) views massage as a limited branch of medicine and therefore massage therapy falls under the jurisdiction of the state medical board. Other states require registration or certification. Some states have no recognized practice acts for massage. In those states, counties or municipalities may employ their own requirements.[22]

## NATUROPATHY

## Definition

Naturopathy is "a system of primary healthcare practice by doctors of naturopathic medicine for the prevention, diagnosis, and treatment of human health conditions, injuries, and diseases that uses education, natural medicines, and therapies to support and stimulate the individual's intrinsic self-healing processes."[29]

## Scope of Practice

Naturopathic practice acts currently exist in Alaska, Arizona, Connecticut, Hawaii, Maine, Montana, New Hampshire, Oregon, Utah, Vermont, District of Columbia, and Puerto Rico. In states with no practice acts, a medical license may be required to practice naturopathy, or licensure in another health profession with a scope of practice including naturopathic methods may be required. The scope of practice for naturopathy may include acupuncture, biofeedback, homeopathy, hypnotherapy, and massage. Some statutes permit naturopaths to perform minor surgeries and natural childbirth. Naturopaths are typically able to use a broad range of adjunctive therapies that include physical agents (air, water, heat, cold, sound, light, electromagnetics), physical modalities (electrotherapy, diathermy, ultraviolet light, manipulation, and therapeutic exercise), natural medicines and therapies for preventative and therapeutic purposes and diagnostic procedures (physical, oral, and x-ray examinations; electrocardiograms; phlebotomy; clinical lab tests; and physiological function tests), nonprescriptive medications, and most diagnostic procedures common to other medical practitioners. In Connecticut, counseling is included in practice acts for naturopaths. Washington, DC, provides that naturopaths "may counsel individuals and treat human conditions through the use of naturally occurring substances."[22]

## Regulation and Authority

Five or more states have independent boards of naturopathy; other states regulate naturopathic practice through a division of a state department and with the assistance of a naturopathy board or advisory committee. Licensure is required in states maintaining authority over the practice of naturopathy. Naturopathy practice acts readily acknowledge that the therapies used in the practice of naturopathy are not the exclusive domain of naturopaths

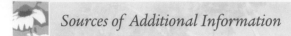

Alaska Department of Community & Economic
    Development
Division of Occupational Licensing, Naturopathic
    Section
PO Box 110806
Juneau, AK 99811-0806
(907) 465-2695
E-mail: P.J._Gingras@dced.state.ak.us

Arizona Naturopathic Physicians Board of Medical
    Examiners
1400 W Washington, Suite 230
Phoenix, AZ 85007
Executive Director: Craig Runbeck, NMD
(602) 542-8242
E-mail: Craig.Runbeck@npbomex.a2.gov

Board of Governors
Association of Naturopathic Physicians of British
    Columbia
409 Granville Street, Suite 218
Vancouver, BC V6C 1T2
CANADA
Executive Director: Carolyn Chiasson
(604) 688-8236
(604) 688-8476 FAX
E-mail: anpbc@msn.com

Connecticut Board of Naturopathic Examiners
Connecticut Department of Public Health
410 Capitol Avenue, MS 12APP
PO Box 340308
Hartford, CT 06134-0308
Contact: Latarsha Sterling
(860) 566-6257

Hawaii Board of Examiners in Naturopathy
PO Box 3469
Honolulu, HI 96801
Executive Officer: Candace Ito
(808) 586-2704

Maine Board of Complementary Health Care
    Providers
35 State House Station
Augusta, ME 04333
Contact: Jerri Betts
(207) 624-8579

Montana Alternative Health Care Board
Department of Labor and Industry
Professional and Occupational Licensing Division
301 S Park
Helena, MT 59620
Program Manager: Cheryl Brandt
(406) 841-2300

New Hampshire Naturopathic Board of Examiners
Department of Health and Human Services
129 Pleasant Street
Concord, NH 03301-6527
Contact: Christine Topham
(603) 271-4688

Ontario Board of Drugless Therapy-Naturopathy
112 Adelaide Street E
Toronto, ON M5c 1K9
CANADA
Office Administrator: Jane Lowe
(416) 236-4593

Oregon Board of Naturopathic Examiners
800 NE Oregon Street, Suite 407
Portland, OR 97232
Executive Director: Anne Walsh
(503) 731-4045
E-mail: obne.info@state.or.us

Puerto Rico Naturopathic Licensing
Department of State
PO Box 9023271
San Juan, PR 00902-3271
Contact: Francis Perez
(787) 725-7303 FAX

Utah Division of Occupational & Professional
    Licensing
Naturopathic Physicians
160 E 300 South
Salt Lake City, UT 84114-6741
Contact: David Fairhurst
(801) 530-6628

Vermont Secretary of State Professional Regulations
26 Terrace Redstone Building
Montpelier, VT 05602
(802) 828-2837

Washington State Naturopathic Physician Licensing
    Program
1300 Quince Street SE
PO Box 47870
Olympia, WA 98504-7870
Executive Director: Tracy Hansen
(360) 236-4941

but are used by a wide variety of other health and medical professionals. Therefore naturopathic enactments are not applicable to persons authorized to practice other health professions by state law. Some states prohibit the practice of naturopathy as a distinct profession. Tennessee law has made the practice of naturopathy a class B misdemeanor but makes this law inapplicable to persons complying with the regulations that apply to their own medical or health discipline. South Carolina also prohibits the practice of naturopathy, subjecting offenders to a criminal fine and imprisonment at the discretion of the court.[23] Direct contacts for licensing boards are listed in the box on p. 410.

## THERAPEUTIC TOUCH

### Definition

*Therapeutic Touch (TT)* is defined as the intentionally directed process of energy modulation with the practitioner using the hands as a focus to facilitate healing. TT may or may not involve actual contact with the client's body, but contact is always made with the client's energy field.[30]

## Scope of Practice/Regulation and Authority

There are no statutory regulations that govern the use of TT as a modality. The term *touch therapy* is used in several statutes to refer to massage therapy and should not be confused with TT, an energy healing system.

## HYPNOSIS

### Definition

Hypnosis is defined as a state of attentive, focused concentration with suspension of some peripheral awareness. Components of hypnosis include absorption, controlled alteration of one's attention, dissociation (ability to compartmentalize different aspects of one's experience), and suggestibility.[31]

### Scope of Practice

There are statutory references to hypnotherapy or hypnosis in legislation related to health occupations.

---

### *Sources of Additional Information*

Nurse Healers-Professional Associates International
3760 S Highland Drive, Suite 429
Salt Lake City, UT 84106
(801) 273-3399
(509) 693-3537 FAX
E-mail: nh-pai@Therapeutic-Touch.org
www.therapeutic-touch.org/

This is the official organization of TT, established in 1977 under the leadership of Dolores Krieger, PhD, RN. The organization serves as an expert resource for information on the Krieger/Kunz model of TT and sets standards for the practice and teaching of TT. The organization facilitates the exchange of research findings, teaching strategies, and new developments in the area of TT.

The American Holistic Nurses' Association
PO Box 2130
Flagstaff, AZ 86003-2130
(800) 278-2462
www.ahna.org

Founded in 1980 by nurses dedicated to the concepts of holism, this organization now boasts an international membership of 4,000.

Pumpkin Hollow Farm
1184 Route 11
Craryville, NY 12521
(877) 325-3583
(518) 325-5633 FAX
www.pumpkinhollow.org

TT workshops are taught at the farm by recognized TT teachers.

When referenced, hypnosis is predominantly within the scope of practice of the psychological disciplines or, in some cases, marriage and family counselors, anesthetists, naturopaths, clinical social workers, mental health counselors, and medical practitioners.

## Regulation and Authority

Statutory qualification and clinical experience vary from state to state. Dentists, optometrists, podiatrists, chiropractors, osteopaths, and MDs are prohibited, in some cases, from using hypnosis for treatment of neu-

 *Sources of Additional Information*

*Organizations/Associations/Boards*

American Board of Hypnotherapy
2002 E McFadden Avenue, Suite 100
Santa Ana, CA 92705
(714) 245-9340
(800) 872-9996
(714) 245-9881 FAX
E-mail: aih@hypnosis.com
www.hypnosis.com/abh/abh.html

American Council of Hypnotist Examiners (ACHE)
700 S Central Avenue
Glendale, CA 91204
(818) 242-1159
(818) 247-9379 FAX
www.hypnosisforhealth.com/ache.html

American Hypnosis Association
18607 Ventura Blvd., Suite 310
Tarzana, CA 91356
(818) 758-2730
www.hypnosismotivation.com/american.html

American Psychological Association
Division 30, Psychological Hypnosis
750 First Street NE
Washington, DC 20002-4242
(202) 336-6013 (division services)
www.apa.org/divisions/div30/

American Society of Clinical Hypnosis
140 N Bloomingdale Road
Bloomingdale, IL 60108-1017
(630) 980-4740
(630) 351-8490 FAX
E-mail: info@asch.net
www.asch.net

International Medical and Dental Hypnotherapy
    Association
4110 Edgeland, Suite 800
Royal Oak, MI 48073-2285
(248) 549-5594
(800) 257-5467
www.infinityinst.com

The Milton H Erickson Foundation, Inc.
3606 N 24th Street
Phoenix, Arizona 85016
(602) 956-6196
www.erickson-foundation.org/

National Board for Certified Clinical Hypnotherapists
1110 Fidler Lane, Suite L1
Silver Spring, MD 20910
(301) 608-0123
(800) 449-8144
(301) 588-9535 FAX
E-mail: nbcch@natboard.com
www.natboard.com/contact.html

Society for Clinical and Experimental Hypnosis
    (SCEH)
SCEH Central Office
Washington State University
PO Box 642114
Pullman, WA 99164-2114
(509) 332-7555
(509) 335-2097 FAX
http://sunsite.utk.edu/IJCEH/scehframe.htm

rotic problems. However, they may be allowed its use for hypnoanesthesia or for reducing treatment-induced anxiety.[32]

## IMAGERY

### Definition

Imagery is the thought process that invokes and uses the senses (vision, sound, smell, taste, movement, position, and touch). Imagery is considered a doorway to conscious reality and can affect how a person feels emotionally and physically. Imagery has been demonstrated to modulate physiological, biochemical, and psychological short-term and long-term outcomes.[2,33]

### Scope of Practice/Authority and Regulation

There are no practice acts for imagery, although the term is included in practice acts for psychiatry, psychology, and social work. Imagery can be considered a component of many physical and psychological interventions. It is often employed by individuals without adequate education and experience in imagery as a medical intervention. Educational organizations and associations are listed in the box below.

## MEDITATION

### Definition

Spiritual forms of meditation have existed for thousands of years. Over the last 25 years meditation has been researched as a medical intervention for a variety of acute and chronic conditions. Technically, meditation forms are classified as concentrative or nonconcentrative. In concentrative methods, stimulus is limited by focusing on a single unchanging repetitive stimulus such as sound, breathing, or a focal point. Nonconcentrative techniques expand the meditator's attention to include the observation, in a nonjudgmental way, of his or her thoughts. There are three forms of meditation that have demonstrated clinical efficacy as medical intervention: Transcendental Meditation (TM), The Respiratory One Method (ROM), and Mindfulness Mediation (MM). Depending on the form, meditation has been observed to reduce healthcare costs, strengthen immune function, reduce symptoms of anxiety and depression, lower blood pressure, reverse some components of cardiovascular disease, reduce frequency and duration of epileptic seizures,

*Sources of Additional Information*

*Educational Organizations/Associations*
Academy for Guided Imagery, Inc.
PO Box 2070
Mill Valley, CA 94942
(800) 726-2070
(415) 389-9342 FAX
www.interactiveimagery.com
Offers 150-hour training course in guided imagery.

International Association of Interactive Imagery (IAII)
300920 Lanes Turn Road
Eugene, OR 97401
www.iaii.org

Simonton Cancer Center
PO Box 890
Pacific Palisades, CA 90272
(800) 459-3424
(310) 457-3811
(310) 457-0421 FAX
www.simontoncenter.com

Nurses Certificate Program in Imagery (NCPII)
(650) 570-5706
E-mail: ncpii@aol.com

### Sources of Additional Information

Center for Mindfulness in Medicine, Healthcare
and Society
University of Massachusetts Medical School
Stress Reduction Clinic
U Mass Memorial Medical Center
Shaw Building
55 Lake Avenue N
Worcester, MA 01655
(508) 856-2656
(508) 856-1977 FAX

Maharishi Vedic University
Fairfield, Iowa 52557
(888) 532-7686
E-mail: info@tm.org
www.tm.org

improve coping skills for chronic pain, and lower rates of substance abuse.[2,34]

## Scope of Practice/Regulation and Authority

There are no practice acts governing meditation. Meditation forms result in beneficial medical outcomes only when properly taught and practiced. The most clinically beneficial forms, MM and TM, require strict training protocols from the instructors who teach these methods to patients. Information on how to access training appropriate to medical environments is provided in the box above.

## References

1. Eisenberg DM, Kessler RC, Foster C, et al: Unconventional medicine in the United States: prevalence, costs, and patterns of use, *N Engl J Med* 328(4):246-252, 1993.
2. Freeman LW: *Best practices in complementary and alternative medicine: an evidence-based approach with CEs/CMEs,* Gaithersburg, Md, 2001, Aspen.
3. Landmark Healthcare: *The Landmark report I on public perceptions of alternative care,* San Francisco, Calif, 1998, Landmark Healthcare. (A summary of the report can be viewed on www.landmark.healthcare.com.)
4. Krauss HZB, Godfrey C, Kirk J, et al: Alternative health care: its use by individuals with physical disabilities, *Arch Phys Med Rehabil* 79:1440-1447, 1998.
5. Astin JA: Why patients use alternative medicine, *JAMA* 280(19):1548-1553, 1998.
6. Freeman LW, Lawlis GF: *Mosby's complementary and alternative medicine: a research-based approach,* St Louis, 2001, Mosby.
7. Weeks J: Licensed CAM practices and their patients: Cherkin study creates needed foundation, *Integrator Bus Altern Med* pp 2-3, Jan/Feb 2001.
8. Milbank Memorial Fund: *Enhancing the accountability of alternative medicine,* Jan 1998 (www.milbank.org/mraltmed.html).
9. Landmark Healthcare: *The landmark report II on HMOs and alternative care,* San Francisco, 1999, Landmark Healthcare. (A summary of the report can be viewed on www.landmarkhealthcare.com.)
10. Weeks J: Landmark Healthcare on HMO coverage of alternatives: report II, *Integrator Bus Altern Med* pp 1, 4, April 1999.
11. Weeks J: A kind of blue: alternative medicine spreads in Blue Cross Blue Shield plans, *Integrator Bus Altern Med* pp 1, 5, June 1999.
12. Weeks J: Licensed CAM practices and their patients: two negotiated HMO-integrative clinic relationships, *Integrator Bus Altern Med* pp 6-7, Jan/Feb 2001.
13. Weeks J: Licensed CAM practices and their patients: Cherkin study creates needed foundation, *Integrator Bus Altern Med* pp 2-3, Jan/Feb 2001.
14. Weeks J: MD regulators and educators position for CAMs infusion, *Integrator Bus Altern Med* p 8, Jan/Feb 2001.
15. Studdert DM, Eisenberg DM, et al: Medical malpractice implications of alternative medicine, *JAMA* 280(18): 1610-1615, 1998.
16. Shames R, Frampton J, Weisblatt R: Credentialing and quality assurance for Harvard Vanguard's Alternative Paths to Health program, *Forum* 19(6), 1999. (www.rmf.harvard.edu/publications/forum/v19n6/article4/index)
17. Sale DM: *Overview of legislative development concerning alternative health care in the United States,* Kalamazoo, Mich, 1999, Fetzer Institute, p 4. (This report can be viewed at www.healthy.net/public/legal-lg/regulations/fetzer.htm.)
18. Freeman LW, Lawlis GF: Acupuncture. In *Mosby's complementary and alternative medicine: a research-based approach,* St Louis, 2001, Mosby, p 312.
19. Mayer DJ et al: Antagonism of acupuncture analgesia in man by the narcotic antagonistic naloxone, *Brain Res* 121:368, 1977.
20. The legal language by state and a list of states with practice acts can be accessed at www.aaom.org/aaomlegis/status.html.

21. Reston J: Now about my operation in Peking, *New York Times* 1971.

22. Cohen MH: *Complementary and alternative medicine: legal boundaries and regulatory perspectives,* Baltimore, 1998, John Hopkins University Press, pp 40-53.

23. Sale DM: Provider practice acts: acupuncture. In *Overview of legislative development concerning alternative health care in the United States,* Kalamazoo, Mich, 1999, Fetzer Institute, pp 5-9, 11-16. (This report can be viewed at www.healthy.net/public/legal-lg/regulations/fetzer.htm.)

24. Freeman LW, Lawlis GF: Chiropractic. In *Mosby's complementary and alternative medicine: a research-based approach,* St Louis, 2001, Mosby, pp 288-295.

25. Freeman LW, Lawlis GF: Homeopathy. In *Mosby's complementary and alternative medicine: a research-based approach,* St Louis, 2001, Mosby, pp 345-359.

26. Freeman LW, Lawlis GF: Massage. In *Mosby's complementary and alternative medicine: a research-based approach,* St Louis, 2001, Mosby, pp 361-363.

27. Tappan FM, Benjamin PJ: *Tappan's handbook of healing massage techniques: classic, holistic, and emerging methods,* ed 3, Stamford, Conn, 1998, Appleton & Lange.

28. Lucy Laws, National Certification Board for Therapeutic Massage and Bodywork, McLean, Va, personal communication, Feb., 2001.

29. N.H. Rev. Stat. Ann § 328-E:2 (IX) (supp. 1994).

30. Freeman LW, Lawlis GF: Therapeutic Touch: healing with energy. In *Mosby's complementary and alternative medicine: a research-based approach,* St Louis, 2001, Mosby, pp 493-506.

31. Freeman LW, Lawlis GF: Hypnosis. In *Mosby's complementary and alternative medicine: a research-based approach,* St Louis, 2001, Mosby, pp 226-259.

32. Sale DM: Provider practice acts: B—other alternative modalities: hypnotherapy. In *Overview of legislative development concerning alternative health care in the United States,* Kalamazoo, Mich, 1999, Fetzer Institute, p 8. (This report can be viewed at www.healthy.net/public/legal-lg/regulations/fetzer.htm.)

33. Freeman LW, Lawlis GF: Imagery. In *Mosby's complementary and alternative medicine: a research-based approach,* St Louis, 2001, Mosby, pp 260-283.

34. Freeman LW, Lawlis GF: Meditation. In *Mosby's complementary and alternative medicine: a research-based approach,* St Louis, 2001, Mosby, pp 166-195.

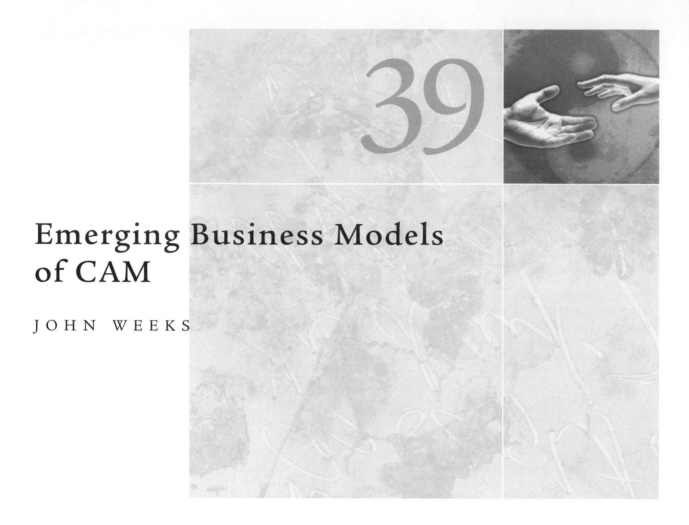

# Emerging Business Models of CAM

JOHN WEEKS

## PREAMBLE: INGREDIENTS SHAPING INCLUSION MODELS

The current business models for the inclusion of complementary and alternative medicine (CAM) in mainstream payment and delivery are shaped by many factors. The label on the side of the container of these influences might read as follows.

**Contents:** consumer demand, marketplace opportunity, scientific understanding, research funding priorities, government requirements, potential increases in employee functionality and productivity, experience data, guild competition, diminished absenteeism, political clout, personal bias, experience of clinicians, shifting belief systems, potential cost offsets, and concerns with abiding structural challenges in mainstream payment and delivery

The diversity of these influences confounds our future forecasting. Changes in one factor, or in a cluster of factors, can reframe or shift the course in the business of future integration.

## CRITICAL CHANGE FACTORS

A few of the change factors that may be expected to play a significant role in the evolution of CAM's role in payment and delivery in the next few years follow.

### Current Research Agenda

Those in the integration field debate whether inclusion should be for a few discrete CAM modalities or should embrace the more philosophical, whole-person–oriented character of the self-description of the CAM movement. The preference of the research community for exploring the "low-hanging fruits" that fit easily into placebo-controlled study designs suggests that most research-driven integration will be through the grafting of a few CAM modalities onto conventional practice. For example, in contradistinction to seeing increased use of traditional Chinese medicine in general practice medicine (as it is used, for instance, in China), we will see increased coverage of the use of acupuncture needles in the treatment of a few conditions, such as nausea. Following this line, selective nutraceuticals from a handful of major manufacturers who agree to stringent manufacturing guidelines will increasingly be used and reimbursed as options to conventional pharmaceuticals.

## The Leading Edge of New Integration and Coverage

Inside the new guidelines for nonpharmacological pain management issued by the Joint Commission on Accreditation of Healthcare Organizations (JCAHO) in January 2001 is a requirement that diverse delivery systems accredited by JCAHO—from in-patient to home care—educate patients to the potential pain-reducing value in an array of CAM treatments. The requirement to increase awareness of patients and providers alike to the existing growing research base for integrative pain management will transform over time into routine clinical integration that will, over time, be routinely paid for by third parties.

Advocates of increased integration will begin to use the JCAHO requirement as leverage to foster changes in conventional practices that have proved difficult to penetrate without the help of such regulatory requirements. Economic support for coverage of integrative pain strategies will grow out of both consumer satisfaction and additional findings that pre- and post-op integrative approaches diminish lengths of stay, pharmacy usage, and the need for additional services. Much of this care will be delivered through cross-trained conventional providers, nurses, and MDs rather than by members of the distinctly licensed CAM professions. Another influence will be the nursing shortage as hospitals begin to sell their holistic dimensions to attract and retain providers. Notably,

pain conditions are already leading drivers of consumer usage of CAM.

## Employer/Purchasers

An odd finding in a year 2000 survey of integrative medicine industry leaders is that the majority believe that, next to the consumer, the employer is the stakeholder who has interests most closely aligned with the emerging industry. Some of the dimensions of the perceived alignment were captured when over 90% of those surveyed agreed that CAM interventions are most likely to look best in research approaches that feature broad outcomes that measure the global costs of a benefit design. Markers of interest to employers are cost offsets; employee productivity, satisfaction, absenteeism, functionality, and health-promoting behaviors; and even diminished costs to hire and replace through enhanced employee loyalty. Concern about uncontrolled escalation in healthcare costs in 2001-2002 will push some employers to explore the role of CAM in helping them with such broad outcomes. The more whole-person approaches to CAM delivery of integrative medicine will have their best chance for being affirmed in this environment.

## Health Plan Coverage

As discount products and distinctly licensed CAM providers become commonplace, some HMOs and insurers will begin to offer covered benefits to distinguish themselves in the marketplace. Licensed acupuncturists, regulated massage therapists, and (in states where licensed) naturopathic doctors will increasingly join chiropractors in coverage schemes. Coverage will continue to be quarantined in the poorly integrated chiropractic model: closely managed by subcontracting provider networks, paid for through stand-alone benefit riders, and involving only a few covered conditions. Internal forces in the distinctly licensed CAM professions will begin to shape education and practice around those approaches and conditions that are first in the door, such as the relative acceptance of low back pain, which has influenced the development of chiropractic. Without a significant alignment of a major stakeholder with the integration effort (see "Paradigm Shifts," following), such coverage of distinctly licensed providers will continue to reflect a very small part of the healthcare dollar (less than 2%). In the meantime, in a second, parallel CAM economy, diverse practices known in 1990 as alternative or unconventional will quietly become accepted, covered parts of the conventional practices in mainstream delivery without reference to their CAM lineage. Insurance equity laws will become a key battleground for CAM provider guilds.

## PARADIGM SHIFTS

The natural tendencies of mainstream payment and delivery promote a stepwise assimilation through which the integrative medicine movement is mined for approved elements that might then be attached to mainstream delivery. In this scenario, the transformative edges of what early advocates of CAM considered a new paradigm of more health-oriented care are reshaped both through the drone of a reductive research agenda and through the selective assimilation of individual modalities. Many CAM practices will quietly be included and reframed.

Whether future business models for integration foster the integration movements, more radical aspirations will be determined by one key issue: resource availability. Most of the parties proactively involved in promoting expanded delivery and third-party payment of integrative care are struggling economically. The financial margins are not there to support the mounting, on their internal resources, of any significant policy or outcomes initiative that seeks to reframe the integration discussion away from how to integrate CAM into the mainstream.

## Integrating CAM into the Mainstream

How can CAM therapies and providers be optimally used in an integrated environment to create health in the populations served? To undertake the challenges

### Resources

Collaboration for Healthcare Renewal
    Foundation
Jery Whitworth, Principal and Co-Founder
PO Box 581, Pomona, NY 10970
(845) 354-2388
www.thecollaboration.org

Integrated Healthcare Policy Consortium
Matt Russell, Executive Director
6890 E. Sunrise Drive, Suite 120, PMB #176
Tucson, AZ 85750
(520) 232-1130
mattrussell@earthlink.net

of developing the business models that might grow out of this question, the integration movement will need a partnership with a significant, well-heeled stakeholder if this more fundamental question is to be engaged. Employers, philanthropic organizations, and perhaps the federal government could be the interested stakeholder partners. A decision from one of these stakeholders to open the integration dialog will need the pincer movement of two influences: (1) ongoing high demand from the consumer as patient, as media influence, and as voter and (2) continuing frustration with soaring increases in the costs of mainstream delivery.

Finally, to attract and hold the stakeholder, those involved in promoting integration will need to catalyze the connection through their own collaborative efforts to define an agenda that flows out of their distinct, health-oriented paradigm. The agenda must be presented in terms that respect the general principles, if not the exact constraints, of conventional payment and delivery. By early 2002, the time of this writing, a few spare signs of such activity have emerged.

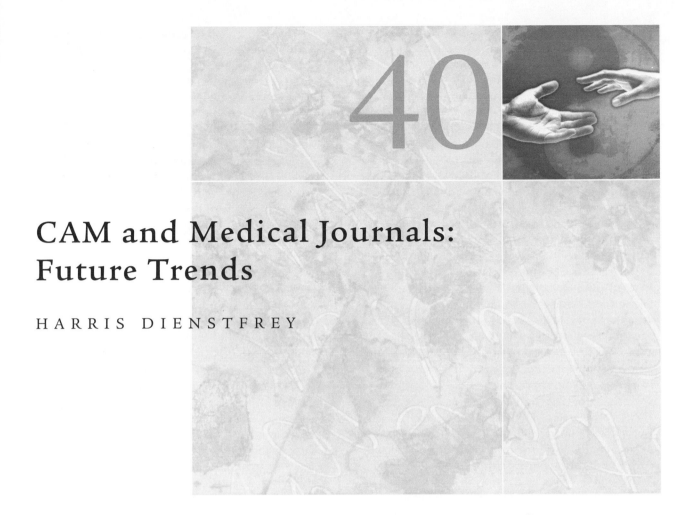

# CAM and Medical Journals: Future Trends

HARRIS DIENSTFREY

For 16 years, ending late in 2001, I was the editor of the quarterly journal *Advances in Mind-Body Medicine.* I suppose that if anyone should have a feel for the coming shape—the advances—of mind-body medicine, I should. But after a decade and a half of editorial involvement in the mind-body enterprise, my strongest impression is one of disorder. The field is a bit like a gold rush. Everyone tracks his or her hunches like prospectors set loose on a scrubby new continent, each person working an individual piece of land with energetic independence.

I should say that virtually no one but myself seems to think this disorder is worthy of comment. Maybe it is not. Maybe mind-body researchers are right to "do" their science as robustly and as elegantly as they can, large understandings and big theory be damned.

Maybe I am too fixed on the hope (the fantasy?) of a new kind of medicine that sets biology within the context of mind.

Disorder or no, mind-body medicine is a work in progress, and where it will end is far from clear. Unlike such fully developed medical systems as homeopathy and Chinese medicine, it offers no organized understanding of the dynamics of the body (or the mind) and no basic armamentarium of treatments. It cannot even claim, as for example biofeedback can, a distinctive intervention to treat the ills that fall within its domain. Actually, it cannot even say that it knows exactly how to define its domain.

As a central perspective, the best that mind-body medicine can offer is the general insight, derived from clinical experience, laboratory findings, and research studies, that feelings and thoughts can affect health and disease. But to what extent, in regard to what ills, with what hope of a "mind treatment" the current congeries of findings about the assorted contributions of thoughts and feelings to good and bad health provides no answers. Will mind-body medicine ever become a full medical system? Or even a subspecialty in the medicine we have? We can only guess.

All this said, where, in the short run, might mind-body medicine be heading? The following are predictions about four likely trends in mind-body medicine for the next decade.

1. The research and the data will become better, more rigorous, and more extensive. I have three reasons for saying this. First, the National Institutes of Health is becoming involved in mind-body research, and one assumes that it will fund substantial, sound studies. Second, mind-body research is attracting a new generation of researchers for whom studying the consequences of thoughts and feelings for physical health no longer carries the stigma of scientific disrepute (or the fervor of a new truth) and who approach the mixed or incomplete evidence for the effects of thoughts and feelings as engrossing scientific challenges to be resolved with clarifying studies. Third, in a medical world that so far is unable to resolve continuing illnesses such as cancer and heart disease (not to mention AIDS), the search for better treatments (or treatments to offset the debilitating effects of accepted treatments) is gradually bringing a heightened scientific attention to relevant mind-body studies, as it has with complementary and alternative therapies.

2. Along with better research and a widening interest in mind-body studies will come a greater receptivity to mind-body research among the highest rank of American medical journals, represented by the *Journal of the American Medical Association (JAMA)* and the *New England Journal of Medicine (N Engl J Med)*, the bête noir (and holy grail) of mind-body researchers. Mind-body studies are already accorded attention in top British medical journals such as the *Lancet* and the *British Medical Journal.* In the United States, the response of *JAMA* and especially the response of the *N Engl J Med*, whose current and recent editors often voice their disdain for mind-body research, has been cool. The attitude will gradually warm. As studies become better and findings mount, the interest of the medical community, driven by the general public and patients and by the desire for results, will grow, and without much fanfare, the pages of the most prestigious medical journals will begin to fall open to mind-body research. Indeed, only a short time ago, in 1999, *JAMA* published a striking study by Smyth et al[1] in which asthmatics and rheumatoid arthritics reduced their symptoms "simply" by writing about stressful events in their lives. *N Engl J Med* will be the last to succumb; quite apart from its fervent defense of the high standards of medical research, it seems to find the whole idea of mind-body studies slightly disreputable. (Oddly, in critiques of mind-body studies, its past and present editors never note that a decade ago, in 1991, the journal published a highly acclaimed mind-body study on stress, Cohen et al's "Psychological Stress and Susceptibility to the Common Cold."[2])

3. As American medical journals become more responsive to mind-body studies, the publications will favor studies that examine the clinical effects of external experience. By definition, effects in mind-body medicine must ultimately come from internal, subjective phenomena such as feelings, thoughts, and expressions of the imagination. But most mind-body research reaches for this internal activity indirectly, through studying the clinical effects of external events and interventions that somehow affect thoughts and feelings, and this line of research will also become the focus of American medical journals in the near future.

I say this because I believe that the dominant view of Western medicine, including most mind-body research, derives from and is largely bound within the perspective of germ theory. Germ theory says that illness and its treatment come from something outside the body. Illness comes from a germ or its equivalent that invades the body and proceeds to wreak havoc with one or another physiological process, whereas the restoration of health comes from a pill or an equivalent that is deliberately delivered into the body to kill the germ or prevent it from setting off the triggers that undermine health. Put simply, Western medicine and medical research look outside the body for the physical troublemaker or the soothing balm.

So too does most mind-body research (perhaps understandably—we are all part of the same culture), though in this instance the outside event is not physical but, as current mind-body jargon puts it, "psychosocial." The work on stress and social support are good examples. In mind-body studies, stress functions as the psychosocial equivalent of a germ, entering the body through the mind to cause havoc, while social support functions as the equivalent of a vaccine or antibiotic, reducing the risk for illnesses of many kinds. In both cases, the psychosocial experiences have an impact on the body/self, and succeeding events then happen, in effect by themselves. As with a germ or a pill they happen, it seems, without intent—or, one could say, mindlessly.

A small number of mind-body researchers do look inside for the features that affect health. Two studies are illustrative. In one study, Jon Kabat-Zinn and colleagues[3] found that when people with psoriasis meditated and visualized while receiving the standard light treatment, their skin cleared 4 times faster than did the skin of patients who received only the light treatment. (This study was fiercely critiqued by Arnold Relman,[4] former editor of the *N Engl J Med,* who, among other things, maintained that it was improperly blinded.) In another study Cunningham et al,[5] following a group of cancer patients in a self-help program (meditation, self-hypnosis, and pain management), found that the patients who were most involved in the self-help work lived the longest. The key for Cunningham was the degree of internal involvement, not the impact of external intervention.

Such inside-directed studies deal with what I like to call the "powers" of the mind. I believe that wherever we are going with mind-body studies of the external, we will get there faster if our research also contains a rich complement of studies of the internal. However, for now I believe that the "mindless," outside-the-body perspective engendered by the germ theory will continue to frame most mind-body research and the outlook of most medical journals, perhaps the most-renowned journals most of all.

4. While all of this is going on—more and better research, a fuller presence in biomedical journals, a continued focus on the effects of external experiences and interventions—health maintenance organizations (HMO's), health insurance companies, and even the government will pick and choose

among mind-body treatments and make them available. The process has begun. About 40 insurance companies offer its members Dr. Dean Ornish's lifestyle program for heart disease, which includes meditation and group support, along with a low-fat diet and yoga, and at this writing, Medicare is paying for 1,800 patients to go through the program. Aetna U.S. Healthcare offers Belleruth Naperstek's guided imagery audiotapes for members hospitalized for coronary problems. Such interventions reduce costs and help make people healthier, and some portion of the paying public wants to try them.

The end result will be a gerrymandered medical system, with mind-body interventions of varying kinds haphazardly stitched into the system. This can go on for years, perhaps for decades, until enough is known (if enough ever is known) to reconceive the assumptions and strategies that have framed medicine since the triumph of the germ theory—which is to say, until the mind is seen as a constant element of biology. This will happen when it happens. Until then (if there is a then), as this and that mind-body understanding is cobbled onto biomedicine, the least that can be said is that the scope of medicine will expand to the benefit of all of us.

## References

1. Smyth J, Stone A, Hurowitz A, et al: Writing about stressful events produces symptom reduction in asthmatics and rheumatoid arthritics: a randomized trial, *JAMA* 281:1304-1309, 1999.
2. Cohen S, Tyrrell DAJ, Smith AP: Psychological stress and susceptibility to the common cold, *N Engl J Med* 325:606-612, 1991.
3. Kabat-Zinn J, Wheeler E, Light T, et al: Influence of a mindfulness meditation–based stress reduction intervention on rates of skin clearing in patients with moderate to severe psoriasis undergoing phototherapy (UVB) and photochemotherapy (PUVA), *Psychosom Med* 60:625-632, 1998.
4. Relman A, Riley D, Kabat-Zinn J, et al: Parsing the data: an examination of a study on meditation and the treatment of psoriasis, *Adv Mind Body Med* 17:66-77, 2001.
5. Cunningham AJ, Phillips C, Lockwood GA, et al: 2000 Association of involvement in psychological self-regulation with longer survival in patients with metastatic cancer: an exploratory study, *Adv Mind Body Med* 16:276-287, 2000.

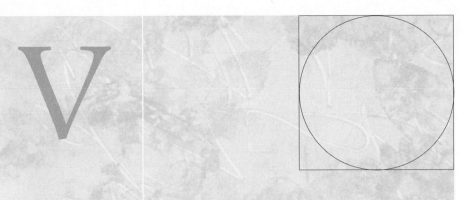

# THE REHABILITATION PATIENT'S PERSPECTIVE

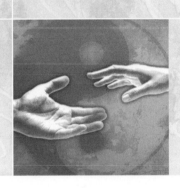

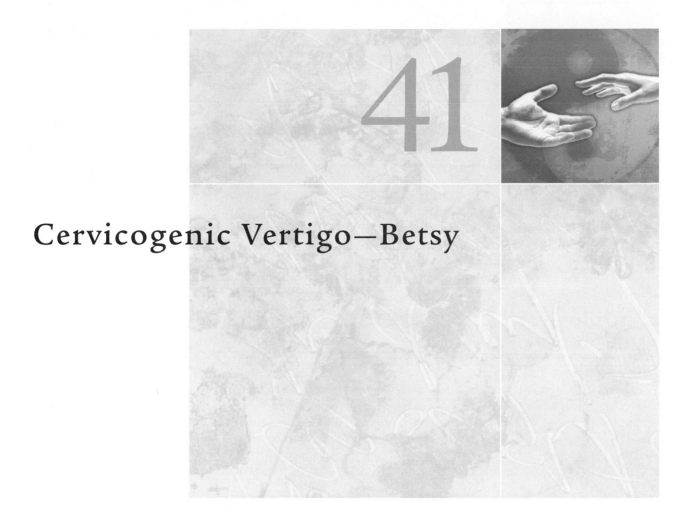

# Cervicogenic Vertigo—Betsy

## EDITOR'S INTRODUCTION

Betsy was a 32-year-old married freelance journalist when she first came to the Spaulding Rehabilitation Hospital (SRH) outpatient clinic in 1998. She described a 10-year history of vague and changing complaints that ranged in focus from neurological to musculoskeletal to psychiatric: weakness, dizziness, fatigue, poor concentration, headaches, anxiety attacks, depression, and others. She had been to a wide range of healthcare practitioners, both mainstream and complementary, and yet she had never been given a definitive diagnosis or an effective treatment plan. Her rehabilitation physician finally made the correct structural diagnosis—cervicogenic vertigo (a misalignment of her neck vertebrae that impinged on neurological and circulatory connections to the brain)—and thus was able to explain the bewildering array of neuropsychiatric symptoms as arising from a physical disorder that impaired brain function. The symptoms were thus somatopsychic rather than psychosomatic in origin—a perhaps less chic version of the mind-body connection, but one which is so often the key in rehabilitation.

As Betsy notes in this essay, her treatment program didn't come together until she found a treatment team that actually worked together as a team. Because all aspects of her care were finally coordinated under one roof, she no longer felt fragmented by the medical system. Ironically, once the healthcare system stopped reflecting back to her own sense of inner fragmentation, she was able to reintegrate herself on all levels and recover the lost sense of inner wholeness.

Her treatment began by focusing on these physical misalignments, which were corrected via cranial osteopathy and physical therapy. She was then stabilized enough to be able to address the emotional crosscurrents that had damaged her over the years. She used her writing skills to help make sense in psychotherapy of a chaotic family background. Her persistence in the face of confusion and defeat speaks volumes about her inner courage, but the lack of coordination and collaboration that she experienced, even among some of her alternative therapists, is also a reminder that there is no magic per se in the use of alternative therapies. For lasting change to occur, the various modalities have to be coordinated, the practitioners have to be tuned in to the patient, and the focus must be multidimensional. It takes more than an exotic technique to make holistic therapy effective. The relationship between the therapist and the patient is still the key, even in the world of complementary and alternative medicine (CAM).

## Betsy

### History of the Symptoms

I am a medical mystery. At least, I used to be. Now I have a diagnosis and lots of doctors and even a treatment plan that won a coveted seal of approval from my HMO. What's that? Treatment covered by my insurance? I must really be sick.

In fact, I've been sick for years. I started complaining to doctors about dizzy spells when I was 16. During my 20s life started to lose its luster—fatigue set in. I had to plan in down time to get through my days. None of this was bad enough to cause concern, though. I made adjustments and life went on, albeit a bit more slowly than it had in the past.

But there was something that wasn't alright, that was never manageable, that I couldn't bear. About once a month, with no warning or identifiable trigger, my heart would start racing and I'd know that the worst was coming: the feeling that my head was exploding, that the world was falling away. It felt like an electrical blowout in my brain. I thought I would either die or go insane every time. These infrequent episodes, which had started out of the blue one day in my senior year of college, filled me with despair. Desperation, I learned, made me both tenacious and incredibly open minded.

Over the past 15 years I have been to at least half a dozen cardiologists, two neurologists, three allergists, five gynecologists, three psychiatrists, a physiatrist, three physical therapists, an occupational therapist and a cranial osteopath. I've seen two homeopaths and four acupuncturists and a naturopath and three massage therapists and someone who does something called "Zero Balancing" and a guy who does chakra-based allergy treatments. I've been to a dowser and a psychic. I've tried tai chi and yoga and a yeast-free diet; for 3 months (though it was supposed to be for 6), based on one of my favorite doctor's recommendations, I rinsed my nose and throat out with a saline rinse that left me gagging. I have even taken grapefruit seed extract, which, rather than purifying my system, gave me reflux. I've had gallons of blood drawn and dozens of ECGs performed. I've been tilted up on a table until I passed out. I've had a roomful of cardiologists fascinated by my case but oblivious to me as I sat on a hospital bed in a skimpy gown, shivering from both cold and fear.

Most of the doctors I'd seen over the years attributed my problems, even the incredibly intense incidents I described, to anxiety and stress. They tested me for all they thought might be wrong and found only a few benign heart disorders; none of these, they said, could explain the intensity of my symptoms. For the record, doctors have told me I have mitral valve syndrome, vasovagal syncope, panic disorder, and a prolonged QT interval. One neurologist claimed with certainty that I have a seizure disorder, despite a normal EEG; when he wanted to stick electrodes under the skin of my temples and have me keep them there under a helmet for 3 days, I walked out and didn't return. I had had enough tests. Having found no identifiable medical cause, the doctors gave a collective sigh, wrote down many referrals to psychiatrists, and told me that, other than Prozac, they had nothing to offer. I'd have to adapt to the quirks of my body.

So I tried. I discarded their prescriptions for drugs and made a grudging peace with my symptoms. Over the next few years, in my late 20's, the big-bang episodes seemed manageable and increasingly rare. I felt safe enough to move forward with my life. I had a child.

Three months post-partum, just after my 30th birthday, my body went wild.

Think of a panic attack or a seizure happening to someone who is trapped on a boat in a storm. In between these daily detonations, I had shaking and tremors. Eye strain, as if I had someone else's too-strong glasses on (and couldn't take them off). Searing muscle pain. Vertigo. Nausea. Disorientation. The feeling that something behind my eyes was melting. Skipped heartbeats, racing heartbeats, palpitations. Loss of breath. Terror. Fogginess. Flu-like exhaustion. I couldn't sleep, I couldn't eat, at times it felt like I couldn't breathe.

Still, my primary care doctor insisted that there was almost certainly nothing physically wrong with me. Despite the severity of my symptoms, my internist, like most of the doctors I'd seen (though not, I must point out, the alternative practitioners), thought my problems were all in my head.

## Getting the Correct Diagnosis

In fact, that was the big joke between me and the first doctor to diagnose me. All those doctors had been right after all—my problems were indeed in my head. Or to be more specific, they were in my neck and head, my spine and hip. It turned out that I had an idiopathic head and neck injury, mild scoliosis, and a rotated hip, all probably 20 years old. I was diagnosed with cervicogenic vertigo, or dizziness originating in the neck. It sounds so benign when you say it that way, so small. It is so very big, though. What's most amazing is that almost all of the sensations that have plagued me originate in the neck. But then I remember that people with neck injuries can die, can lose the use of their limbs. I try not to think about this too often.

My body has been twisted for many years, probably since I was in my early teens. My head and neck looked (but only to the highly trained eye) as if I was always peering around a corner: head perpetually cocked, one shoulder sloped down toward the ground, one hip higher than the other. The pressure on nerves in my neck and head caused the neurological, cardiac, and digestive symptoms that had plagued me for much of my adult life. Childbirth shattered the last fragile remnant of balance that my beleaguered body had, until then, managed to preserve.

What caused all of this to happen? I'll never know. I'm a freak. I saw a famous neurologist who specializes in vertigo. He listened to my story and sternly told me, "You don't have a neck injury unless you've had an accident." He then took me into his examining room and, seconds after actually touching my neck, shook his head and said with disbelief, "You have a neck injury."

Okay, I had thought at first, there's finally a diagnosis—a head and neck injury. So let's just fix this old head and neck and I'll be on my way. I'll see an osteopath, do my physical therapist's exercises, lie still while my physiatrist sticks dizzying therapeutic needles in my neck. I'll see the occupational therapist to learn how to wash the dishes, pick up my child properly and, in fact, experience my body in a way I never have. I'll look at the world in a new light if these doctors and therapists tell me to, and I'll even pray if I must. But let's get on with it. I want my life back.

## Becoming Attached to Your Illness

Fortunately, my caregivers understood the challenges of rehabilitation better than I did. They knew that it doesn't matter what the affliction is, whether it's a bum leg, cancer, or unresolved grief. Healing is hard. There's no quick fix. Because once you've been sick (or disillusioned or addicted or despairing) for just long enough, you see that everything you'd known before has disappeared. Wellness, I realized, would necessitate a whole new life. Reality shifted.

The problem was, I had taken my doctors' advice to heart: I had adapted to illness. They had tacitly told me that I was frail, and after a while I believed them. One neurologist was not so subtle: he told me I was a canary—the kind people used to send into mines to see if they died from the fumes. Believing my doctors' perspective had slowly changed me. Over time I had become fearful, less trusting of life and people and, of course, my own body. My expectations of life diminished. A diagnosis meant that I could hope again. After spending my entire adult life conforming to the requirements of sickness, I suddenly had to switch directions and think about life growing bigger, not smaller.

Strange as it sounds, I wasn't elated when I finally received the correct diagnosis. Indeed, by the time I finally found the right doctors, I had actually grown attached to illness. Becoming healthy, I knew, might even feel like the death of an old friend: a way of life, a world view, the place where my soul thought it had grown roots. It's not easy to give up old habits, even ones like vigilance, fear, and self-pity. They're my bad habits, damn it; who will I be without them? I wonder if an alcoholic feels sadness about becoming sober, a drug addict about becoming clean, an obese person about losing weight.

I knew I would need help to make it through this transition, but over the years I had grown wary of doctors. In fact, I've learned that doctors can be detrimental to my health.

Eric Leskowitz, my psychiatrist, once said that many doctors teach their patients how to fear death rather than how to embrace life. He's right, though I'm not sure why they do this. I suspect it's something much deeper than just the threat of lawsuits, though this is a real concern for healthcare practitioners, I know. Regardless of the reason, though, the results of this conveyed fear can be damaging indeed.

## Learning Fear from Doctors

For example, I saw a psychiatrist once who insisted I didn't have vasovagal syncope (a tilt-table test later proved her wrong), that I definitely had panic disorder, and that I had three types of drugs I could choose from. When I asked about mind-body programs, she said I could try one if I wanted but it wouldn't be enough to help. As our time was up and I was on my way out she said, almost gloating, "I'm just letting you know that left untreated, panic disorder only gets worse." I give her credit for the massive panic episode I had the next day at work.

I went to see an allergist about long-standing food allergies—not dangerous, but irritating. He tested me for nuts, which I have been eating my whole life, and it turns out my crazy body tested positive for every single one. So he told me I should never eat nuts again and that he wanted me to watch a video "that would scare me." I wisely didn't watch his horror movie, but I idiotically went to another allergist. This one dispensed with saying he wanted to scare me and simply waved a death announcement in front of me—a young man had recently died eating a bag of pistachios—to prove that I could be next.

Death and misery, they wanted me to know, awaited me with every beat of my heart, every morsel of food that passed my lips. And they wondered why I was anxious.

I assume that most doctors go into medicine wanting to help people. As a frequent (if reluctant) user of the American healthcare system for a decade and a half, I have a pretty informed opinion about what makes an effective doctor. I used to be a big believer in MD's with degrees from fancy schools. I know better now. Now I want more from my doctors. If they don't deliver what I need and I have any choice in the matter, I leave.

## Holistic Techniques Vs. Holistic Doctors

As is to be expected at the dawn of a new era in medicine, there seems to be some confusion about what "alternative" or "complementary" medicine is. Some of these alternative modalities are acupuncture, Chinese medicine, homeopathy, Therapeutic Touch, and many more. As far as I'm concerned, though, it's not just these tools themselves that transform medicine, it's how they're applied. For example, I recently switched primary care physicians. I chose someone who professes to practice holistic medicine. The first time I saw her she "prescribed" tai chi or yoga for me. Fantastic, I thought, a doctor who knows about alternative approaches to healing!

The only problem was, I hate tai chi and yoga. I've tried them both a number of times and they're just not for me. But this doctor didn't know that because she hadn't taken the time to talk with me. So when I saw her again, still feeling unwell and admitting that I didn't want to take yoga or tai chi, she whipped out her prescription pad. When I balked, she got stern and told me that if I didn't control my anxiety I would get lupus, cancer, multiple sclerosis. "I mean, you might get those things," she weakly amended. I took the piece of paper from her but never filled the prescription. I have my reasons for disliking drugs, though she never took the time to learn them. And by the way, I now have a new primary care physician.

In contrast, when my physiatrist told me for the umpteenth time he wished I would take tai chi, and I said, "I don't want to," instead of just shaking his head, or threatening me, or pulling out his prescription pad, he sat and talked with me. We came up with another plan. My team of doctors and therapists, the ones who have done infinitely more good than harm, includes physical and occupational therapists, a physiatrist, a homeopath, an acupuncturist who does zero balancing, a psychiatrist, and a psychotherapist. These are the people who have offered me their skills gently and kindly. They all work in different ways—some use their hands, some are better with words, and some can soothe with just their eyes—but they have each, in their own way and at different times, alleviated the very worst part about being ill: overwhelming loneliness and despair. To save my own life, I had to feel it was worth living. Severe chronic illness made me question whether it was. My doctors gave me their assurances that, while they didn't have all the answers, they were certain I could find my way back to myself. Because they had earned my trust, I believed them. I fought for my life.

Still, as much as I grew to love them over time, my doctors made me a little nervous at first. Unlike the cocky physicians I had grown used to, these practitioners offered no guarantees that they fully understood what was wrong with me. They never promised they could make me feel better. What they did insist, though, was that miracles do indeed happen, and that no matter what direction my own path through life took, they would remain by my side for as long as I needed them. Sometimes their methods were standard textbook, while at other times they used "alternative" or energy-based methods like acupuncture. Regardless of what they did, though, what sets them apart is that from the very beginning, they all seemed to believe that the shaking, terrified shadow of a person in front of them was, in fact, whole and lovable. They accepted imperfect me long before I did.

## The Importance of Uncertainty

When I met them, these doctors I now claim as "mine," I wasn't sure what I thought of them. What I really wanted in a doctor was someone who knew exactly what was wrong with me and could make me well immediately. In short, I wanted God in the office with me. They would not act the part, but guess what? I've met more than a few doctors who would. When a patient and her doctor share this same fantasy, it's a match made in heaven—except for the small matter that the relationship is based on a lie.

And there's the problem: When both doctor and patient buy into the myth that doctors can make miracles happen, healing can't take place, because ultimately, healing is the patient's privilege and responsibility. Any doctor who forgets this is usurping his patient's power. Yes, in the beginning I wanted my life to be in my doctors' hands because I ached for life to be that easy. Besides, it's what I'd been taught doctors were for: saving lives, curing illness. Then I got sick, and I found out that illness, like infancy or old age, rendered me dependent. Healing required me to take back authority over my life no matter if I was sick or well. Asking for help is not the same as having someone else take the wheel. My life is mine. I had forgotten that.

Now I understand that no doctor can heal me. The best ones—the ones I found at the Spaulding—understand this, too. Yes, they offered gold-standard medical care, and just as important they provided hope so that I could find the path back to myself. Almost without ego, they have rejoiced as I have slowly gotten better. But they never claimed to have saved me. We all know that I have saved myself.

Many doctors—perhaps those who have cut themselves off from the heartache and holiness of their work—don't seem to have mastered the art of compassion. But mine have. These are people who know they aren't God, but who try their best anyway. Well-trained clinicians who aren't clinical, but who are brave enough to make connections to those of us desperately in need of help. In other words, they are imperfect human beings like the rest of us, acting from the only human impulse that serves life: love.

I'm sure that it's not easy to care deeply about lots of patients while keeping yourself safe. But I've noticed that those who are open to life's mysteries, including alternative modes of healing, find this balance more easily than their counterparts across the ideological divide.

I've also noticed that doctors who don't at least make the effort to be open minded can get mean. When I told my internist that an osteopath was making my heart feel better, she said sarcastically, "Aw, isn't that sweet." Why did my saying this make her angry? From what I understand, my vagus nerve had been compressed in all the torque of my body, causing many of the disturbing cardiac symptoms I'd had for over a decade; as this doctor helped my body release the tension, the nerve was no longer compressed and the symptoms lessened. I thought my internist might find my improvement interesting, not to mention important. I was wrong.

## Suggestions for Doctors

We patients are smart—we know what our doctors think of us, whether they express their opinions overtly or not. People in need are especially sensitive to nuance. If only more doctors—more people—could remain open to the possibility that there is so much about life that we simply don't understand! Maybe then they would surrender the false belief that they are responsible for another person's life. And maybe then they would remember that all any of us can ask of others is that they do their best with loving intent. For doctors especially, forgetting this often translates into overestimating their power. Then, when people are human, imperfect, undiagnosable, these same doctors take their frustrations out on the one skewing their world view. Being ill becomes an affront, and the patient becomes the enemy.

Those of us who are ill need doctors, but doctors need us patients, too, and not just to meet quotas.

Being sick means we don't have the energy to pretend we care about anything except what's absolutely essential in our lives; our mere presence can remind others of what matters most. Our job as patients is to take on the incredible challenge of reclaiming our lives, reinventing ourselves. Your job as doctors is to expect the best both from us and from yourselves be-cause you have the strength for optimism, whereas we may not. With a little faith on both sides, we can all be bettered by having come together.

*(Editor's note: As this book went into publication, Betsy gave birth to her second child after a relatively uneventful pregnancy, labor, and delivery. Mother and child are both doing very well.)*

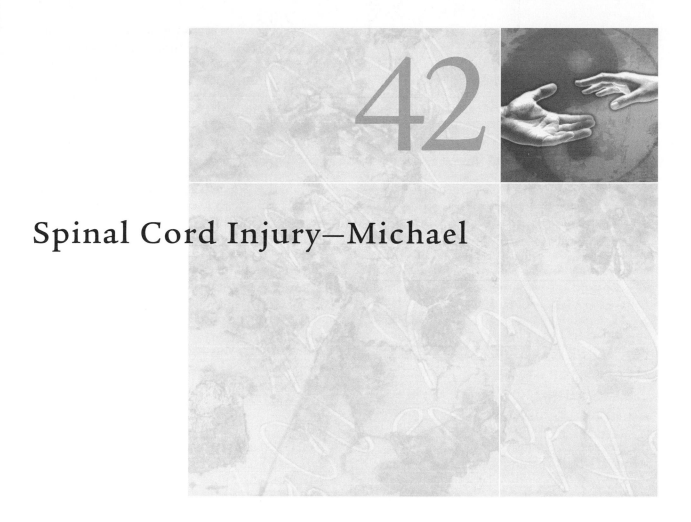

# Spinal Cord Injury—Michael

## EDITOR'S INTRODUCTION

Michael was a 35-year-old married male construction worker when he first entered the Spaulding Rehabilitation Hospital (SRH) Inpatient Pain Program in 1995 to taper off his opiate pain medications and to learn self-management strategies for his chronic pain. He had been injured in 1990 while working as a roofer when he fell onsite while carrying a 150-pound load and suffered a traumatic compression of the cervical spine that left him with a C5-6 root injury. Even after a decompressive laminectomy, he had a severely restricted range of motion (ROM) and limited weight bearing capacity that prevented even minimal tasks beyond ADLs. His story is typical of chronic pain patients—fragmented medical care (allopathic and complementary and alternative medicine [CAM]), misuse of inappropriately prescribed medications, legal obstacles and poor insurance coverage, and ever-worsening levels of function.

Unexpectedly, despite a blue-collar background that was firmly rooted in traditional American and Catholic "male" values, Michael became fascinated by his first exposure to traditional Chinese medicine. He became an avid student of the martial arts, initially attracted by the macho aura of combat and self-defense. He later saw it as a tool for self-healing, and ultimately as a path toward self-knowledge and spiritual understanding. His current level of function shows full ROM with no residual neuropathic pain. He has recovered full strength in his upper extremities and is pursuing training as a martial arts instructor. I have seen him in outpatient psychotherapy approximately every 4 to 6 weeks since he came to SRH.

His story is remarkable for the persistence with which he pursued his vision of self-healing via martial arts training. He sought out, and eventually outgrew, a series of teachers that included the leading practitioners in the Boston area, in his quest to forge his own philosophy of health and wellness. His story is a cautionary tale about the power of so-called subtle energy techniques because, unfortunately, the same fervor to excel that made him a good worker also triggered intense psychological side effects from his overly intensive practice of healing techniques. These symptoms were in marked contrast to the initial numbness—both physical and emotional—he experienced due to nerve damage and medication excess. At times earthy, at times poignant, his story is a remarkable example of rehabilitation at all levels—physical, emotional, and spiritual. (At the patient's request, the names of key people and places have been altered.)

## The Work Injury and Initial Symptoms

*Dr. Leskowitz:* Talk a little about your injury.

*Patient:* The first thing for me was, I was blown away that they couldn't fix it. I just figured I threw my back out and they'd cut a disk out and I'd be back to work in a month. Then I realized nobody knew how to fix it. What happened was my arm and leg went dead. I kind of downplayed it, thinking I'd just bounce back. But it kept getting deader and deader, so I went to the Carney Hospital emergency room. They told me to stop working for 2 weeks and then come back to Orthopedics. I went into Orthopedics a few weeks later and I was starting to get, you know, real bad pain and they kind of like blew me off, but a woman doctor come out in the hallway and said "You know, that's a sign that this could be real serious."

*Dr. L:* So when you fell at work, you didn't think that it was that serious?

*Patient:* No I didn't, but my arm and leg went dead. I actually worked out that night and I just blocked it out, but it got to a point where it got so dead my leg started falling over and I couldn't hold things in my hand. That's when I said "Oh, #$*!" and I went to the Carney. But I actually thought they were

saying "this guy'd be back to work in a month." I didn't think *$#! of it. And then the pain just got incredible and I kept getting blown off, but then I'd get warnings and my hand was dead so I went to the Mass General (Hospital). They said it was anxiety and they gave me Valium.

Then I actually called Arnold (my lawyer). I said, "I screwed my neck up," so he sent me to this doctor across the street, he's a retired surgeon. So the surgeon was just milking me for money. Arnold was paying him and finally after a few months of that, I mean I could hardly walk and knew I was flipping out with pain. I called Arnold back up. I said "This guy's an idiot," and Arthur sent me to (Dr. Murphy). I goes to Murphy. Murphy says, "Jesus Christ, you know this should have been done a long time ago." He gives me a prescription for Percs [Percocet, a narcotic painkiller] and he sends me down to get an MRI. They couldn't find *&#! on the MRI so I had to get them myelograms and they found out my spinal cord was flat, so they said, "We got to cut you right away," so I got cut [the laminectomy], and then I was even in worse pain. And it just went on from there, with drug addiction.

## Drug Addiction

*Dr. L:* How did the drug addiction develop?

*Patient:* Well, for me, I couldn't do nothing. I was like in insane pain so what I would do was, I'd eat pills and I'd try to work out. Hit the speed bag (punching bag) and do pushups and sit-ups (laughs). That didn't work so I started doing pills heavier and heavier, so then I started snorting the morphine. I found out if you mix morphine and Klonopin you get a super buzz. I actually snorted 'em. I'd take a Heineken's and blast it down my nose cause I knew I'd get that feeling. You actually got to a point, or I did, where I knew how to mix the drugs. So I actually tried to lift weights again, hit the speed bags but it didn't help (laughs).

*Dr. L:* What were you hoping to do by lifting the weights after your injury?

*Patient:* I was hoping that my body would get strong enough so I'd heal and I wouldn't need the pills, but the pain was so insane, I needed the pills really to do the workout.

*Dr. L:* Why don't you say a little bit about your workout habits before you got hurt.

*Patient:* Oh, I was a nut. I'd do like 50 pushups just to wake up in the morning and then I'd roof (i.e., go to work as a roofer) and then I'd lift weights. I'd work out every day. I always thought of the body as a weapon. Now I kind of think of it as a tool instead of a weapon. I actually thought of it as disposable—yeah (laughs) I was wrong (laughs). You know, I always thought I could fix it. I never in my wildest dreams ever thought. . . . Oh !#%*—I get all choked up (voice cracks). It blew me away. It couldn't be fixed. I've been in motorcycle accidents, I was burned, I've broken things, I've roofed with broken shoulders knowing that I could get through it. But this . . . To be honest, though, the drug addiction was the worst.

*Dr. L:* How so?

*Patient:* Oh, !#%*—self-esteem, pride, everything bad. You stop working and if you didn't take the pills, you get violently sick, and then you know you're a junkie. On one level I knew, and on another level I wouldn't admit it 'cause I kept thinking I could be strong and I could work on the body, work on the body. Wrong! And then I got bummed out, bottomed out. A lot more fear. I had two more kids after that. One was born and then I had another one. How do you support the family? Then you realize you been nailed, and nobody gives a !#%* about you. The lawyers, doctors, insurance companies—scumbags. You realize how corrupt and filthy the world is. You know you're a pawn. You've waited years. You wait for hours in the doctor's office and then you . . . (silence).

*Dr. L:* When did you hit bottom with that whole process?

*Patient:* Probably after Murphy said he couldn't help me. I went in to Carney and they put me on a morphine drip through my spine. They put a catheter and ran it through my spine but it didn't work. I spent a week in the hospital, and they said, "You'll probably never get it back." And I went, "Oh !#%*." And I said "!#%* them." I always thought I could get stronger but the pain was insane.

*Dr. L:* So how did you get from there into the rehab process?

*Patient:* Well Mahoney said "What are you going to do?" I said, "What the !#%* are my choices?" (laughs). I actually did my own research, so I knew I had to get off drugs. I kept trying myself to go cold turkey but it was insane. It felt like somebody was scratching my brain. I was flipping out, I'd hallucinate. I'd feel like

you wouldn't believe. So I says "Spaulding"—it was in the freakin' Yellow Pages! (laughs)

## Starting the Rehab Process

Yeah, so I told him (Dr. Murphy), and he says, "Whatever you want to do." I called up and he did the thing (to get me registered) and I went in and had an initial interview (for the outpatient pain rehab program). What happened was, I was snorting morphine and I was still trying to get stronger with the drugs to mask the pain and one of the women, I forget who it was, asked me what I was doing and I told her. She said, "Well, you better tell the doctor." So when I told (Spaulding Rehabilitation Hospital's Dr.) Makowski, he said you better come in to the hospital, and then I had the big fight with Social Security. Nobody would pay for the inpatient program. Workers' comp wouldn't. So that was a 2-year battle trying to get in and get off drugs.

What happened was, when I got hurt it was negligence. A crane was broken so they didn't clean the rooms where we worked. There was *%#! everywhere—that's how I fell, on spilled glue. So what I did is, I got five letters from guys I used to work with and I had Arnold file a thing for double compensation because it was negligence. So I went in before the judge and we bartered off. If I dropped that claim for double damages, they'd pay for the inpatient rehab program. So that's how I got into Spaulding—I bartered off the double comp case to get off the drugs.

*Dr. L:* Then what happened at the Spaulding program?

*Patient:* Well I got off drugs and actually you told me about chi kung. So then I went and looked in the yellow pages (laughs) and I saw Woodville (Martial Arts Training Center) and I went in there and I did three courses and they stopped it. I learned about Interface (a local holistic education center). So I went over there and I did insight meditation and I did a yoga class and then I did Mimi Ferrara's tai chi. That was once or twice a week, I'm not sure, but it was like a 3-month deal, so there was no progression (to advanced courses). And then I got called by Woodville and they started a satellite program and I went in and I did that. I did a burning meditation and a real strong inverse breathing [powerful energy mobilizing techniques]. They sent me to A.K. Tang's father [a respected elder in the Chinese marital arts community]. And what happened was, I'd go to him twice a week and I actually got relief from pain without drugs, but it wore off in the morning. So I used to go there and I'd do chi kung and I'd feel good 'til about the middle of the night, and I'm frigging back over there in the morning (laughs) waiting for them to open up. They'd do acupuncture and moxibustion and A.K.'s father would do some kind of *%#! with me, and they'd let me sleep there for a few hours. And then I did the herbs for about 2 or 3 years, and every couple of weeks they changed my bag of herbs and I went over there 2 days a week. I never really talked about this (voice cracks).

*Dr. L:* What's that feeling you have now?

*Patient:* It's a relief, it's been a rough journey.

*Dr. L:* And that phase is over now?

*Patient:* Whew. To go in that much pain and *%#!. I always felt like I was dying. I remember driving to Boston thinking I'm going to die. It was like torture, but I did it anyhow. I don't even know why (voice cracks). I knew somewhere in that *%#! I could heal.

*Dr. L:* How did you know?

*Patient:* When I worked out, I used to cry it hurt so much. Woodville was too hard, when I went to their temple. So A.K.'s father said, "What are you doing?" He kept saying "I fix, you break. I fix, you break," (laughs). So I told him and he says, "No, that's how soldiers train." I didn't know there was a healing chi kung and a martial chi kung. So he actually invited me to his house and I went to his house and he taught me a healing chi kung. Then I ended up with Wang Lu and I learned that hot herb treatment. That helped me unbelievable. Wang was kind of a selfish ego man, but that treatment helped me unbelievable. It helped me do kung fu. I'd be just about crying, flipping out with panic attacks. "Put me on a table. Let's do the herbs." It was like letting air out of a ball. So I was actually doing his and this other guy Dr. Po's herbs, and A.K.'s and Wang Lu's chi kung, all at once. Both of my shoulders used to be frozen. One of them opened up in Woodville. The other one opened up when Yang worked on me. I'd be crying but something told me to keep going. I knew once I got past that crying and the fear, I'd get warmth in the parts that didn't have warmth. I *know* I can move energy now. I was in a lot of pain this morning and I can get into a tolerable state.

## Overdoing the Energy Practices

Another time, I was doing the breathing and I got rushed to the Carney Hospital. My whole body started convulsing. Tightened up so hard I couldn't breathe. The air was sucking out of me. My wife took me to the hospital. The doctors were afraid to touch me. It looked like something from *The Exorcist!* My whole body was just sucked in. I was sitting in the waiting room for about a half an hour and it (the energy blockage) released, so I left. I goes in (to Boston) and I was telling A.K., and he starts laughing. He says, "Oh Jesus, I should have told you. That's part of the chi kung." He says sometimes it does that if you're injured bad. And I used to wake up in my frigging own bed, for almost 2 years, I'd wake up at night and my sheets would be like pouring sweat and it stunk like chemicals. A.K. said it was from all the drugs and the radiation treatments I've had, coming out of my body.

Another time I thought I had a urine infection 'cause my pee was a funny color and it stunk. So I goes down to Dorchester House and there's this woman doctor with a Q-tip (laughs) (for a urethral culture). The deal was, my kidneys and liver were purging. I goes in and I tell A.K.—they were in convulsions laughing. He says, "Oh, I should have told you" (laughs). So it's kind of crazy. The training helps you but the *%#! you got to go through is unnecessary. If you got warned beforehand and you knew, it'd be easier to handle than if you're going nuts or got kidney disease or something.

I had tons of crazy stuff happen to me. The worst are the night terrors. I haven't had any in a while. I'd be sound asleep and all of a sudden I'd wake up frigging feeling like I never had in my life. It could last for days. Or I was having unbelievable nightmares and I couldn't tell if I was awake or asleep or couldn't wake up. I've had them last 2 days. It's unbelievable. I'd be shaking. The workouts (laugh). I don't know why (I kept doing them). You know, it's friggin' insane. Then I'm thinking, "Am I insane?" But then something says, "You're not insane." It's, like, crazy.

## The Need for a Guide

*Dr. L:* What did you learn in the Broadmoor School of Tai Chi phase of things?

*Patient:* Bob (the program director) helped me a lot. What I got from Bob is, he charged me a lot of money but it was my only option and I got a lot more mobility out of it. I mean there's no friendships there and it was definitely busy and I paid him a lot and he showed me a lot. He held back a lot but I did get some guidance and it was kind of like an anchor. I had someplace to go and someplace to train. So what I did get out of it is, "I have to do everything myself." Everybody's too busy with their own business and their own lives. I always thought I'd find somebody who thought I was worth training.

I didn't know the energy *%#! existed. There was like a veil. I just didn't have the education (to see through it). It bothered me that energy is marketed. It's molded to somebody's interpretation of it, and that ain't correct. There shouldn't be a market on it—energy is free. It bothered me how people hoard information and they make money off it and there's a lot of embellishing. It is true you gotta do the work yourself and I don't understand why it ain't in rehab programs to learn *%#! about gentle movements.

*Dr. L:* What did you learn about pain by going through this whole process?

*Patient:* Whew, pain. Pain is demons, man (laugh). I know on some level pain is a blockage. I still don't comprehend that fully. Pain's a mother*%#!#%. It's still a big blockage. It blinds you. I think it (the blocked energy) backs up and goes up into the head or something. I actually felt a pain that felt like shocking nerve pain. It actually burns and it's sharp, but it left through my fingers and I actually noticed at that time that the back of my spine stopped hurting. But I didn't feel the direct current going from the pain out the fingers, I actually felt (the pain) in the fingers and then at the same time I realized that the spot on my spine stopped hurting. So I'm thinking that must have been pain leaving. I don't know if I'm correct on that yet. But I do know that certain pains I can handle very well. Other pains still freak me out.

## Spiritual Aspects of Rehabilitation

*Dr. L:* How did you get into the spirituality part of it?

*Patient:* I've always wanted that. What it comes down to is I think everybody knows that it's just fear, of not living up to the "I"—what you're supposed to do. For me, it was "Kill or be killed" (growing up in the

projects). I know I got injured because of my lifestyle selling drugs and being a mother*%#!#%. Every action has a reaction (laughs)—you're still going to get it. What I've noticed too, a lot of people that screw over people for wealth—their bodies are trash, they're obese, they're alcoholics, they're drug addicts. I believe it's fear, conditioned fear of poverty, of powerlessness, that's so overpowering to everybody that they lose sight of spirituality. I don't think it's "Spirituality is better than anything." I think spirituality is just nature. You harm and you'll be harmed. I don't know that much about it. I'm always waiting for my path and I'm realizing now, that's why I suffer. I'm suffering because I want something. I still want. I'm aware of the pitfalls of titles and fame but I still fear poverty.

I can't understand the link between spirituality and energy, unless you're just more connected to everything in nature with your energy. If you're connected enough and balanced enough, you'll just know. You'll recognize the fear. I think for me it's just accepting life as it is. Stop waiting for that teacher.

*Dr. L:* Where do you see your process going in the future?

*Patient:* I'd love to get a way to deal with the pain. I think there is a way. I've had people touch me. A.K.'s father and Wang Lu could do it, a couple of other people. I'd be in flipping out pain and they could end it. I don't know how they did it. I don't know if they took it, or if they neutralized it, or if they ran it out my body—I can't get an answer from anybody. I'd love to get rid of my fear of poverty but from what I'm starting to see from Krishnamurti [the Hindu philosopher] and everything, it's part of our conditioning. Accept it, get so it don't affect you, acknowledge it for what it is and accept it. I think that would be a big part of training because your body must tense on fear, so your energy ain't gonna flow good and you're not going to be content.

I'd love to have a way to help other people. Can I do that? I give some treatments 'cause I know it will help my circle, and I'm giving people treatments and I like the feeling it gives. It ain't to be a friggin' saint. I'll get something out of it, which I don't see nothing wrong with that. They feel good, I feel good. Nobody's screwed. It's strictly a business deal. I think that's spirituality—being honest. Not "I'm above you." That's why I don't like titles, I'm afraid of titles. To be honest I don't think I've done anything great. Forget how I look now. I knew I was !#%*ed. A lot of emotions came out (during the healing process), but it was like reading it in a book. Bob says the memories lost their energetic charge.

I don't get upset anymore like I used to. I don't know if its maturity. What is maturity? Not blaming others? But blaming others is just your conditioned mind being stronger than your heart. I start all my martial or nonmartial (practice sessions) by opening my heart. I'm a little leery of the people that don't. I'm just calling a spade a spade. I believe everything has to go that way (through your heart) or you're gonna be a killer, you're gonna be arrogant. I'm looking for my path but everybody else is confident I'm on it (laughs). I don't see it.

I know tons of people with back injuries. I offer treatment—nobody comes. My personality changed a million percent getting over my fears, but it was fear. The drugs and alcohol didn't help it either. How do you get somebody to get over fear? How do you help somebody even acknowledge their fears? They'll fight you on that or they'll kill the messenger. I think what I'd like is a way to convey, without a school, "This will help you, this won't help you." Some people need martial arts; some shouldn't have martial arts (laughs).

I think a lot of people are afraid to be helped. They're afraid to change. Most guys I know who drink won't quit drinking because they'd be looked at as a sissy buddy. What it comes down to is you have no social life (if you give up drinking to train hard). I have no peers. Not even in working out for martial arts. I have nobody to work out with me. Everybody talks but when it comes down to doing serious training, they don't want to do it for some reason. I can't understand why they're there. It's like a stutter step—they're half doing it. Like they're pretending they're doing it but they're really "!#%* that, I ain't changing." I think it's putting the mirror up (when I'm there). They don't want to look at themselves.

## Change in Self-Image

But who the hell am I to say that? Who the hell is anybody else to? I'm just a broken construction worker. Everybody will pretend (laugh), "Let's all pretend we're good people and we're doing serious !#%*," but it's not so in those classes, and I don't think there's a set way to be spiritual. I just think it's very simple—you receive what you get. Don't harm, man, try to be good. And it's hard. When I was driving in here I was in pain and a guy would cut me off and my mind's going "!#%*ing mother*%#!#%." Where now, thank God, I'm starting to not act on that stuff. I can see it—whoa! (laugh). I always see ways I could be a shyster. The money's tempting. For some reason I can't do it. I don't see no gain to harm people for money or false hope. I don't want to give anybody false hope. That's why people don't want me to say, "Chi kung hurts, and if you don't want to do it you're better off doing meditation and breathing." People don't tell the truth for cash.

I made the choice to hurt myself but something inside me told me to. I look at it as my body, the parts that really hurt were dried up. They were all stiff and hard. I felt like sandstone, dried like a brick, but it wasn't a hard stone, it was a brittle stone. And when the energy moved in there it hurt a real lot and it affected my mind a real lot. I was depressed, want to cry. Something told me to keep going, keep going, and I did.

*Dr. L:* What was it that told you to keep going?

*Patient:* My inner voice, and I think that's my tool. I have no problem getting hurt. The injury, it kind of opened my eyes and I think it happened because of my lifestyle. I have no problem with that. You know, it's kind of like "You play, you pay." I think the energetics and the meditation are the same way. I think everything's the same way. I used to think everything's complicated, but it ain't complicated. It should be simple 'cause it is simple. The ego, whatever that is, doesn't think it's simple. It has a phony sense of things. You know—I don't know. I don't know (laughs).

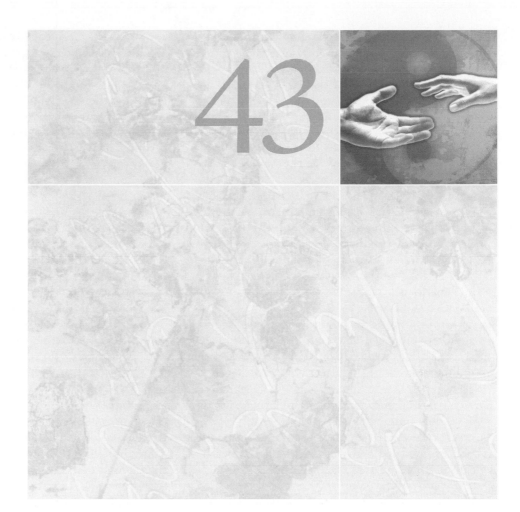

# Stroke*

RAM DASS

## EDITOR'S INTRODUCTION

In 1967 Richard Alpert was a promising young academic psychologist at Harvard University when he was dismissed from the faculty for his involvement in Timothy Leary's early experiments with LSD. He travelled to India soon thereafter and recorded his experiences with his spiritual teacher, Maharajii in the international best-seller, *Be Here Now.* This book placed the newly christened Ram Dass in the forefront of the movement to bring Eastern Philosophy to the West. In subsequent years, he wrote and lectured widely and established several non-profit organizations devoted to serving others. In 1997, he suffered a stroke just as he was completing

his most recent book, *Still Here.* The following essay first appeared as the chapter entitled "Stroke Yoga" in that book. In it he describes the experience of "being stroked" and rehabilitation from the perspective of someone who has spent a lifetime cultivating moment-to-moment spiritual awareness. As such, this essay is a profound blend of the sacred and the mundane, with much to teach us all about the process of rehabilitation—physically, psychologically, and spiritually.

So here I am, some two and a half years after the stroke. The stroke gave me what I was looking for that day in February: it gave me the ending for my book. It gave me an encounter with the kind of physical suffering that often accompanies aging; it gave me a brush with death; it gave me the firsthand experiences I was lacking back then. I can write about aging now.

*From Dass R: *Still here*, New York, 2001, Riverhead Books.

Having the point of view of a disabled person, having come through a catastrophic physical event, I can write about aging in a way I couldn't have before.

I've always gone through experiences and then shared my wisdom about them. That's been my role. I was part of the "advance scouting party" for the psychedelic movement in the Sixties. I was part of the advance guard in the Seventies for people who were opening to Eastern religions. In the Eighties, I explored the ways we might use services as "karma yoga," as a spiritual practice—a practice that's more available to us Westerners than monastic life or other traditional methods might be. In the Nineties, as a kind of "uncle" to the baby boomers, being a little older than they are, I've been leading the way into an experience that lies ahead of most of us—the experience of aging. In the Nineties, the stroke is the learning experience that I have to share.

Of course, a stroke isn't identical to aging; I didn't get any older because I had a stroke. But it is a new chapter in my aging process. The final stage of aging is cuddling up to death, and the stroke gave me some experience with that. Aging in your 60s? That's nothing. Aging in your 90s? That's a different thing. Death is much more imminent then. The stroke moved my counter forward on the board. It gave me the chance to spend some time contemplating life and death, which is usually part of the later stage of aging, when aging itself forces the issue.

The stroke was like a samurai sword, cutting apart the two halves of my life. It was a demarcation between two stages. In a way, it's been having two incarnations in one; this is me, that was "him." Seeing it that way has been an important part of my practice, part of the way I've worked with the stroke. Seeing it that way saves me from the suffering of making comparisons, of thinking about the things I used to do but can't do anymore because of the paralysis in my hand. In the "past incarnation," I had an MG with a stick shift, I had golf clubs, I had a cello. Now I don't have any use for those things. New incarnation!

Before I had the stroke, I was full of fears about aging, and one of my major fears was about the sickness that might be lurking ahead. Gandhi says that before you can get to God, you've got to confront your fears. The stroke took me through one of my deep fears, and I'm here to report that "the only thing we have to fear is fear itself."

This chapter is an antidote to fear because reading what this experience has been like for me will give you

a map. It's like you're on a rafting trip, and you're about to hit some rapids. I've just been through one of those sets of rapids, and maybe my experiences can help you figure out how to handle the rapids when you encounter them.

I'm explicitly making my life a teaching by expressing the lessons I've learned through it so it can become a map for other people. Everybody's life could be like that, if they choose to make it so; choose to reflect about what they've been through and to share it with others.

I call sickness and death "the rapids" because it's an experience of change, change, change—and change is the mantra of aging. I couldn't get a closing for this book because I had never been through an experience of fierce, dramatic change like that. I had *anticipated* what changes like that might be like, but I'd never gone through them.

Over the years, I've done practices to confront my fear of change, of which the fear of death is the foremost. In Benares, I visited the cremation grounds at the *ghats*. I sat there in meditation on the side of the Ganges, a sacred river. Bodies were being burned all around me; I smelled the burning flesh, watched the eldest son break open the father's skull with a stick to release his spirit. I'd overcome a lot of fears about death and change through practices like that, but there was still an undercurrent of fear in my mind; I was in my 60's, I was "getting up there."

Now, having come through this stroke, I am less afraid. The stroke cleaned out some of the pockets of fear. It's happened, and here I am—closer to Maharajji than ever. What more could I ask?

The stroke happened to me for many different reasons, including karmic and spiritual ones. But on the physical level, one of the reasons for the stroke was that I had been ignoring my body. I had spent most of my life keeping my Awareness "free of my body," as I thought of then; but I can see now that I was also ignoring my body, pushing it away. By forgetting to take my blood pressure medicine, I showed how I was disregarding my body. By ignoring the early signs that something was wrong when I was diving in the Caribbean, I was disregarding my body. By overcommitting myself, never saying "no" no matter what my body was telling me, I was disregarding it.

So then came the stroke.

For some days after the stroke, I was just observing. Not thinking, just observing. A friend described me during those first days as being wide-eyed, watching everything that was taking place with a kind of wonderment.

Perceptions from the outside and from the inside were sometimes very different. At one point, I was in what doctors called a "nonreactive state," and they thought I might die. From the outside, I was an object of concern and a cause for apprehension. But inside, I was just floating peacefully. My body was present, but it was irrelevant. It was like I was looking through a window, and the scene through the window had in it the hospital, and me, and the doctors, and everybody else—but I was outside looking in. I was really floating out there!

After awhile, as I started to become aware of the symptoms of the stroke, my thoughts began to come in on me. I worried for awhile about what had happened: Where had the stroke gone in my brain? How bad was it? I didn't know the answers to those questions for a long time, and that was scary. How long would the domino effect of the symptoms go on? As one thing after another "went out" on me after the stroke—my knee, my hip, my shoulder, my ankle— I didn't know that would go next. How long would the pain go on—would it be days, or months, or years? I worried what the effect would be of just sitting in my wheelchair all the time, unable to move around and exercise in the usual way. That flood of questions carried strong elements of fear with it.

To work with the fear, I turned to my practices. The stroke called on all the practices I'd learned over the years: *Vipassana* meditation, *jnana* yoga, *bhakti, guru kripa*—at different points and in different situations I used them all. But in that particular crisis I found that I turned to Ramana Maharshi's practice of "I am not this body." I would note each part of my body, and I would say, "I am not my arm. I am not my leg. I am not my brain." That helped me avoid getting caught in the mind's fears and the body's sensations.

In the months that followed, though, I came to appreciate that however wonderful it is as a practice, "I am not this body" is only half the truth. The stroke brought me squarely in touch with the fact that, although I am certainly *more* than my body, I also *am* my body. The stroke brought my Awareness into my body in a powerful way, with an array of physical symptoms: paralysis, aphasia, pain. The stroke "grounded" me, in both meanings of the word: it brought me in touch with the earth plane, with my body, and it made me stay at home. I used to be traveling constantly, but when you're traveling

in a wheelchair, planes aren't much fun. So this illness "grounded" me and taught me what everyone else already knew: that it's nice to be at home.

Motels had often been my home before. I even had a story I used to tell: I was nearing the end of a sixty-city benefit tour for the Seva Foundation, and I'd been on the road for many, many weeks. In my motel room one night, I found myself thinking, "Just one more week and I'll be home!" Then I caught myself; I saw how thinking that way was a sure path to suffering— being unhappy where I was, chafing to get someplace else. So I fixed up a little *puja* on the plastic motel coffee table, with pictures of Maharajji and all. And then I took my key, walked out of the room, and closed the door behind me. I walked down to the end of the hallway, and then I turned around and walked back to my room. I unlocked the door, stepped into the room and called out, "I'm home!"

I was trying to change my way of looking at the situation, to make "home" be wherever I was at the moment. It was a sophisticated concept that home was the universe. And it was a useful device then, when I had to be traveling so much of the time. But my home now is an emotional haven, a center. If an animal needs to lick its wounds, it retires to its cave; it looks for a protected space. I had never known that before—that a motel room isn't a "protected space" in that way.

It's true that being "grounded" by my wheelchair has its downside. Not traveling as much deprives me of visiting the old friends I used to see in Boston, New York, all the places I used to visit on tour, and I miss that. But mostly I find that I'm very comfortable having the wheelchair. I can even see why I cling to it. Who wouldn't rather ride than walk? Or always have a seat at parties? When I do travel, I whiz through the airport at the speed of light in my wheelchair, going "Beep-beep! Beep-beep!" to warn the pedestrians. The wheelchair is my palanquin.

Nowadays, there's a certain status in our society in being disabled. It's a political movement. I've gone to demonstrations in my wheelchair—a May Day marijuana march, and a "Dignity Day" march for the homeless, where I rolled along side-by-side with Ron Kovic (whose life was portrayed in the film *Born on the Fourth of July*). It's a new kind of role, rolling along in a wheelchair. It's made me into a different kind of symbol because disability carries powerful symbolic values; negative ones (like *dis*-abled), but also positive ones: the blue sticker I get for parking, the accessibility issues I raise.

It's interesting the way these things work. I went to a conference at a retreat center run by conscious people who are very sensitive to accessibility problems. It tuned out, though, that although I could get my wheelchair into the bathroom of the room they'd assigned me, I couldn't get my wheelchair into the shower stall; the shower door wasn't wide enough. They apologized profusely and fixed me up with a special bathtub chair—and then right after the conference, they called in an architect to begin redesigning the bathroom. That's the way it works, the way an understanding of problems spreads among people.

There are funny moments with the wheelchair. I was invited to a cocktail party one evening; it was one of those "stand-up" affairs—for everyone except me, that is. So, I found that everyone else was "up there" talking to one another, and I was "down here" at chair level. Occasionally some thoughtful person would crouch down next to my chair and talk to me for awhile, and then I'd get to see a face. But for the most part, as far as I could see, the party was largely attended by a gathering of assholes.

Besides putting me in a wheelchair, the stroke gave me aphasia—a difficulty in finding the words for things. Just when the Age of Communication arrives, I get aphasia! For someone who's made a living giving lectures and writing books, that was quite a change. I'm in the word business, and for a word merchant like me to have this particular sickness—boy, oh boy!

From the inside, the aphasia doesn't seem like a breakdown of concepts, but like an undressing of the concepts. It's as if there's a dressing room where concepts get clothed in words, and that's the part of my brain that was affected by the stroke. It took me awhile after I'd had the stroke to figure out what was going on. I had to sort out that distinction between words and concepts.

Initially, before I grasped that difference, I started to mistrust my judgment, my thinking mind (which I'd always mistrusted anyway, but on different grounds); because the concepts were divorced from words, I could *experience* the thought-forms but I couldn't *symbolize* them. It took awhile for me to realize the difference between my thinking mind—which is clear—and my verbal ability—which is sometimes iffy.

The aphasia has introduced silences to my conversation, and many of the people I work with use those silences to make contact with the silence within themselves. We surf the silence together, and in it they find their own answers. I've got to treat words as if they're precious now, but that's teaching me what can be conveyed with silence. When the words don't come as easily, it requires that what I say be as much "essence" as possible. I don't have the energy for all the digressions I used to run through.

I had training for this kind of thing when I was with Baba Hari Das in India. I was *mauna* (in silence) for a period of time, and he and I wrote to each other on tiny slates that we wore around our necks. When that's your way of communicating, you have to go right back to the root of things. A few words were better than many. Terse!

I've noticed something interesting: when there's not such a rush of words, the imagery gets subtler. The slower pace sometimes seems to give more poetry to my words than they used to have. I've also wondered if that's an effect of the change in balance that the stroke brought about in my brain. With the left brain—the verbal, analytical half—less dominant since the stroke, maybe the right brain is just freer to come out and play.

Besides the wheelchair and the aphasia, one other physical consequence of the stroke was the heavy encounter with pain that it precipitated. The stroke brought me into intimate contact with pain, and I found pain to be a worthy adversary for my spiritual practices. Working with constant pain pushed my practices to their limits.

I had experienced plenty of pain before—with hepatitis, kidney stones, a torn Achilles tendon. So why was this different? Partly it was the situation. In a hospital, the doctors and nurses freak out about pain, so they give you pills to get rid of it. But they don't know when to give the pills, so they ask you all the time, "Are you in pain? Are you in pain?" and that keeps focusing your attention on it. And partly it was the duration of the pain. The experiences of pain I'd had in the past were intense but relatively brief, lasting only a few day at the most. With the stroke, the pain was less severe, but it went on naggingly, day after day, on one part of my body after another.

Pain is a potent attention-getter. A pain will call to you very strongly to be the experiencer, and you stay stuck in the experience until you can find a way to create some space around it. It took all the practices I could muster, but in the long run they worked. Practices that allowed me to jump into the Soul often worked for me—watching the pain versus experiencing the pain. I had long conversations with Maharajji about the pain. I used the practices I'd learned in my Vipassana training for making the pain the primary object of my meditation.

I still use my Vipassana techniques at night because it's when I'm trying to sleep that I notice the pain the most—my arm, my shoulder, my foot. I can't turn over easily, or shift my position, so my muscles start to cramp up and hurt. But I have a breathing apparatus that I wear to correct a problem of sleep apnea; it magnifies the sound of my breathing, and I use that as my primary object and meditate on it until I'm in a place where I'm just quietly witnessing the pain.

One of the things I've learned in the course of all this is that I'd had some misconceptions about medical marijuana. Because I had always used marijuana (like all psychedelics) in a spiritual context, I hadn't fully appreciated its medical value. Previously I'd thought of it only for its consciousness-changing ability, but that's actually just a side effect to its use for pain relief. I live in California, a state where the use of medical marijuana is legal, and I am a "carded" patient. Marijuana has been one of the treatments that has helped me the most with the spasticity and pain I've experienced as my stroke-damaged muscles contract.

What I've learned from all this is what a delicate game it is to work with intense pain. Like all the experiences of an incarnation, pain has to be experienced fully by the Ego in order to be an effective learning experience for the Soul, but plunging in like that locks you into pain. The only solution is to be on two planes at once; you have to enter the pain fully, and yet be in the Soul level at the same time. That's fierce! You feel the full intensity of pain, and at the same time you transcend it by being in the Witness state. Pain demands that you establish yourself simultaneously in Ego and Soul. What an incredible teacher it is.

The stroke has given me a lot of experience with the medical world. I had no idea how many different kinds of doctors and therapists there are out there! I've learned a lot from the people who have been treating me. Dr. Zhu, my acupuncturist, has been a great teacher for me. His practice takes place in a setting that is a little unlike our usual Western clinical scene. All the patients sit together in a big waiting room on chairs arranged along the walls. Dr. Zhu and his assistants go from patient to patient, asking questions, placing needles, making adjustments. It's all very public.

On my second visit to Dr. Zhu, I was rolled in in my wheelchair. After he had worked with some of the other patients for awhile, Dr. Zhu stepped across to the side of the room opposite me. He looked directly at me, crooked his finger, and motioned me towards him. I pointed to my wheelchair questioningly, but he gestured no. Clearly he meant for me to walk all on my own. Walk all the way across the huge room? And with all those strangers watching me besides? But I thought, "He's the doctor!" The strength of his determination got me up out of my chair, and I walked—tottering like a baby—across the room to where he stood. Therapists and doctors believe it's their *techniques* that make the difference, but I've come to realize that it's much more the power of their certainty that counts. It's their heart-to-heart resuscitation.

I have all kinds of therapies these days: speech therapy, occupational therapy, physical therapy, aquatherapy. All the therapies call upon me as an Ego: Try harder! Don't you want to get better? Exert your will! I've fought that; I fought it because it was pegging me as an Ego. The stroke became a playing field for a whole new level of achieving: How much "progress" has there been? Can you walk yet? More gold starts to be won. Instead of will, I've found in myself a peaceful surrender to the karmic unfolding of life—an unfolding that's like a tree growing or a flower blooming.

Many of my doctors have been curious about me. They were curious about the fact that I wasn't reacting the way they expected me to. One doctor said to me, "How can you be happy when you've had a stroke?" I said, "Because my Awareness is on another plane." My Awareness isn't material; it's not part of the brain. Thoughts are in the brain, but Awareness isn't. That didn't seem to mean much to the doctor, but it was what was making all the difference to me.

Another doctor came into my room and said, "It's funny—I'm the head of this hospital, and where I find I most want to be is right here in this room. It's so peaceful!" It was because I was using the stroke to reflect about Awareness and had recognized through that reflection that my Awareness doesn't have a locus and so my consciousness isn't trapped in my body. I had *experienced* that—not as an abstract understanding, but as a real event. I was feeling the sense of peace that comes from that, and the doctor was picking it up from me.

There are people around me who trust my Awareness, and they say, "Well, *his* Awareness won't get stuck!" That's the devotion—they're the ones who assume I won't get caught, and that helps me stay unstuck. There are other people who assume that my mind will be stuck because they know theirs would be in that situation. That's most of the medical establishment—and that makes hospitals a hard environment to work in. The hospital environment identifies me with my body, and the body has been "insulted." If I buy into that, it's the root of suffering. For a long time I've fantasized about how nice it would be if we could have a hospital that also functioned as an ashram, where patients and staff would all be satsang and would all be doing whatever they were doing—being sick, being caregivers—as a spiritual practice. Now that I was experiencing hospital life firsthand, I *really* wished such a place existed.

Besides all the physical problems I faced with the stroke, there were some interesting psychological changes. All the roles I'd been playing, all my attitudes, were affected. The stroke took all the games I was playing and allowed me to re-perceive them. It put my games into perspective; they seem much less important now because I'm not so attached to the fruits they have to offer. I'm not as easily caught in wanting to be this or that for other people, to play their games. I don't feel I have to please people all the time by putting on an act for them and so my consciousness is a little freer. For example, I always wanted power—worldly power. That was one of the things that motivated me. For years, I was a member of organizations because they played on the desire for power, fed it in me. Now I don't find those institutions very interesting.

One of the hardest psychological hurdles I had to deal with after the stroke was the loss of independence. Getting into and out of bed. Going to the bathroom. Going someplace in the car. Preparing my meals. I need help with every one of those things. I'm embarrassed by having to ring my bell and summon my attendant for trivial things: "Would you close the window?" "Would you tie my shoes?"

Dependency has been so fierce because I used to be a super-independent person. I've always prided myself on my independence. I've come to appreciate, from my new perspective, just how much "independence" is revered in our culture, and how humbling we consider dependency. I can see the way I had absorbed those ideas from the culture, how deeply I shared them, and how much they influenced my values.

I can also see that part of the appeal of independence was not to be vulnerable. When I became dependent, I was immediately much more vulnerable. But what I discovered was that it was my vulnerability that opened me to my humanity. I saw how I had pushed away my humanity in order to embrace my divinity out of fear of my vulnerability, and I saw the way the stroke was serving me, by opening me to that human vulnerability.

I can see now that I got my power from helping. These days, I'm helped; these days instead of *How Can I Help?* I'd have to write a book called *How Can You Help Me?* I've gone from being the helper to being the helpee. It's a whole new role.

I see myself reflected through the minds of the people who take care of me. To one of them, I'm a job. To another, I'm a buddy. To another, I'm a sick person. To another, I'm a famous person. To another, I'm an interesting case. To another, I'm a grouch. I see the way my caregivers' personalities get reflected in their serving. Some of my caregivers hold onto an image of me right after the stroke: very fragile, they're protective, they don't want me to try anything new. Others are of the "You can do it!" school and push me for all they're worth.

What I see in all our interactions is that from the Soul perspective, we're just hanging out together. Both helper and helpee are serving—they're the complementary roles in a dance. Two Souls are serving each other, honoring each other, mirroring each other's hearts. Without us helpees, what would the helpers have to do?

Since the stroke, I've found that the psychological stuff like dependency has ceased to have so much importance for me. It's not only because those things are minor in contrast with the stroke, but also—even more—because I'm more in my Soul level, where it's just, "There's independence, there's dependence, beautiful tapestry!"

That's why the stroke hasn't turned out to be as bad as I once would have anticipated—because it's pushed me up to a higher level. The "I" I am now isn't experiencing things the way the "I" I was then would have. I identify more with my Soul now, and to the Soul, things like disability and pain and dependence are just . . . poignant.

If I look at the stroke, I can interpret it at a number of different levels. There's the physical level—it was a hemorrhage in my brain. There's the karmic level—it happened because it was my karma to happen. And there's the bhakti level—it was given to me by my compassionate guru as a spiritual teaching. It's that last one that I find most interesting. When I ask myself, "If this is a teaching from Maharajji, what am I supposed to be learning?" I come up with a number of interesting answers.

One answer is that I've had an opportunity to practice a deeper form of karma yoga. In the Bhagavad Gita, Krishna (God) tells Arjuna (the devotee) how to use the battles of life to come to God. My stroke is one of those battles. It's hard stuff. The stroke raised the bar because it entailed so much suffering, but greater suffering elicits higher consciousness. It was Maharajji turning up the pressure for me to "get it," and it moved the game to a different league.

The stroke gave me the chance to appreciate in a much deeper way the preciousness of the love that surrounds me. The stroke created more love than I had ever seen before. Even people who don't like me sent me their good wishes! There were prayer networks, healing circles, meditation groups—I saw all these hearts opening all around me. I had tried to do that, to open hearts, through my lectures and my tapes and all, and here it was, happening all by itself. I felt love coming at me from all directions.

The love comes to me from more than just one place, too. My shaman shows me beings of compassion on other planes. He sees them and communicates with them, and he makes me aware of all these beings who are surrounding me with love. There seems to be a whole network, reaching out with love and compassion.

I want to be part of that network of compassion that brings the multitude of beings back to the One, to love, to consciousness, to all of it. I'd like to bring myself and everyone else to that Awareness—that's always been my central purpose. The stroke took away a lot of Ego distractions and brought me back to my Soul's purpose.

That's what healing is really all about. In the distinction that I make between healing and curing, healing is what brings us closer to God. Curing means bringing you back to what you were—but if "what you were" wasn't closer to God, then you haven't been healed. I haven't been cured of my stroke, but I have definitely been *healed by it*. Healing moves us closer to the One, and if you're the One then you're whole. That's the ultimate in healing—"making whole"—because there's no longer anything left out, including the sickness.

When people ask about me, they often say, "Is he all right?" That always makes me think of a story about Maharajji. He was surrounded by a group of people, and he said, "Somebody's coming." They said, "Nobody's coming, Maharajji." "Yes, yes, somebody's coming." Just then a man entered the ashram—the servant of one of Maharajji's old devotees. Maharajji looked at the man and said, "I know—your master had a heart attack, but I'm not coming."

"He's been calling for you, Maharajji," the servant said, "and he's been your devotee for so many years."

"No, no, I'm not going to go," Maharajji said. Then he picked up a banana and handed it to the servant and said, "Here. Give him this. He'll be all right." Now in India, when the guru gives you a piece of fruit, it's like the wish-bestowing tree; anything you want happens. So the servant rushed home with the banana. They quickly mashed it up and fed it to the man. And as he took the last bit, he died.

So what's "All right?" We at least have to consider the possibility that dying at that moment was the most "all right" thing that could have happened to that man—that Maharajji's banana opened him to his death, and brought him closer to God. That's healing, not curing.

Because the stroke brought me all these teachings from Maharajji, brought me into my Soul level, I call it grace. But it's not the "easy" grace I'd known from Maharajji in the past. It took me right to that edge between Maharajji's love and the ferocity of the stroke, so I call it "fierce grace."

In the time right after the stroke, as I started to assess what it had done to my body, to my plans, to my expectations, I felt a flash of anger at Maharajji. It reminded me of an experience I'd had with my stepmother, Phyllis, some years before. Phyllis was a wonderful, feisty woman, and I'd come to love her a lot. She had developed cancer, and the question was whether it had metastasized to her liver, which would be fatal. They had done a biopsy, and they were going to call with the results.

Phyllis had asked me to be on the phone with her. I was in the bedroom, sitting on the floor, doing some writing, and the phone rang. I picked up the phone and Phyllis picked up hers and the nurse on the other end said, "Just a minute—the doctor is coming." I looked up at a picture of my guru, and I said to Maharajji, "Look—I don't ask you for anything because you know how things are, and how things have to be, so what am I asking for? But if you could just slip it through, karmically, without any trouble, would you . . ." At that moment, the doctor came on the line and said, "Mrs. Alpert, I'm sorry to tell you this, but the cells in your body show the worst kind of malignancy. The cancer has spread. You only have about 6 months to live."

I felt my heart close, and freeze; and I looked at the picture of Maharajji and I said, "You son of a bitch!" It shocked the hell out of me—I mean, I *never* spoke to him like that! But I was *furious!* And then a moment later, I felt a flood of love filling my heart. I realized I was meeting Shiva, I was meeting change personified, and I said, "Yeah, that too!" And I was that much closer to Maharajji. We had just cut through, he and I, another level of the kind of "goody-goody" part of the devotion trip, and had moved into a place where we were recognizing each other across the universe, with *all* of its chaos and *all* of its horror and *all* of its changes.

The same thing happened with the stroke. There was a surge of anger—the feeling, "How could you let this happen to me?!" And then as I turned on Maharajji with all my fury, I felt his love just pouring into me, and I felt closer to him than ever. I was learning the lessons of fierce grace.

At that point I realized that I had been dealing with a very "refined" sort of grace in the past—the loving kind of grace, the grace of the good things that kept happening to me. "Fierce grace" means I've now been given a fully rounded understanding of grace. Now I have a full view of what grace is all about. But it's like learning to love Shiva or Kali—two deities who represent destruction and ferocity. It's learning to love *whatever* it is that brings me closer to God.

We suffer because of a desire, an attachment, a clinging, so our suffering points the way to where the work is. With suffering, there's suddenly a lot of motivation to rid yourself of the desire, and not much motivation to hang onto it—and the more desires I let go of, the freer I become. So as Maharajji would say, "See? That's the way it works. Suffering does bring you closer to God."

What was changed through the stroke was my attachment to the Ego. The stroke was unbearable to the Ego and so it pushed me into the Soul level also because when you "bear the unbearable," something within you dies. My identity flipped over and I said, "So that's who I am—I'm a Soul!" I ended up where looking at the world from the Soul level is my ordinary, everyday state—not an occasional experience with psychedelics or for some other reason, but my everyday reality. And that's grace. That's almost the definition of grace. And so that's why, although from the Ego's perspective the stroke is not much fun, from the Soul's perspective it's been a great learning opportunity.

There's a paradox here because although I'm more in the spirit now, I'm also more human. Before, I was always protecting myself from the desires of the Ego. To a renunciate, the material world represented temptation so I was busy pushing it away. Now I can risk going deeper into my incarnation because I'm feeling more secure in my identity with the Soul. When you're secure in the Soul, what's to fear? There is no fear of death, of anything your incarnation can bring. And it's interesting the way it works in both directions because the very fact of entering my incarnation more fully than ever brings me more fully into my Soul.

I'm taking more risks with my consciousness these days. I can let the kite string out a lot farther. It's scary sometimes; it's like going into outer space, and you're afraid of getting lost out there. Sometimes I'll find my consciousness someplace and I'll ask myself, "Now how did I get here?" I let myself get farther away from home plate than ever.

More and more I'm becoming an appreciator of silence. For many years, I have been attracted to the teachings of Ramana Maharshi, who gave me most of his teachings without ever saying a word. He would sit in silence, and the people who sat with him would come away with the answers to their questions. Just a couple of months before my stroke, I had narrated a video about Ramana Maharshi. The video was released during the time I was at the rehab center, and two of my friends brought a copy of it to the hospital for me to see. At one point in the narration, I heard myself saying, "Ramana Maharshi usually taught in silence." Watching that moment, there in my post-stroke state, I smiled and nodded. "In silence" . . . I understood that place much better now.

I speak fewer words outside these days, and I also have fewer words inside. My mind is much quieter than it used to be. Instead of an urge to be busy all the time, I'm the happiest just sitting at home, watching the trees, watching the clouds, watching the birds. I don't need to schedule every minute—birds don't have schedules, why should I?

I'm much closer to Maharajji that I've ever been. I spend much more time hanging out with him every day than I used to. The stroke brought me closer to Maharajji because it brought me closer to my center—

the hot center, the life-and-death issues. I have been able to open to this stroke, to go along willingly on the journey, because I saw that it was another unfolding of Maharajji's plan.

My link to Maharajji is very strong. He's the very context of my existence. He's my friend, my constant imaginary playmate. He's an imaginary playmate who's wise, loving, understanding, rascally—all the things I like in a playmate. What's wonderful is that that kind of playmate is available to each of us because it's inside.

The guru is the ambassador of Awareness. The guru helps us unite the Soul with Awareness, with God, by helping us connect with the part of ourselves that is already divine. Guru kripa is the path to this union. In this practice, we begin seeing the events of our lives as acts of grace—because each event is an opportunity for practicing devotion. It's a method of trust, of seeing Maharajji as showing compassion toward me. It's a method of the heart, of how much I love him. And his kripa, his grace—fierce or otherwise—is his love back to me. It's a heart-to-heart connection.

Guru kripa is a form of bhakti, of devotion, in which love is at the root of the faith. Love God, love guru, love your own inner being—any of them will take you through, and eventually will show you that they're all the same thing. In the *Ramayana,* Hanuman says to Ram—to God—"When I don't know who I am, I serve you; when I know who I am, I am you." That's the Soul's destination in the journey—to become that statement.

The Soul wants only God. Because the Soul's single motive is merging with God, it doesn't value its own individuality. The Ego clings desperately to identity—the Soul is trying to get clear of individuality in order to merge into the One.

The stroke was Maharajji's lightning bolt to jolt me into a new place in my consciousness. The ferocity of the method tested my faith, but in the end my faith held. My bond with Maharajji was strong enough to outweigh everything else.

Maharajji is what opened my heart to that kind of love and faith. He's just my "special example" of faith—yours is whatever it is for you that represents God or Spirit or that larger screen of things.

My relation with Maharajji is one of faith: that what come to me from him is grace. If I have faith in that, then there is no place in my life, no event in my life, where that grace isn't, and all the suffering of the stroke is just the honing of my faith.

This book *(Still Here)* is more of my "advance scout" role. These days I'm the advance scout for the experience of aging, and I've come back from the scouting party to bring good news. The good news is that the spirit is more powerful than the vicissitudes of aging. My stroke was a good test for my faith; the bar was high. I came away from the stroke firm in my faith, and I know now that my faith is unshakable. That assurance is the highest gift I have received from the stroke, and I can say to you now, with an assurance I couldn't have felt before, that faith and love are stronger than any changes, stronger than aging, and, I am very sure, stronger than death.

# Afterword

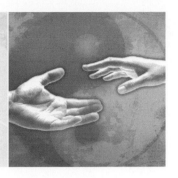

I'm sitting down to write this Afterword nearly 3 years after initially developing the idea of a text in CAM/rehabilitation as part of the series, *Medical Guides to Complementary and Alternative Medicine.* Not only has it been a long editorial journey, but also the target of CAM in rehab has moved (if I may mix metaphors a bit). The field of CAM is so rapidly changing that the terrain looks very different today than it did in 1998. For one thing, acceptance of CAM has risen to the point where a majority of medical schools now offer formal exposure in classrooms; the first Fellowship in Integrative Medicine has been approved; national Board Certification in Holistic Medicine is now available; and NIH funding for CAM is now over $70 million dollars annually. In rehabilitation, the national PM&R conference has a section devoted to CAM, while medical students and residents, at least at my institution, are often coming into medicine cross-trained (as PTs, DCs, LMTs, and more) or taking training in CAM modalities in tandem with their medical training. OTs and PTs now routinely incorporate many of the modalities from Section I of this book into their clinical work.

The target is moving in the sense that all of the preceding chapters on specific treatment techniques and clinical conditions will all be revised and updated to incorporate ongoing trends and movement in the field. There will someday need to be a second edition to this text, but in the meantime the message to me has been that this is truly a field in flux: no text can hope to encompass it all. I'm even more aware now of how many important topics simply did not fit into this edition: entire subspecialties like sports rehabilitation, integrative treatment plans for major syndromes like traumatic brain injury or stroke, and a long list of important therapies that could not be even be mentioned here, due to space considerations. My hope is that this compendium has at least intrigued and inspired you to take the next step in learning more about CAM from your own colleagues and teachers in the community, not only because it will enhance your own clinical work, but also because it will lead you further along on your own path to greater health and greater fulfillment in life.

**Eric D. Leskowitz**

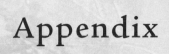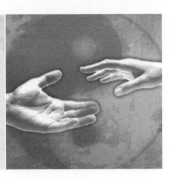

# Appendix

## Case Studies by Diagnosis

# Index

Page numbers with *f* indicate figures, and those with *t* indicate
tables.